# An Atlas of African Dermatology

Barbara Leppard

Regional Dermatology Training Centre
Kilimanjaro Christian Medical Centre
Moshi
Tanzania



RADCLIFFE MEDICAL PRESS

**Radcliffe Medical Press Ltd**
18 Marcham Road
Abingdon
Oxon OX14 1AA
United Kingdom

**www.radcliffe-oxford.com**
The Radcliffe Medical Press electronic catalogue and online ordering facility.
Direct sales to anywhere in the world.

---



British Library Cataloguing in Publication Data

A catalogue record for this book is available from the British Library.

ISBN 1 85775 544 8 (limp)
1 85775 975 3 (cased)

Typeset by Advance Typesetting Ltd, Oxon
Printed and bound by Alden (Malaysia)

# Contents

CONTENTS

CONTENTS

# Preface

The cover picture shows some of the students at the Regional Dermatology Training Centre. They come from five different African countries (Cameroon, Kenya, Malawi, Swaziland and Uganda) and illustrate that the African skin is not a uniform colour but infinitely variable.

I would like to thank all the patients and their relatives for allowing me to use their photographs in this atlas. I also thank the following colleagues and friends who kindly allowed me to use their photographs – Coopers Animal Health (Figure 480), Dr Anthony du Vivier (Figure 213), Dr Adrian Ive (Figures 169, 184, 401), Mr Pak Sang Lee (Figure 260), Dr John Masenga (Figures 595, 600), Professor Ben Naafs (Figures 108, 362, 472, 654), Dr Gabriele Poggensee (Figure 577), Professor Peter Stingl (Figures 185, 470, 476, 477) and Dr Michael Waugh (Figures 259, 596).

There are very few books about dermatology in the African skin. This atlas has been prepared with the aim of helping in the diagnosis and treatment of skin diseases in an African context. The diseases are arranged in alphabetical order to make them easy to find and the treatments are those which are currently available in Tanzania.

Barbara Leppard
*October 2001*

**Dedicated to the past and present students at the Regional Dermatology Training Centre at KCMC, Moshi, Tanzania whose enthusiasm and willingness to learn have encouraged me over the years.**

## ABSCESS

**Figure 1** Collection of pus in the dermis and subcutaneous fat usually due to *Staphylococcus aureus*.

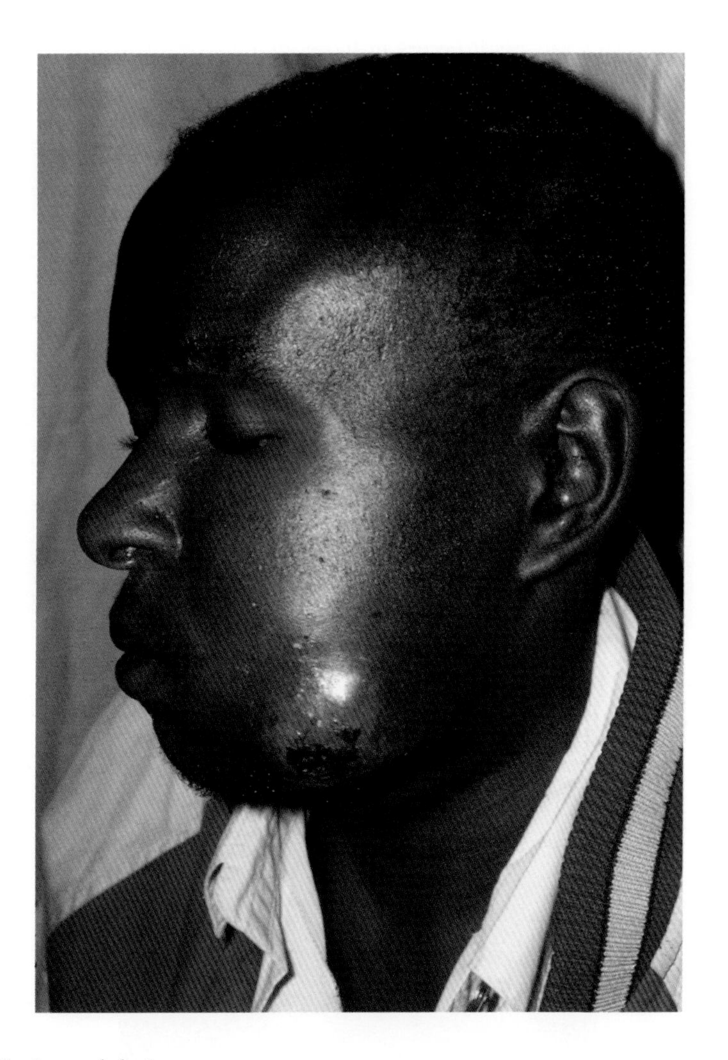

*Treatment:* Incise and drain.

## ACANTHOSIS NIGRICANS

**Figures 2, 3** The skin of the neck and flexures becomes hyperpigmented and thickened with a velvety, slightly papillomatous surface. There may or may not be skin tags within and around the acanthosis nigricans. After the age of 40 years it may be due to an underlying malignancy. In younger patients it occurs in those who are overweight (pseudoacanthosis nigricans) and will disappear if they lose weight.

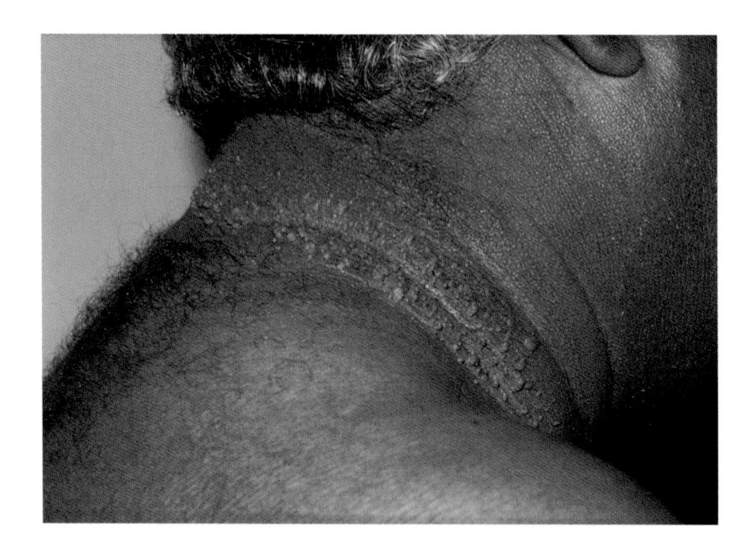

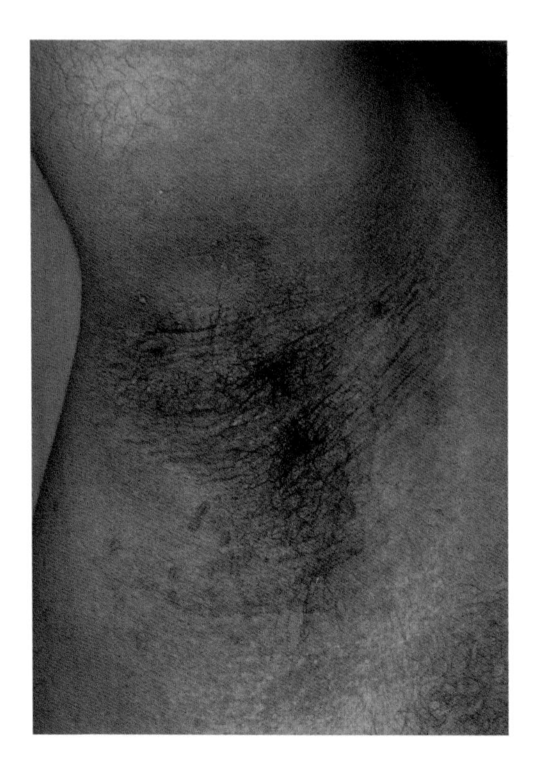

## ACCESSORY AURICLE

**Figure 4** Present from birth. Small skin-coloured papule containing cartilage in front of the ear.

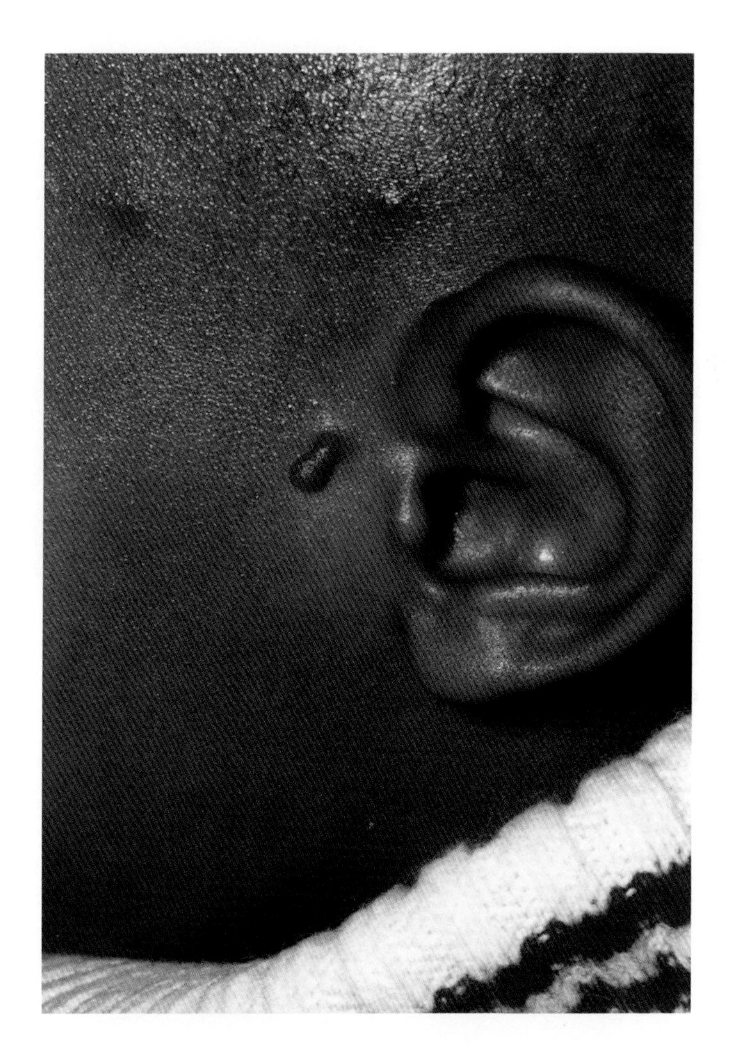

*Treatment:* None needed.

## ACCESSORY DIGIT

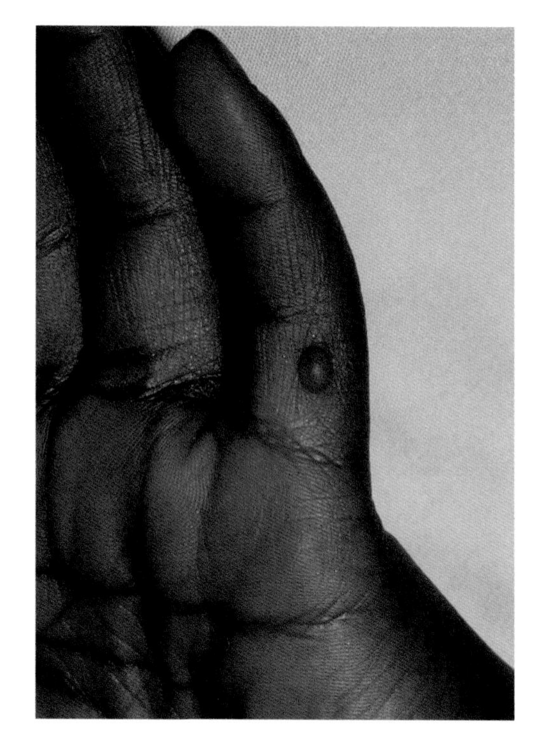

**Figure 5** Present from birth. Unilateral or bilateral papule most commonly at the side and base of the little finger. May run in families; inherited as an autosomal dominant trait (*see* Figure 295). Can be confused with a digital fibrokeratoma (*see* Figure 181).

*Treatment:* Can be snipped off with a pair of sharp scissors soon after birth.

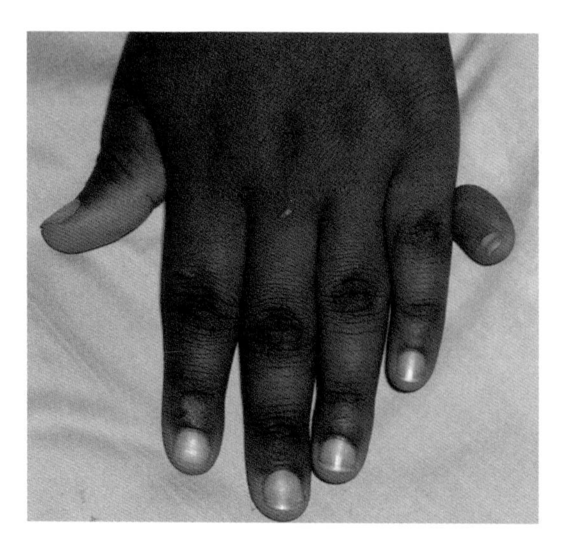

**Figure 6** If not removed at birth it may grow into an extra finger.

## ACCESSORY NIPPLE

**Figure 7** Present from birth. Single or multiple small papule(s) in the nipple line. Can be confused with a compound naevus (*see* Figure 66) but if you look carefully you can see both nipple and areola.

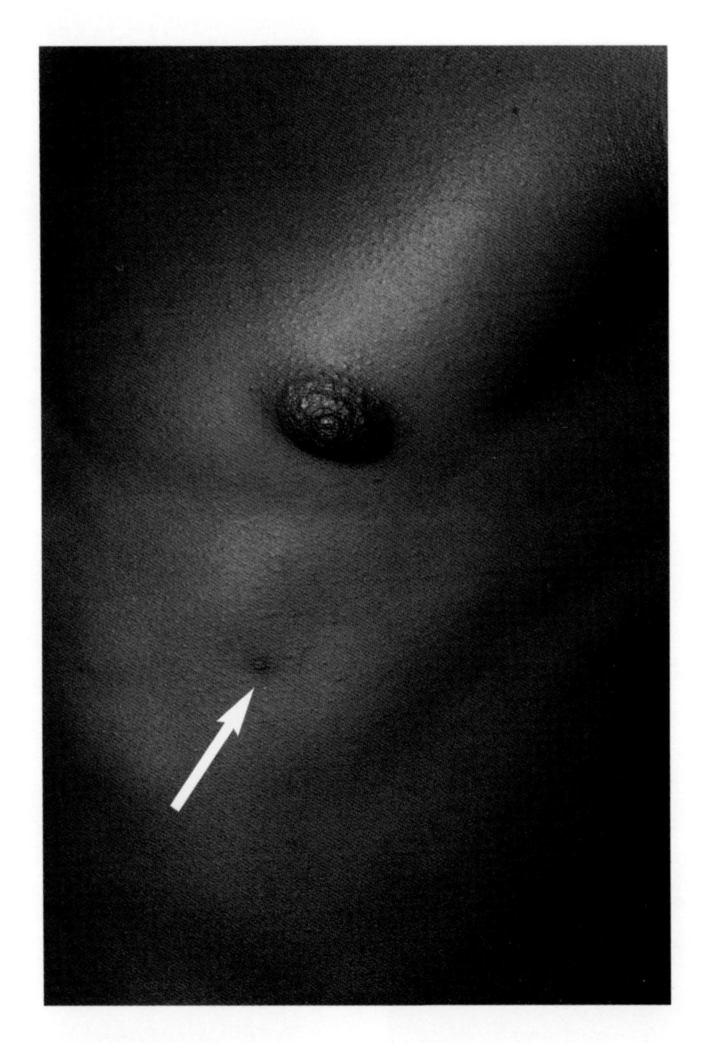

*Treatment:* None needed.

## ACNE

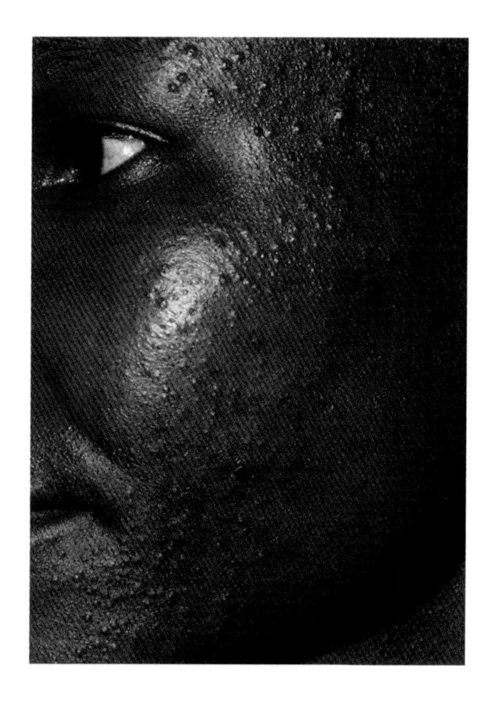

**Figure 8** Greasy skin with open and closed comedones (blackheads and whiteheads). Begins at or after puberty on the face, chest and back.

*Treatment:* Stop applying greasy ointments like Vaseline. Wash with soap and water and get out in the sun as much as possible. If this does not work apply 5% or 10% benzoyl peroxide at night.

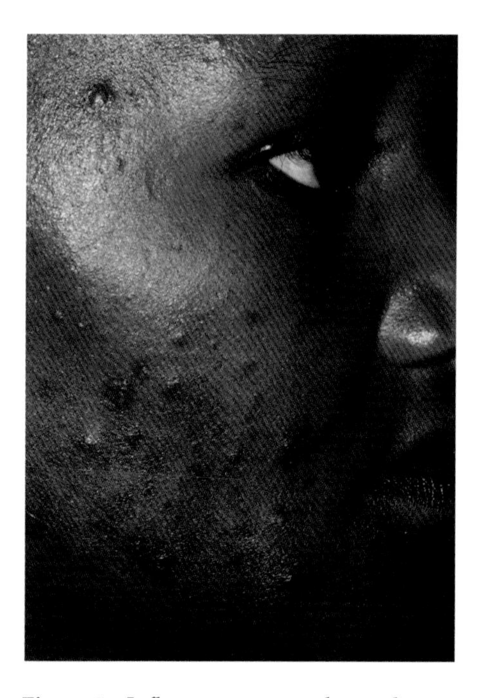

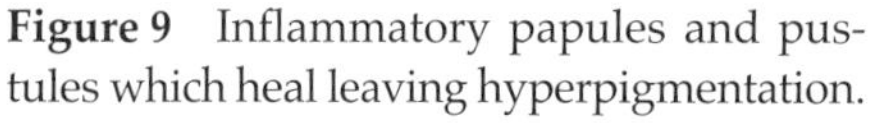

**Figure 9** Inflammatory papules and pustules which heal leaving hyperpigmentation.

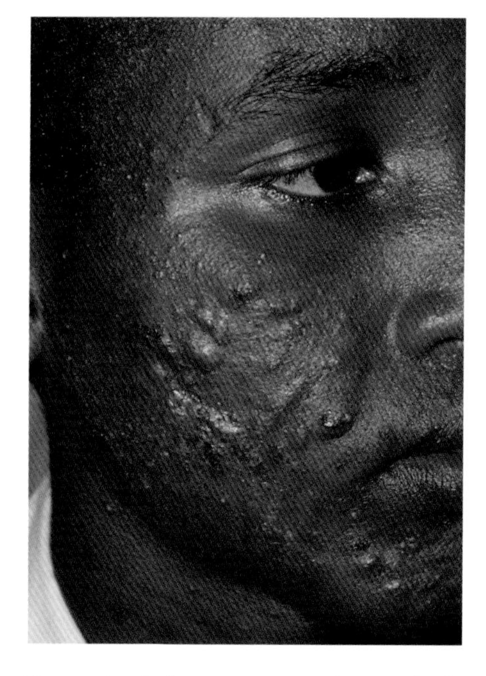

**Figure 10** Inflammatory nodules which heal leaving scars.

*Treatment:* Stop applying greasy ointments. Wash with soap and water and get out in the sun as much as possible. May need long-term (6 months to several years) low dose tetracycline orally (250mg bd), but it must be taken regularly and on an empty stomach.

## ACNE KELOID

**Figure 11** A disease of young men. Begins with small pustules in the occipital region which are often not noticed until they become firm, uncomfortable (sometimes itchy) papules.

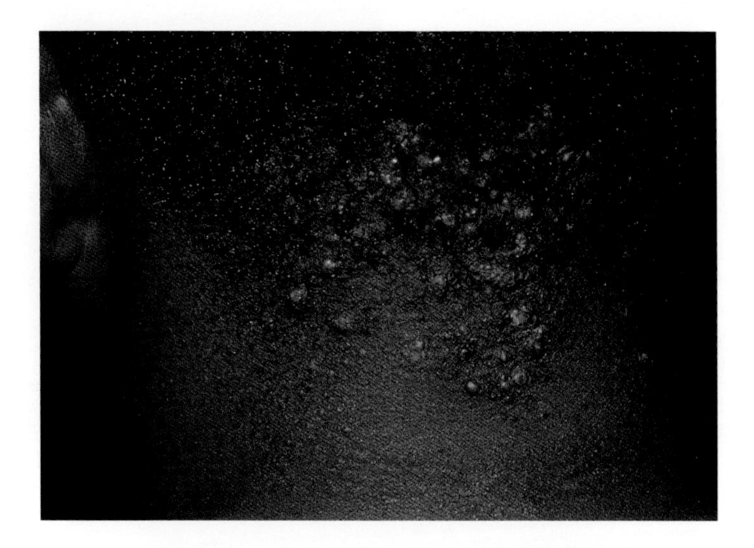

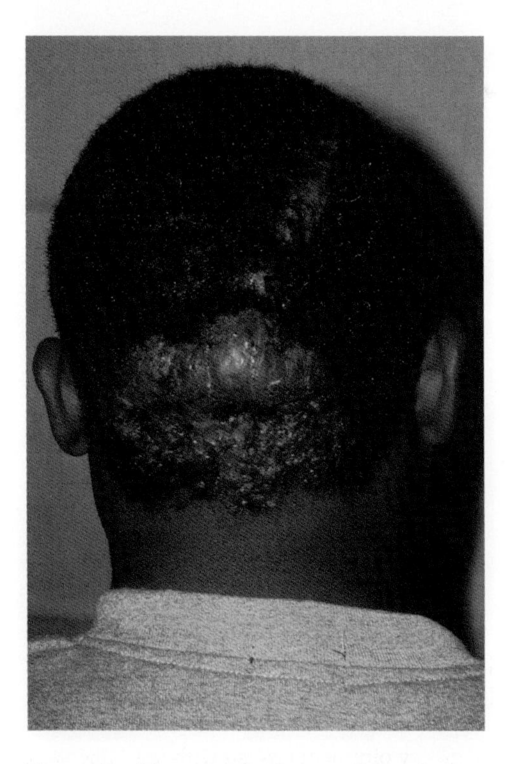

**Figure 12** May extend to become large plaques.

*Treatment:* Unsatisfactory. Can inject triamcinolone (10mg/ml) intralesionally once a month until it flattens, or excise widely.

## ACRODERMATITIS ENTEROPATHICA

**Figures 13, 14** Rare disease due to congenital deficiency of zinc absorption. It is inherited as an autosomal recessive trait (*see* Figure 18). Four to 6 weeks after weaning the child becomes withdrawn, develops diarrhoea, hair loss and a blistering rash on the hands and around the orifices (mouth, genitalia and anus). The blisters break leaving erosions. The same rash can be due to nutritional zinc deficiency and is associated with kwashiorkor (*see* Figures 345–6) and the rare glucagonoma syndrome.

*Treatment:* Oral zinc sulphate, 2mg/kg body weight/day.

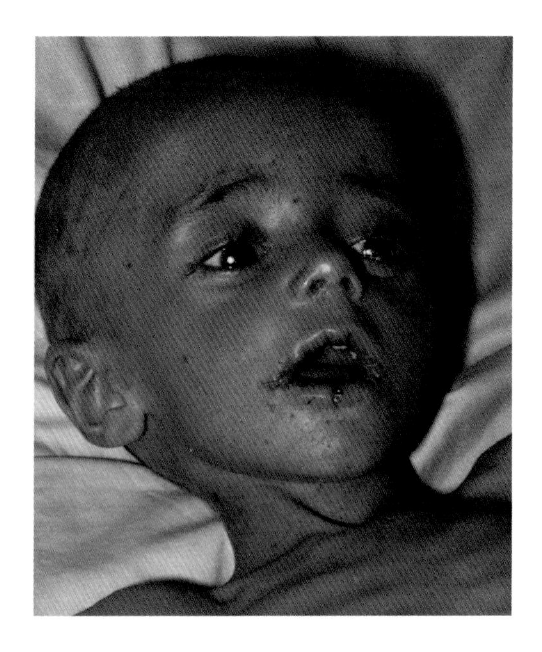

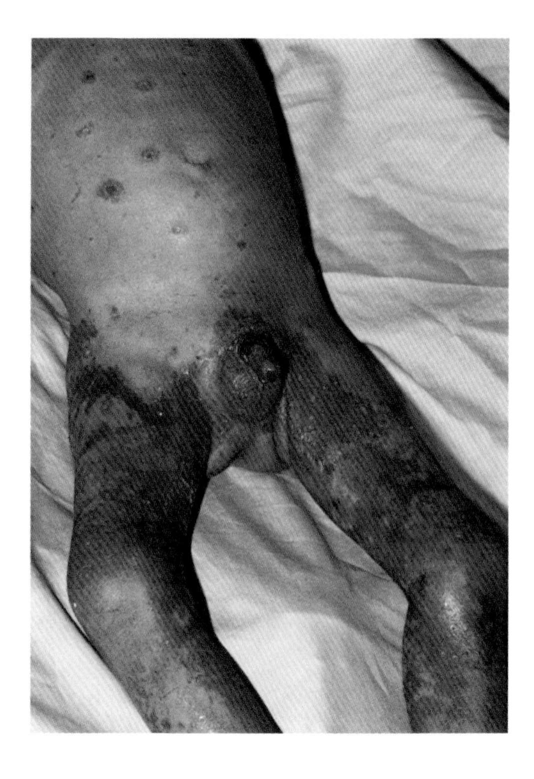

## ACROPUSTOLOSIS OF INFANCY

**Figure 15** Crops of small blisters on the palms and soles of infants. It resolves spontaneously usually before the age of 3 years. It can be confused with scabies in infants (*see* Figure 571).

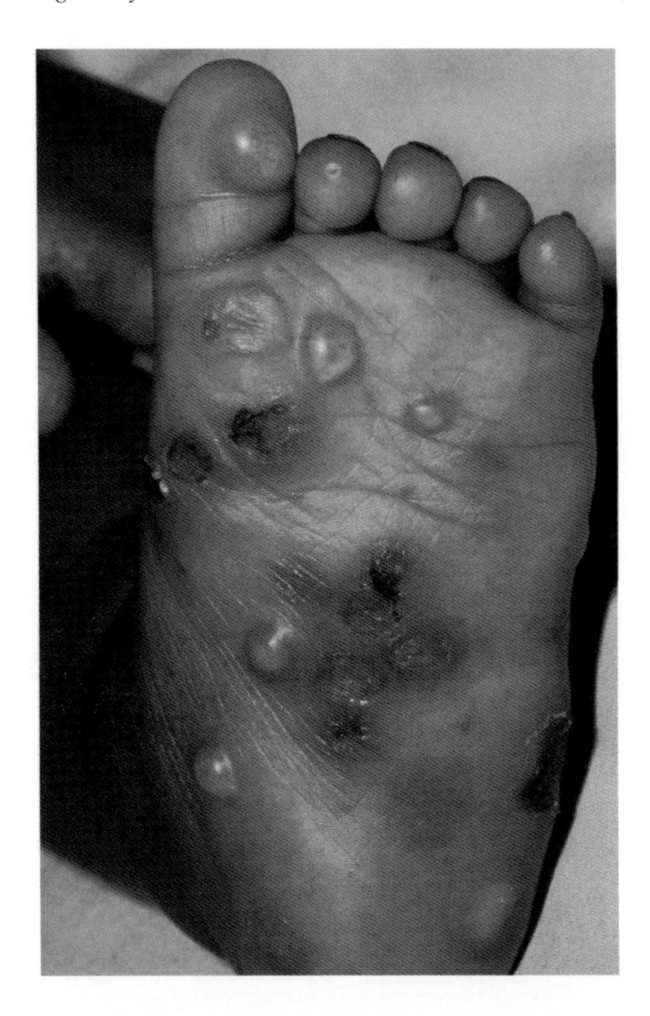

*Treatment:* Dapsone 2mg/kg body weight/day orally until it gets better spontaneously.

## AINHUM AND PSEUDO-AINHUM

**Figure 16** Ainhum is a painful constriction band (groove) around the fifth toe leading eventually to auto-amputation. Similar constriction bands can occur on other toes or even fingers (pseudo-ainhum) as in this picture.

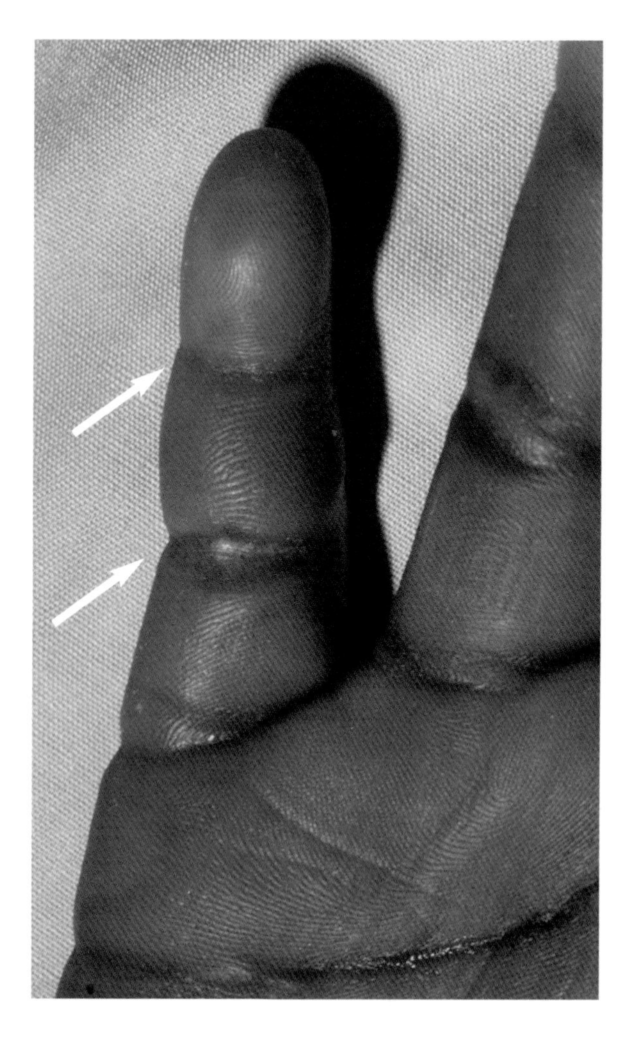

*Treatment:* Control secondary infection. If it is obvious that amputation will occur, remove the toe or finger surgically.

## ALBINISM

**Figure 17** A group of inherited conditions in which there is lack of melanin in the skin, hair and eyes. An individual with albinism is called an albino. Most African albinos belong to the OCA2 group which is inherited as an autosomal recessive trait (*see* Figure 18). It is obvious at birth – the baby is white instead of black, the hair is blonde or yellow and the iris is blue or hazel.

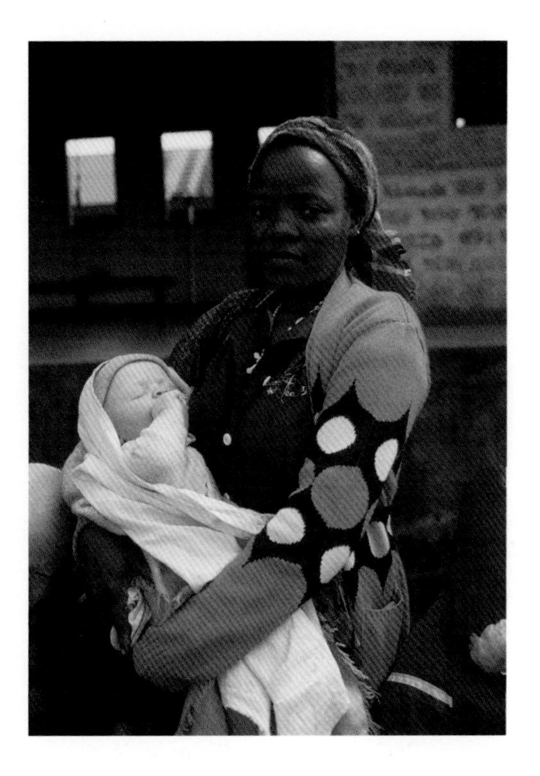

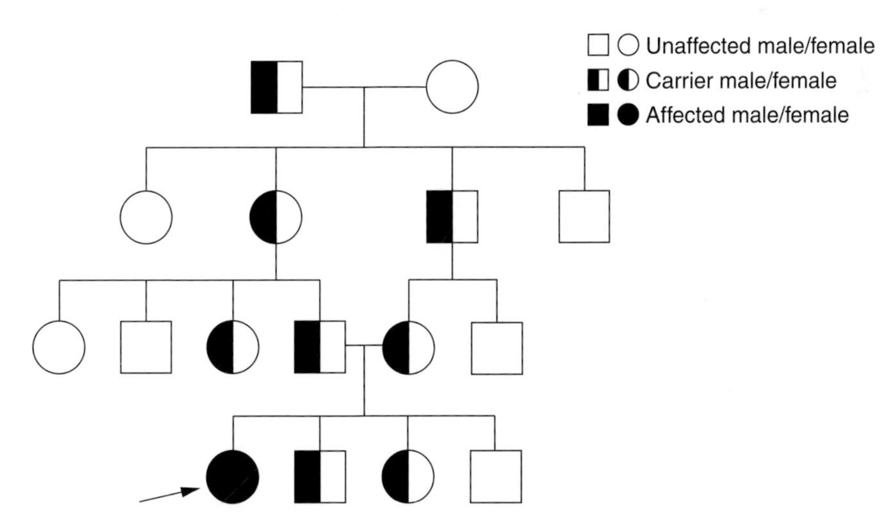


**Figure 18** Autosomal recessive mode of inheritance. The condition is only apparent in the homozygous state which means that the child must receive the abnormal gene from both parents. The parents themselves are usually normal (*see* Figure 17) but each child will have a 1 in 4 risk of being an albino. It is more likely to occur in families in which there is consanguinity.

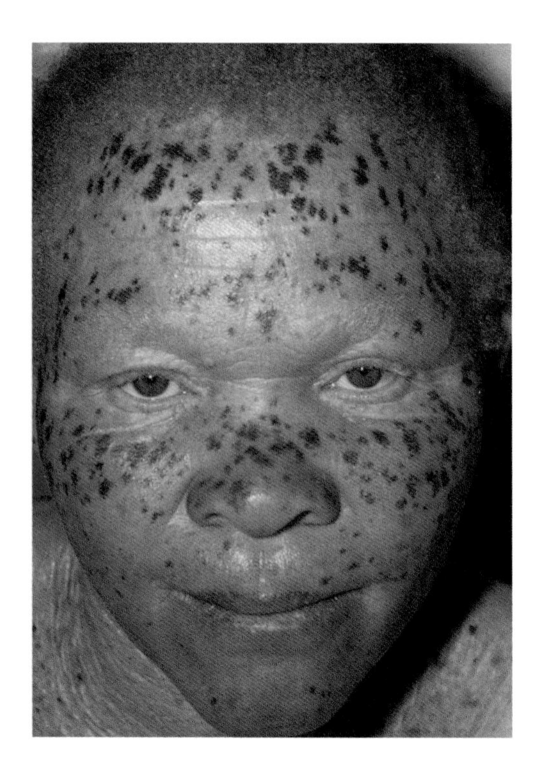

**Figure 19** Some albinos are not completely white but have multiple lentigoes (dark brown macules and patches) on sun-exposed parts of the skin.

Because of the lack of melanin, the sun causes the following problems in the skin of albinos:

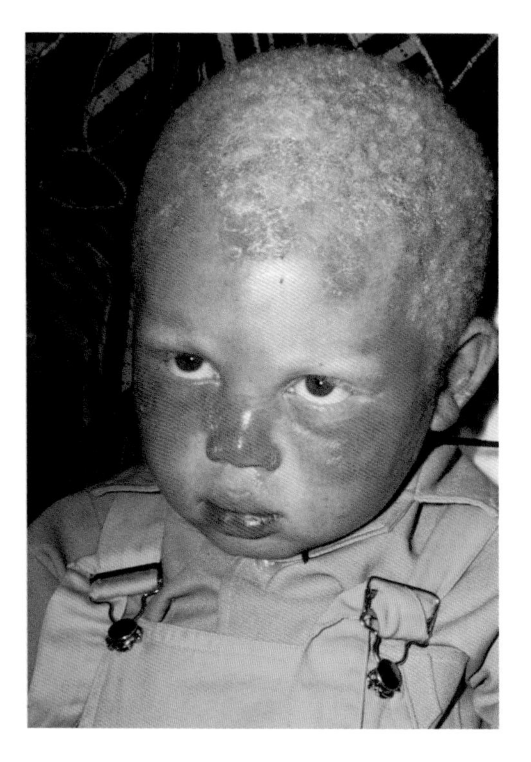

**Figure 20** Sunburn. Redness and soreness of the skin, and if severe, blistering.

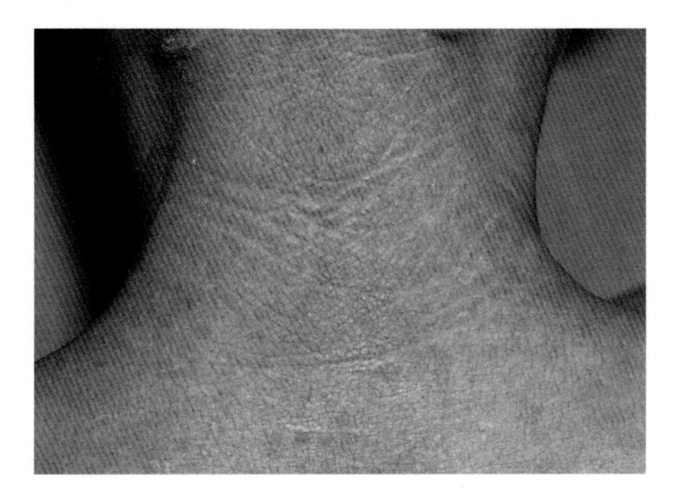

**Figure 21** Solar elastosis. Yellowish discolouration of the skin with increased skin markings is the earliest sign of sun damage and is present in most albino children on the back of the neck by the age of 12 months. Seen here in a 15-year-old girl.

**Figure 22** More extensive solar elastosis in a 37-year-old lady. The sun damage can occur not only on exposed skin but through thin clothing as seen here. Where there are two layers of clothes (e.g. under her bra) the skin is normal.

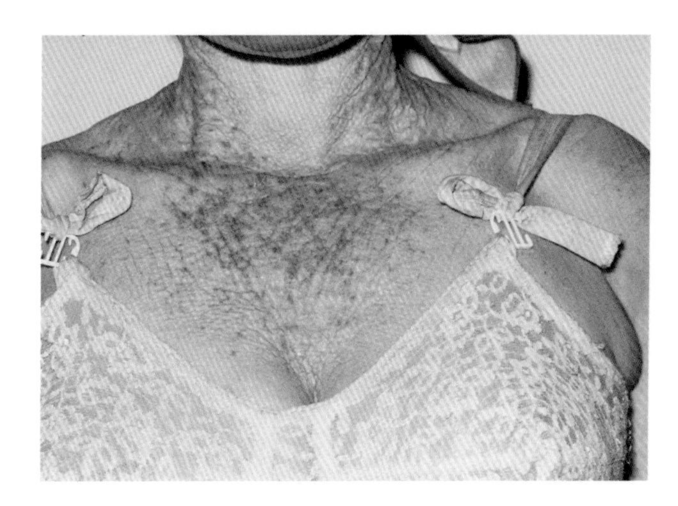

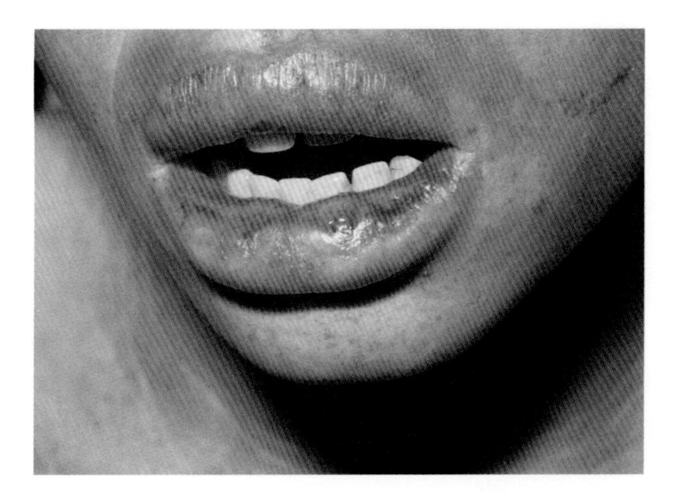

**Figure 23** Actinic cheilitis. Dryness and scaling of the lips due to sun damage.

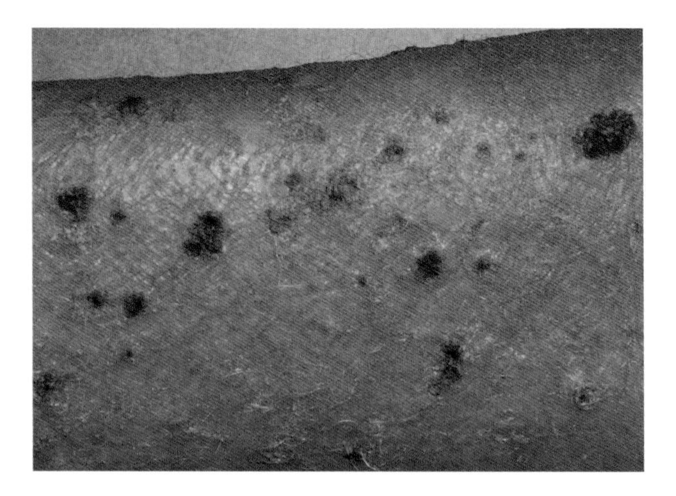

**Figure 24** Solar keratoses on the arm of a 39-year-old lady. These are skin-coloured or hyperpigmented papules which are rough to the touch. They are premalignant and can become squamous cell carcinomas. They begin to occur in childhood (age 8 years and upwards) and are universally present by the age of 20.

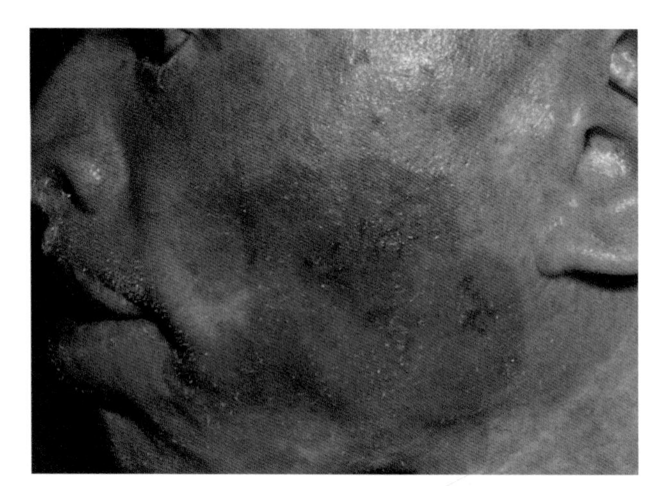

**Figure 25** Bowen's disease (intraepidermal squamous cell carcinoma). This is a premalignant condition. It presents as a red scaly plaque which slowly extends. Four years later this man developed an invasive squamous cell carcinoma on the left cheek within the area of Bowen's disease.

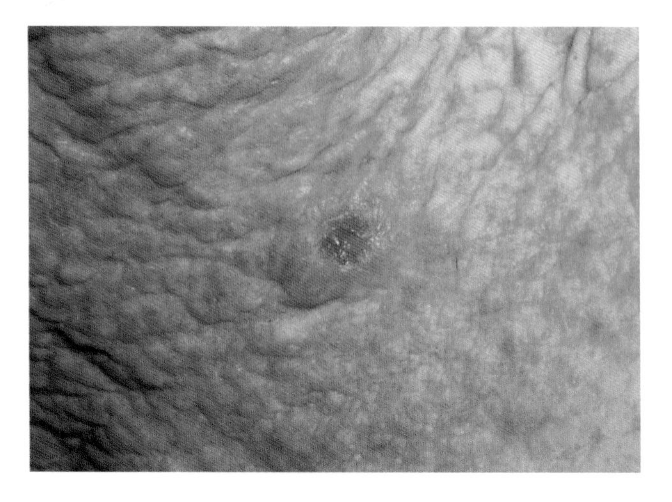

**Figure 26** Basal cell carcinoma on the neck of a 53-year-old man (note the surrounding solar elastosis).

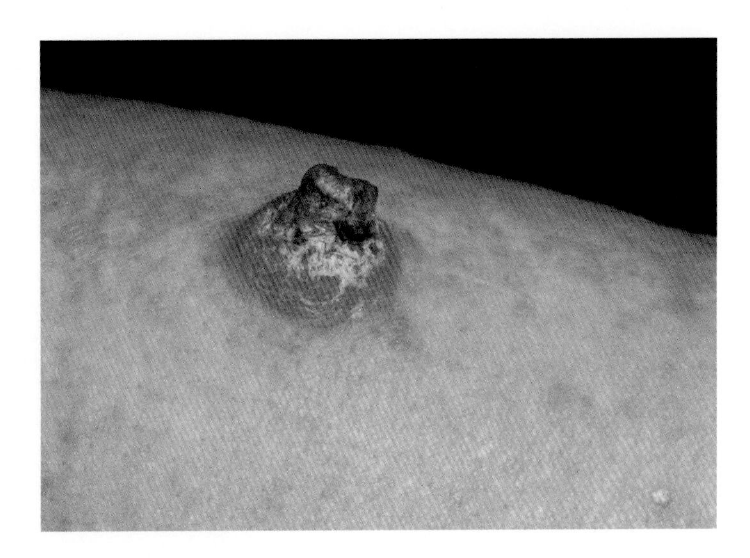

**Figure 27** Kerato-acanthoma on the upper arm (*see also* Figure 118).

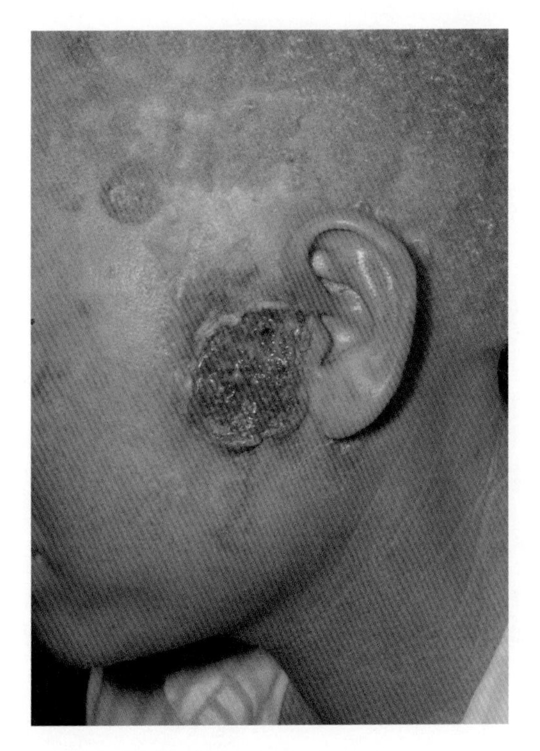

**Figure 28** Squamous cell carcinoma just below the hair margin and a second larger one in front of the ear of a 26-year-old man.

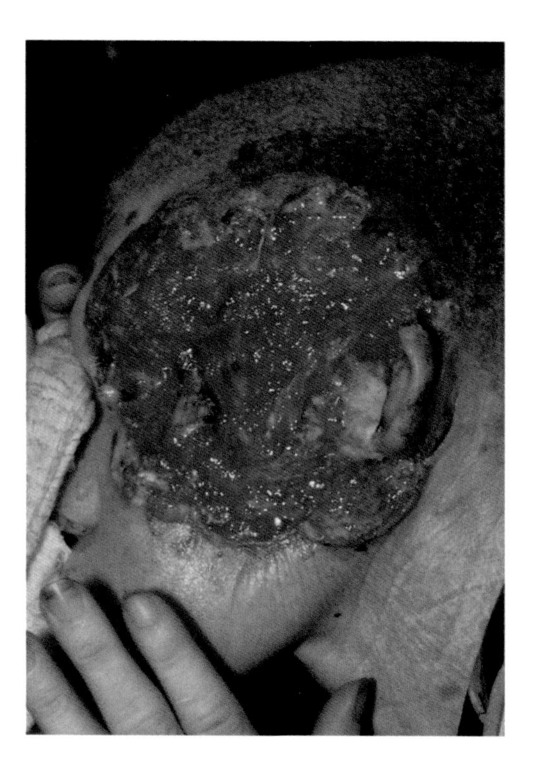

**Figure 29** Very extensive squamous cell carcinoma on the face of a 32-year-old lady.

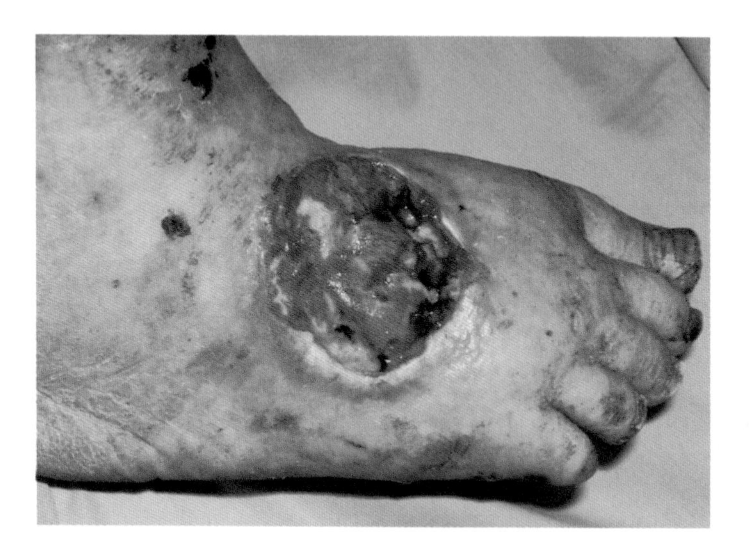

**Figure 30** Squamous cell carcinoma on the dorsum of the foot. This bled causing the man's haemoglobin to drop to 5mg/100ml, making surgery hazardous. Skin cancer can occur on any sun-damaged site.

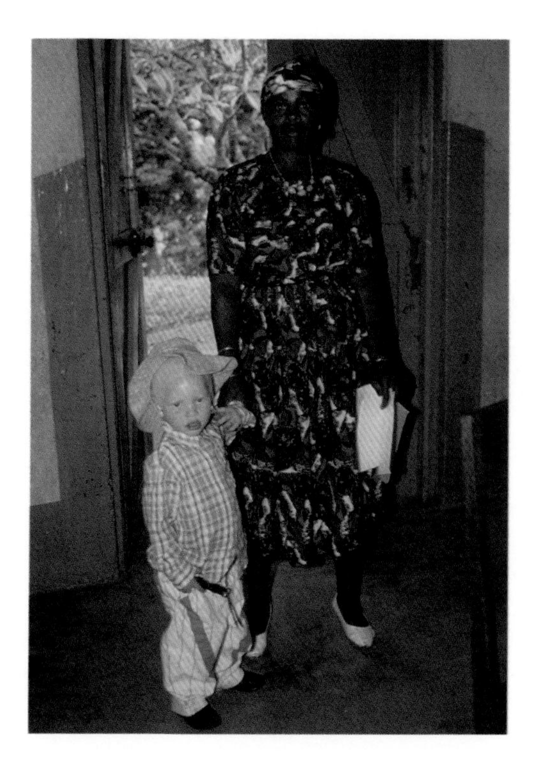

**Figure 31** With proper protection from the sun (wide-brimmed hats to protect the face, ears and neck, long-sleeved shirts, blouses or dresses, long trousers, long skirts and shoes and socks) albinos can live out a normal life span.

Because of the lack of melanin in the eye, albinos also have nystagmus, squint, poor central vision and photophobia.

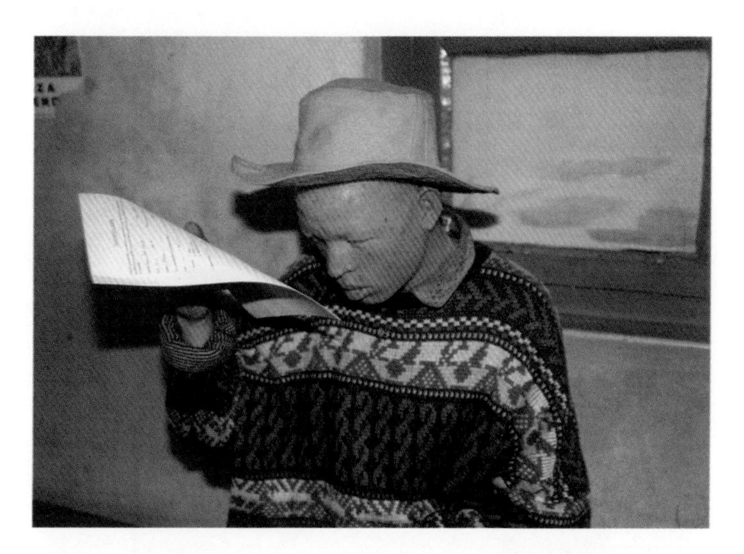

**Figure 32** Poor vision can be compensated for by holding a book or paper up close to the eye to read.

# ALOPECIA

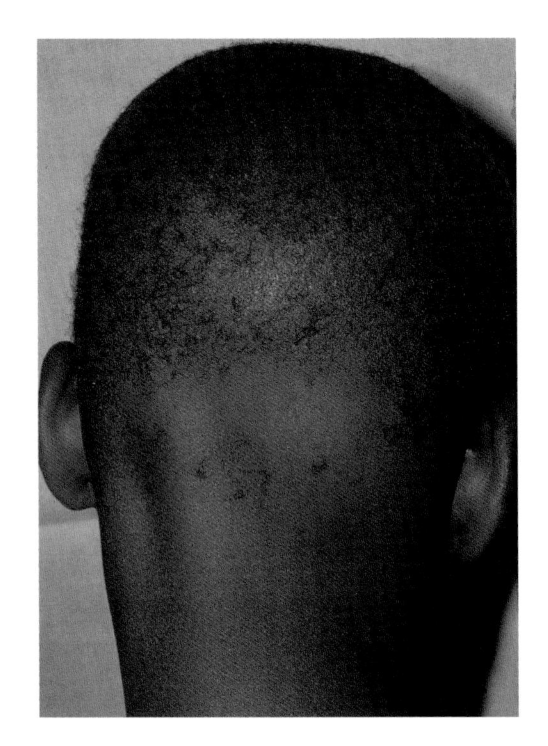

Alopecia means hair loss. There are many different causes and patterns of hair loss.

## Alopecia areata

**Figures 33, 34** Discrete bald patches which can be single or multiple. The skin in the bald patches is normal and not scaly as in tinea capitis (*see* Figure 621). It is a harmless condition and the hair usually regrows without treatment in 3–6 months. When the hair regrows it regrows white initially (*see* Figure 36) but returns to a normal colour after a few weeks.

*Treatment:* Reassurance that the hair will regrow.

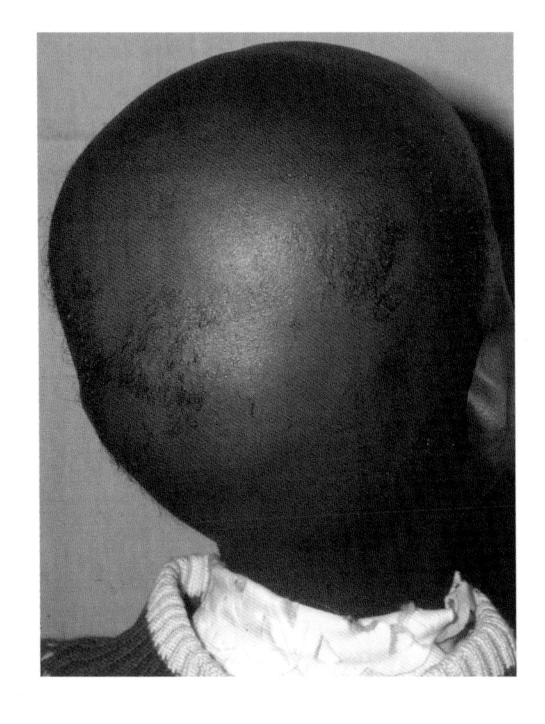

**Figure 35** Any hairy area can be involved. Here there is loss of eyebrows and eyelashes.

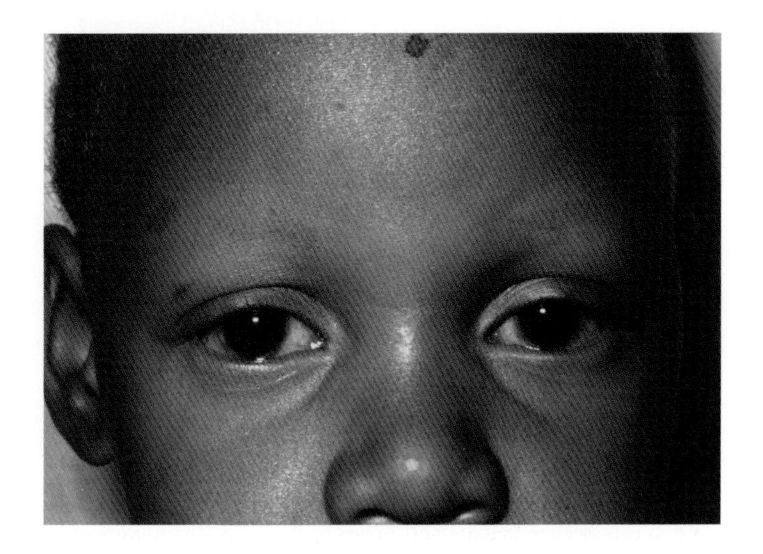

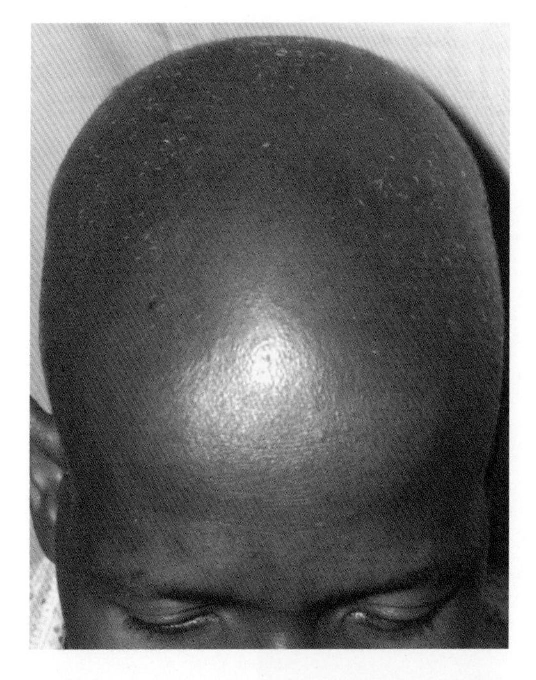

**Figure 36** If alopecia areata affects the whole scalp it is called alopecia totalis. Here a few white hairs are regrowing.

## Diffuse hair loss

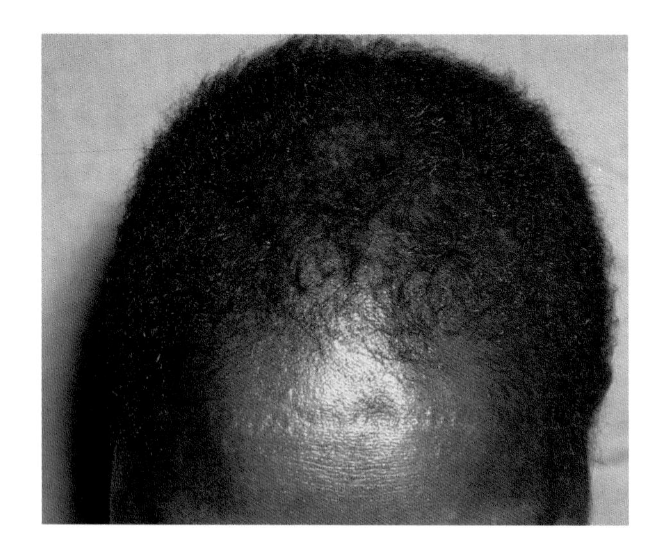

**Figure 37** Diffuse hair loss can be due to iron deficiency anaemia, hypothyroidism, secondary syphilis, systemic lupus erythematosus and drugs such as anticoagulants or those given to treat thyrotoxicosis. The hair density decreases as people get older, so a degree of diffuse alopecia is common in the elderly.

*Treatment:* Treat the underlying cause.

## Diffuse hair loss due to cytotoxic drugs

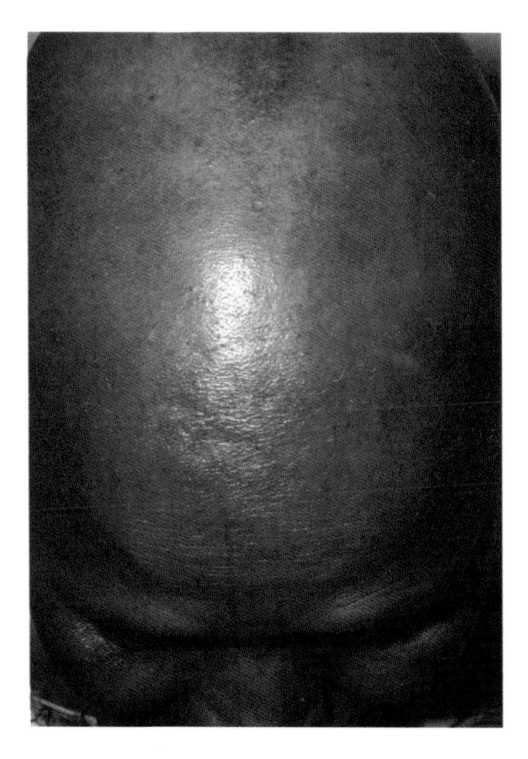

**Figure 38** Cytotoxic drugs stop the cells of the hair matrix from dividing, so all growing hairs are lost. This is called anagen effluvium. It causes virtually complete alopecia, but the hair will regrow when the drugs are stopped.

## Male pattern alopecia

**Figures 39, 40** This is not a disease but a normal pattern of hair loss in adult males due to the presence of androgens. It begins at the temples and crown and the two areas may join up. The hair is never lost from the occiput or around the sides of the scalp. A similar pattern of hair loss, but usually less extensive, can occur in females. This is called female pattern alopecia.

*Treatment:* None is needed other than an explanation of what is happening.

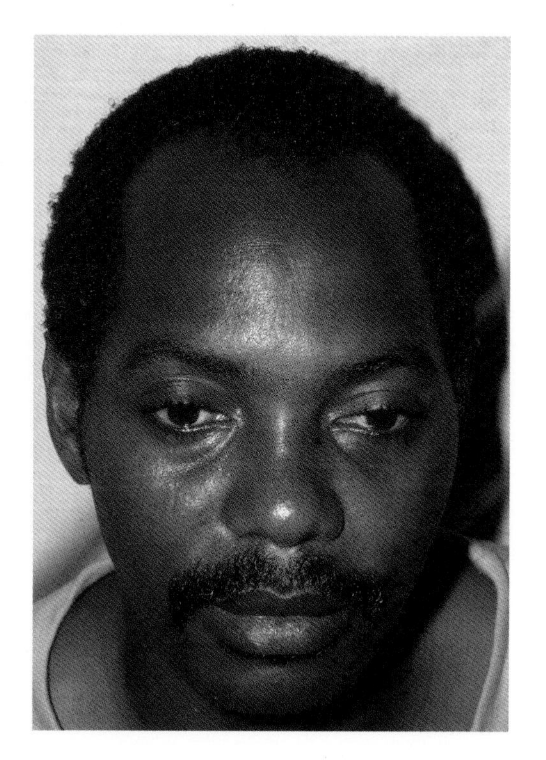

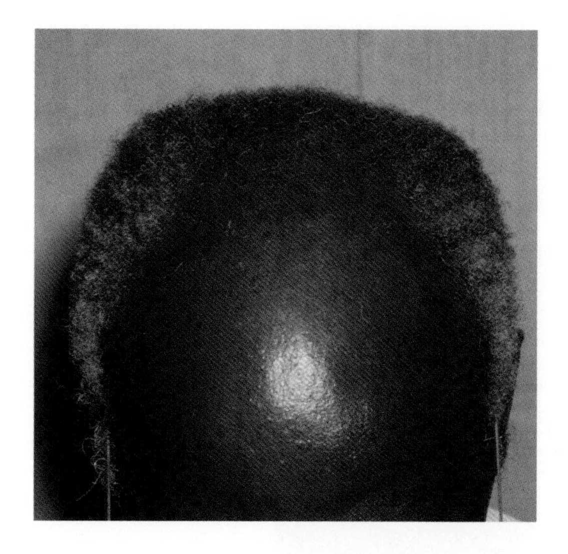

## Scarring alopecia

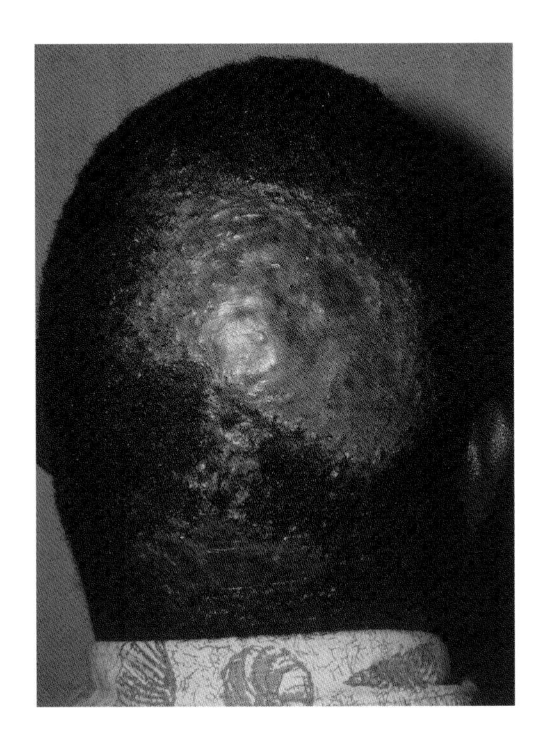

**Figure 41** Here the hair loss is permanent. The hair follicles are destroyed and replaced by scar tissue. Very often the cause is unknown but it can be due to burns, discoid lupus erythematosus (*see* Figure 403), lichen planus or an infection such as a chronic infection with *Staphylococcus aureus* (folliculitis decalvans), or after a kerion (*see* Figure 622) or herpes zoster. In children, localised areas of scarring alopecia can be due to congenital abnormalities such as aplasia cutis or naevus sebaceous (*see* Figure 76).

*Treatment:* Usually nothing can be done.

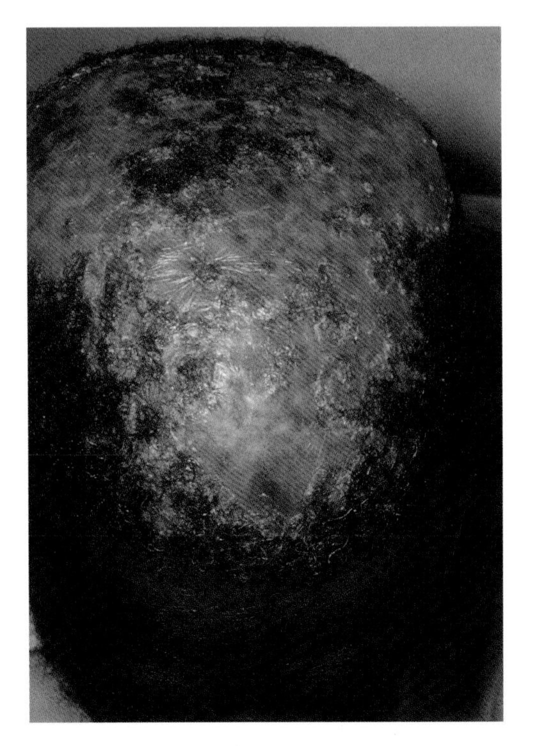

**Figure 42** Folliculitis decalvans.

*Treatment:* Long-term antibiotics. Sulphamethoxazole-trimethoprim 960mg bd is usually the drug of choice.

## Telogen effluvium

**Figure 43** This is a physiological type of hair loss that occurs in all women 3 months after childbirth. The hair comes out by the handful and all the hairs are resting or telogen hairs. The same phenomenon occurs 3 months after any severe illness (high fever, major surgery, starvation). The hair loss lasts only a few weeks and the hair will then regrow.

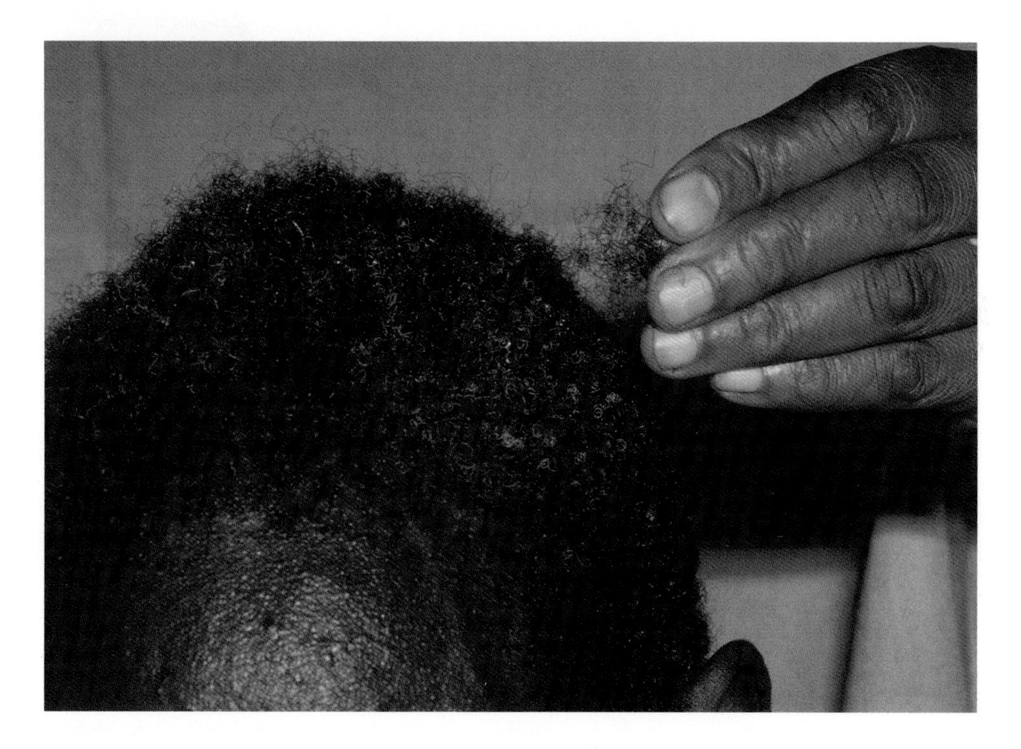

*Treatment:* Explanation and reassurance are needed. The hair will take about 6 months to get back to a normal length.

## Traction alopecia

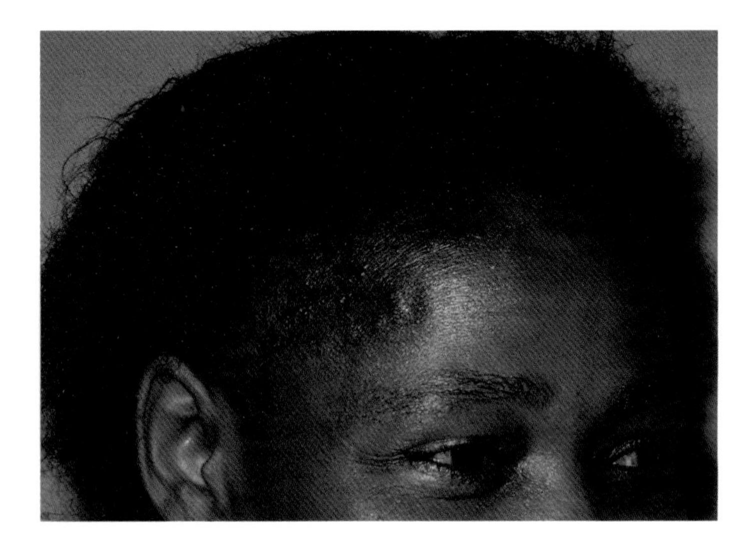

**Figure 44** This is due to the hair being pulled tightly back or tightly plaited. The hair loss is from around the margins of the scalp.

*Treatment:* Stop the pulling or plaiting.

## Trichotillomania

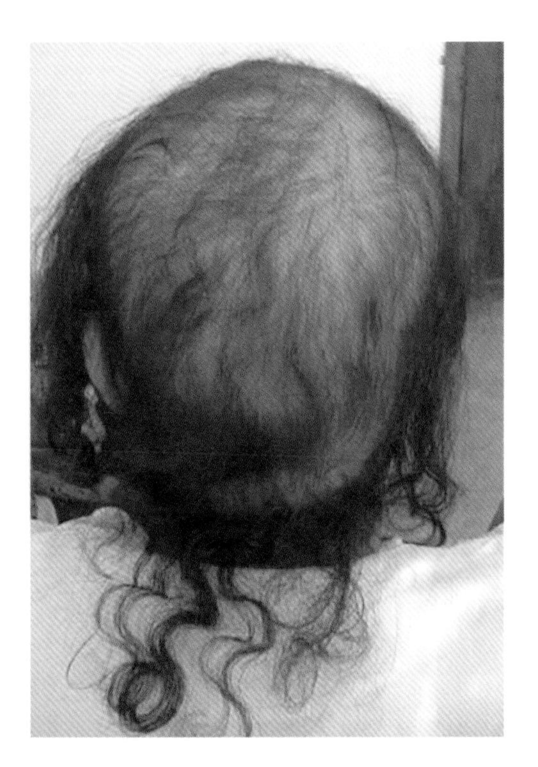

**Figure 45** This condition is caused by an individual pulling the hair out, usually at a time of severe emotional upset. The hairs are removed by twisting them around the finger and pulling. The hair loss is usually a well defined area on the centre of the scalp. The area is not completely bald, but contains short hairs which are too short to twist around a finger.

*Treatment:* The help of a psychiatrist is usually needed.

## ANTHRAX

**Figure 46** Primarily an infection of animals (goats, sheep, cows or dogs). Transmitted to humans by inoculation through traumatised skin, usually directly from a sick animal. A few (1–5) days later a small vesicle appears at the site of trauma. This enlarges, becomes haemorrhagic and is often surrounded by a ring of vesicles +/– oedema. The centre necroses causing the characteristic black eschar. This is the so-called *malignant pustule*. It is usually painless.

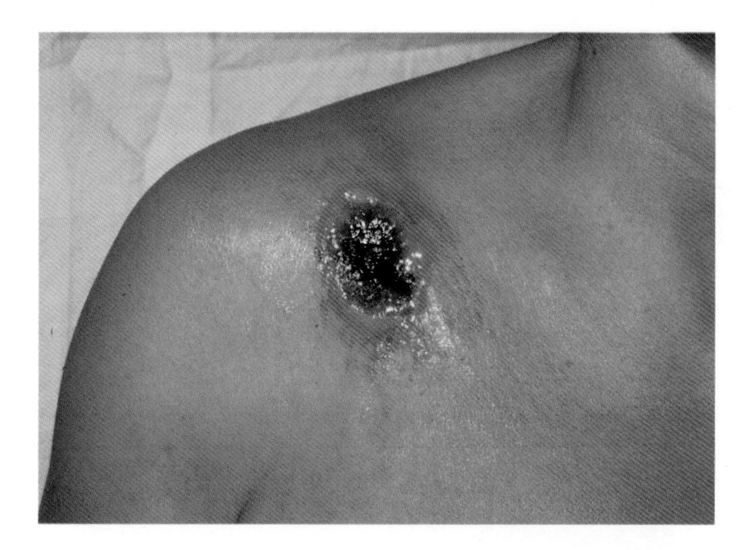

**Figure 47** Marked oedema around the eye. Note the original malignant pustule on the lower eyelid.

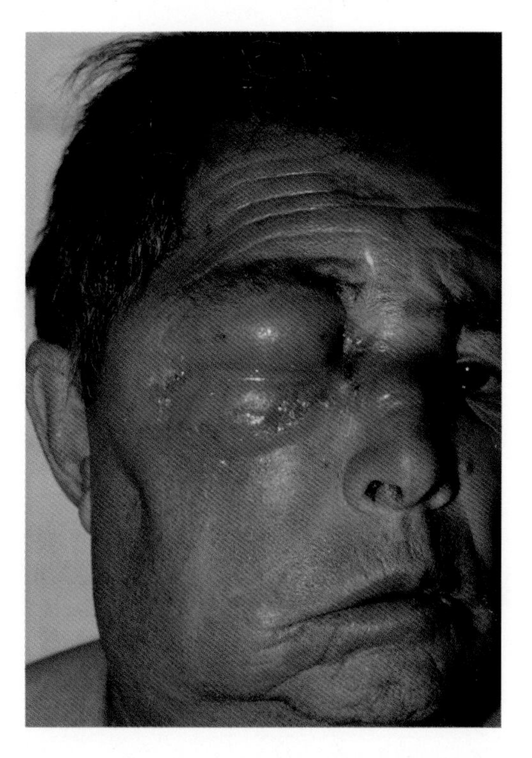

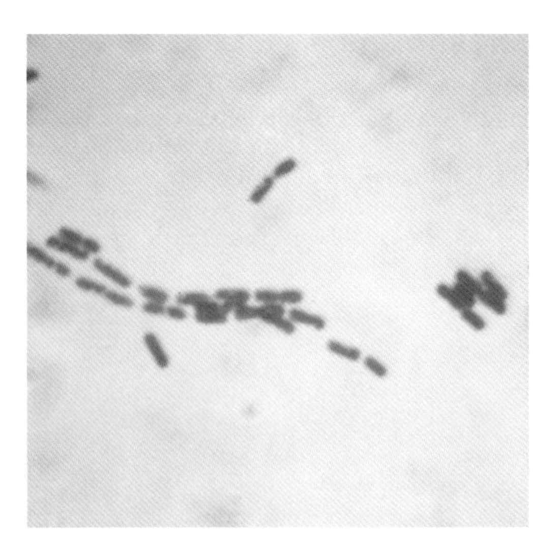

**Figure 48** Identify the organism, *Bacillus anthracis*, from scrapings from the ulcerated base of the lesion. Gram staining shows Gram positive rods in short chains.

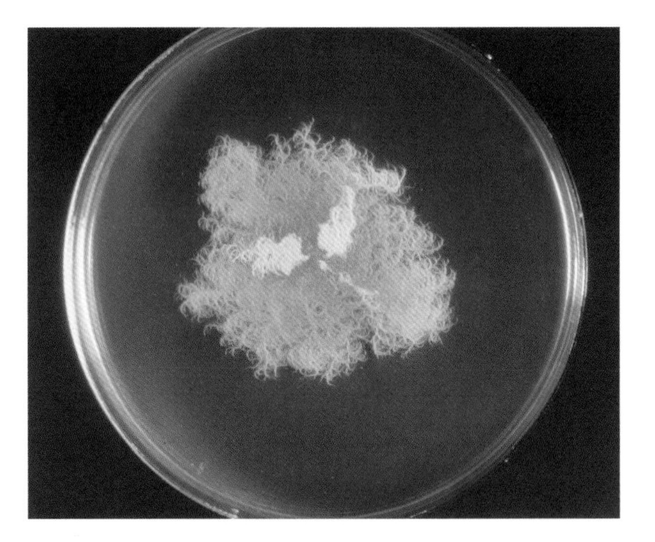

**Figure 49** Culture of the organism on blood agar. Grey hairy colonies (likened to a medusa head) develop after 24 hours.

*Treatment:* Intramuscular or intravenous benzyl penicillin, 1 mega-unit 6 hourly for 7 days. Animals with anthrax should not be eaten as they cause ulceration of the stomach and small bowel in humans (and often death). Dead animals should be burnt because the organisms form spores in the soil which can survive to infect other animals for many years.

# BALANITIS

Balanitis is inflammation of the glans penis. There are many different causes.

## Circinate balanitis

**Figure 50** Erosive balanitis with a serpiginous pustular edge. Part of Reiter's disease (urethritis, conjunctivitis and arthritis).

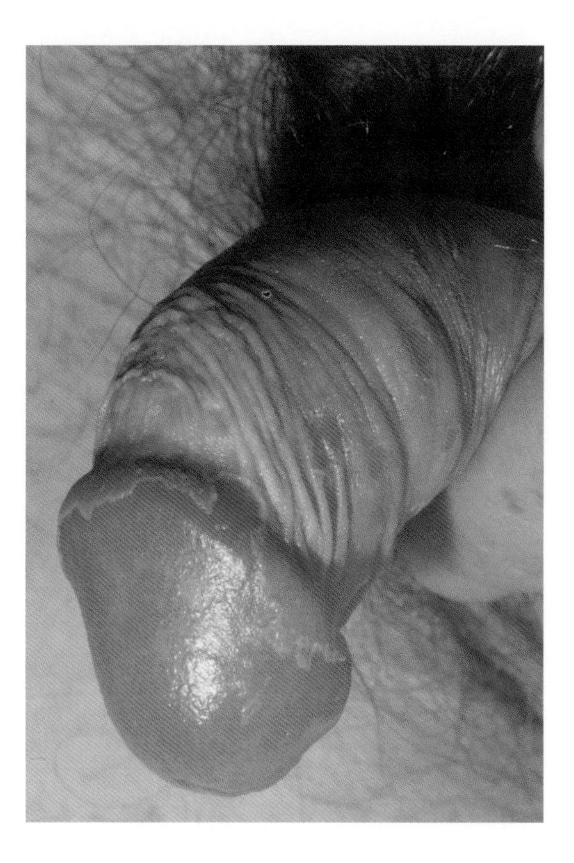

*Treatment:* Treat the urethritis with doxycycline 100mg bd for 10–14 days and the arthritis with a non-steroidal anti-inflammatory drug. The balanitis can be improved with saline soaks (1 tablespoon of salt in a pint of water) for 10 minutes bd +/− 1% hydrocortisone cream bd.

## Balanitis xerotica obliterans (lichen sclerosis et atrophicans)

**Figure 51** White macules or papules on glans penis +/− haemorrhagic blisters. If the urethral meatus is involved urine may spray in all directions. A common cause of needing circumcision in both children and adults.

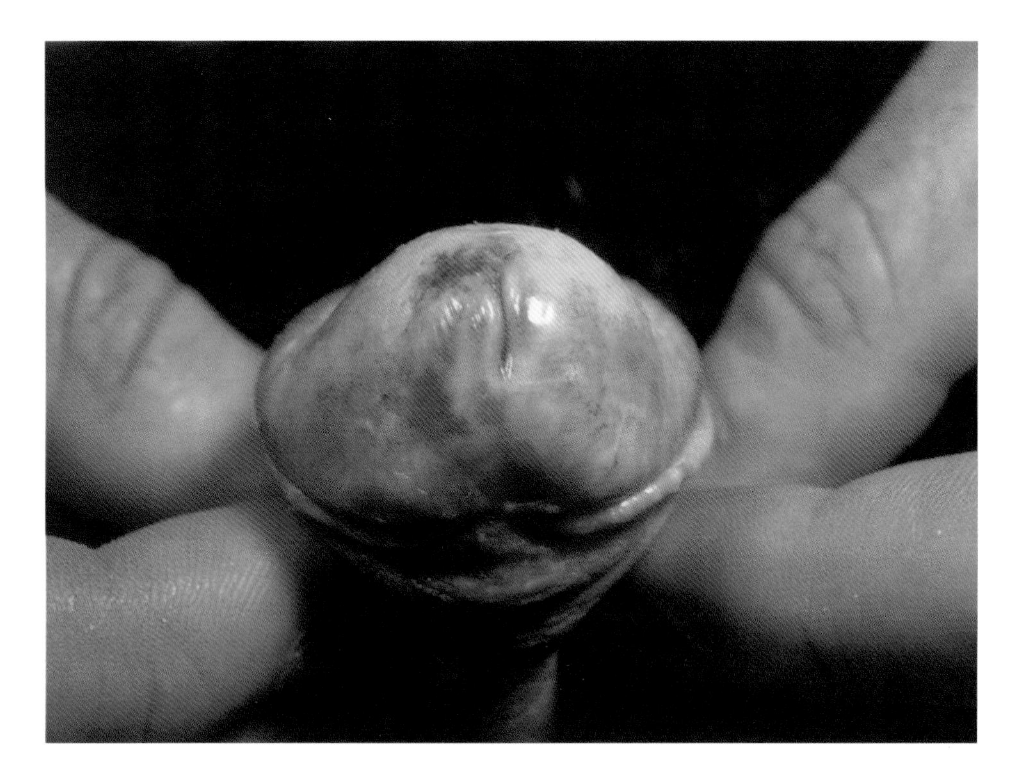

*Treatment:* Potent or very potent topical steroid (e.g. 0.1% betamethasone 17-valerate ointment or 0.05% clobetasol propionate ointment) applied twice a day until symptoms subside. Then use a weaker topical steroid such as 1% hydrocortisone ointment indefinitely.

## BED BUGS

**Figure 52** *Cimex lectularius* (approximately 4 × 3mm in size) lives in the walls and woodwork of houses and in old furniture (e.g. mattresses and cushions). They come out only at night (in the dark) and bite their host on any part of the skin sticking out of the bed clothes to obtain his/her blood. The bites are very similar to flea bites (*see* Figure 86), often in rows, but differ in appearing only on exposed parts of the body. New lesions are present each morning.

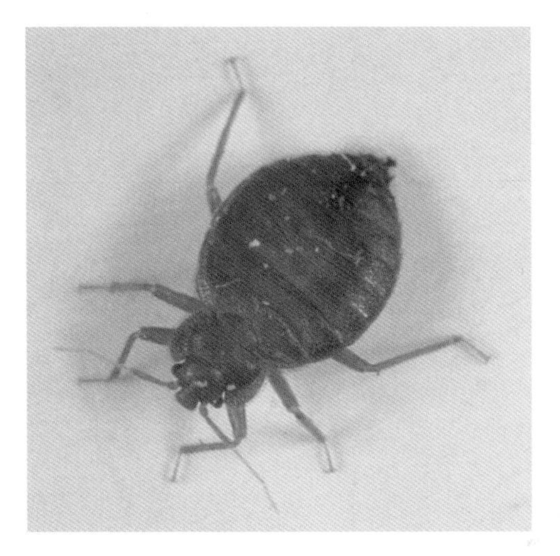

*Treatment:* Spray the walls and bedding with a residual insecticide (i.e. one that persists after evaporation of the solvent) such as 2% malathion, 0.9% dichlorvos or 0.5% d-phenothrin. Use a mosquito net in the future to stop them getting into the bed.

## BED SORE (Pressure sore)

**Figure 53** Patients lying in one position in bed are likely to develop bed sores, especially those who are unconscious or have paraplegia. They begin with erythema and oedema at the site of pressure between the skin and the underlying bone, then necrosis occurs which may extend deep into muscle.

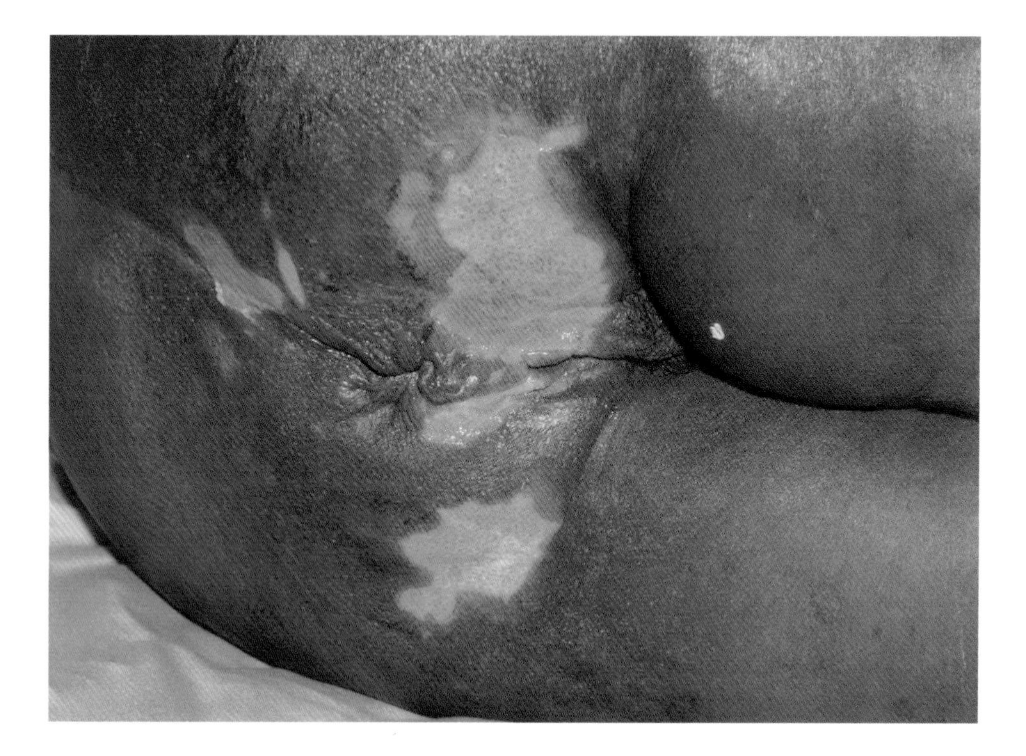

*Treatment:* Remove pressure by regular turning of the patient and keep the wound clean until it heals. Good nursing care is more important than topical agents applied to the sore itself.

## BERI BERI

**Figure 54** Gross oedema of the legs, sometimes up to the waist +/– polyneuropathy due to thiamine (vitamin $B_1$) deficiency.

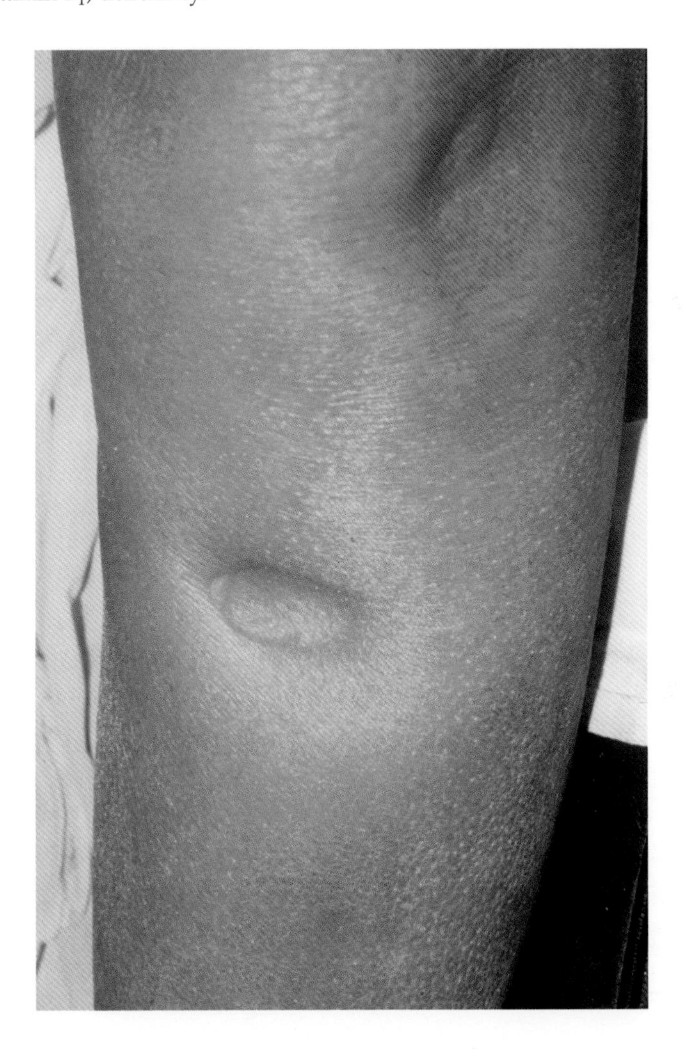

*Treatment:* Thiamine 2–3mg tds and improve the diet.

## BIRTH MARKS OR NAEVI

These are either non-neoplastic malformations (hamartomas) or benign tumours which are mainly present from birth. They can arise after birth in early childhood. Mostly, they do not need treatment. Some of those that are very large or unsightly can be excised.

### Becker's naevus

**Figure 55** Hyperpigmented patch with increased hairs. Most common over the shoulder or on the upper trunk, but it can occur anywhere. Not usually seen until the mid-to-late teens.

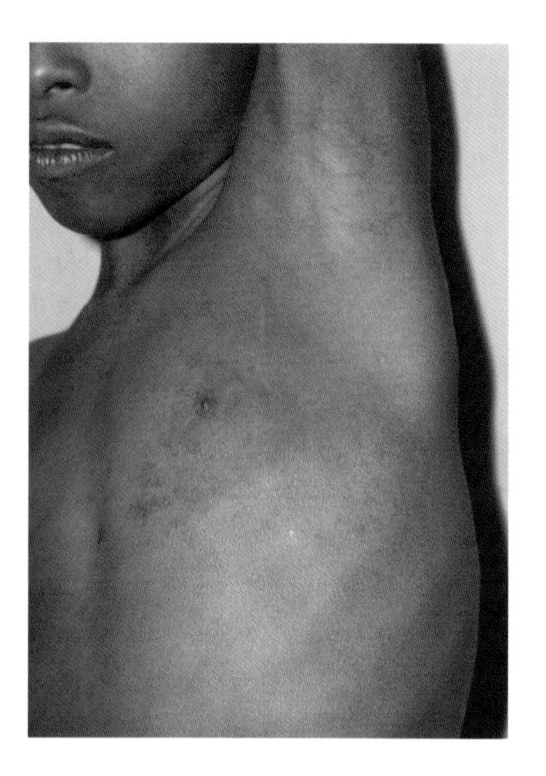

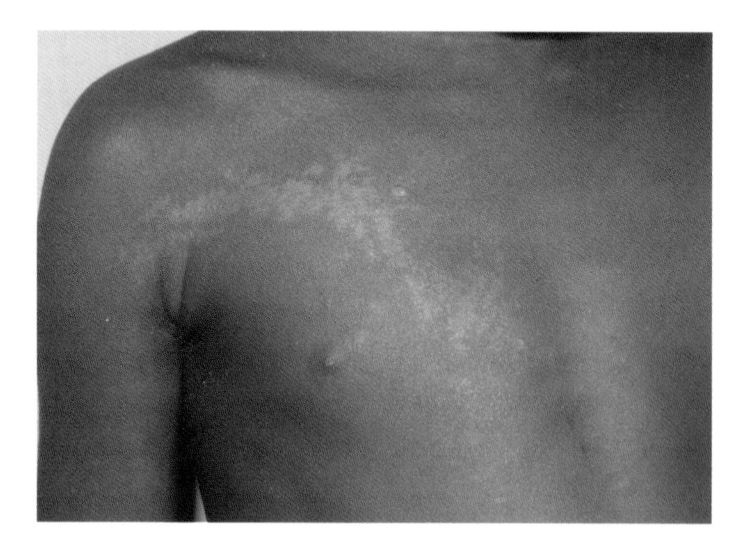

### Epidermal naevus

**Figure 56** Linear skin-coloured, hypo- or hyperpigmented, hyperkeratotic plaque. Often looks like a row of viral warts but is present from birth. Can be small (1–2cm) or extend down the whole length of a limb or around the trunk.

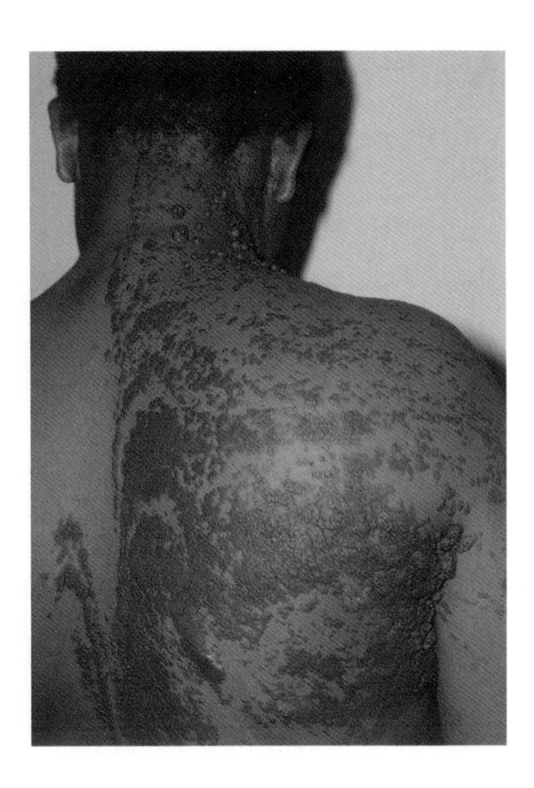

**Figure 57**
Very extensive epidermal naevus.

## Inflammatory, linear, verrucous, epidermal naevus (ILVEN)

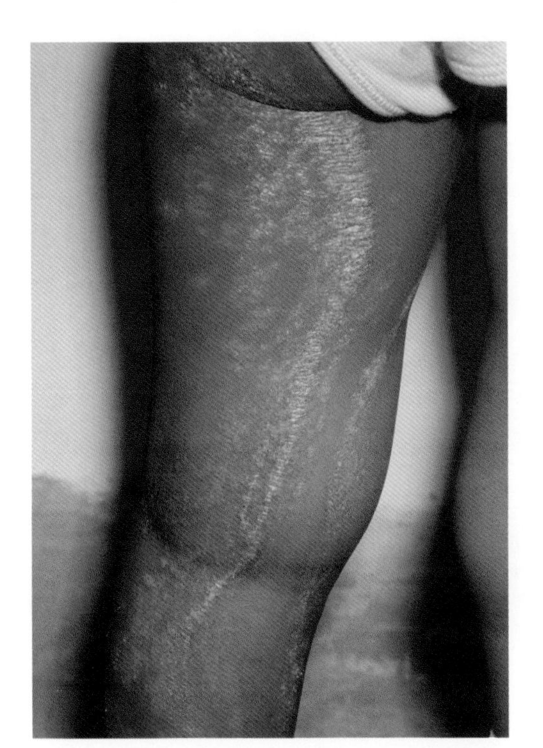

**Figure 58** This is a linear lesion like an epidermal naevus but it is red in colour and very itchy. The surface is scaly so that it looks like a line of eczema or psoriasis. It appears during the first 5 years of life.

*Treatment:* Application of a moderately potent topical steroid will help the itching.

## Lymphangioma circumscriptum

**Figures 59, 60** Grouped vesicles looking like frog spawn. Can be found anywhere on the skin and are present from birth. It is thought they occur because the embryological lymph sacs fail to connect to the lymphatic channels.

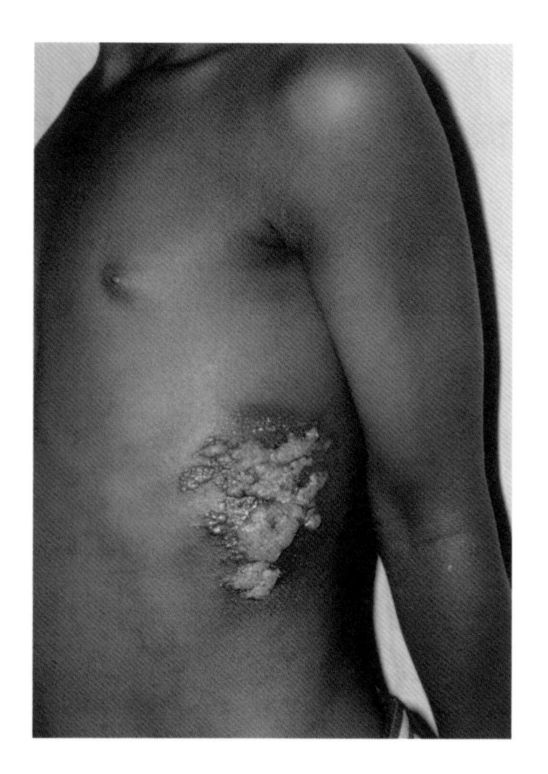

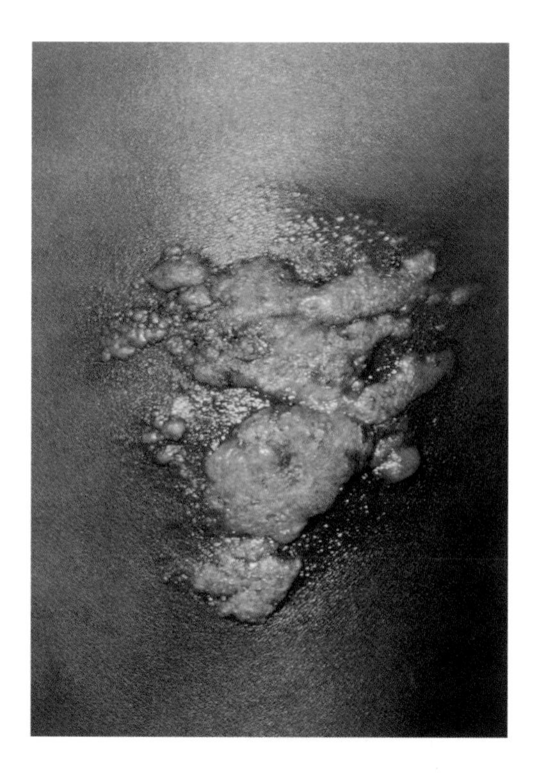

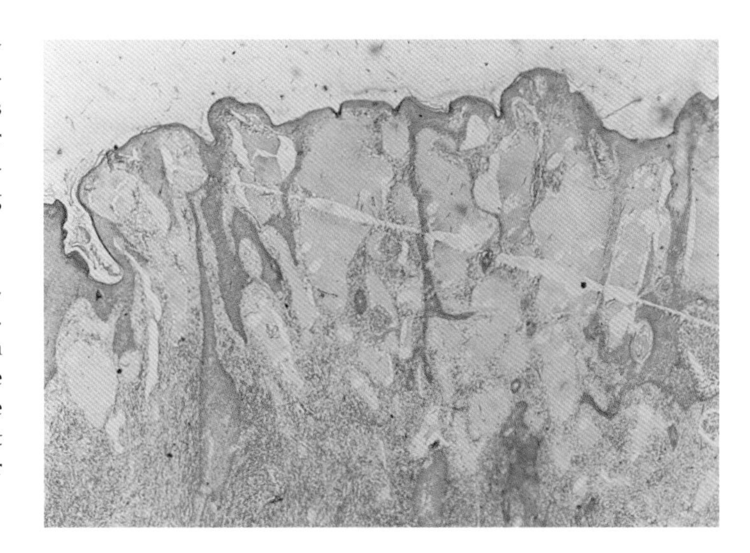

**Figure 61** Histology shows dilated lymphatics in the dermis with a muscular pump in the subcutaneous fat feeding them.

*Treatment:* If small, leave them alone. If large, they can be excised, but the muscle pump in the subcutaneous fat must also be excised or they will recur.

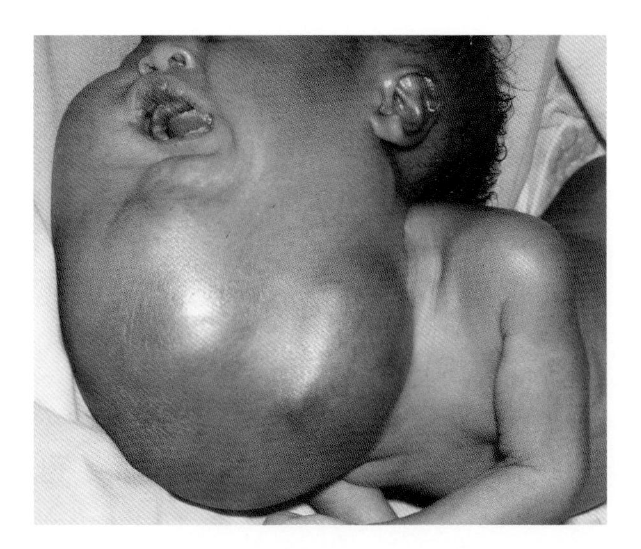

## Cystic hygroma

**Figure 62** This is a large cystic mass, most common in the neck, which is present from birth. It develops from a defect in the formation of lymphatic vessels and is histologically very similar to a cavernous lymphangioma. May cause death by interfering with breathing if very large.

*Treatment:* Surgical excision, if feasible.

## Melanocytic naevi

Apart from the giant melanocytic naevus these are not present at birth but begin to appear in the first 5 years of life. They can continue to develop into adult life. They are commonly called 'moles'.

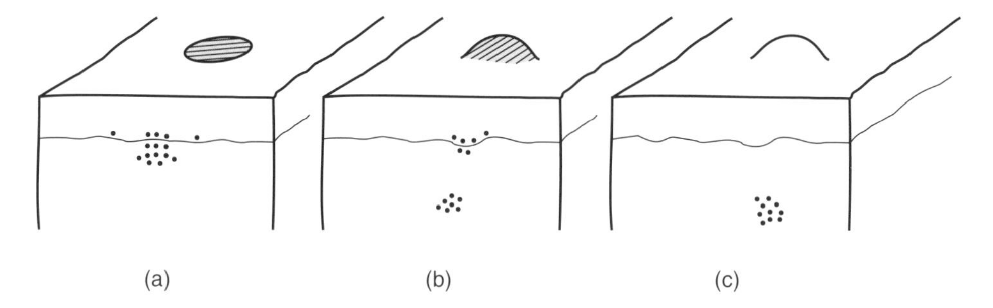


**Figure 63** Pathology of melanocytic naevi. (a) Junctional naevus – the naevus cells are at the dermo–epidermal junction. (b) Compound naevus – the naevus cells are at the dermo–epidermal junction and also in the dermis. (c) Intradermal naevus – the naevus cells are only in the dermis. The natural history of a melanocytic naevus is to progress from junctional naevus to compound naevus to intradermal naevus over time.

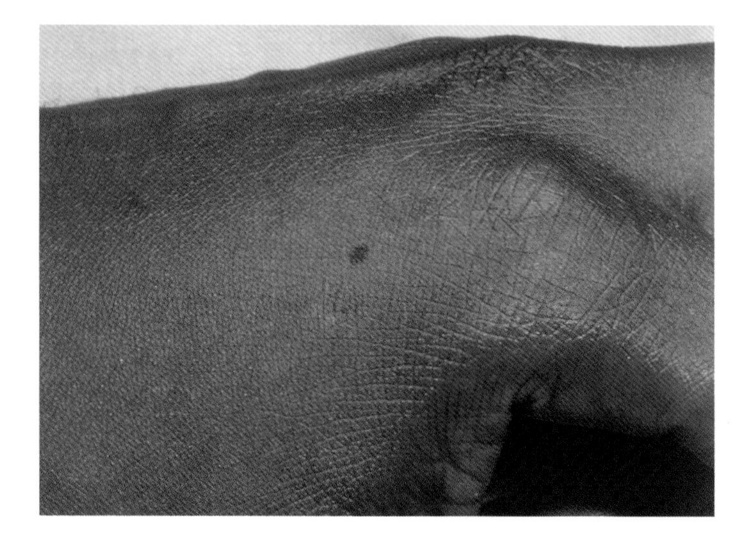

## Junctional naevus

**Figure 64** Small round or oval hyperpigmented macule found anywhere on the skin surface.

**Figure 65** Junctional naevi on the palms and soles usually remain throughout life. Those arising in the nail matrix appear as a brown line going down the nail (*see* Figure 455).

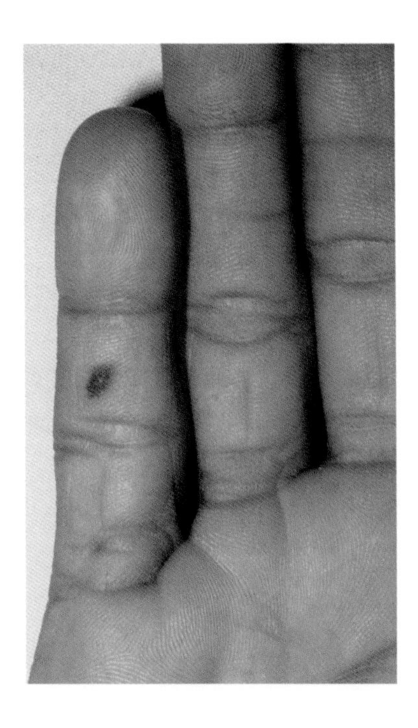

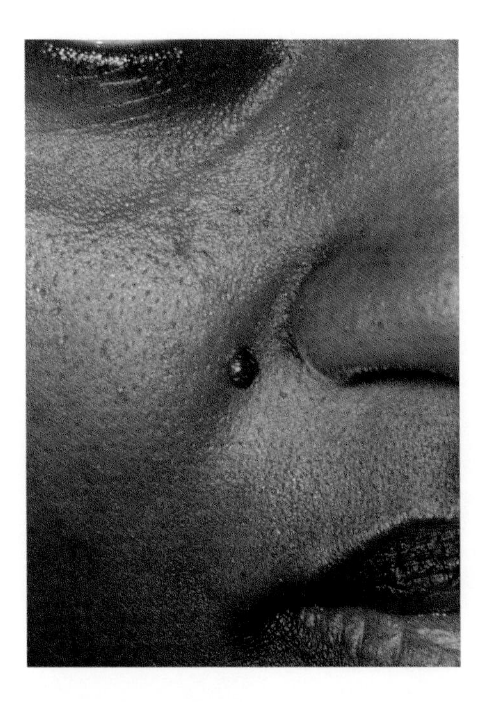

## Compound naevus

**Figure 66** Most people have several of these hyperpigmented papules scattered over their bodies.

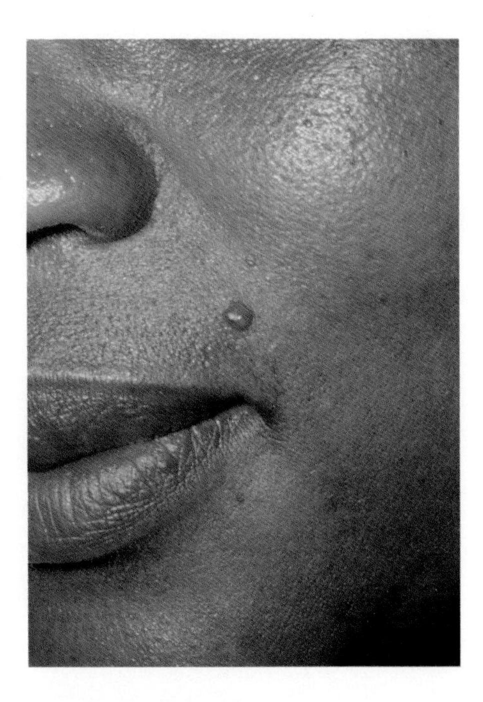

## Intradermal naevus

**Figure 67** Similar to a compound naevus but skin-coloured rather than hyper-pigmented.

## Congenital melanocytic naevus

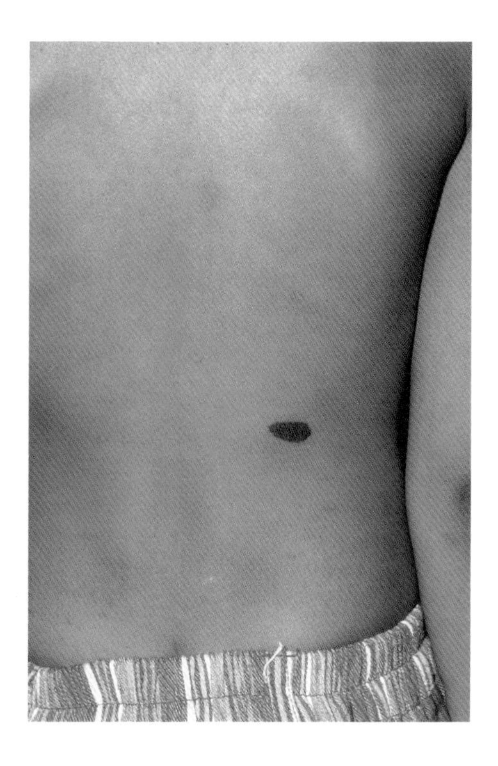

**Figure 68** Larger than an ordinary compound naevus and present from birth. They are usually both hyperpigmented and hairy.

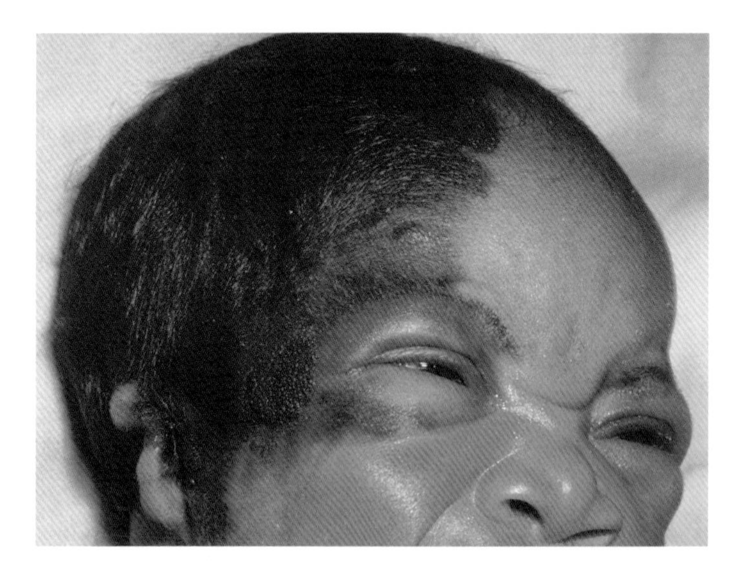

**Figure 69** Vary in size from a few centimetres to up to half the body surface. The larger ones are called giant pigmented (hairy) naevi (or bathing trunk naevi if they occur on the lower trunk). They are usually hairy as well as hyperpigmented. Histologically they are compound naevi. For the very large naevi there is a 9% lifetime risk of malignant melanoma, the risk being greatest before puberty.

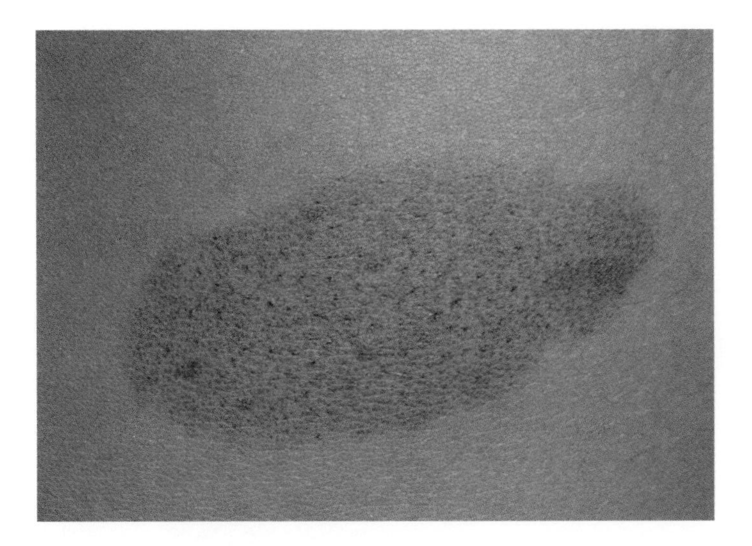

## Naevus spilus (spotty naevus)

**Figure 70** Flat hyperpigmented patch with darker macules or papules within it.

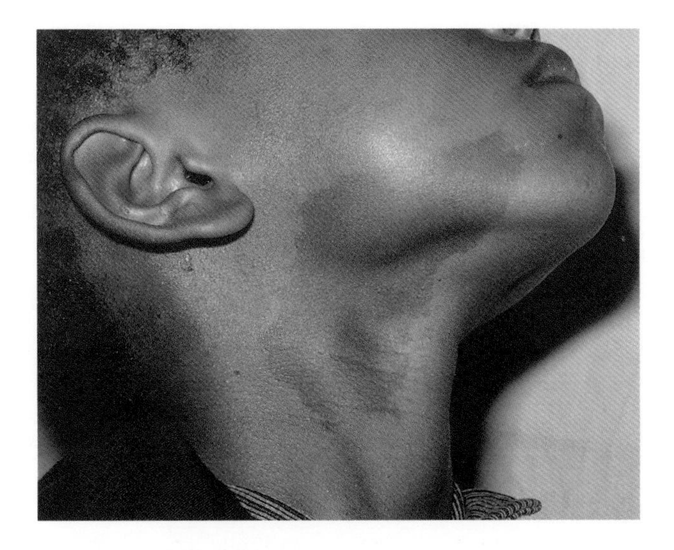

## Lentiginous naevus

**Figure 71** Hyperpigmented patch found anywhere on the skin. Present from birth.

## Dermal melanocytic naevi (blue naevi)

**Figure 72** The common blue naevus looks like a compound melanocytic naevus but is bluish-black in colour rather than dark brown (compare with Figure 66).

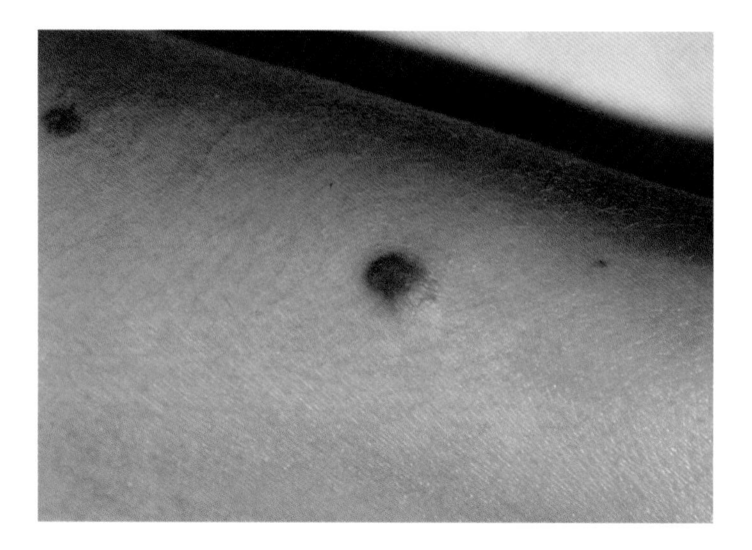

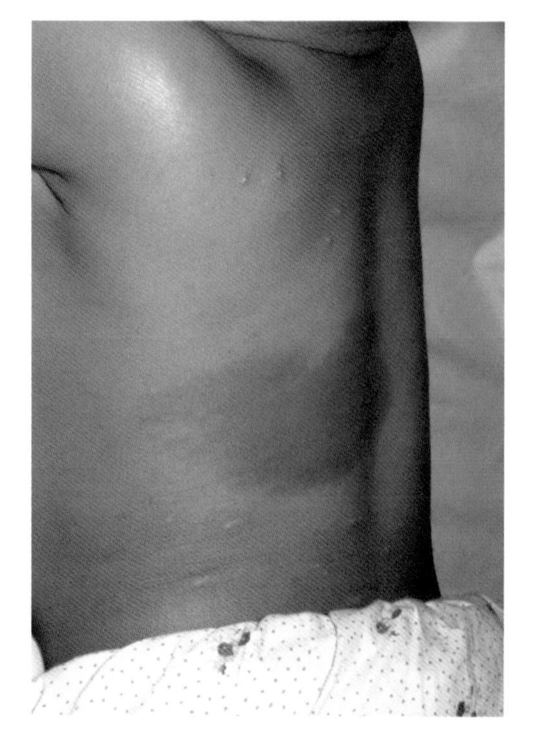

**Figure 73** The Mongolian spot is a large bluish patch on the lower back at birth. Disappears spontaneously usually by the end of the first year of life.

**Figures 74, 75** A naevus of Ota is similar in appearance to a Mongolian spot. A bluish patch on the face around the eye and involving the sclera. The same lesion over the shoulder is known as a naevus of Ito.

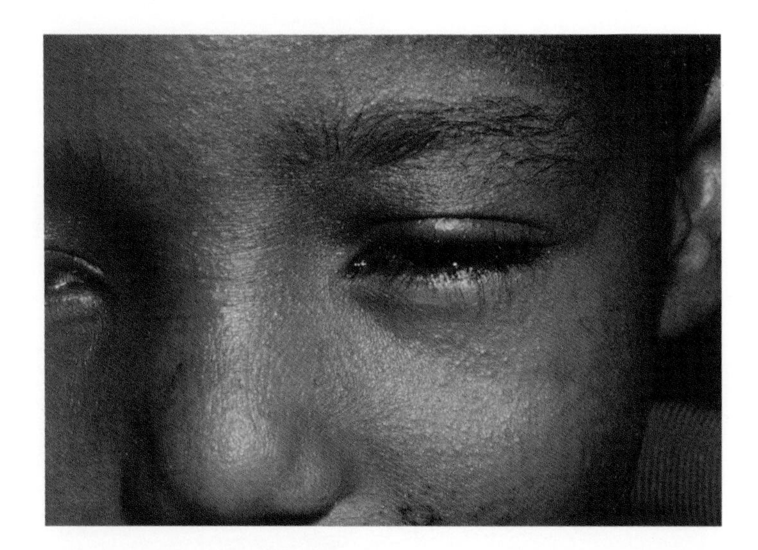

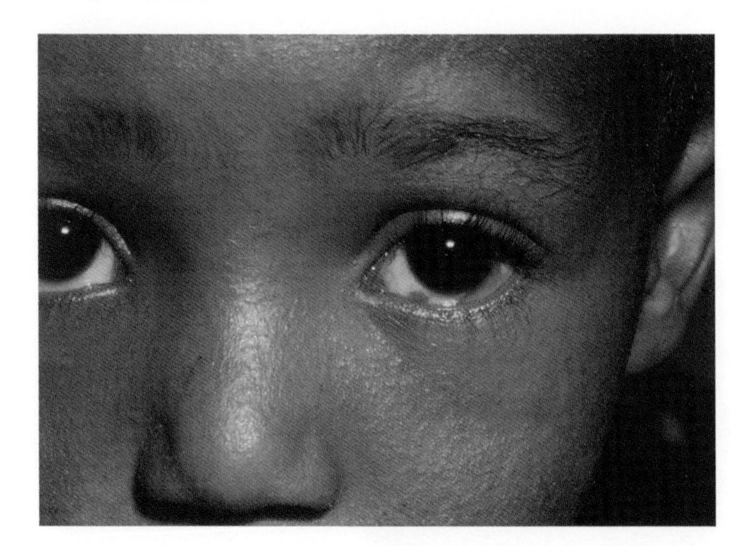

## Naevus sebaceous

**Figure 76** Complex congenital malformation involving the hair follicles, sebaceous glands, eccrine and apocrine glands. Appears as a linear or oval warty plaque at birth. Frequently found on the scalp where it causes alopecia, but it can be found anywhere on the body.

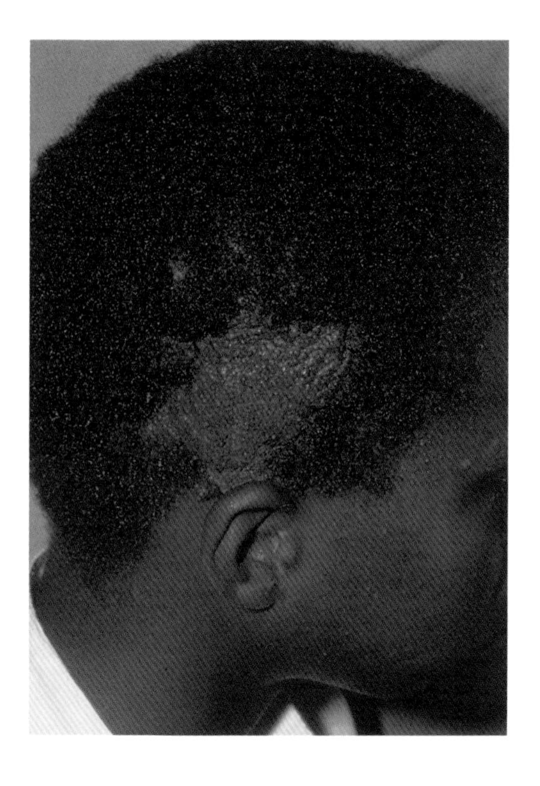

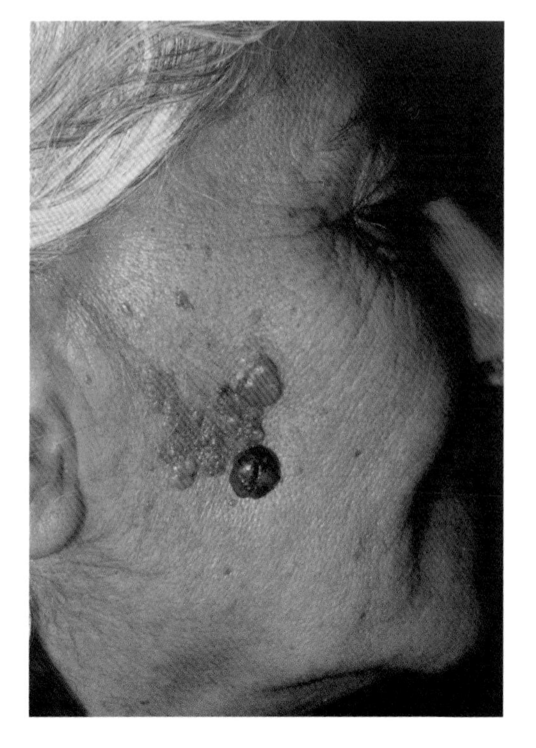

**Figure 77** In middle age it can develop tumours within it, e.g. a basal cell carcinoma or one or more benign or malignant adnexal tumours. Here, three basal cell carcinomas have arisen from the naevus in a 60-year-old lady.

*Treatment:* Do nothing unless it develops a tumour, then excise.

## Vascular naevi

These are divided into haemangiomas and vascular malformations. Haemangiomas are vascular tumours that have a period of active growth followed by a period of inactivity, and then spontaneous involution (e.g. strawberry naevi). Vascular malformations are structural abnormalities representing an error in development *in utero* (e.g. port wine stain).

## Capillary haemangioma (strawberry naevus)

**Figures 78, 79, 80** Appears after birth but during the first 4 weeks of life. Bright red nodule or plaque which grows rapidly for 12–15 months and then involutes spontaneously over the next 4 or 5 years. Left to its own devices it will disappear without scarring.

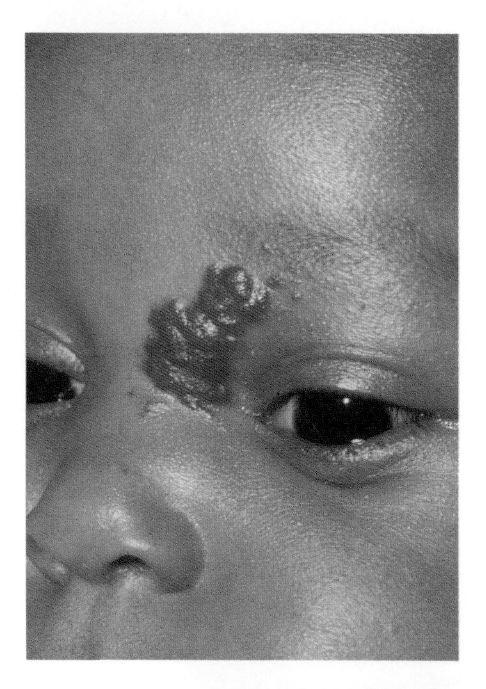

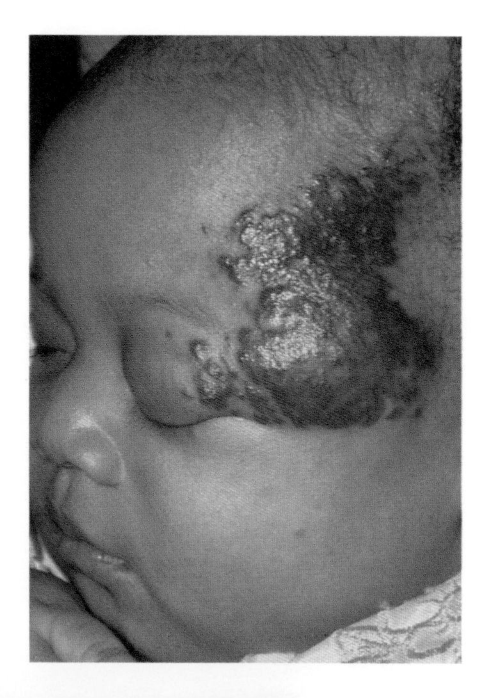

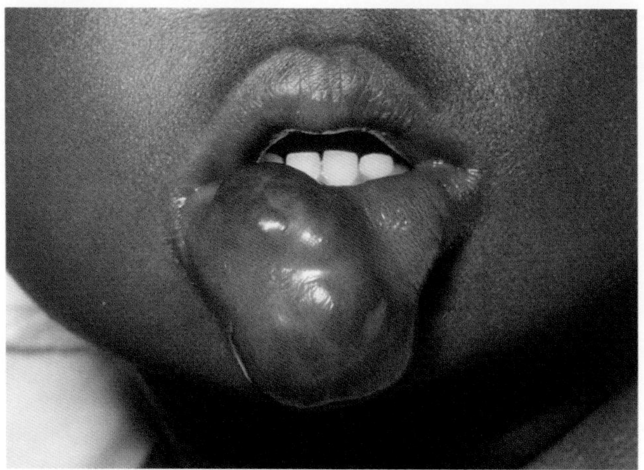

*Treatment:* Reassure the parents that it will disappear on its own.

## Naevus flammeus (salmon patch)

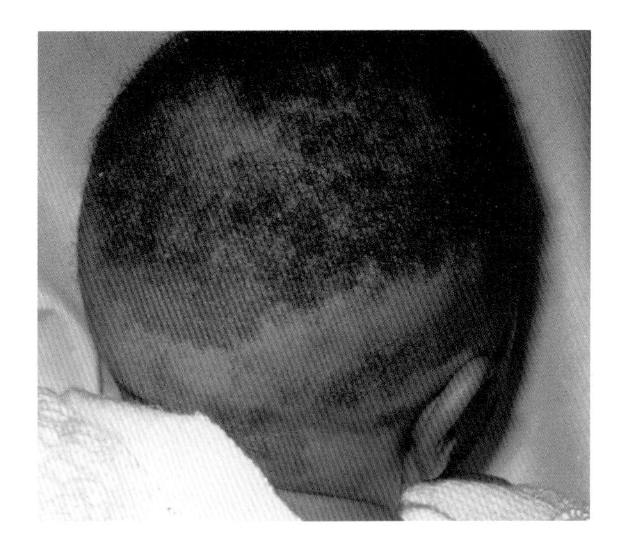

**Figure 81** Flat red patch on any part of the head and neck at birth. If it is on the face it will usually disappear spontaneously by the end of the first year of life. If it is on the occiput it will remain throughout life but will not usually be seen because it will be covered by hair.

## Port wine stain

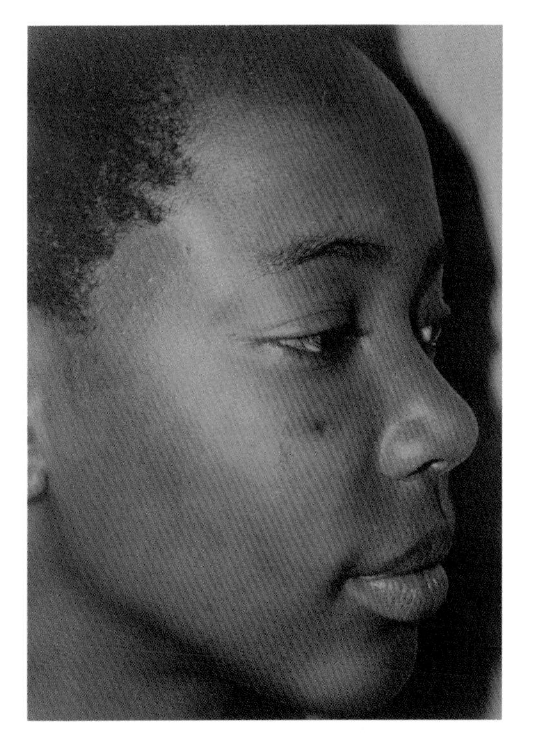

**Figure 82** This is similar to the salmon patch but more extensive and darker in colour. It is present from birth and remains throughout life. It is difficult to see in the African skin and is therefore not usually a cosmetic problem.

**Figure 83** In individuals with a paler skin a port wine stain can be very unsightly. When it involves the forehead it may rarely be associated with cerebral or meningeal vascular abnormalities (Sturge-Weber syndrome).

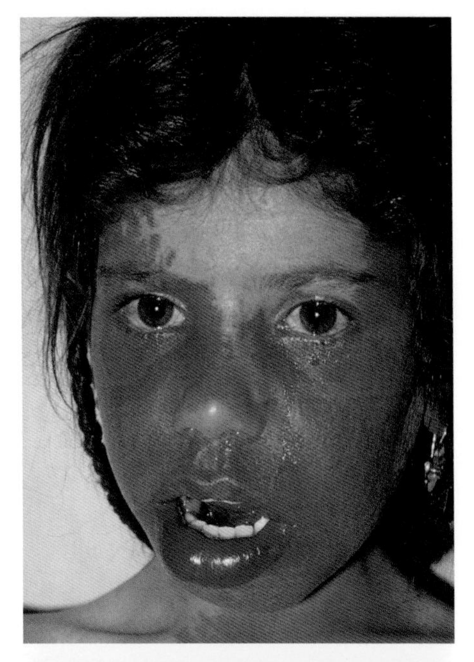

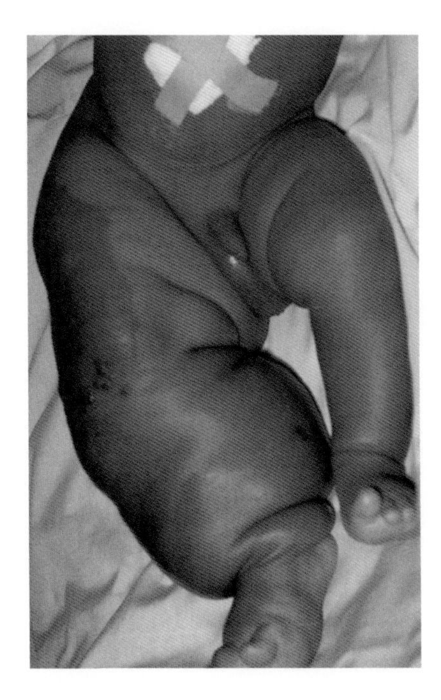

**Figure 84** Klippel-Trenaunay-Weber syndrome. A port wine stain on a limb may rarely be associated with multiple arterio-venous communications causing hypertrophy of the limb.

*Treatment:* Nothing can be done for this.

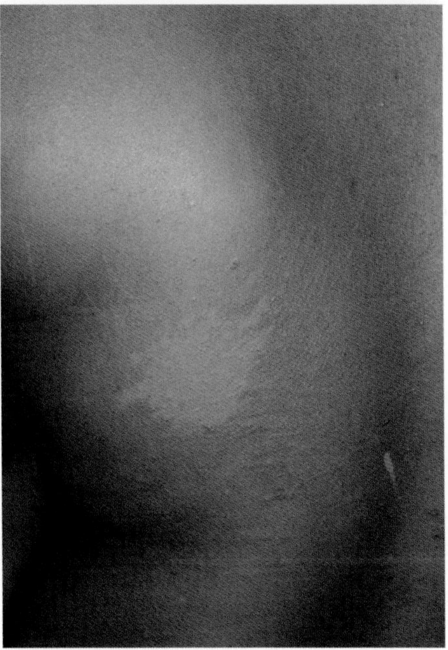

## Naevus anaemicus

**Figure 85** This is a pharmacological naevus. The abnormally pale patch of skin with a geographic outline is due to a localised area of hyper-reactivity to catecholamines. By pressing a glass slide over the edge of the patch the edge will disappear as the pressure causes vasoconstriction of the normal skin.

# BITES

All kinds of creatures can bite the human skin either to obtain blood or as a form of defence or aggression.

## Insect bite

**Figure 86** Flea bites on the foot of a 2-year-old child. These are small grouped papules each with a central punctum.

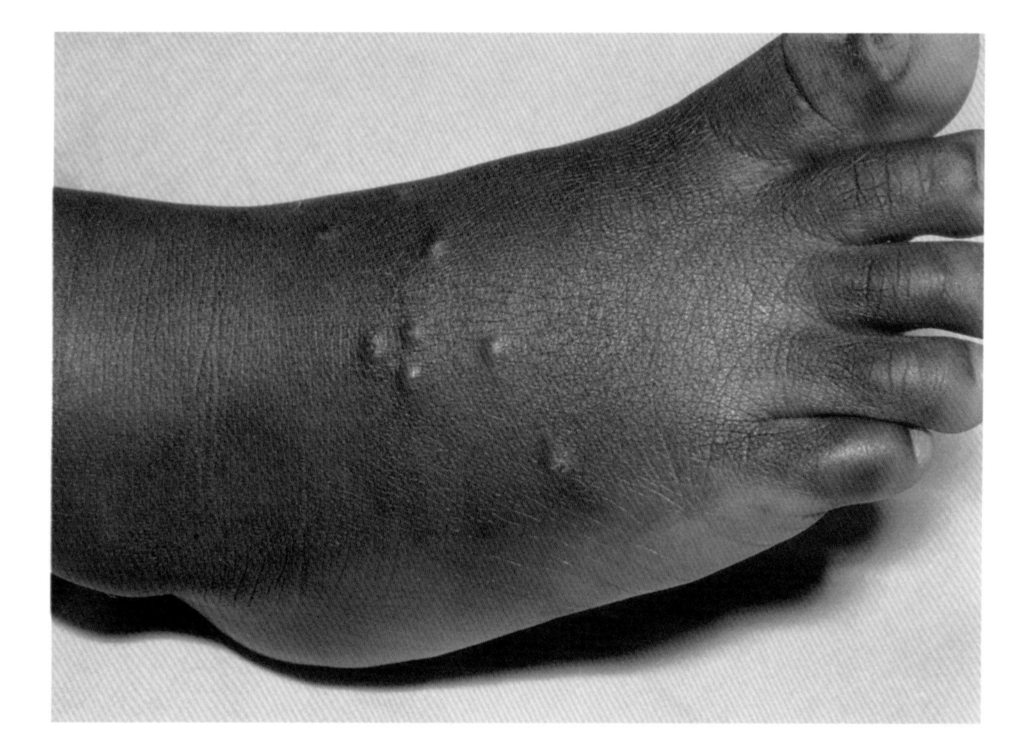

## Snake bite

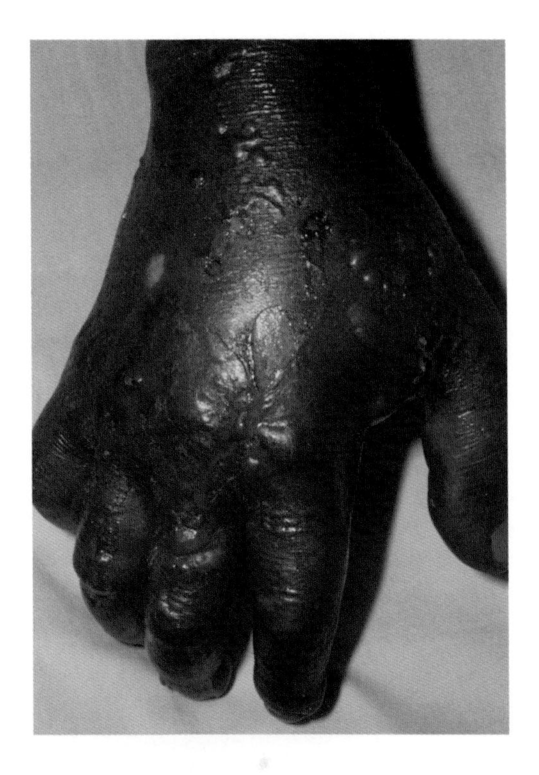

**Figure 87** Snake bites are an occupational hazard of farmers. An individual may not even know that he has been bitten but may present like this with a grossly swollen limb and blistering due to a massive increase in vascular permeability.

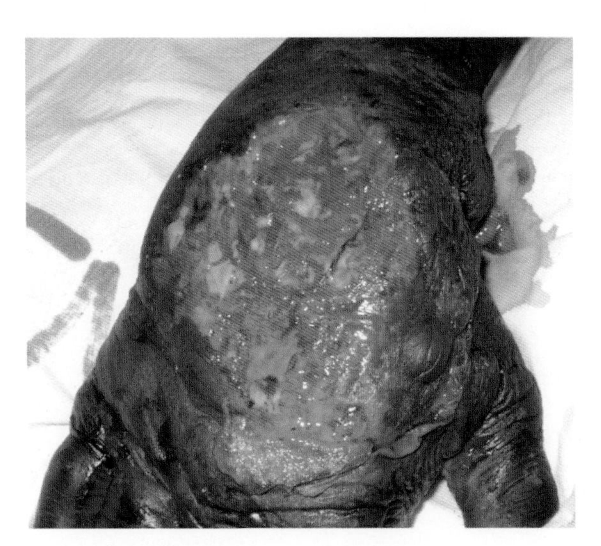

**Figure 88** Later there is tissue necrosis.

*Treatment:* At this stage it is too late for any specific anti-venom. Reassurance, raising of the limb, fluid replacement and prevention of secondary infection are now necessary.

## BLISTER BEETLE DERMATITIS

**Figure 89** *Paederus cerebri punctatus*, known locally in East Africa as 'Nairobi fly'. These blister beetles come down from the mountains during the rainy season and enter houses. When they land on the skin they cause no harm unless crushed when they release cantharidine causing an irritant dermatitis.

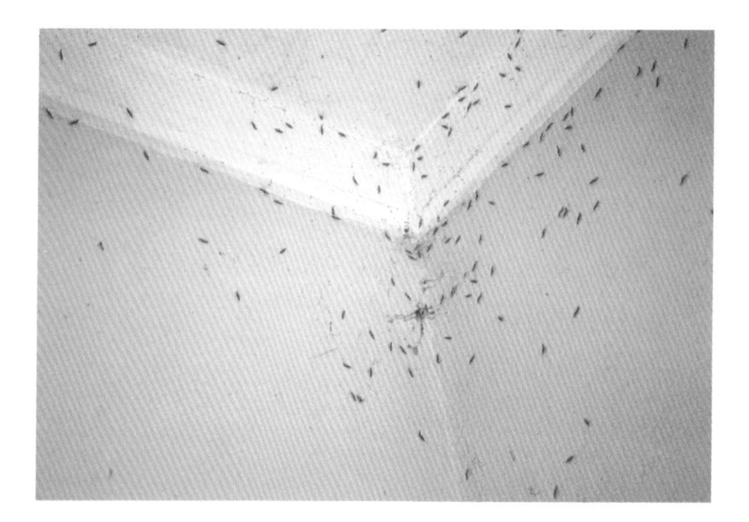

**Figure 90** Cantharidine rash caused by release of this chemical from the mid-gut of the blister beetle. Mostly occurs at night when the beetle is inadvertently brushed away by someone who is asleep. The rash is caused by crushing the blister beetle, not by a bite.

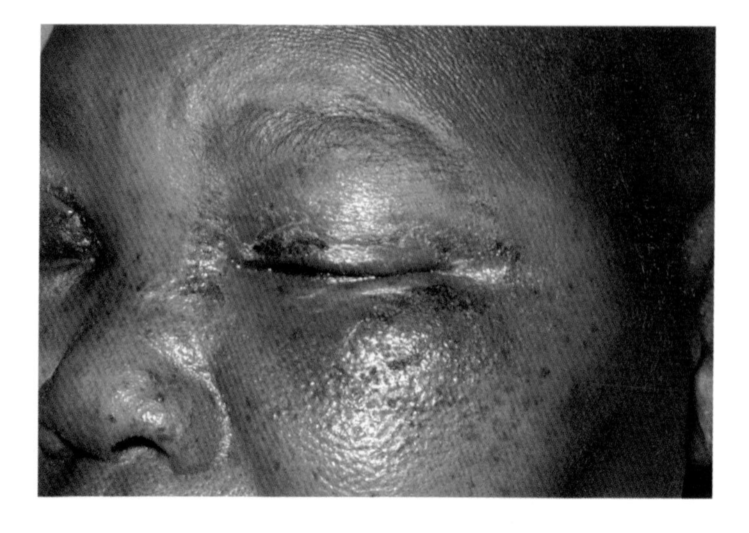

*Treatment:* Leave alone. It will heal spontaneously after 5–10 days.

## BOIL

**Figure 91** Abscess of a single hair follicle due to *Staphylococcus aureus* (*see* Figure 309). A carbuncle is an abscess of several adjacent hair follicles. If boils are multiple and / or recurrent, think of HIV infection.

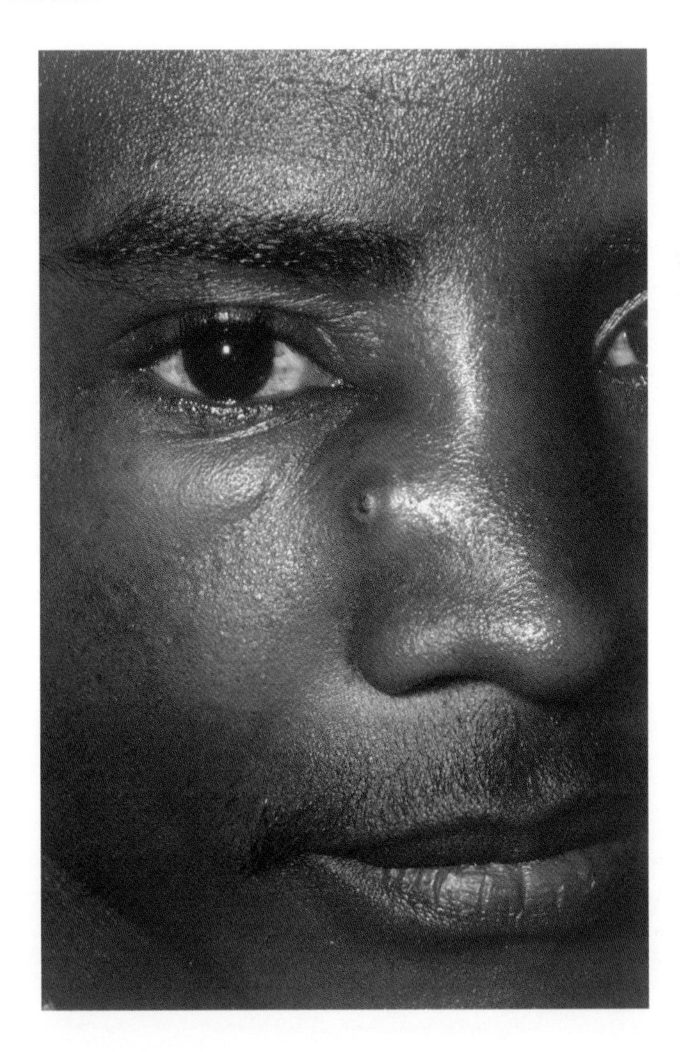

*Treatment:* Oral cloxacillin 500mg qds for 5 days.

## BOTRIOMYCOSIS

**Figure 92** A chronic granulomatous reaction to infection with *Staphylococcus aureus*.

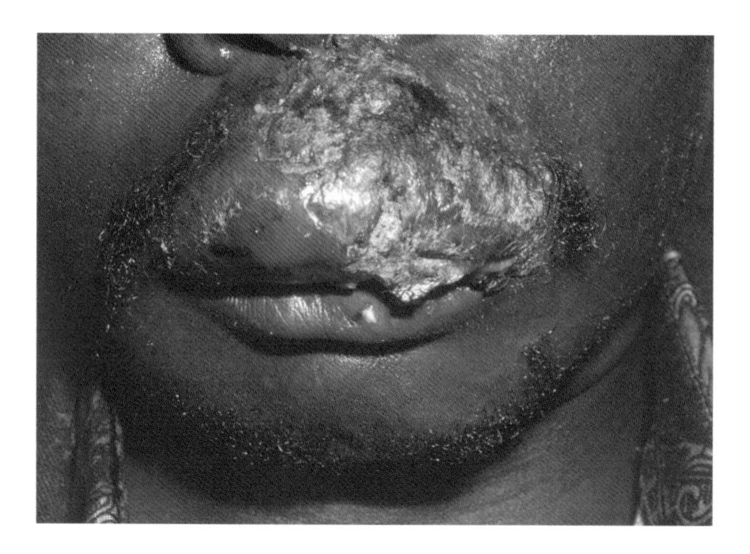

**Figure 93** Same patient as in Figure 92 after the crusts have been removed. It now shows multiple discharging sinuses mimicking a deep fungal infection.

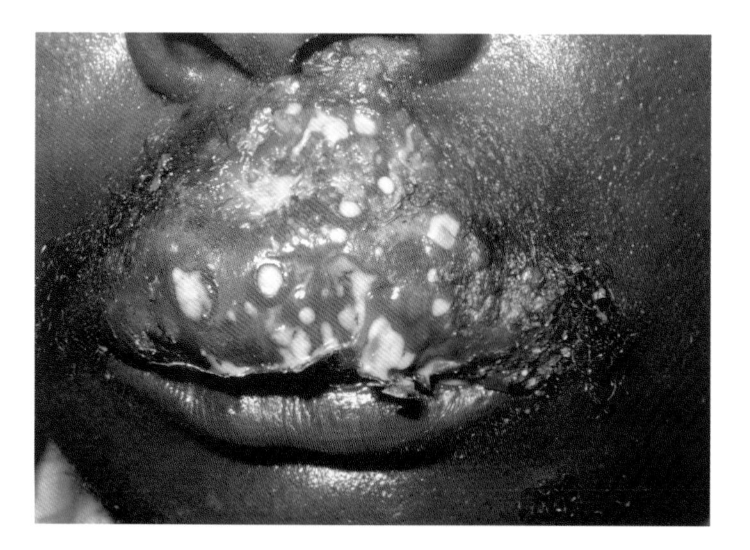

*Treatment:* Oral cloxacillin 500mg qds for 10–14 days.

## BOWENOID PAPULOSIS

**Figure 94** Flat warty lesions on the perianal skin or shaft of the penis due to infection with HPV 16 or 18. Looks like genital warts but has a different pathology.

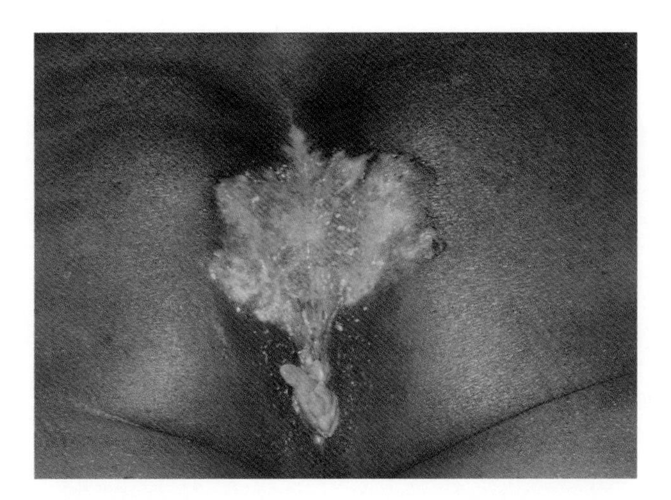

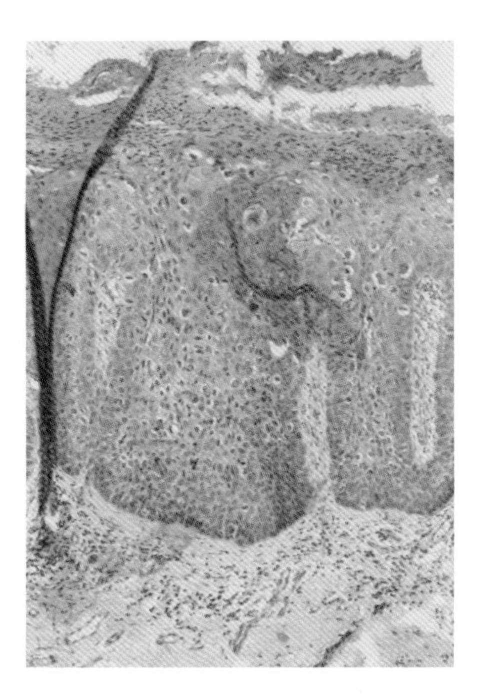

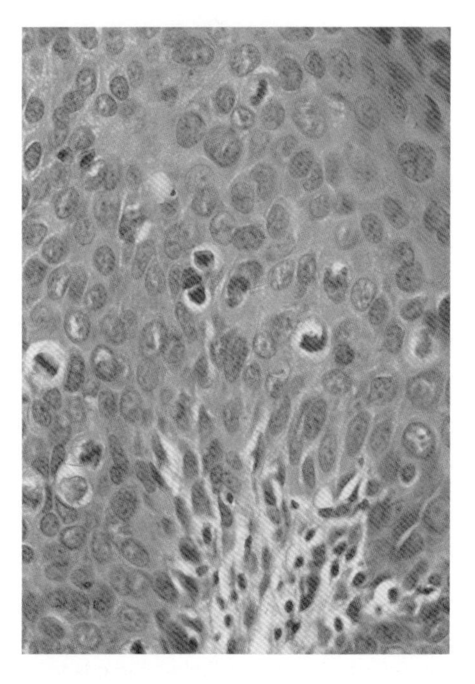

**Figures 95, 96** The pathology looks like an intraepidermal squamous cell carcinoma with very numerous mitoses. Transformation to an invasive SCC is rare (approximately 2%).

*Treatment:* Topical podophyllin once a week as for genital warts (*see* Figures 675–7), or 5% 5-fluorouracil cream once a day for 1 month.

## BULLDOG SCALP (Cutis verticis gyrata)

**Figure 97** Acquired thickening of the scalp causing folds in the skin which run in an anterior-posterior direction. Appears from the mid-teens onwards. Sometimes associated with mental retardation or chronic schizophrenia.

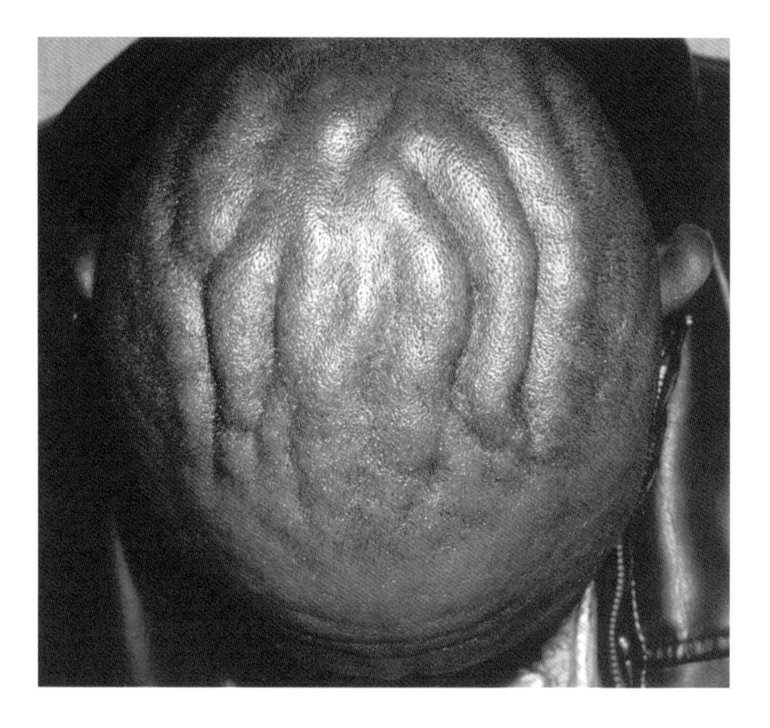

*Treatment:* Plastic surgery if wanted.

## BURN

**Figure 98** Heat injury from boiling liquids being spilt on the skin or from falling in a fire. Classified as superficial (epidermis only), partial thickness (down to mid-dermis) or full thickness (dermis down to fat). Superficial burns are the most painful. If the cutaneous nerves are destroyed no pain is felt.

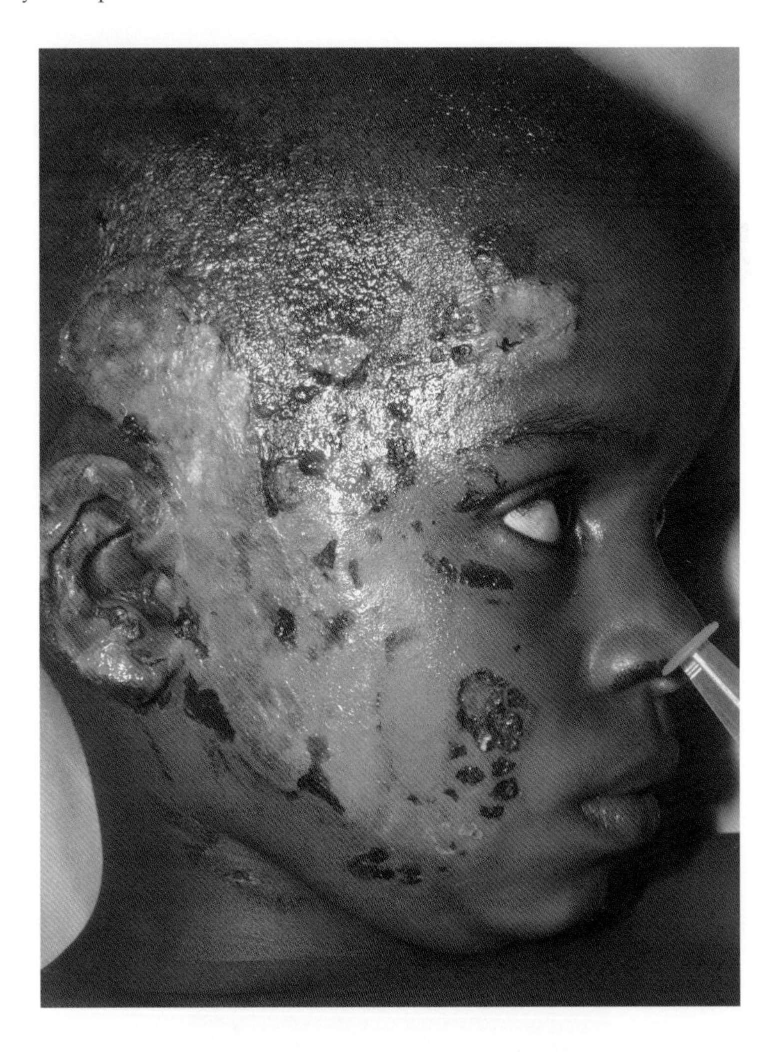

*Treatment:* Immediately immerse the affected part in cold water to lower the temperature. Protect the burnt area from flies and other sources of infection. Skin grafting for partial or full thickness burns.

## CALCINOSIS CUTIS

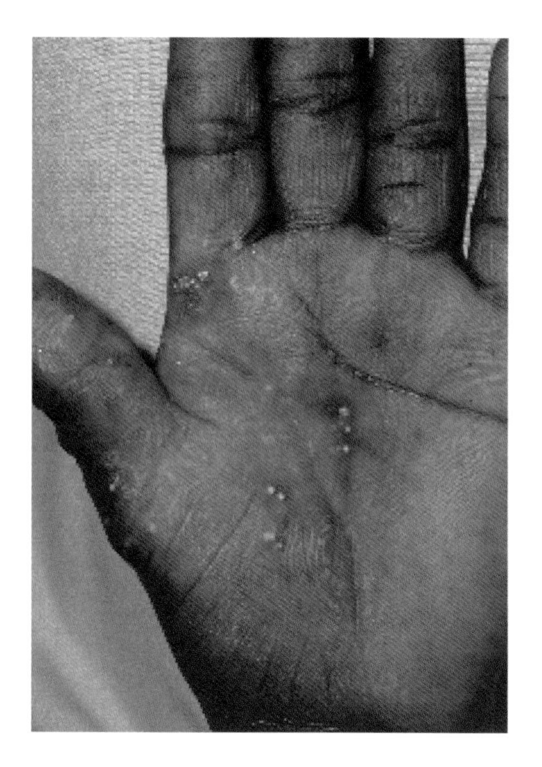

**Figures 99, 100** Deposition of calcium in the dermis or subcutaneous fat due to hypercalcaemia (hyperparathyroidism or chronic renal failure), local injury or connective tissue diseases such as dermatomyositis (*see* Figures 176–8) or systemic sclerosis (*see* Figures 578–81).

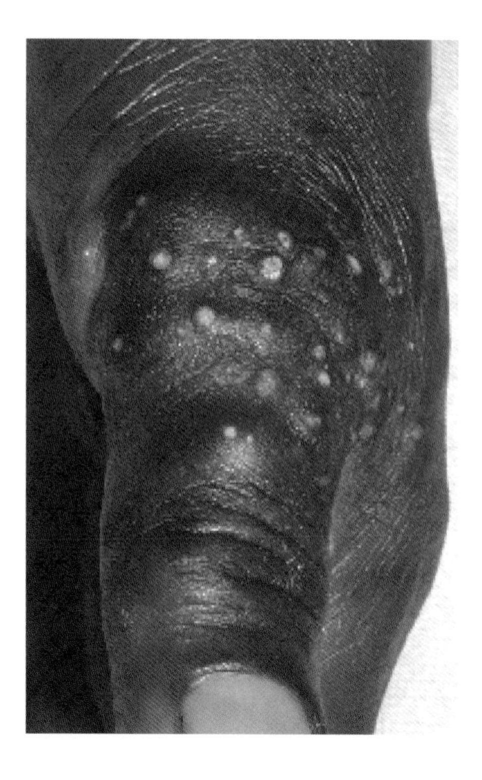

## CANDIDIASIS

Candidiasis is an infection with the yeast-like fungus, *Candida albicans*. It is a normal commensal organism found in everyone's gut and in the female genital tract as a budding yeast. Under certain circumstances it becomes pathogenic, producing hyphae (*see* Figure 110) and causing disease. There is always a reason for this which should be looked for. Possible causes are recent antibiotic ingestion, diabetes mellitus, pregnancy, or immunosuppression (due to HIV infection, cancer, systemic steroids or cytotoxic drugs). It is usually the skin and mucous membranes which are affected.

**Figure 101** Candida of the tongue. White, curd-like papules which are easily scraped off with a spatula.

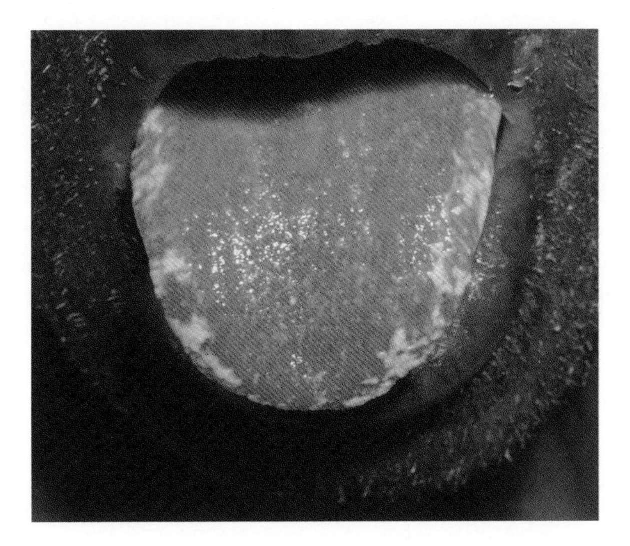

**Figure 102** Extensive candida of the tongue in a patient with HIV infection.

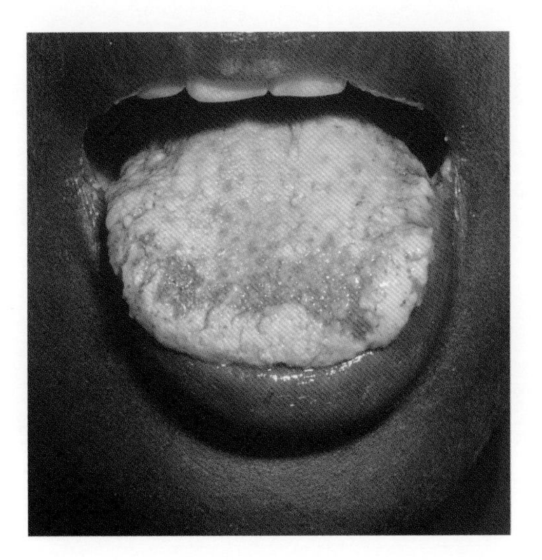

**Figure 103** Candida of the palate. Infections of the oral cavity may also extend down the oesophagus.

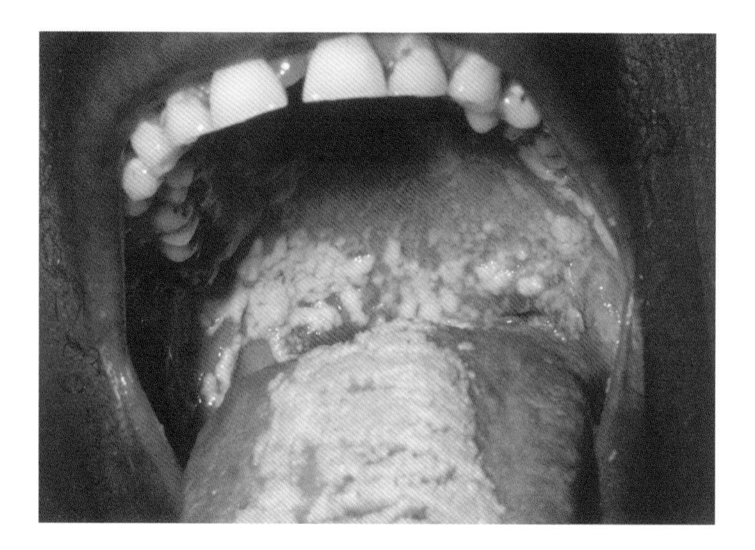

*Treatment of oral candidiasis:* Mouthwash with a 0.5% aqueous solution of Gentian Violet three times a day. Alternatives are 1ml of nystatin oral suspension (100 000 units/ml) swished around the mouth three times a day after meals and then swallowed, or in young children, miconazole gel applied by the mother with her finger qds.

**Figure 104** Angular cheilitis. This is usually from candida infection under a denture, although in patients who are HIV positive it can occur in those who do not wear dentures.

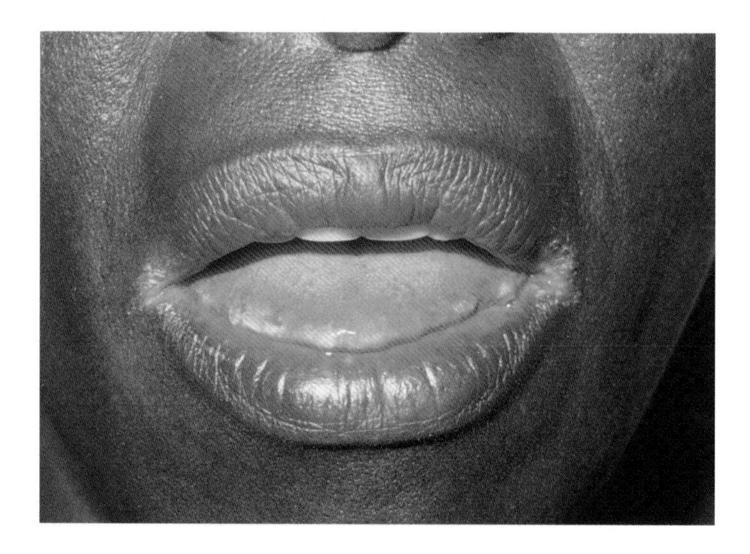

*Treatment:* Take the dentures out after every meal and scrub them with a hard toothbrush and soap.

**Figure 105** Candida of the lips in a patient with HIV infection.

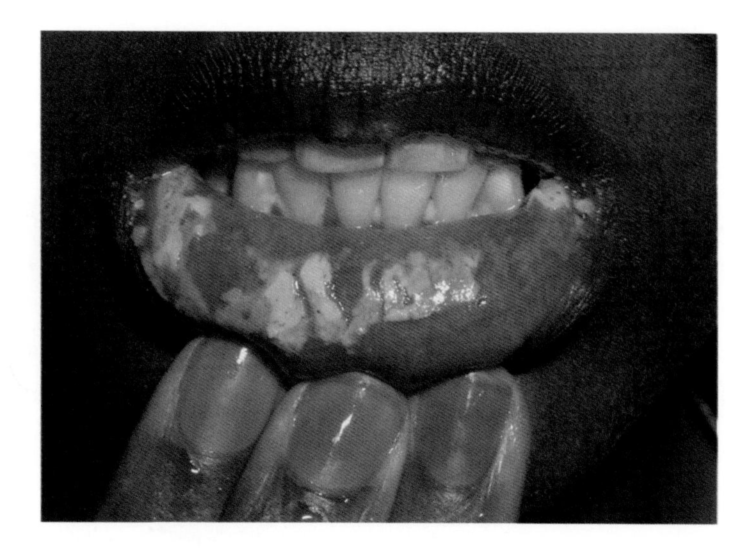

*Treatment:* Apply a 0.5% solution of aqueous Gentian Violet twice a day and treat the inside of the mouth too (*see* Figure 103).

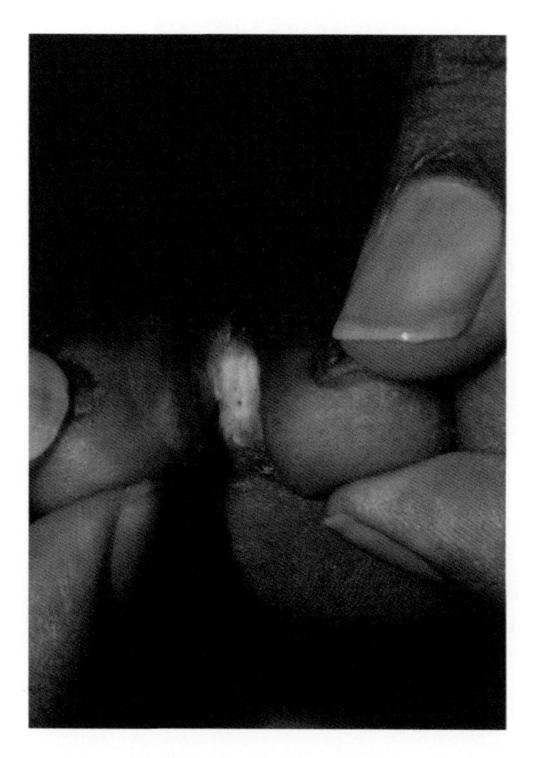

**Figure 106** Candida of the toe webs or finger webs. White maceration of the lateral toe webs which looks very similar to tinea (*see* Figure 625) but is whiter in colour and usually bilateral and symmetrical. The finger webs can also be involved, especially in individuals who have their hands in water a lot.

*Treatment:* Paint the finger webs or toe webs with 0.5% Gentian Violet paint bd and keep the hands and feet dry.

**Figure 107** Chronic paronychia. This is an infection of the soft tissues around the nail; one fingernail or several can be involved. It occurs mainly in ladies who have their hands in water a lot. The cuticle is first softened and then lost. *Candida albicans* enters where the cuticle has left a gap between the posterior nail fold and the nail (*see* Figure 441). The inflammation over the nail matrix can cause pitting and transverse ridging of the fingernail.

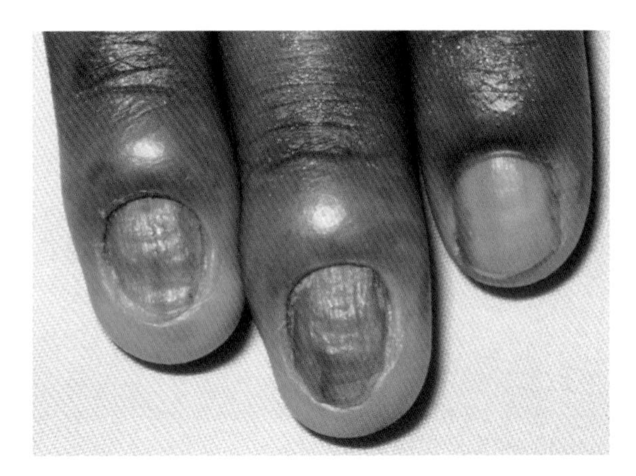

*Treatment:* Keep the hands dry at all times to allow a new cuticle to grow. No specific treatment is needed for the candida; it will disappear once the gap has been plugged. Note that it takes 5–6 months for the cuticle to regrow and a normal nail to grow out.

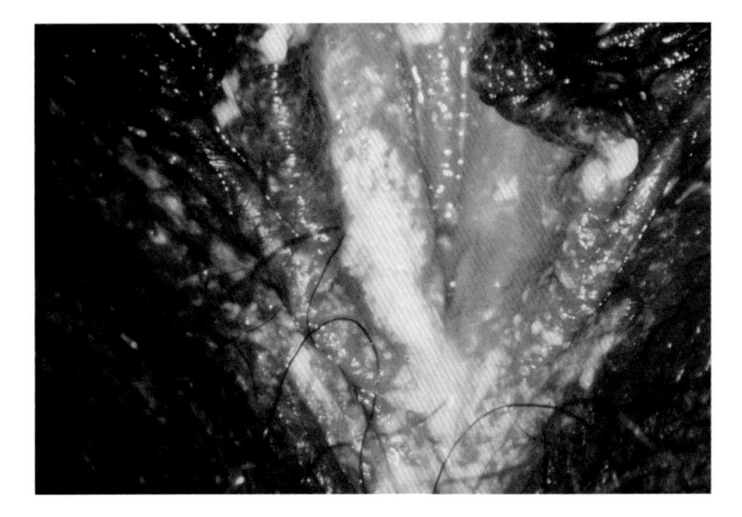

**Figure 108** Vaginal candidiasis. The patient presents with a thick white vaginal discharge. There may be itching or soreness of the vulva +/– vulval oedema.

*Treatment:* 0.5% aqueous solution of Gentian Violet applied with a thick cotton wool swab on a stick to the vagina bd is the cheapest treatment but it is very messy. Alternatives are clotrimazole (500mg) or miconazole (1200mg) pessaries applied high in the vagina at night, once only, or nystatin pessaries (100 000 units) for 14 successive nights.

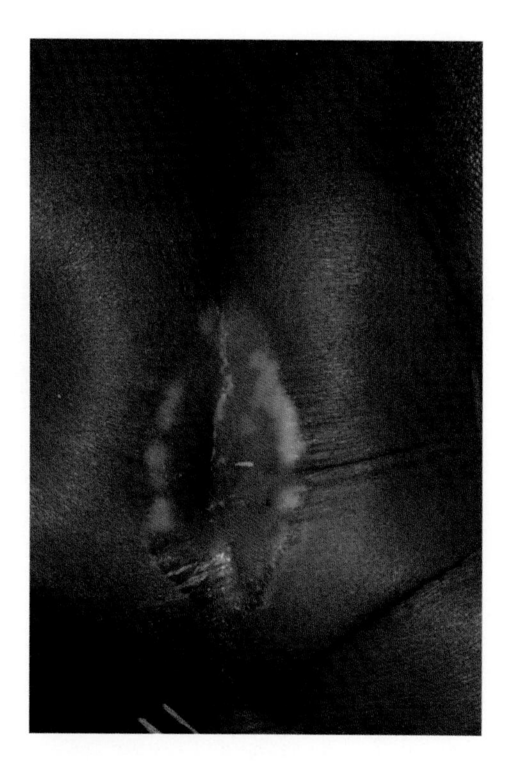

**Figure 109** Perianal candidiasis in a child who has been taking broad spectrum antibiotics. Symmetrical red plaques around the anus with a thick white discharge. There may or may not be outlying satellite lesions (vesicles, papules or pustules) – not seen here.

*Treatment:* Oral nystatin suspension, 100 000 units/ml; 1ml four times a day to clear the gut, plus 0.5% Gentian Violet paint topically bd until it is clear.

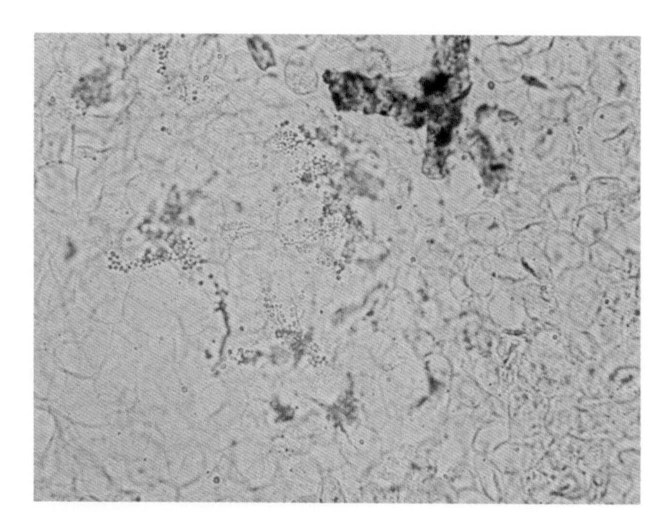

**Figure 110** Direct microscopy of *Candida albicans*. Take sample onto a glass slide and mix with 20% KOH solution. Both spores and hyphae are seen with pathogenic candida.

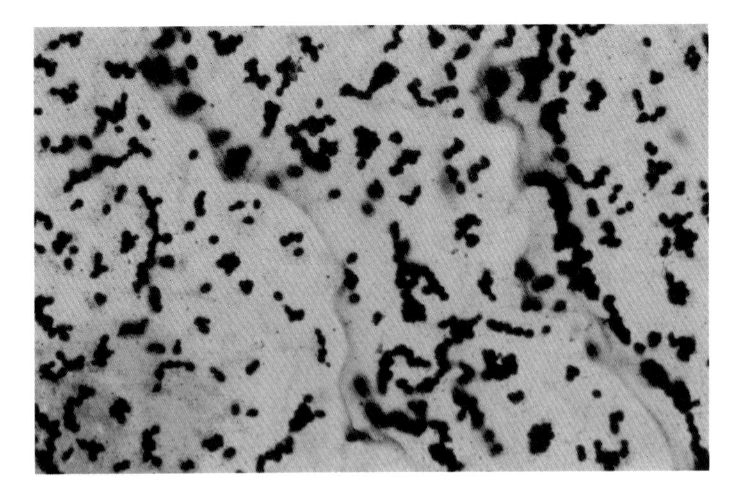

**Figure 111** Gram stain: the budding spores of *Candida albicans* are seen to be Gram positive.

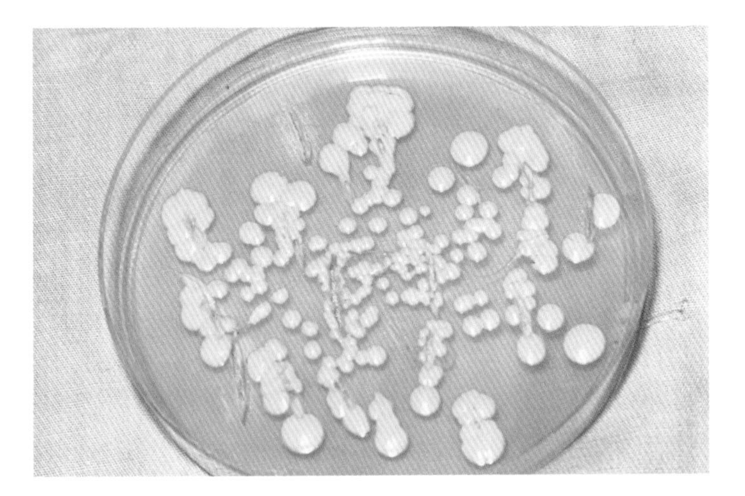

**Figure 112** Culture of *Candida albicans* on Sabouraud's dextrose agar without cyclohexamide. Creamy-white round colonies appear after 48 hours.

# CARCINOMAS

Skin cancers are almost all due to ultraviolet light; a few occur in chronic ulcers. Because of the protective effect of melanin they are not very common in Africans in spite of the constant sunshine.

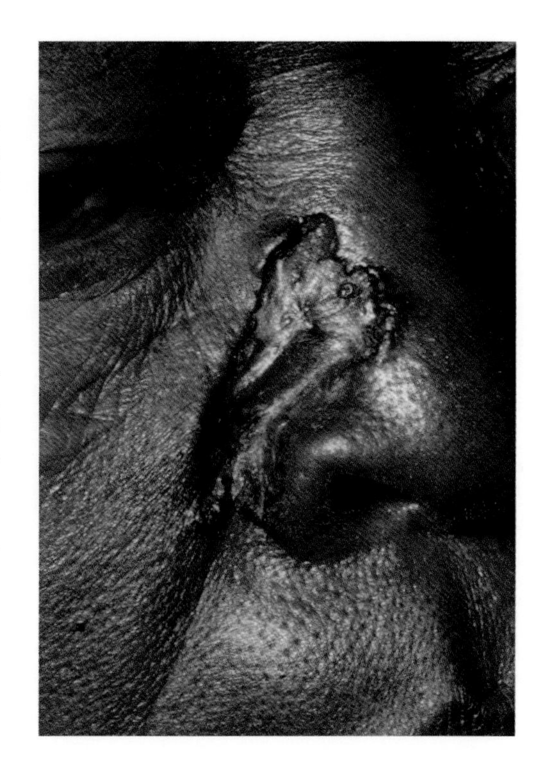

## Basal cell carcinoma

**Figure 113** Slow growing tumour with rounded, thread-like edge. It grows to a size of about 1cm in diameter over 4–5 years. It may be heavily pigmented as here.

*Treatment:* Surgical excision or radiotherapy, whichever is available.

## Squamous cell carcinoma

**Figure 114** A faster growing tumour than a basal cell carcinoma. It reaches this size in only 6–9 months.

*Treatment:* Surgical excision or radiotherapy, whichever is available.

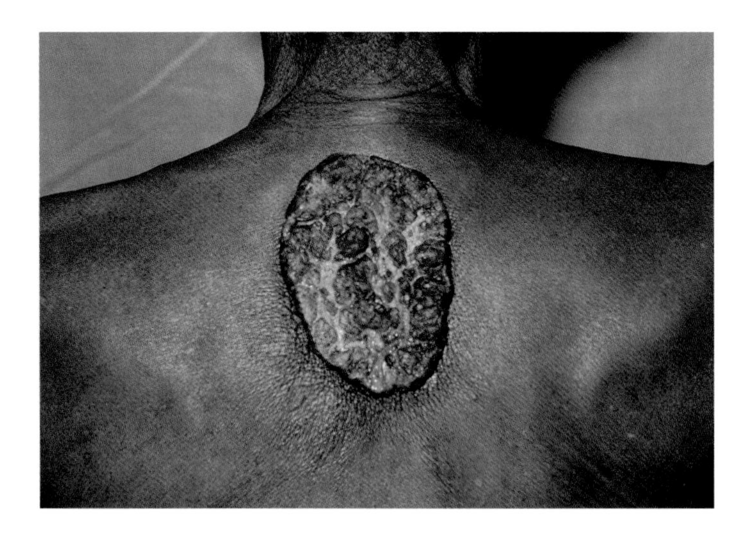

**Figure 115** If a tumour is hyperkeratotic, it is a squamous cell carcinoma.

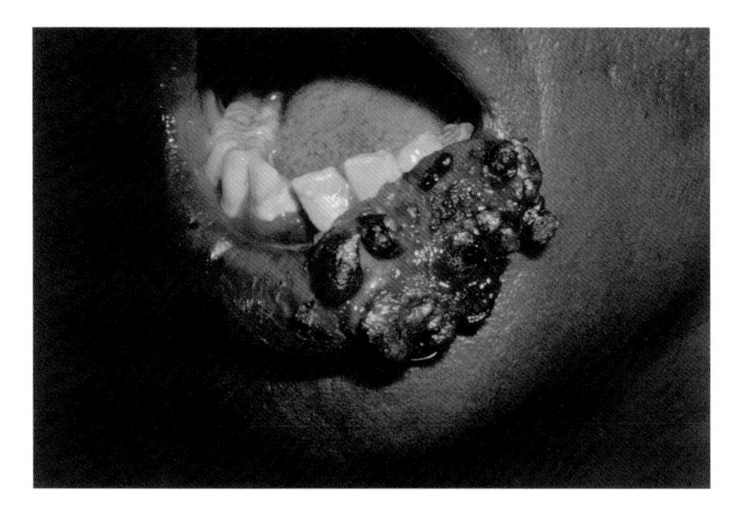

**Figure 116** Tumours on the lower lip are almost always squamous cell carcinomas.

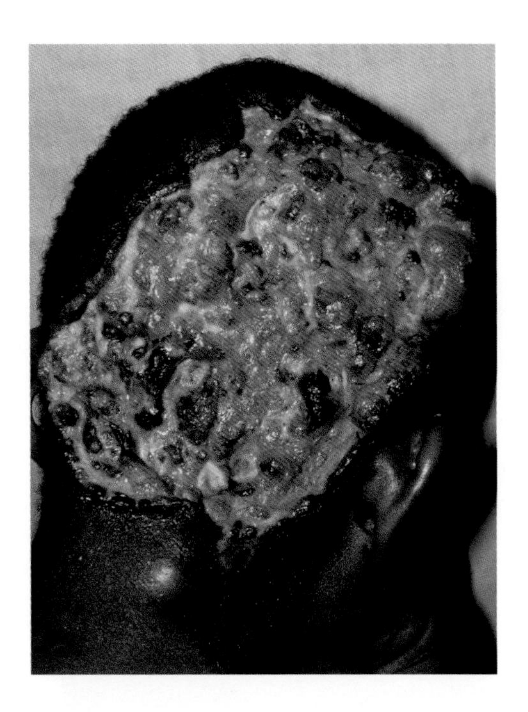

**Figure 117** Some squamous cell carcinomas behave aggressively, metastasise and cause the patient's death. This one is invading the skull and has already metastasised to the local lymph nodes.

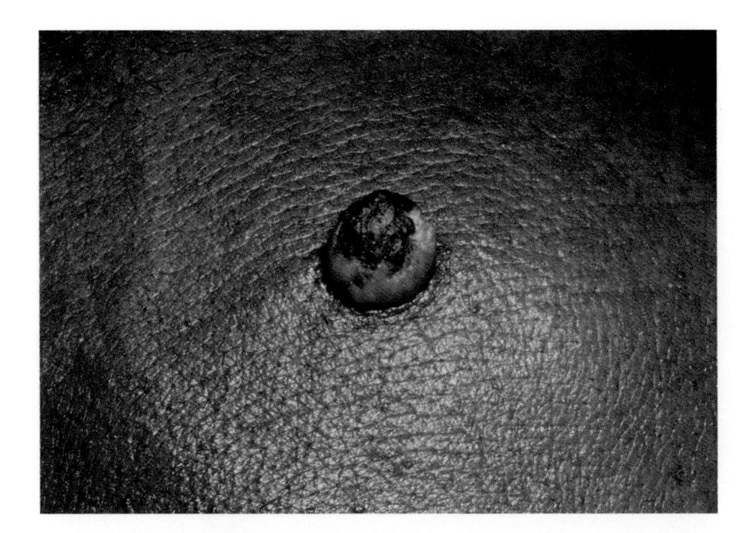

## Keratoacanthoma

**Figure 118** Rapidly growing tumour which looks like a basal cell carcinoma but with a central keratin plug. Grows rapidly for 3–4 months and then regresses spontaneously. Not common in Africans; much more common in albinos (*see* Figure 27).

*Treatment:* Remove by curettage and cautery or by excision.

## Malignant melanoma

Malignant melanoma is a rare tumour on pigmented skin. Most are found on the soles of the feet in the elderly. They are usually black in colour.

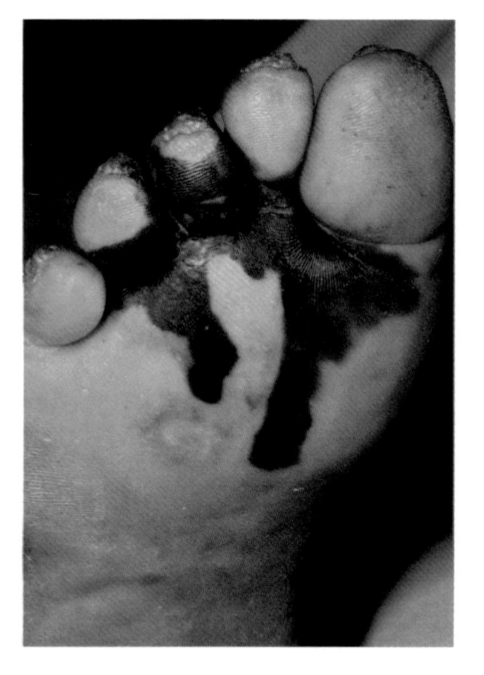

**Figure 119** Superficial spreading malignant melanoma in an 83-year-old man.

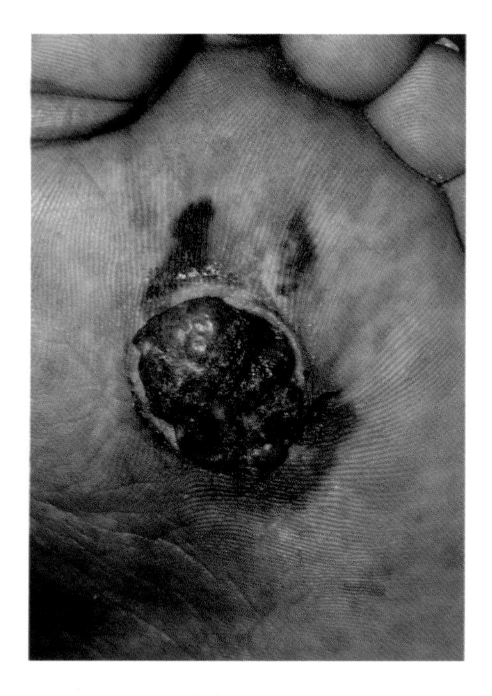

**Figure 120** Nodular malignant melanoma.

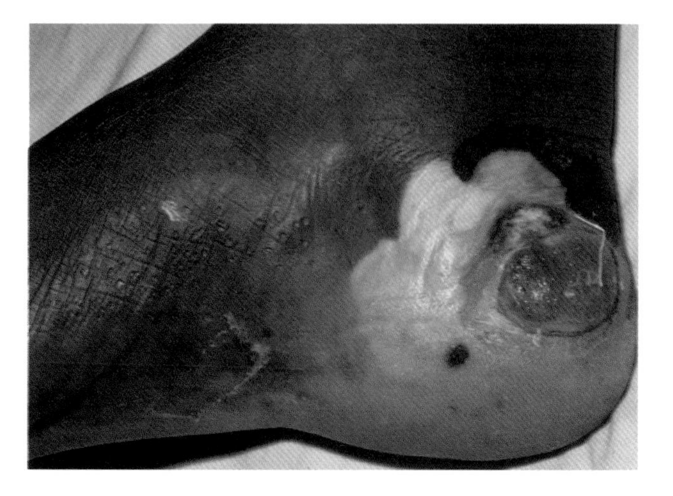

**Figure 121** Amelanotic melanoma on the heel of an 80-year-old woman. In spite of the fact that the nodule is red rather than black, there is a black satellite nodule nearby to give a clue to the diagnosis.

*Treatment:* Surgical excision.

## Secondary carcinoma

**Figure 122** Nodules of secondary breast cancer in a mastectomy scar and further afield.

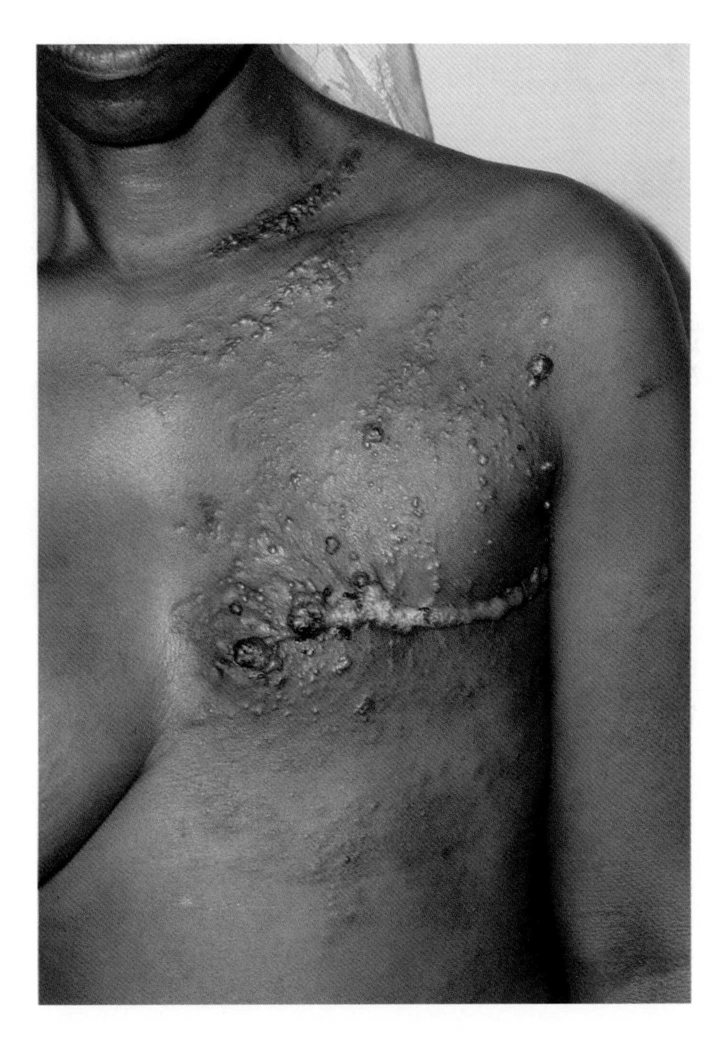

*Treatment:* Nothing can be done at this stage.

## CAROTENAEMIA

**Figure 123** Orange discolouration of the palms and soles. It is due to eating a lot of carrots and other vegetables which raise the blood level of beta carotene. Not to be confused with pityriasis rubra pilaris (*see* Figure 516) which causes hyperkeratosis as well as orange discolouration of the palms and soles.

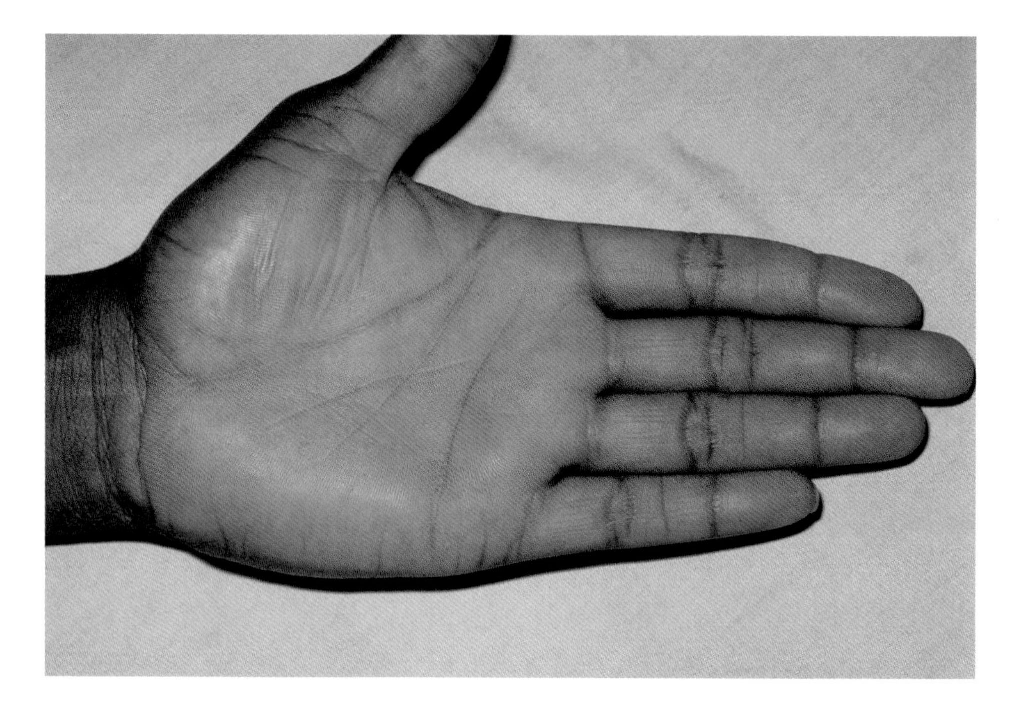

*Treatment:* It is completely harmless and does not need treatment.

## CELLULITIS

**Figure 124** Diagram to show sites of infection with *Streptococcus pyogenes*. Cellulitis is an infection of the lower half of the dermis.

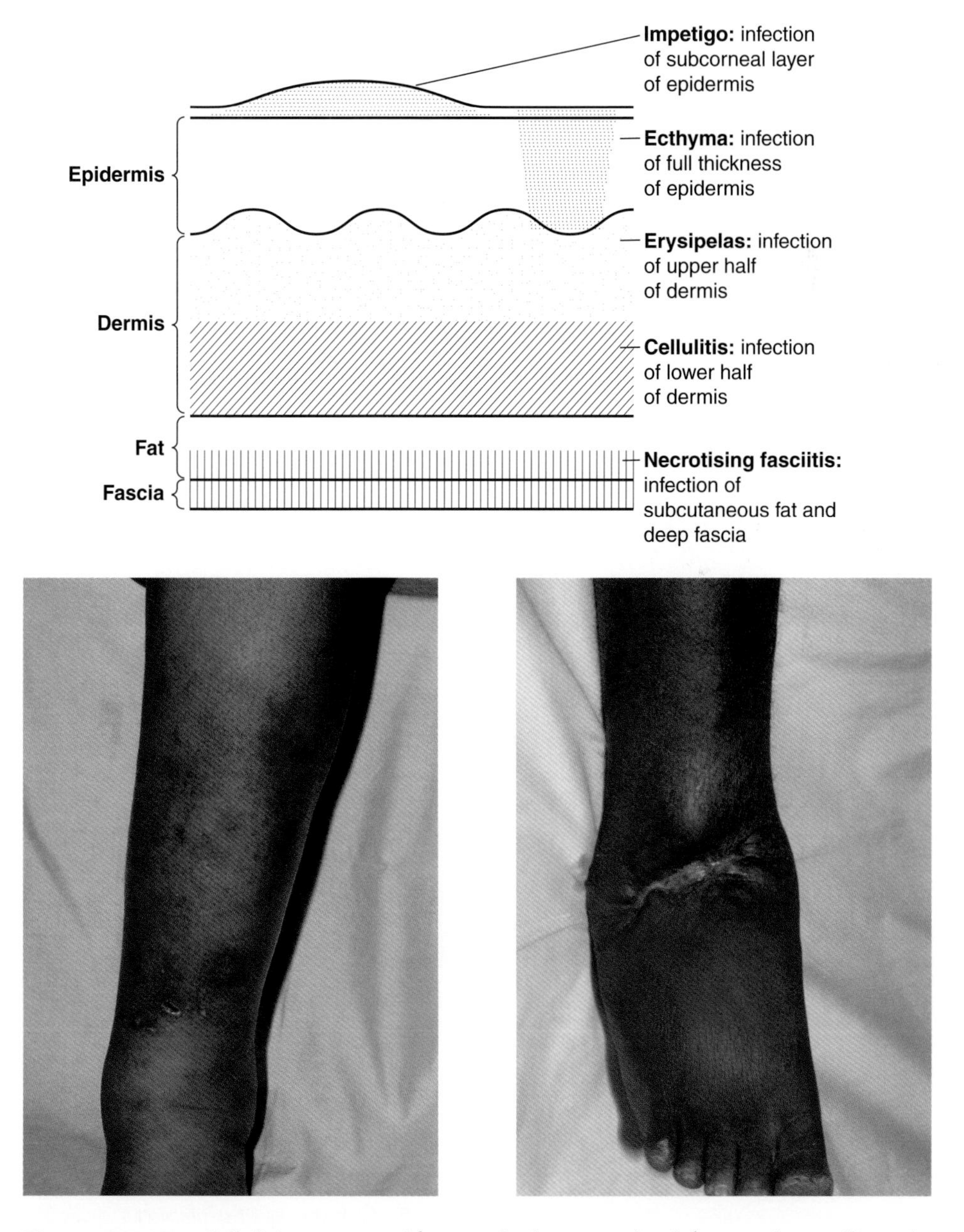


**Figures 125, 126** Cellulitis presents with a poorly demarcated red, hot, tender swelling of a limb together with lymphangitis and lymphadenopathy. There is usually an obvious portal of entry such as an ulcer (as in both these patients), eczema or tinea.

*Treatment:* Intramuscular or intravenous benzyl penicillin, 1 mega-unit, 6 hourly until it settles. It may take 10–14 days. The underlying disease (ulcer, eczema or tinea) which allowed entry of the streptococcus must also be treated or the cellulitis will be recurrent.

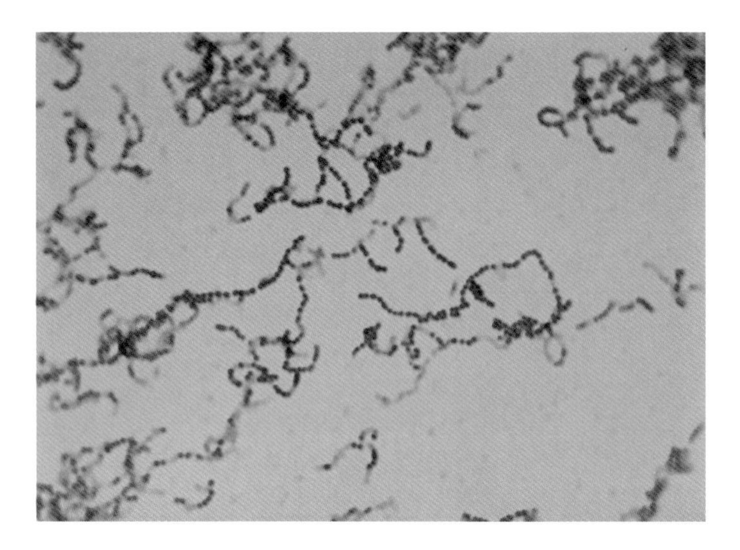

**Figure 127** Gram stain of *Streptococcus pyogenes*. Gram positive cocci in chains.

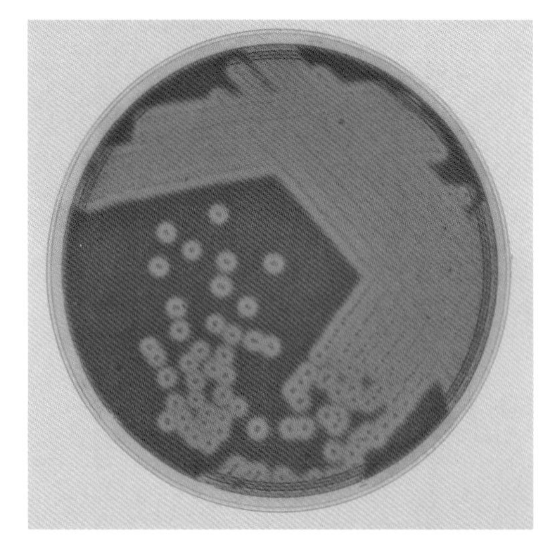

**Figure 128** Culture of *Streptococcus pyogenes* (group A beta-haemolytic streptococcus) on blood agar.

## CHANCROID

**Figure 129** Sexually transmitted disease due to *Haemophilus ducreyi*. It begins with a painful erythematous macule on the genitalia 2–3 days after sexual contact. It then becomes a pustule which ulcerates. The ulcer is soft and painful with an irregular ragged base covered with a thick purulent exudate. Characteristically, the ulcers are multiple from autoinoculation (kissing ulcers). One week after the ulcer appears unilateral lymphadenopathy (bubo) occurs. If an ulcer and a bubo are present together the most likely diagnosis is chancroid.

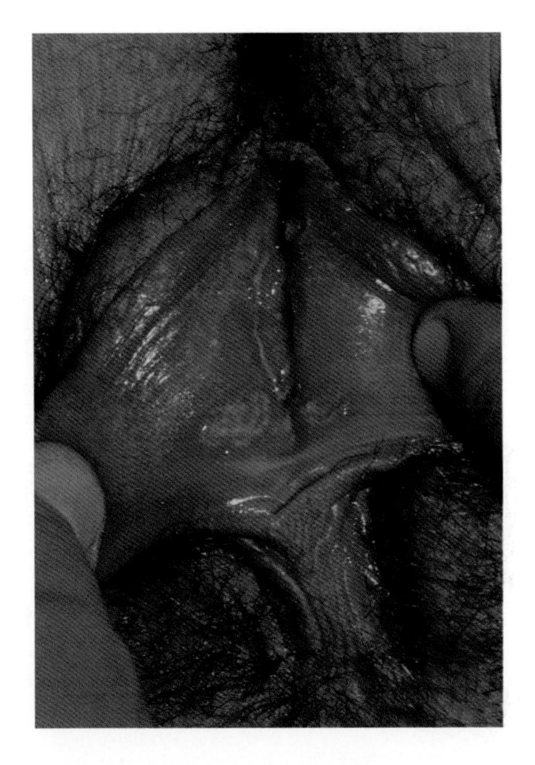

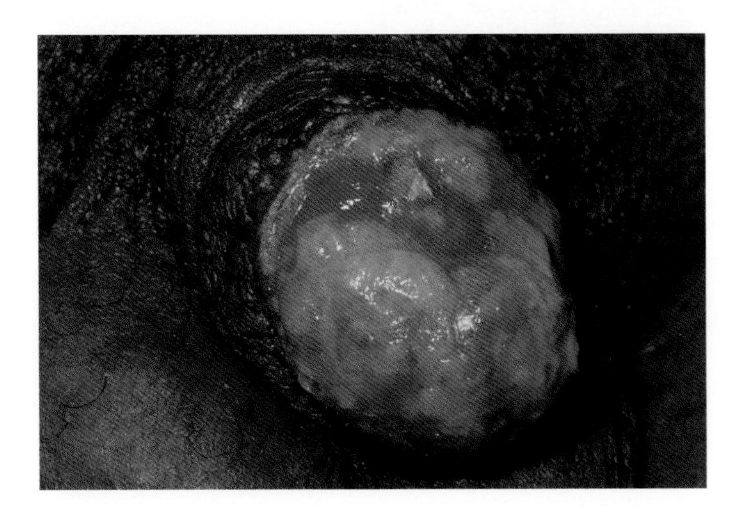

**Figure 130** Phagadenic chancroid. Here the rapidly growing ulcer can lead to auto-amputation of the penis. Always do several biopsies to check the diagnosis because it can be difficult to distinguish chancroid from a squamous cell carcinoma.

*Treatment:* Doxycycline 100mg twice a day for 10–14 days. Clean the ulcer and soak in dilute potassium permanganate, aspirate the bubo and give analgesics for the pain. Rule out syphilis by checking the RPR or VDRL. Check for HIV infection.

## CHEILITIS (Actinic cheilitis)

**Figure 131** Red scaly plaque on lower lip. Most commonly seen in HIV infection in black Africans. It is a common problem in albinos (*see* Figure 23).

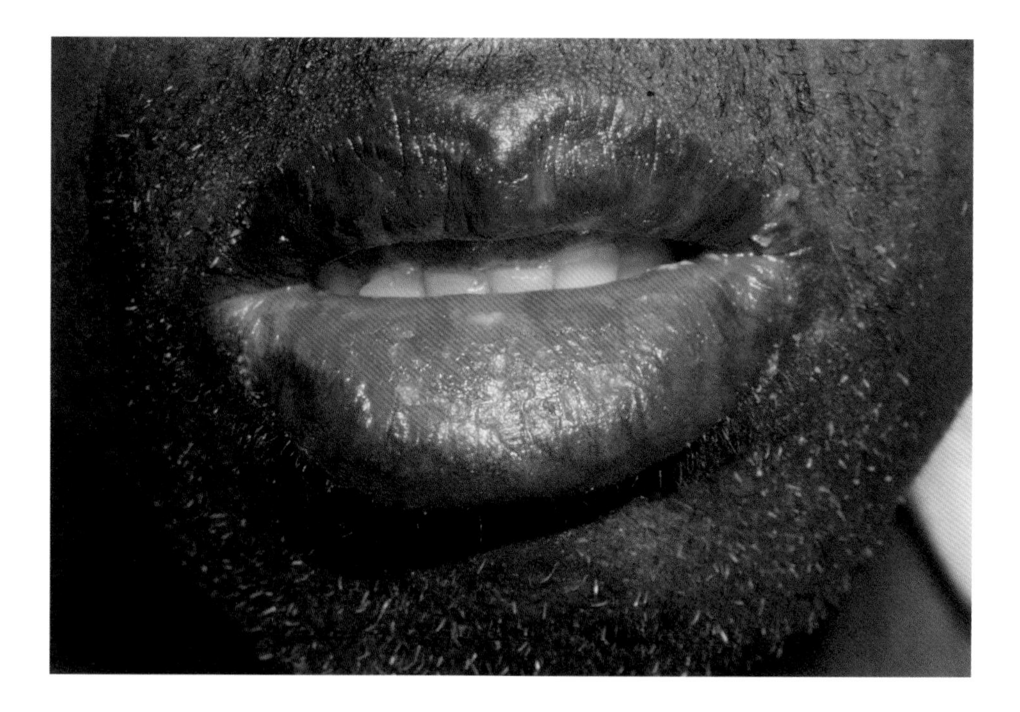

*Treatment:* Sunscreen applied to lip(s). Check for HIV infection.

## CHICKEN POX

**Figure 132** Common viral infection of children due to *Herpes varicella zoster*. The incubation period is around 14 days and the child is infectious for 2 days before the rash appears and for about 5 days afterwards. An itchy rash mainly on the face and trunk, with lesions at different stages of development all visible at the same time – macules, papules, vesicles, pustules and crusts. The most characteristic lesion is a vesicle looking like a drop of water on the skin.

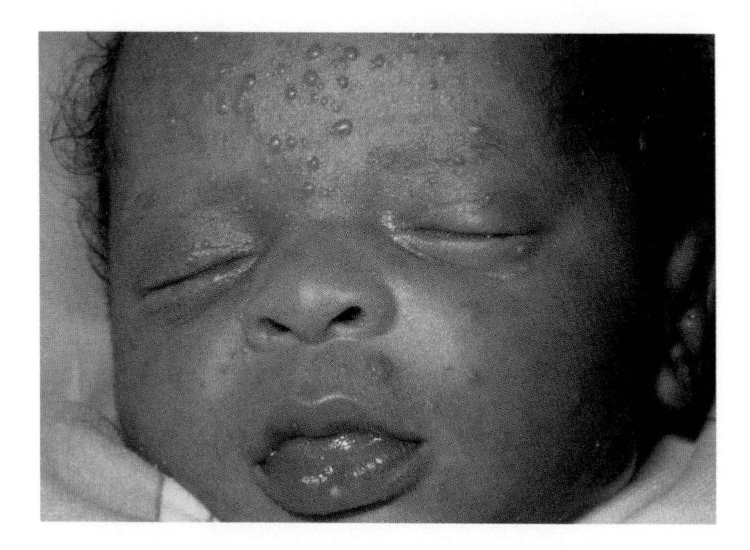

**Figure 133** If the lesions are scratched and secondarily infected they may heal leaving hypopigmentation and/or scars.

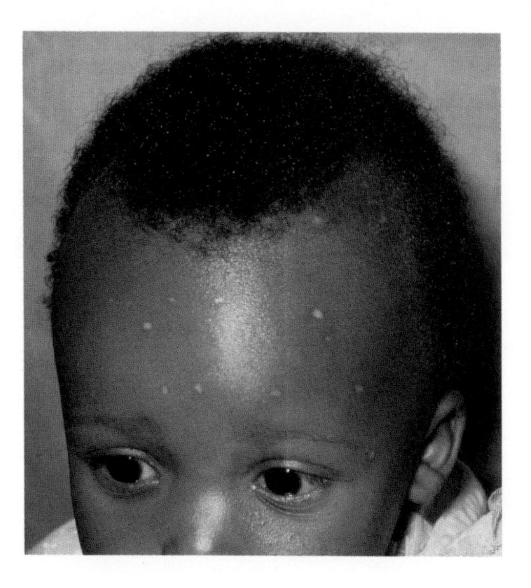

*Treatment:* Usually a mild illness in children which needs no treatment. Possibly apply calamine lotion to alleviate the itching. If it occurs in an adult check for HIV infection.

## CHLOASMA

**Figure 134** Symmetrical hyperpigmented patches on the forehead, cheeks and moustache area of women. It characteristically occurs during pregnancy or when taking the oral contraceptive pill. When it occurs at other times it is called melasma.

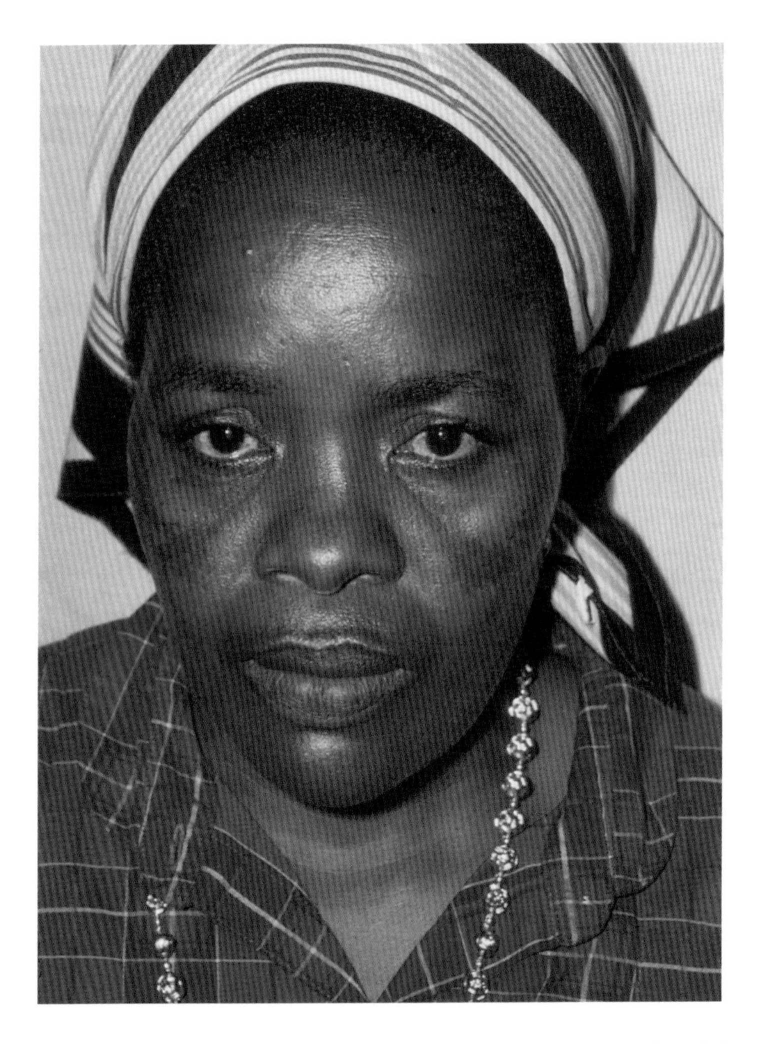

*Treatment:* Reassurance that it is harmless and will often disappear after delivery or on stopping the contraceptive pill. Since it worsens in sunlight, sun exposure should be avoided if possible. 2–4% hydroquinone cream applied twice a day for 3 months (but no longer) may help.

## CHRONIC BULLOUS DISEASE OF CHILDHOOD

**Figure 135** Usually begins at age 3–5 years with grouped blisters around the genitalia, umbilicus and face. It is not itchy. It gets better spontaneously after 3 or 4 years. Histology shows a sub-epidermal blister and direct immunofluorescence, a band of IgA along the basement membrane zone. *See also* linear IgA disease (Figure 397) which is the adult version of the same disease.

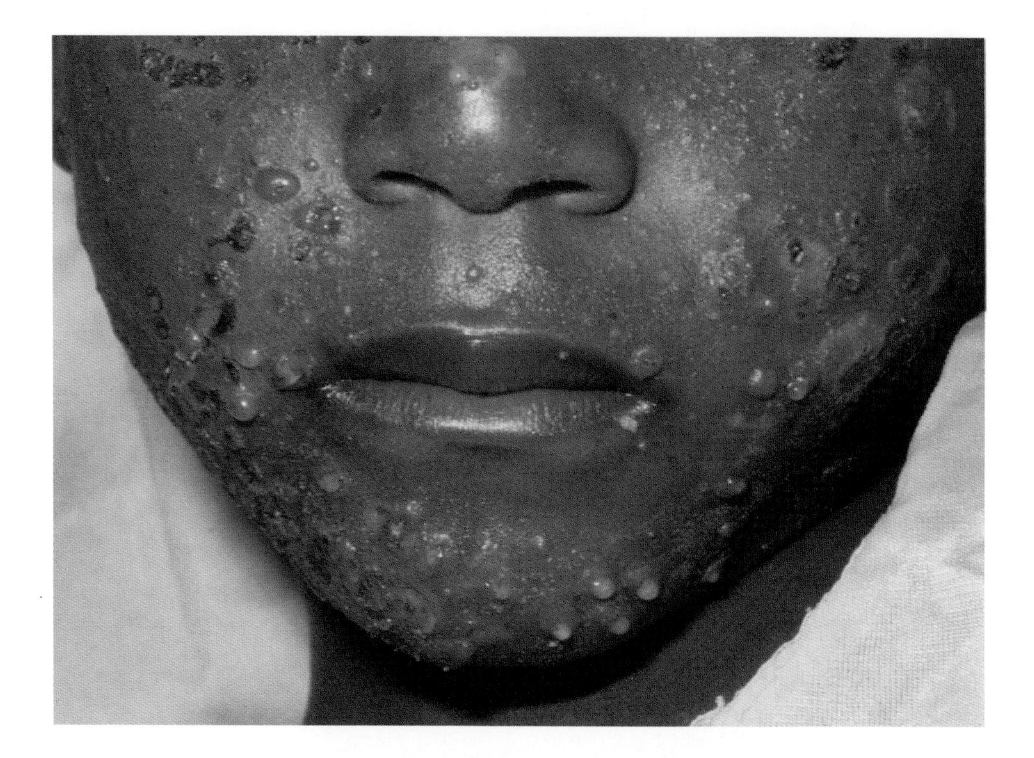

Figure 135

*Treatment:* Oral dapsone 25–100mg/day until it remits spontaneously.

## COCKAYNE SYNDROME

**Figure 136** This is a rare syndrome inherited as an autosomal dominant trait (*see* Figure 295) characterised by short stature, mental retardation, photosensitivity and disproportionately large hands, feet and ears. The face is triangular in shape with large ears and is sometimes described as being like 'Mickey Mouse'. Not to be confused with progeria (*see* Figure 532).

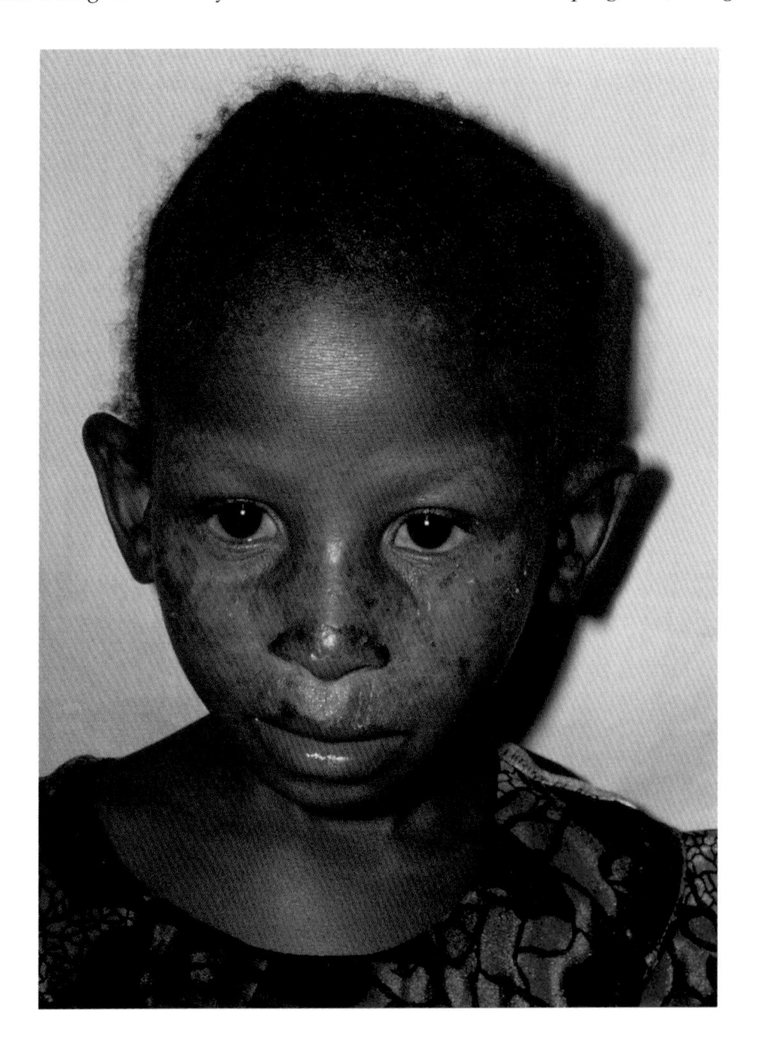

*Treatment:* Sunscreens may help the photosensitivity, but otherwise nothing can be done.

## CONFETTI DEPIGMENTATION

**Figure 137** This is due to the topical application of the monobenzyl ether of hydroquinone. The depigmentation is permanent once it has occurred and may spread beyond the area it was applied to. This chemical should never be used as a skin lightening agent.

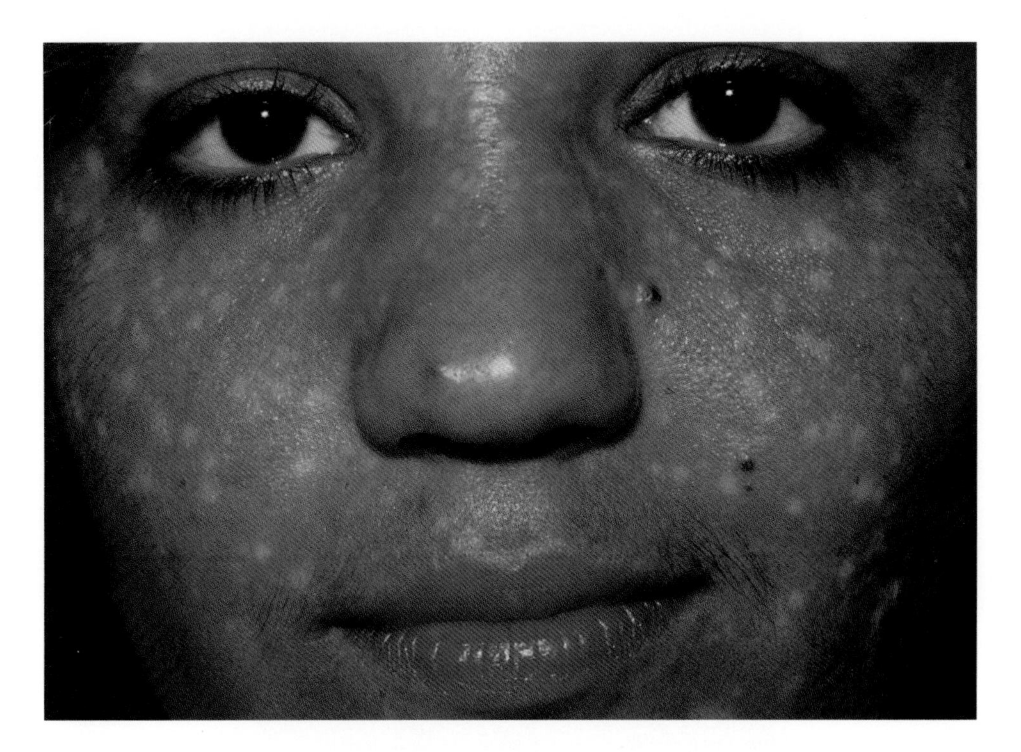

## CORNS AND CALLOSITIES

**Figure 138** Corns are localised areas of hyperkeratosis over bony prominences, usually on the feet.

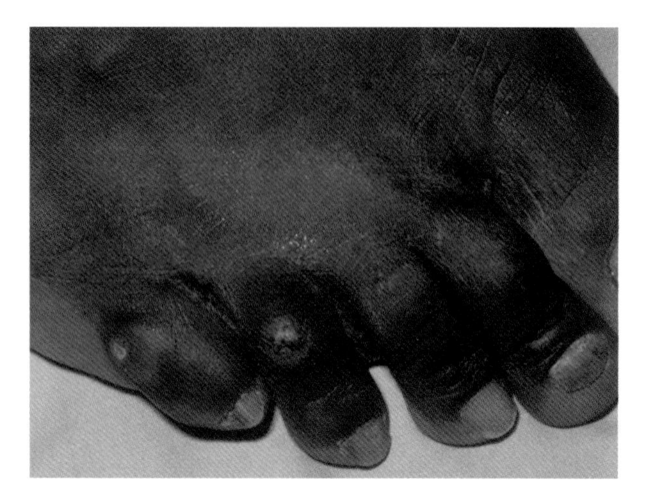

*Treatment:* If painful, rub them flat with a pumice stone. Wear proper fitting shoes.

**Figure 139** Callosities are areas of hyperkeratosis due to recurrent friction, often on the hands from manual labour.

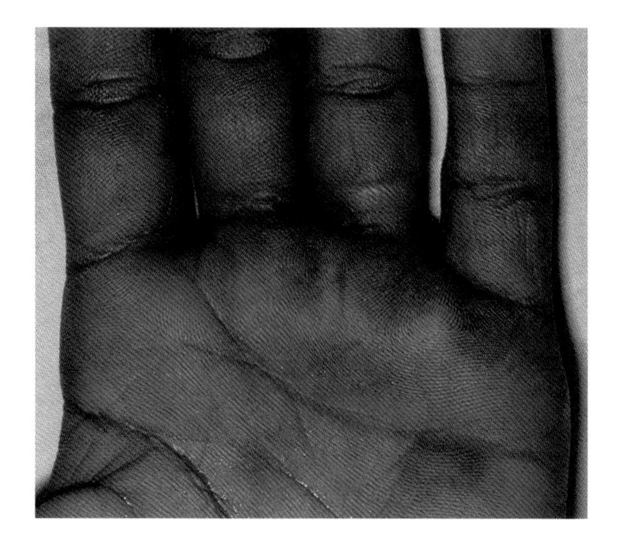

## CRYPTOCOCCOSIS

**Figure 140** Systemic fungal infection involving the skin, meninges and lungs. The skin lesions mimic molluscum contagiosum (*see* Figures 430–1), chicken pox (*see* Figure 132) or acne (*see* Figures 9, 10), but they may grow rapidly and ulcerate. Most commonly found in patients with AIDS. Due to the encapsulated yeast, *Cryptococcus neoformans*, which is found in soil where there are a lot of pigeon droppings.

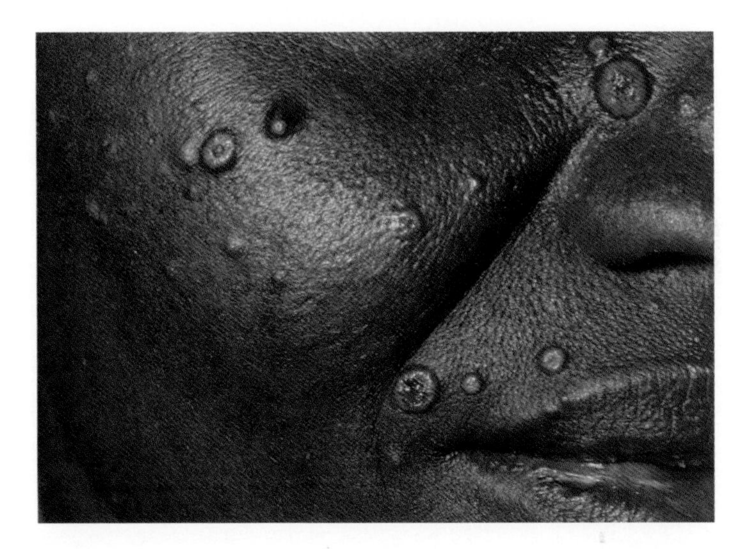

**Figure 141** The diagnosis can be confirmed by removing a lesion with a scalpel and wiping the underside on a glass slide. Add one drop of Indian ink and examine under a microscope. The encapsulated spores are easily visible and look like shiny poached eggs.

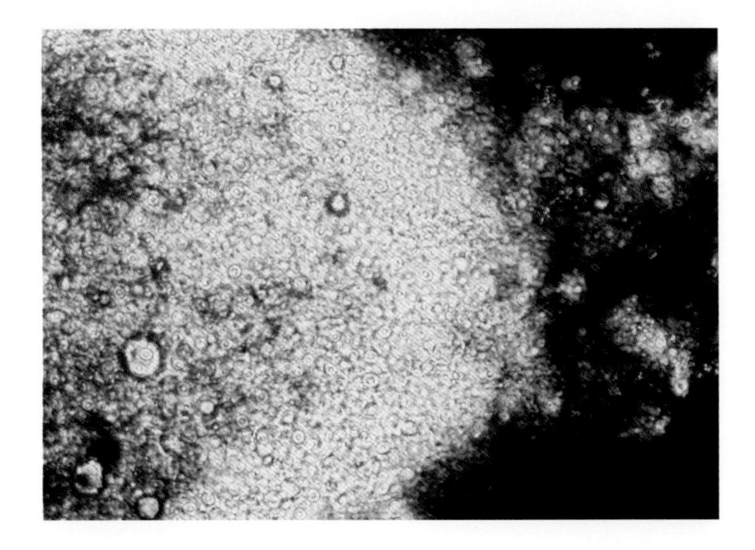

*Treatment:* Oral fluconazole 400mg/day for 12 weeks and then lifelong maintenance with 200mg/day. This is very expensive.

## CUSHING'S SYNDROME

**Figure 142** Moon face, buffalo hump and trunkal obesity due to taking large doses of systemic steroids. Will disappear when the steroids are stopped or the dose is reduced.

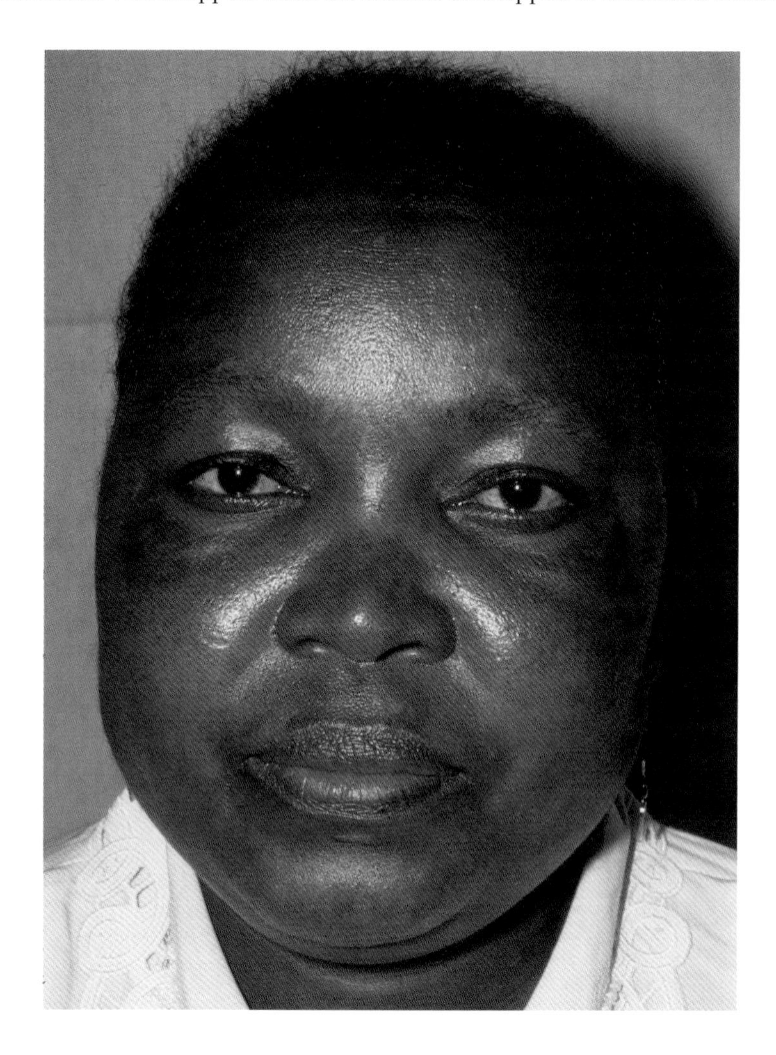

## CUTIS MARMORATA TELANGIECTATICA CONGENITA

**Figure 143** Present from birth. A flat reticulate erythema giving a marbling effect. Similar changes can occur in normal infants due to the cold (cutis marmorata).

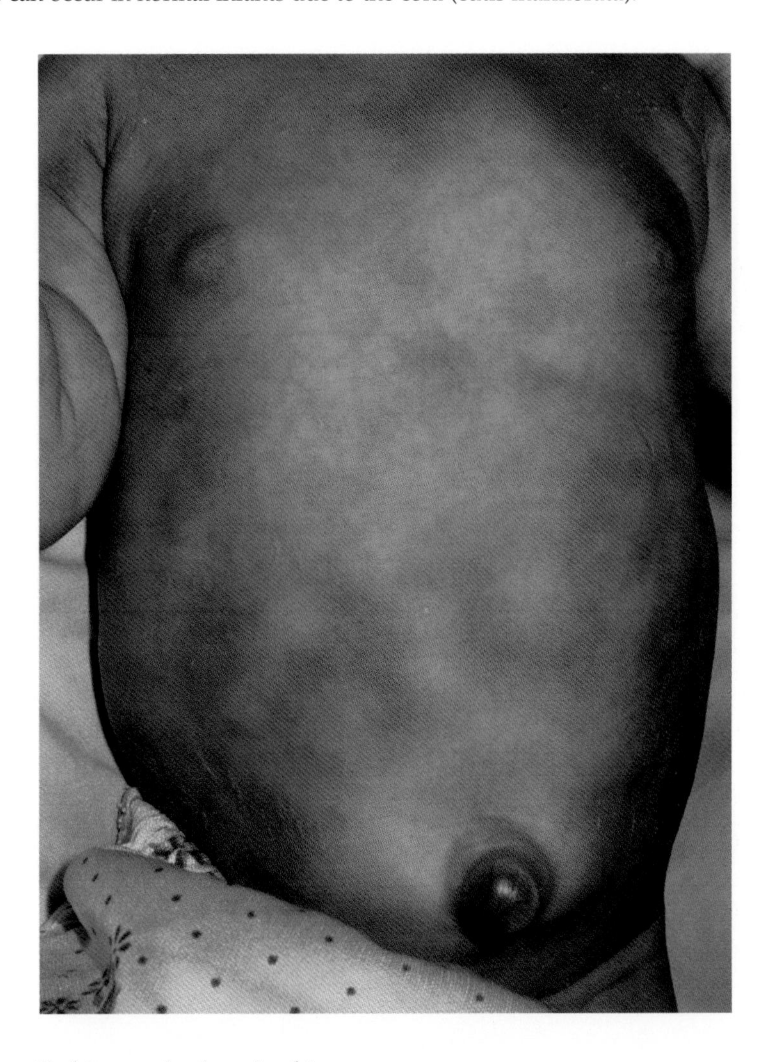

*Treatment:* Nothing can be done for this.

# CYSTS IN THE SKIN

## Dermoid cyst

**Figure 144** Cyst in the midline present from birth. It can also occur at other sites of embryonic skin closure (e.g. at corner of eye). It may have hairs protruding from it.

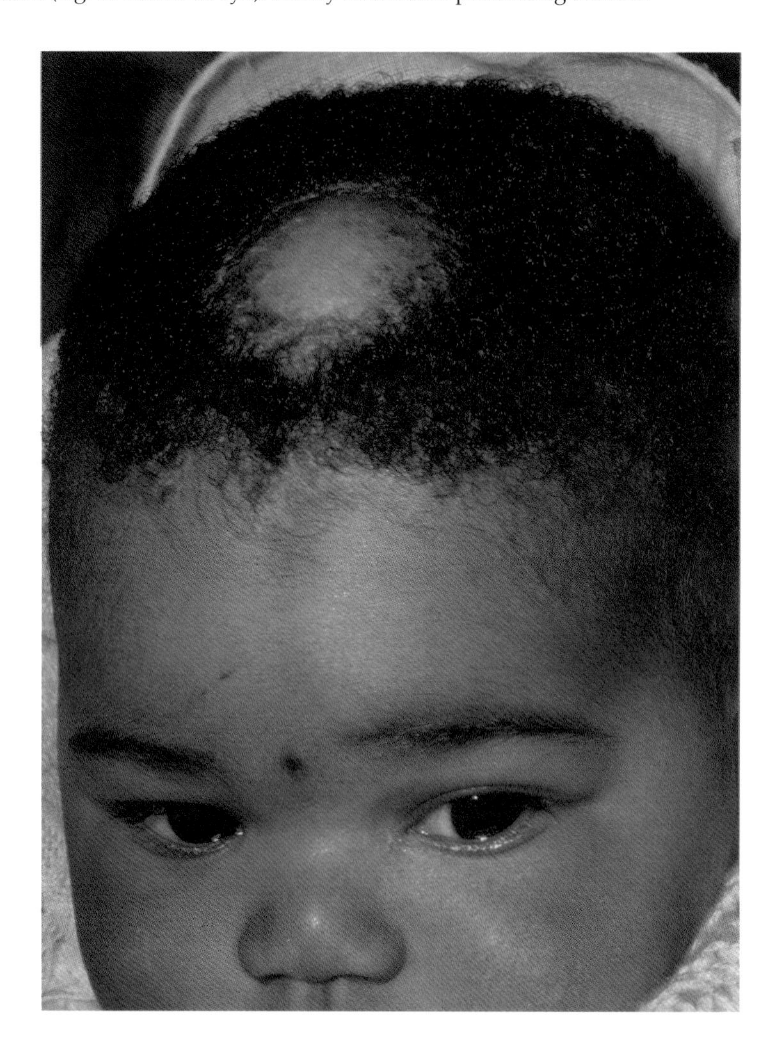

*Treatment:* Excise if unsightly.

## Epidermoid cyst

**Figure 145** Single or multiple cysts with a central punctum occur anywhere on the body except the palms and soles. They may become secondarily infected. Run in families, inherited as an autosomal dominant trait (*see* Figure 295). They do not appear until after puberty (except in Gardner's syndrome).

*Treatment:* Excise if unsightly or if there is recurrent infection.

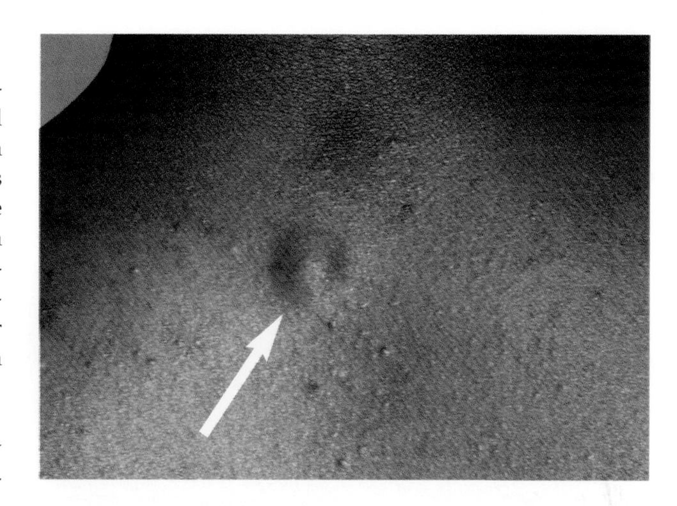

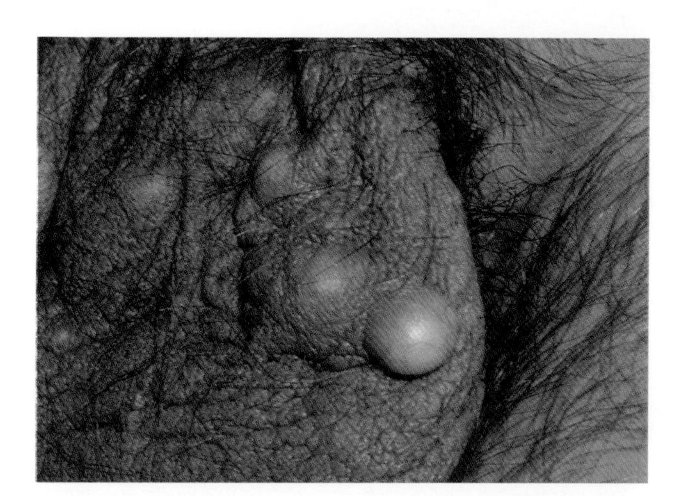

**Figure 146** Epidermoid cysts may occur on the genitalia in both sexes.

**Figure 147** X-ray of lesions that looked like epidermoid cysts on the scrotum, but these are calcified. They are probably calcified epidermoid cysts, but they are often called idiopathic calcinosis of the scrotum.

*Treatment:* They are not a problem; the patient can be reassured that they are harmless and can be left alone.

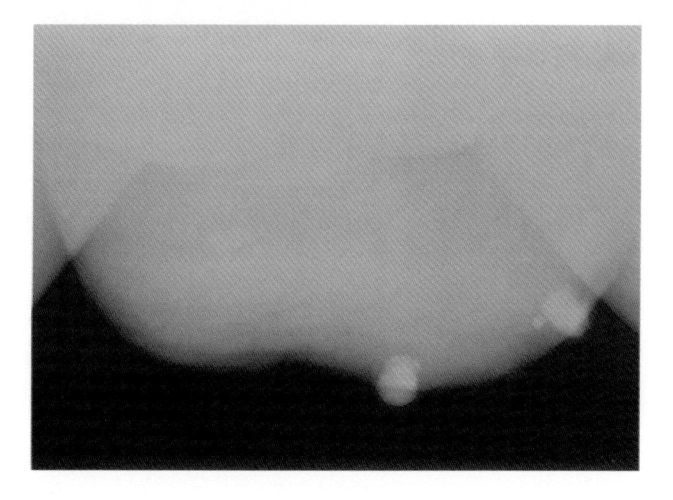

## Pilar (trichilemmal) cyst

**Figure 148** Most occur on the scalp. Single or multiple cysts occurring after puberty. Run in families, inherited as an autosomal dominant trait (*see* Figure 295).

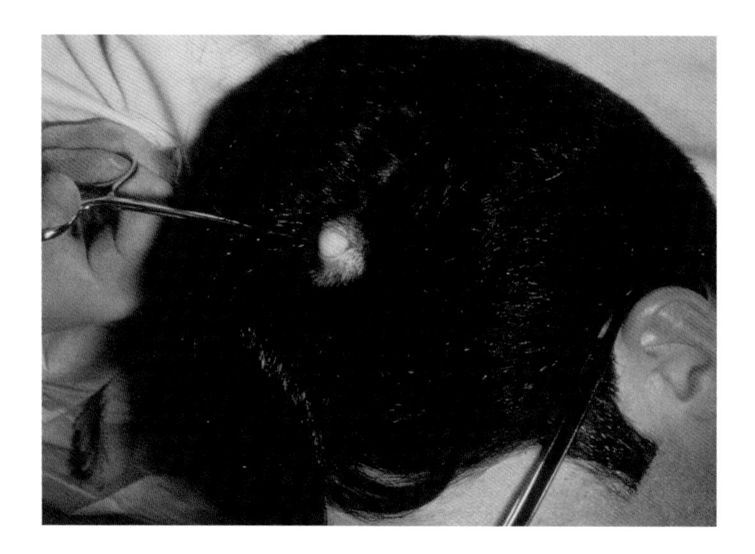

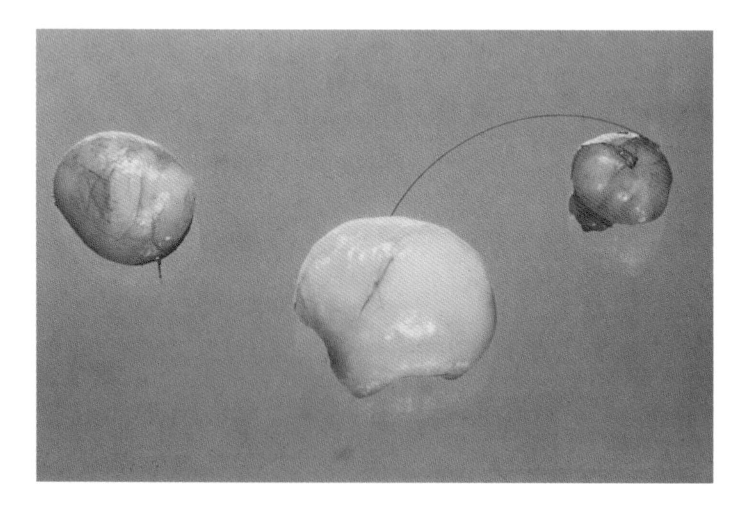

**Figure 149** Easily removed because they are encapsulated.

## Steatocystoma multiplex

**Figures 150, 151** Multiple small cysts on the trunk in males and in the flexures in females. They appear after puberty. Run in families, inherited as an autosomal dominant trait (*see* Figure 295).

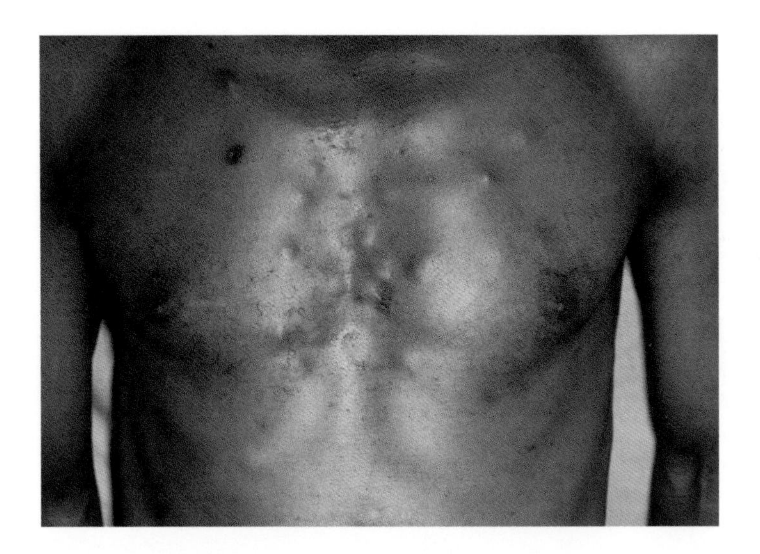

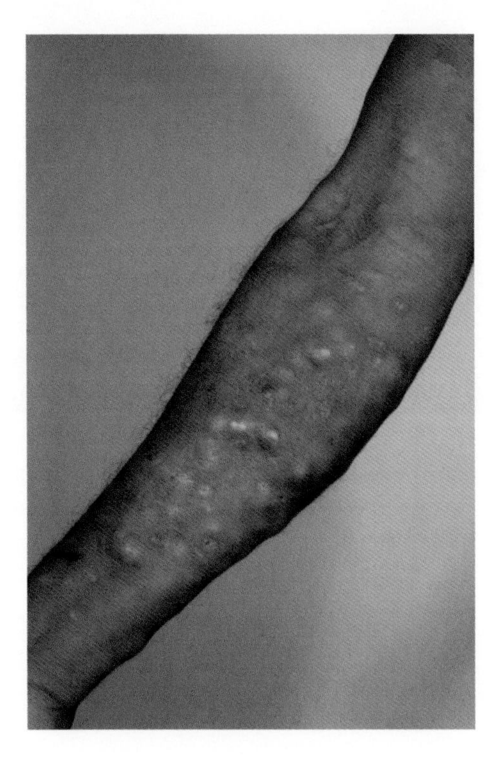

*Treatment:* Reassurance only. Usually there are too many to excise.

## DARIER'S DISEASE

**Figure 152** Genetic disease inherited as an autosomal dominant trait (*see* Figure 295). Begins in the early teens with greasy crusted or warty papules in a seborrhoeic distribution (face, trunk and anogenital region).

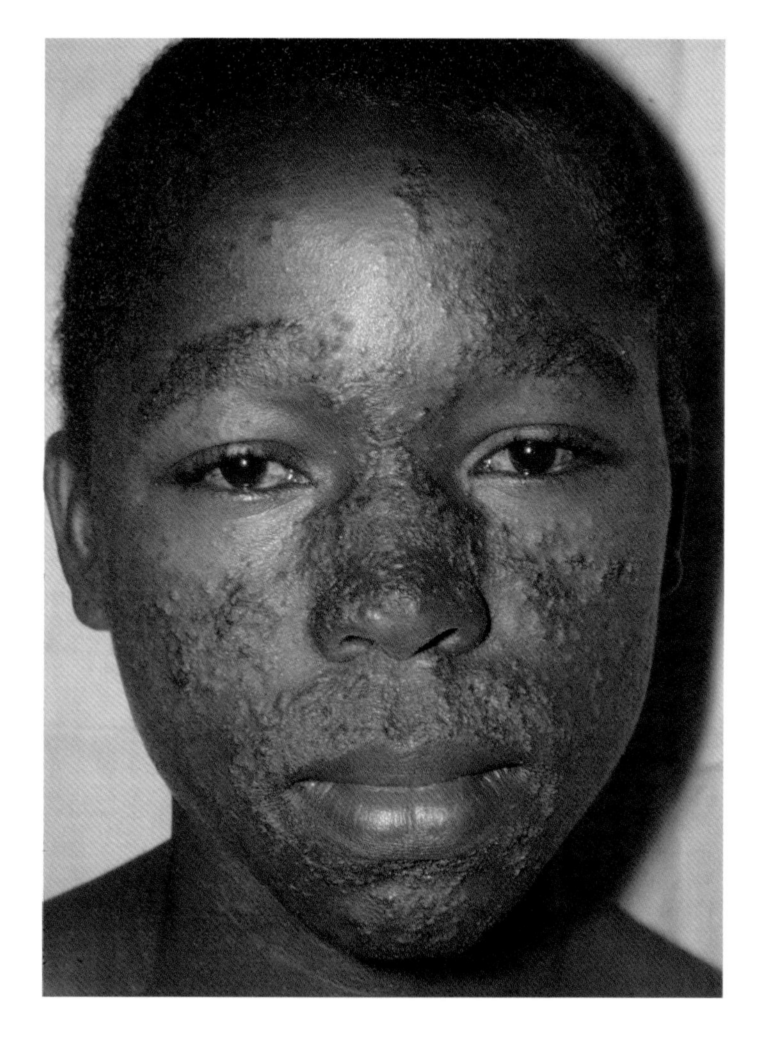

*Treatment:* Explain the disease to the patient and give genetic counselling. Systemic retinoids are helpful if the disease is extensive. Acetretin 0.5mg/kg body weight/day is used but it is teratogenic so should not be used in young women. It is also very expensive.

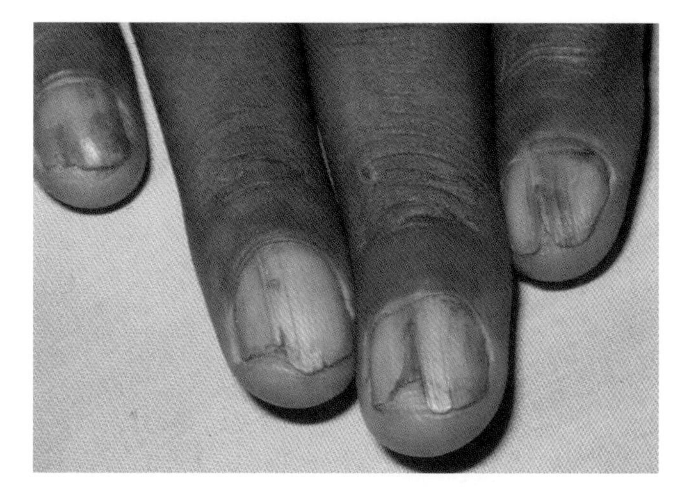

**Figure 153** Nails show longitudinal ridges with 'V' shaped nicks at the ends.

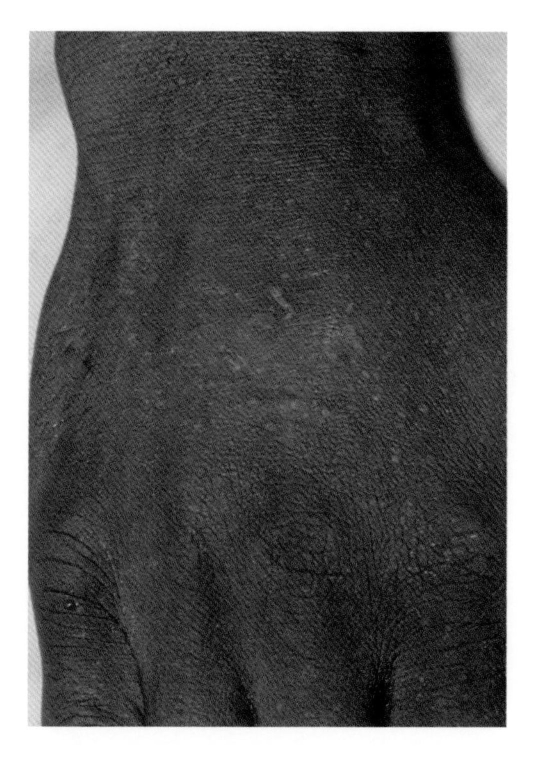

**Figure 154** On the dorsum of the hands and feet are small flat topped papules resembling plane warts, which are called acrokeratosis verruciformis. In addition, there are small pits on the palms and soles.

## DCPA (Dermatitis cruris pustulosa atrophicans)

**Figure 155** This is a folliculitis on the lower legs of teenagers and young adults (mainly females). It is due to the practice of applying Vaseline or other greasy ointments to the legs allowing *Staphylococcus aureus* to multiply in the mouth of the hair follicles (*see* Figure 309).

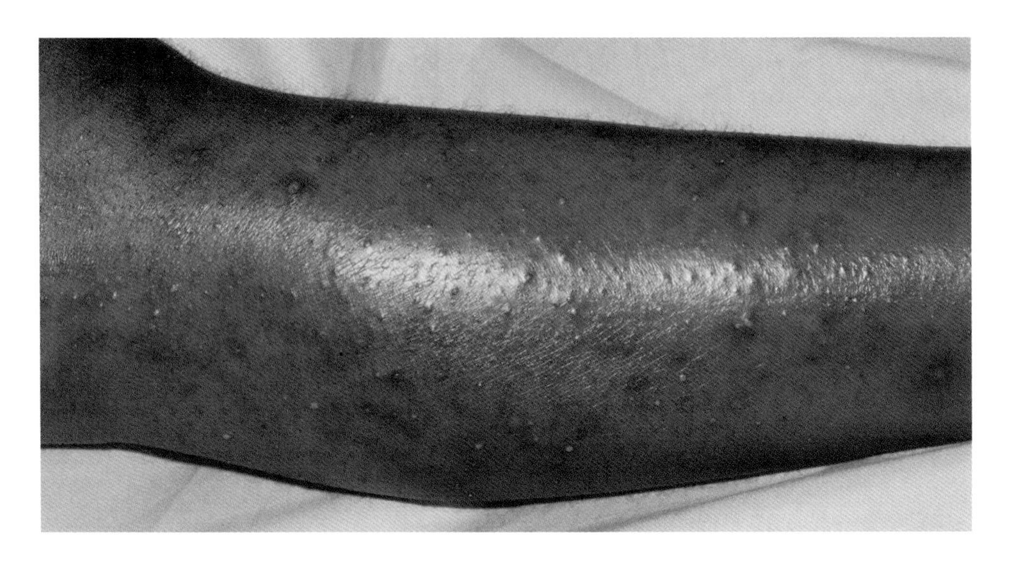

*Treatment:* Stop applying greasy ointments.

# DEEP FUNGAL INFECTIONS

## Mycetoma (Madura foot)

This is a chronic infection of the dermis and subcutaneous fat caused by various species of fungi which occur as saprophytes in the soil (eumycetoma), or by bacteria (actinomycetoma).

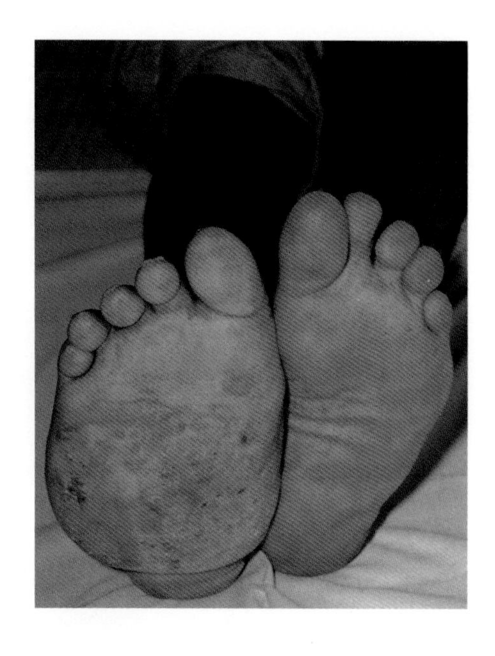

**Figures 156, 157** Mycetoma due to fungus. Infection usually follows a penetrating injury from walking around bare footed. The most common site is the foot. The foot is swollen and there are multiple sinuses which discharge granules (black, white or yellow depending on the specific fungus).

*Treatment:* Surgical excision if at all possible. Long-term treatment with systemic antifungal agents such as itraconazole (200mg bd) for 9–12 months is prohibitively expensive.

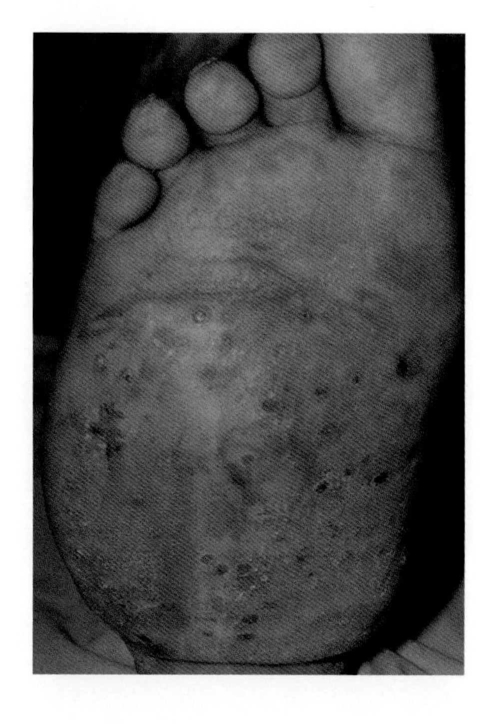

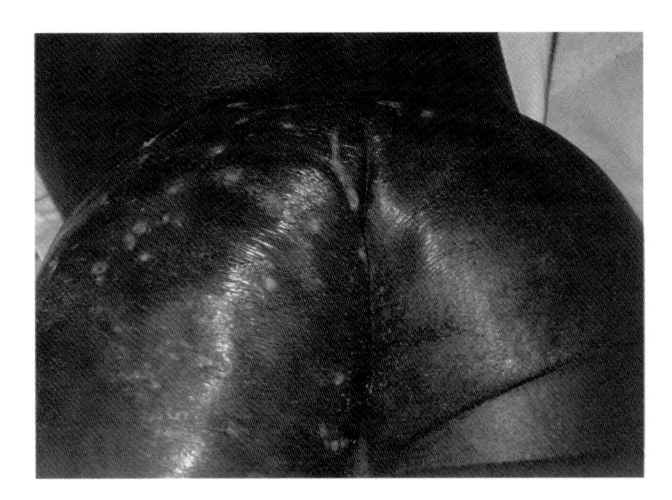

**Figure 158** Mycetoma on the buttocks.

**Figure 159** Black granules of *Madurella mycetomatis* in surgical excision specimen. White or yellow granules are due to *Pseudoalleschia boydii, Neotestundina rosatii, Aspergillus nidulans* and various fusarium species.

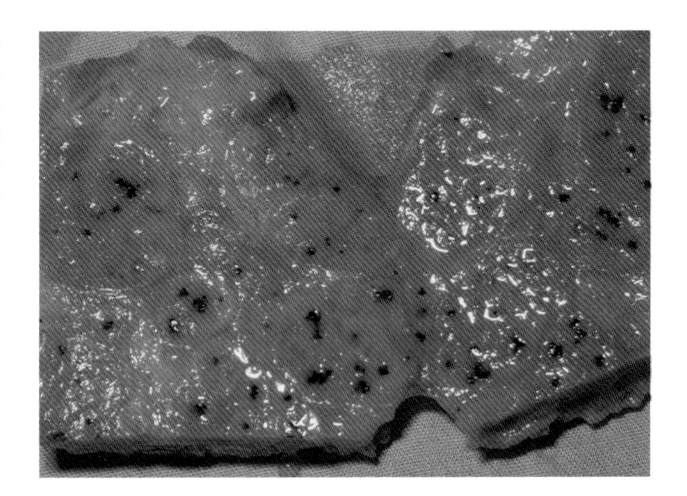

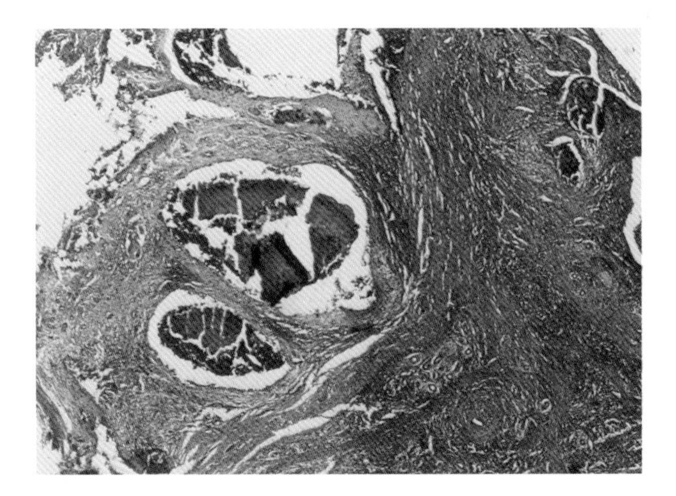

**Figure 160** Histology specimen. Granules of *Madurella mycetomatis* are easily seen on H&E stain (stained brown).

**Figures 161, 162** Mycetoma due to actinomycetes. This is a bacterial infection rather than a fungal infection but it looks very similar to the fungal mycetoma. The granules may be white (due to *Actinomadura madurae* or *Streptomyces somaliensis*) or red (due to *Actinomadura pelletieri*).

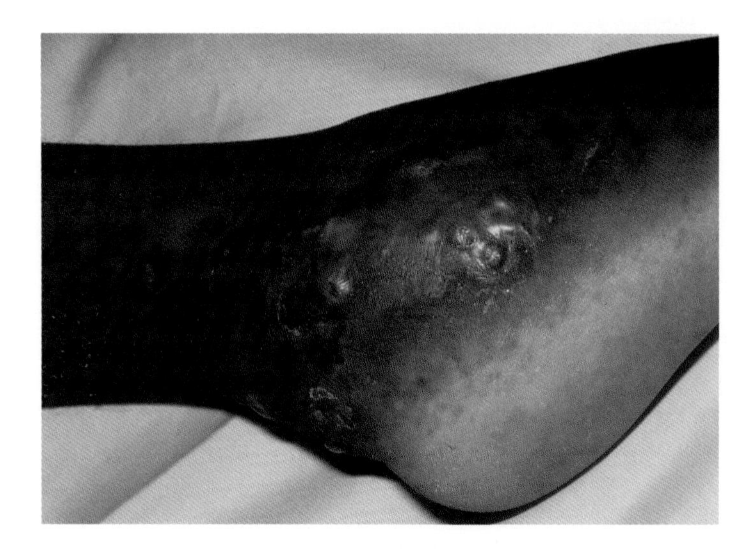

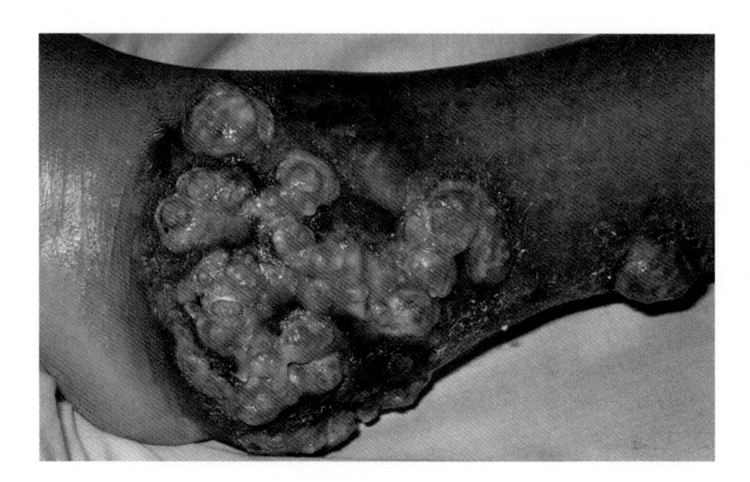

*Treatment:* Surgical excision if possible. If not, long-term treatment with oral sulphamethoxazole-trimethoprim 960mg bd for up to 2 years.

**Figures 163, 164** Histology of actinomycetoma shows the organism within an area of pus.

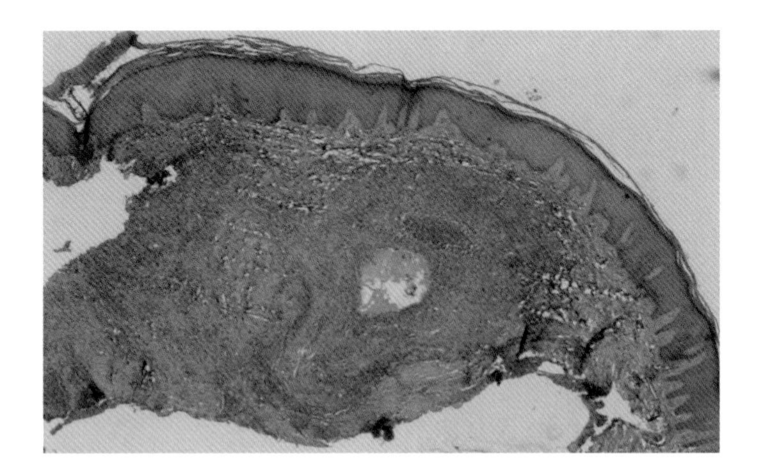

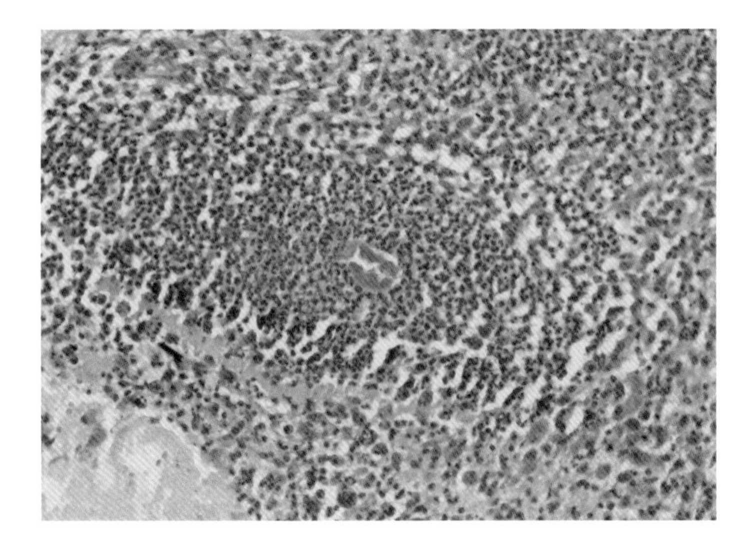

## Chromoblastomycosis

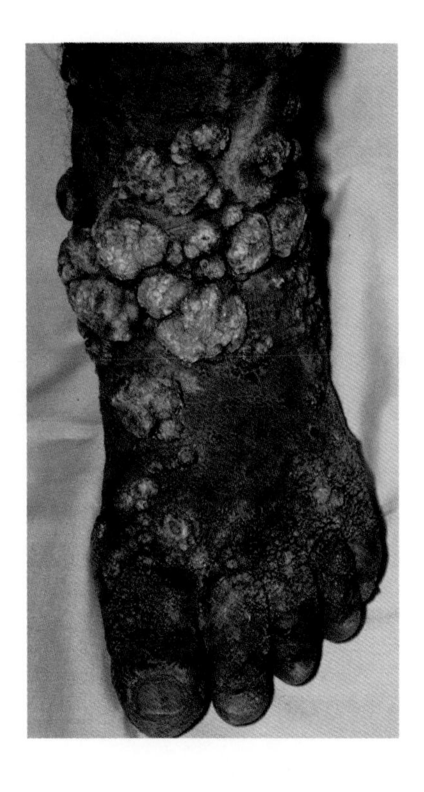

**Figure 165** Chronic deep fungal infection due to a number of organisms such as *Phialophora verrucosa, P. pedrosa, P. compactum, Wangiella dermatidis* and *Cladosporium carrionii.* The organism is found in decaying wood and soil. Most infections follow a penetrating wound to the foot or lower leg with a splinter of wood or a thorn. Warty papules or nodules are characteristic; they develop slowly over many years.

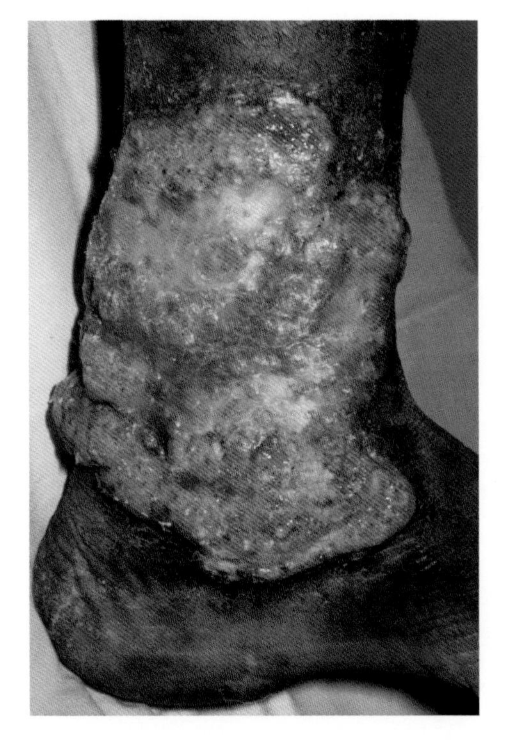

**Figure 166** Sometimes there are large red scaly plaques which mimic psoriasis.

*Treatment:* If the patient presents early (which is unusual), surgical excision is the treatment of choice. If presenting late give oral itraconazole 200mg twice a day for 9–12 months. It works well but is very expensive.

**Figure 167** The diagnosis of chromoblastomycosis can be confirmed by biopsy. Within the granulomatous infiltrate in the dermis and subcutaneous fat you can see the organisms which look like 'copper pennies' (H&E stain).

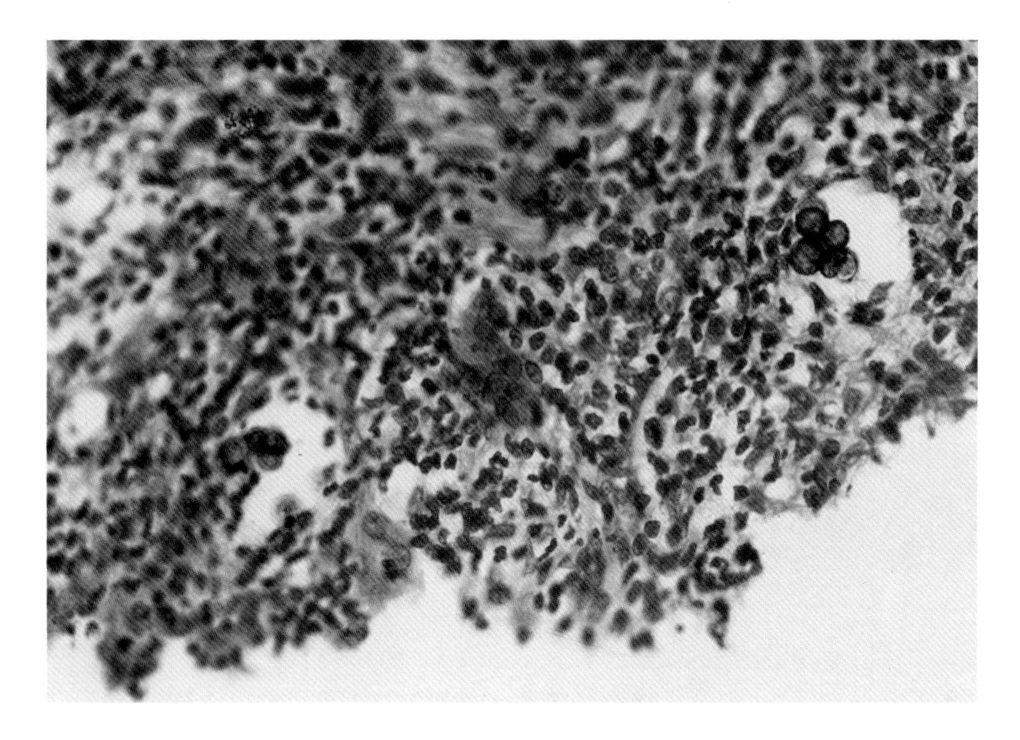

## Phycomycosis

**Figures 168, 169** This is a fungal infection due to *Entomophthora coronata* and usually affects the face and nose. The fungus extends deeply through cartilage and bony ostia.

*Treatment:* Surgical excision if feasible, but it may be difficult if it extends through the skull. Otherwise, treatment for 6 months or more with oral itraconazole 200mg/day.

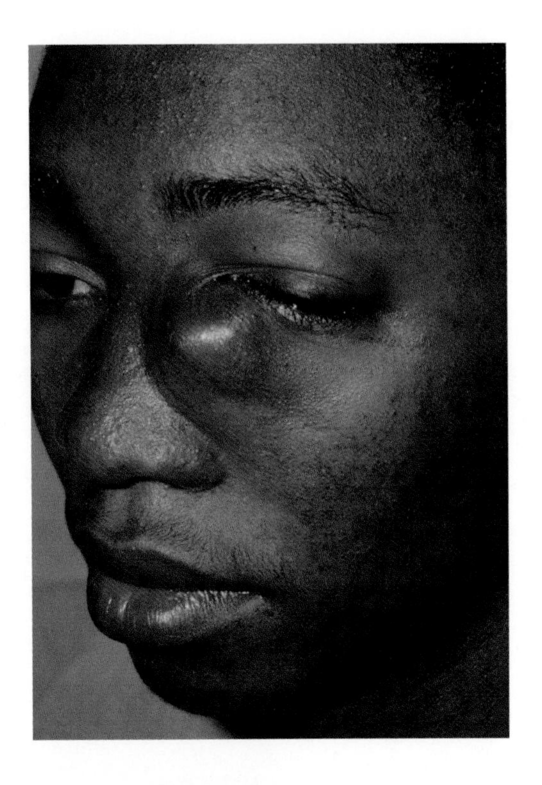

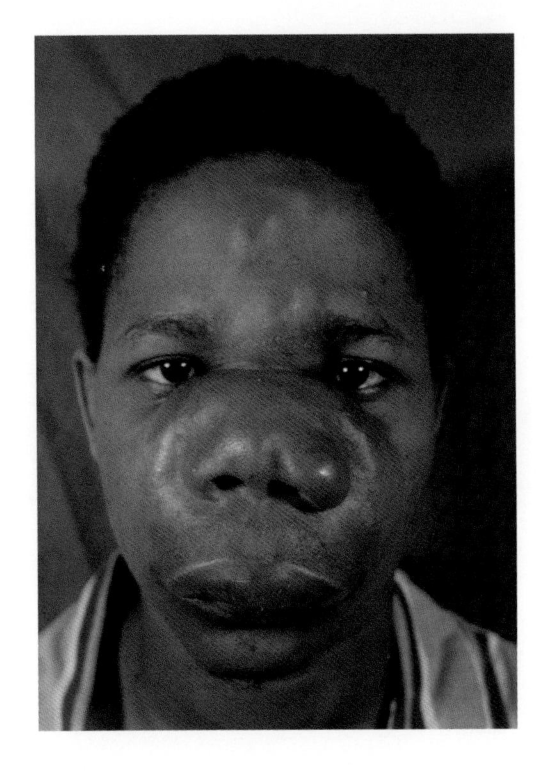

**Figures 170, 171** The pathognomonic feature of phycomycosis histologically is the presence of large irregularly branched hyphae within an inflammatory reaction or in giant cells (PAS stain).

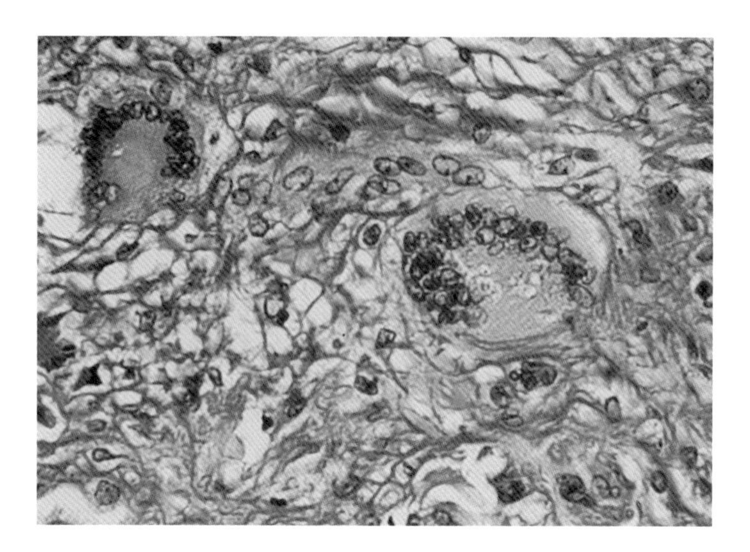

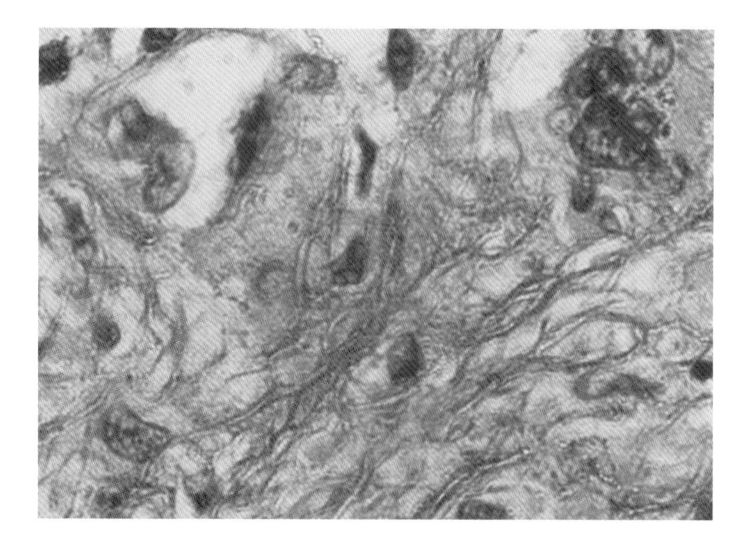

## Sporotrichosis

**Figure 172** Infection due to *Sporothrix schenckii*, a fungus which is found in the soil and in plants. Infection is acquired through a superficial laceration or prick with a thorn. A small papule appears at the site of injury, slowly enlarges and then ulcerates. The regional lymph nodes enlarge and after a few weeks more nodules appear along the line of the lymphatic drainage.

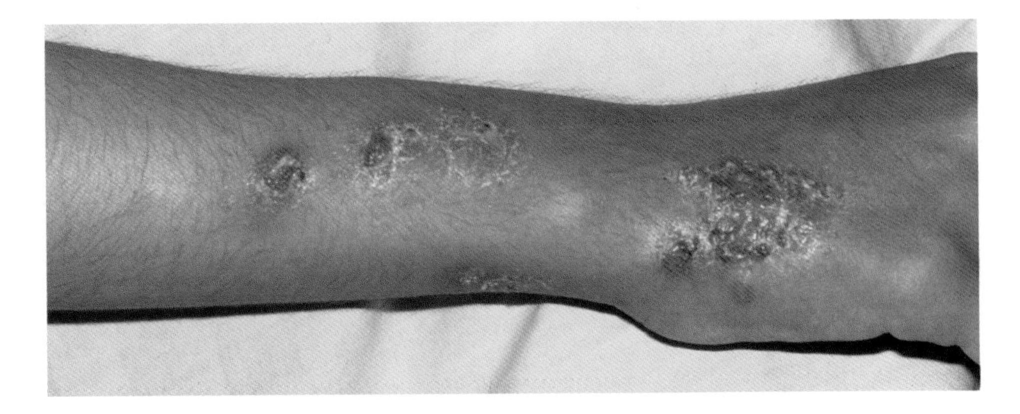

*Treatment:* It heals spontaneously with scarring after several weeks. Healing can be speeded up by using oral itraconazole 200mg/day, but this is very expensive.

## DENTAL SINUS

**Figure 173** Sinus opening onto the skin from an underlying dental abscess.

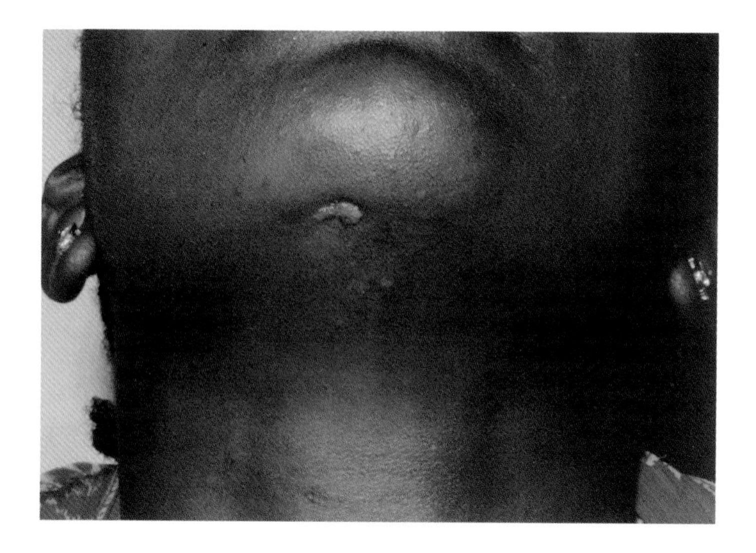

**Figure 174** Same patient as in Figure 173 to show origin of the sinus.

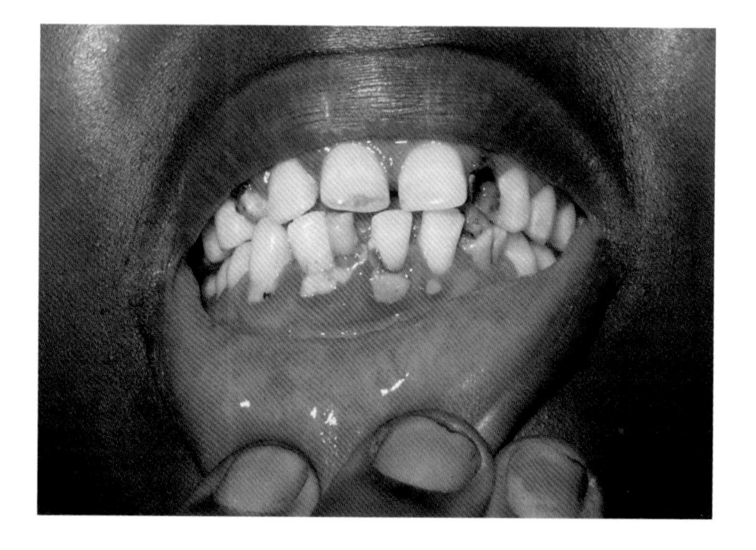

*Treatment:* Remove the offending tooth or teeth.

## DERMATITIS ARTEFACTA

**Figure 175** Self-induced lesions, often linear or bizarre shapes.

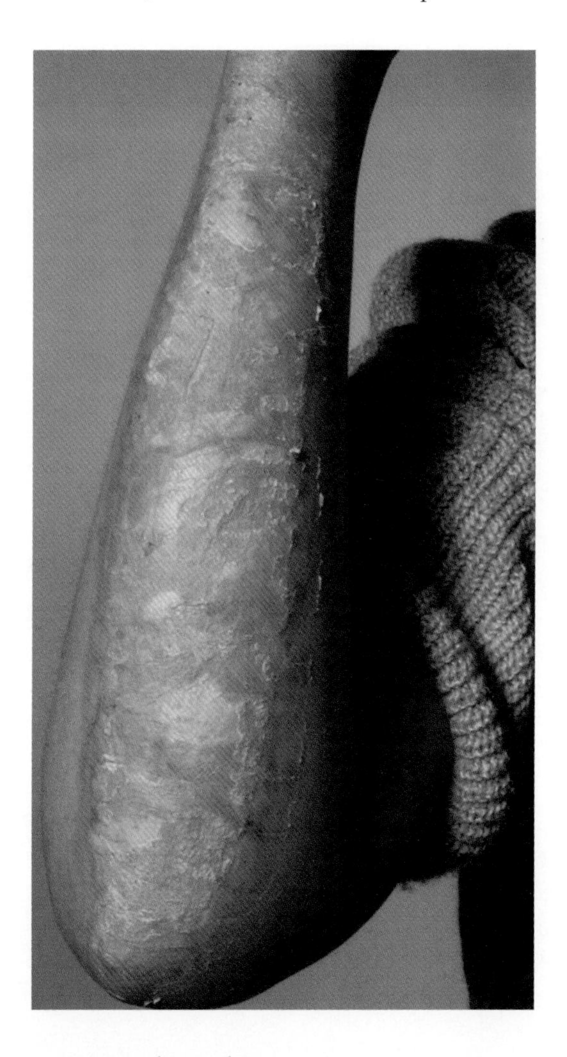

*Treatment:* The patient needs psychiatric help.

## DERMATOMYOSITIS

**Figures 176, 177** Erythema and oedema on sun-exposed skin (face, arms and 'V' of neck) and upper eyelids, together with proximal muscle tenderness and weakness. In patients over the age of 40 years there may be an underlying malignancy. In younger patients there may be calcification in the soft tissues (*see* Figures 99, 100).

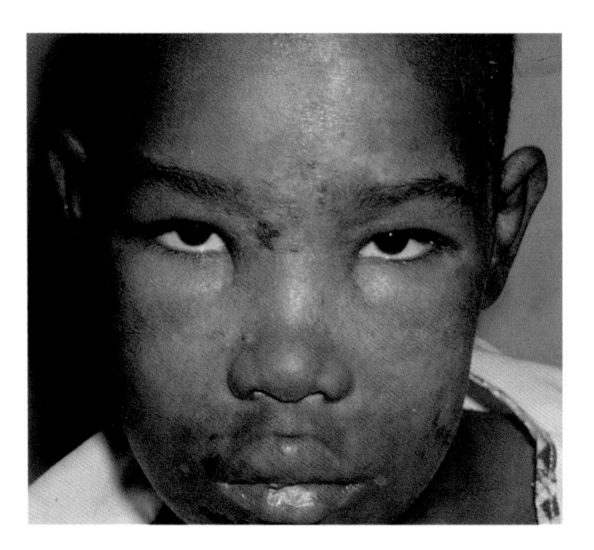

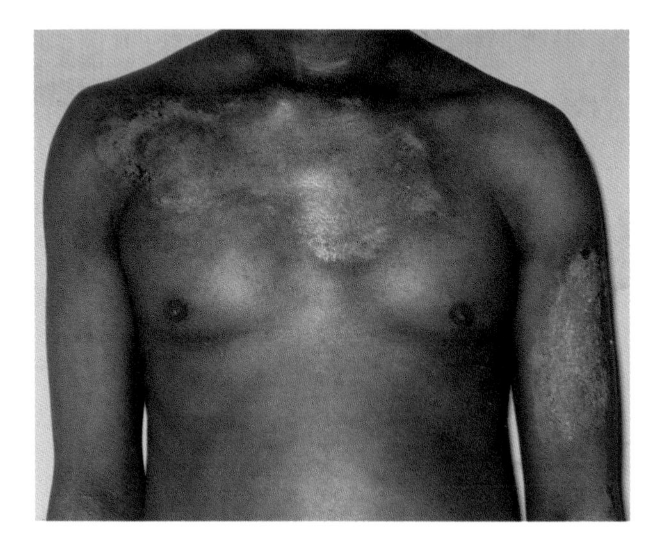

**Figure 178** On the dorsum of the hands and down the length of the fingers there may be linear erythematous plaques or Gottron's papules (small, flat-topped, erythematous papules). Nail fold telangiectasia is a common finding but also occurs in systemic lupus erythematosus (*see* Figures 404–5) and systemic sclerosis (*see* Figures 578–81).

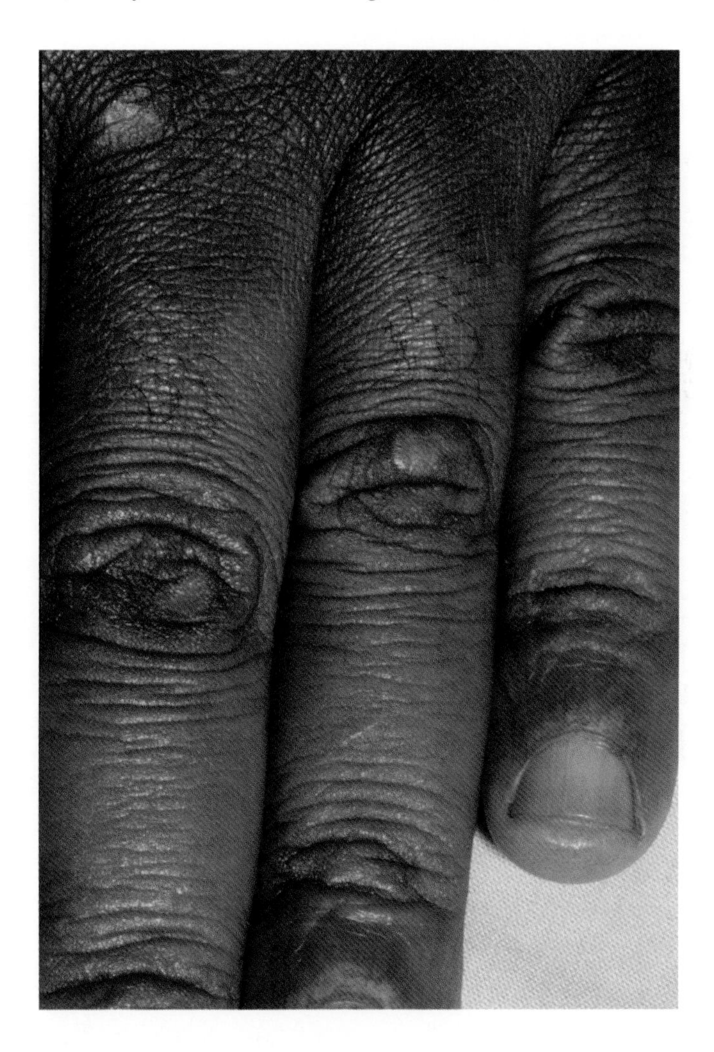

*Treatment:* High dose systemic steroids, starting with 60mg prednisolone daily, gradually decreasing as the disease comes under control. If it is due to carcinoma of the breast, lung or stomach, removal of the tumour will bring about a cure.

## DERMATOSIS PAPULOSA NIGRA

**Figure 179** Small seborrhoeic warts on the cheeks which appear in childhood and gradually increase in number with age. This condition runs in families, being inherited as an autosomal dominant trait (*see* Figure 295).

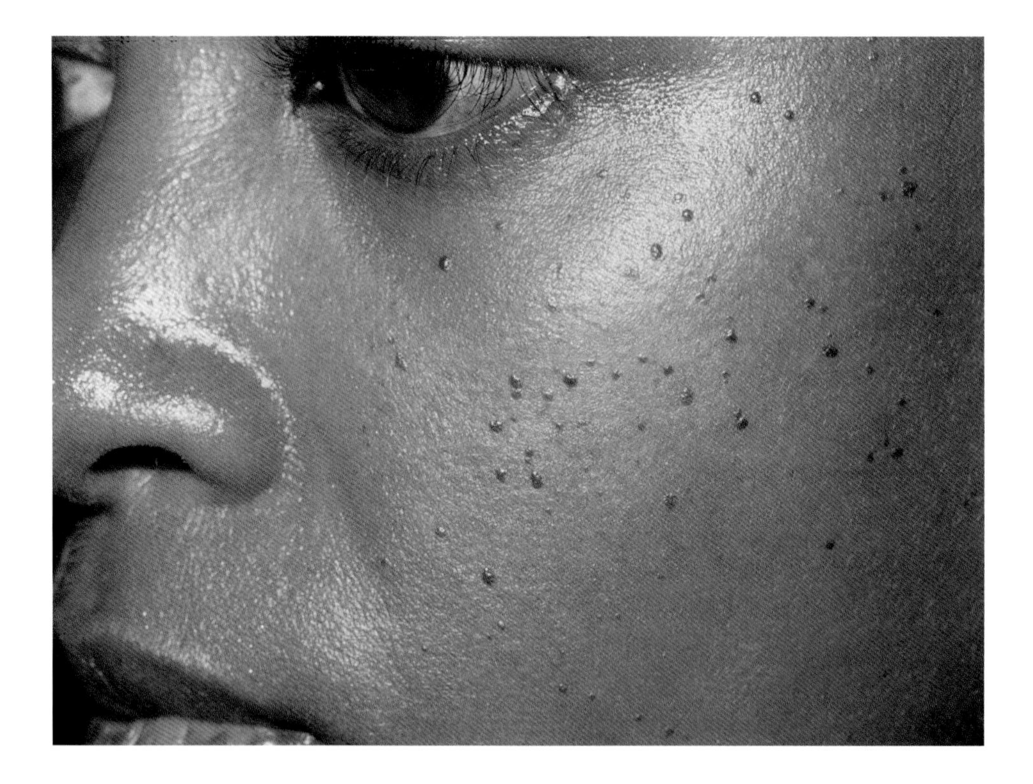

*Treatment:* Reassurance that the condition is harmless is all that is required.

## DERMOGRAPHISM

**Figure 180** This is urticaria induced by trauma or scratching of the skin. The clinical features are due to histamine release, i.e. Lewis's triple response – localised erythema followed by oedema and flare.

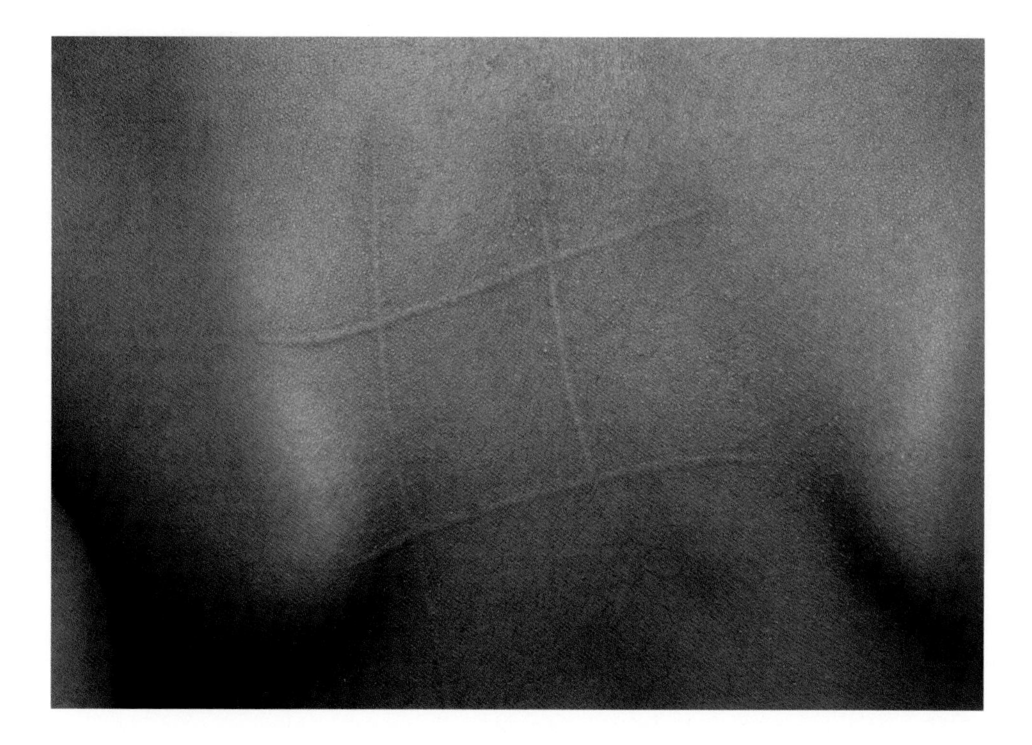

*Treatment:* Often does not require treatment. If it is very itchy a systemic antihistamine taken regularly will help, e.g. promethazine 25mg nocte.

## DIGITAL FIBROKERATOMA

**Figure 181** Small papule arising from the side of a finger at one of the joints. It appears after trauma and it can be distinguished from an accessory digit (*see* Figure 5) by the fact that it occurs in adult life.

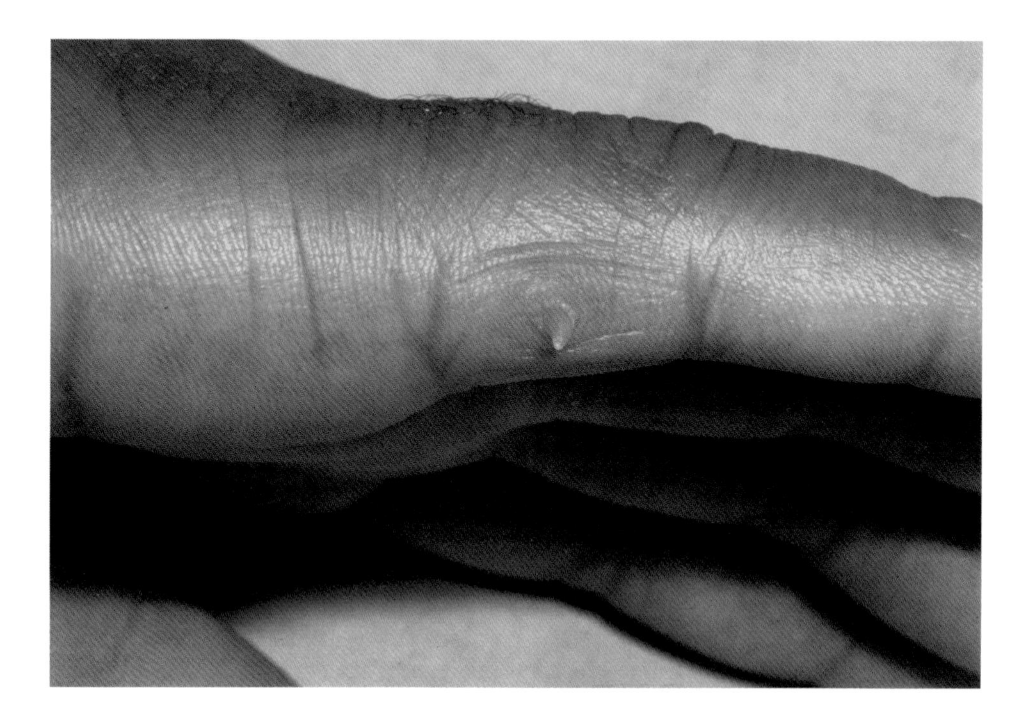

*Treatment:* Excise if it is unsightly or causes a nuisance.

## DISSEMINATED INTRAVASCULAR COAGULATION (DIC)

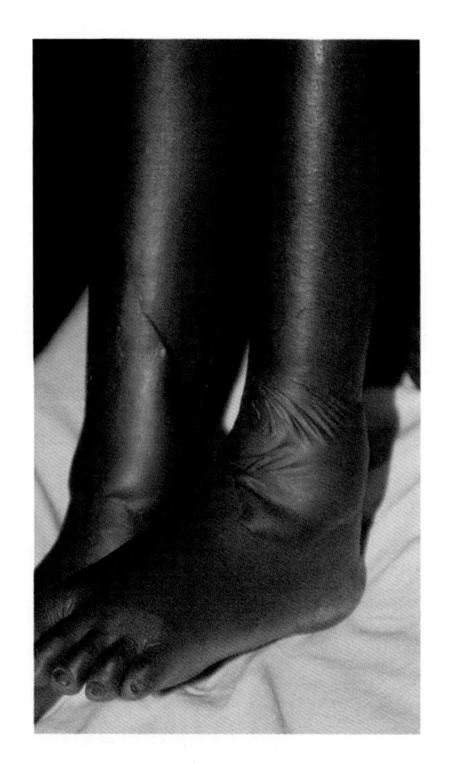

**Figure 182** A combination of bleeding and thrombosis due to a widespread activation of haemostasis. It is usually a reaction to massive infection, e.g. streptococcal or Gram negative septicaemia, or to an obstetric catastrophe. Easy bruising, bleeding from intramuscular injection and venepuncture sites, together with microthrombotic lesions in the skin which lead to purpura fulminans (extensive necrosis of the skin). Similar lesions in the kidneys lead to renal failure and often death. The diagnosis can be confirmed by finding thrombocytopaenia, an increase in fibrin degradation products, and prolongation of the prothrombin time, the activated partial thromboplastin time and the thrombin time.

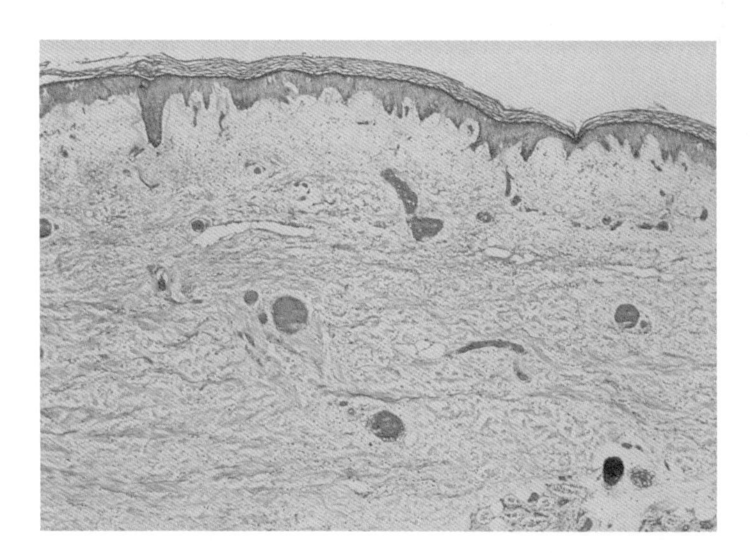

**Figure 183** A skin biopsy will show thrombosis of the small blood vessels in the skin.

*Treatment:* Treat the underlying cause. Fluid replacement +/– fresh frozen plasma if it is available.

## DRACUNCULOSIS (Guinea worm)

**Figure 184** Due to the nematode worm, *Dracunculus medinensis*. The female worm (40–50cm long) lives in the connective tissue of the lower legs. After about 12 months it moves to the skin surface causing a burning sensation. When this part of the skin comes in contact with fresh water, a blister develops on the skin and the worm comes out through the blister.

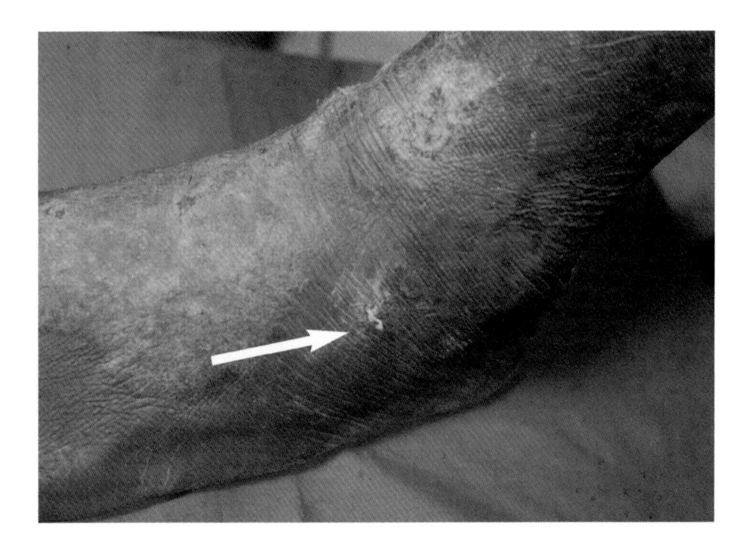

**Figure 185** Larvae of *Dracunculus medinensis*. The female discharges larvae into the water, which are taken up by tiny crabs of the genus *Cyclops*. Humans become infected when they drink water containing the tiny crabs. In the stomach the larvae develop into adult worms which migrate down to the legs. The diagnosis is made when the adult worm is seen coming out through the skin (*see* Figure 184).

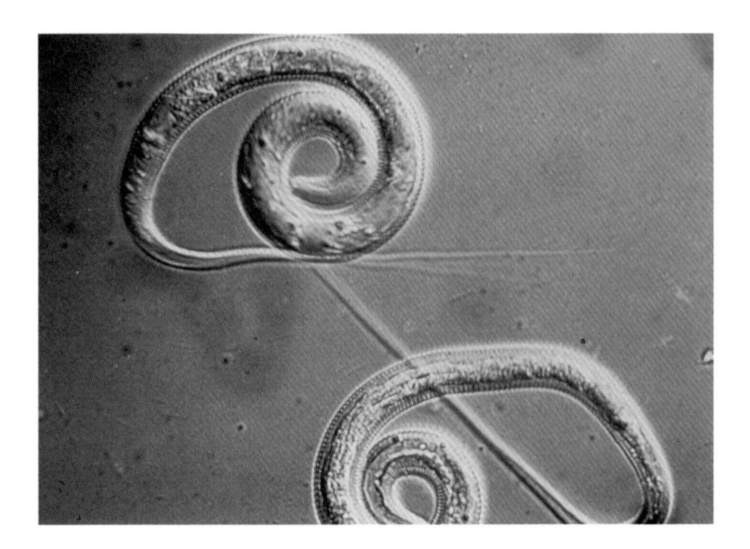

*Prevention:* Prevent people from dangling their legs in, or walking in, water which will be used for drinking. Install village hand pumps or filter drinking water through a piece of cotton.

## DRUG RASH

### Erythema multiforme

**Figure 186** This is a symmetrical rash on the dorsum of the hands and feet (+/– elsewhere) consisting of round papules made up of rings of different colours (or different shades of brown). The lesions are all uniformly small, 1cm in diameter or less. The rash occurs about 14 days after a viral infection (any, but especially herpes simplex), a bacterial infection (any, but especially a streptococcal sore throat) or taking a drug, especially a sulphonamide (most commonly sulphamethoxazole in the sulphamethoxazole-trimethoprim mixture).

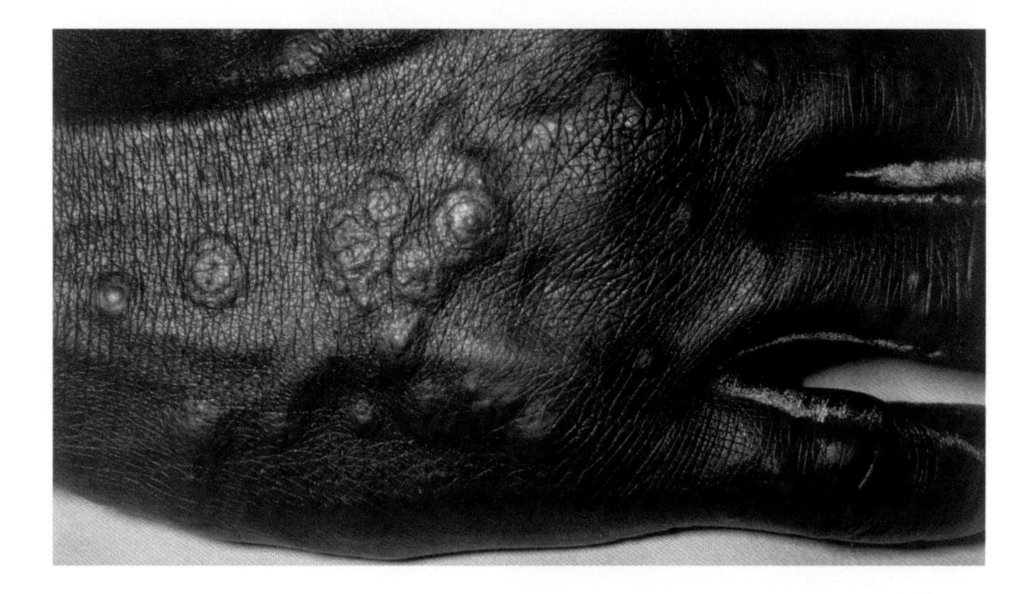

*Treatment:* Whatever the cause it gets better spontaneously in 10–14 days. If it is due to a drug, that drug and any related drugs should be avoided in the future.

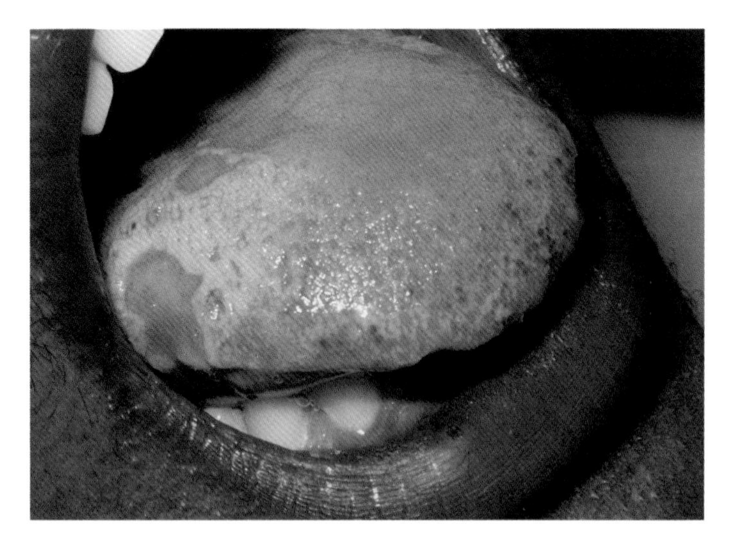

**Figure 187** Erythema multiforme frequently involves mucous membranes causing erosions or ulcers in the mouth. These are usually asymptomatic.

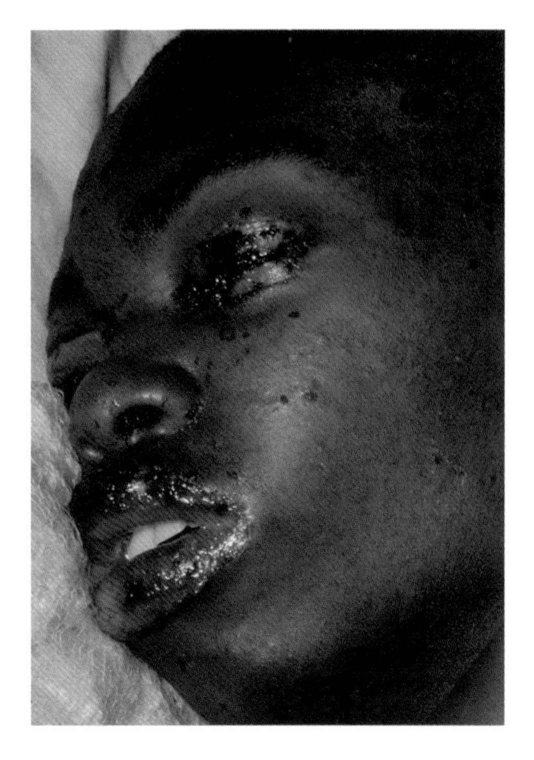

**Figure 188** Erythema multiforme with extensive involvement of mucous membranes is called Stevens-Johnson syndrome. This is frequently due to sulphonamides. It is more common in individuals who are HIV positive.

*Treatment:* Care of mucous membranes: frequent mouth washes, liquid food, artificial tears to the eyes, intravenous fluids if the patient is unable to drink enough. Avoid sulphonamides in the future.

## Fixed drug eruption

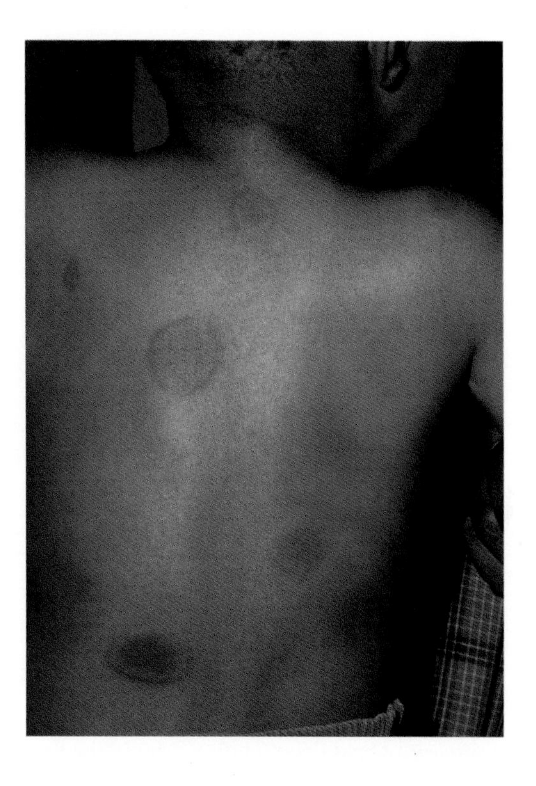

**Figure 189** Perfectly round or oval erythematous plaques (+/– blisters) occurring within 24 hours of taking the offending drug (usually within 1–2 hours). Lesions can be single or multiple.

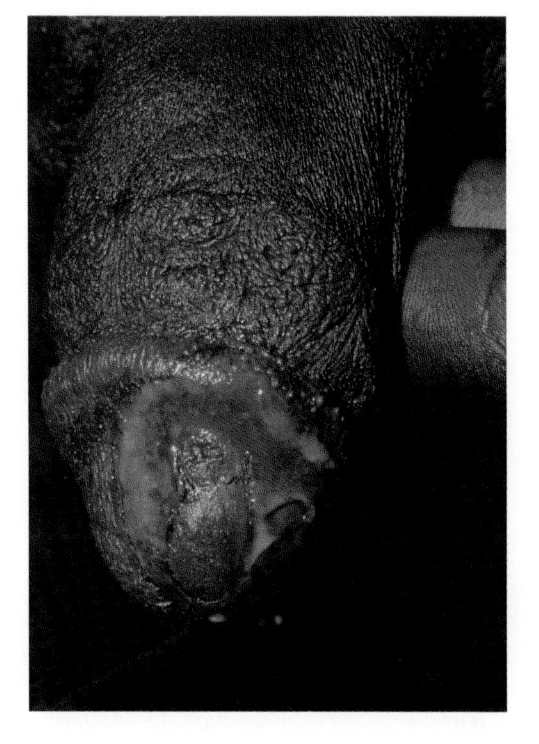

**Figure 190** In the mouth or on the penis (as here) blisters ulcerate. Such ulcers can be confused with those due to sexually transmitted diseases (*see* Figures 129, 276, 595).

**Figure 191** Fixed drug eruptions heal in about 10 days leaving hyperpigmented patches. Every time the drug is taken the rash recurs at the same site. Sulphonamides are the most likely cause. Fixed drug eruption may be a manifestation of HIV infection in both children and adults.

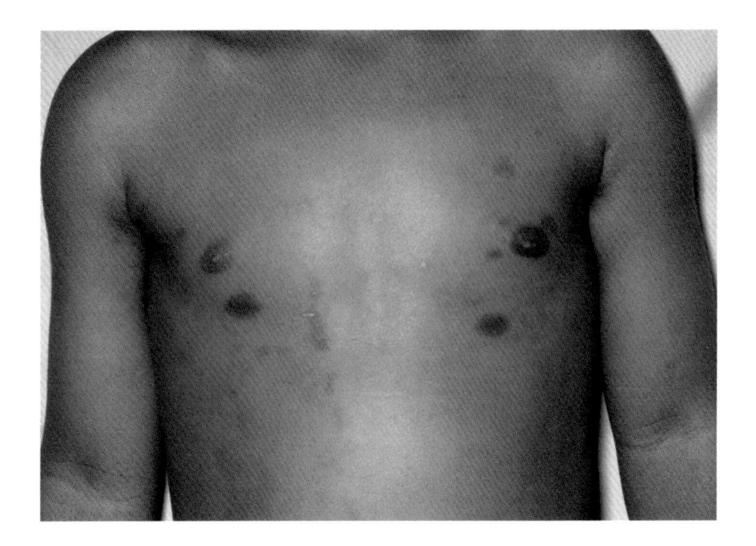

*Treatment:* Avoid the offending drug in the future.

## Morbilliform drug eruption

**Figure 192** This is the common type of drug eruption that occurs after taking antibiotics and diuretics (although any drug can cause it). It is usually not serious.

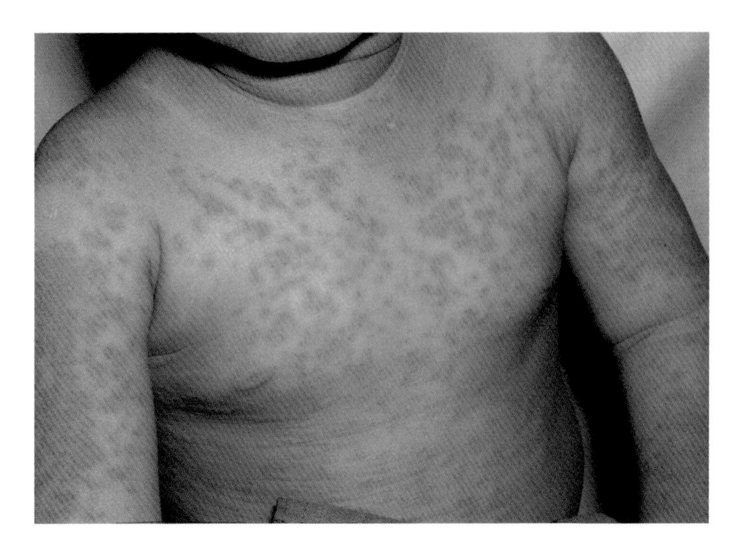

*Treatment:* Symptomatic. If it is itchy, apply calamine lotion prn. Whether to stop the drug or not will depend on the severity of the rash and how essential it is for the patient's well being.

## Toxic epidermal necrolysis (TEN)

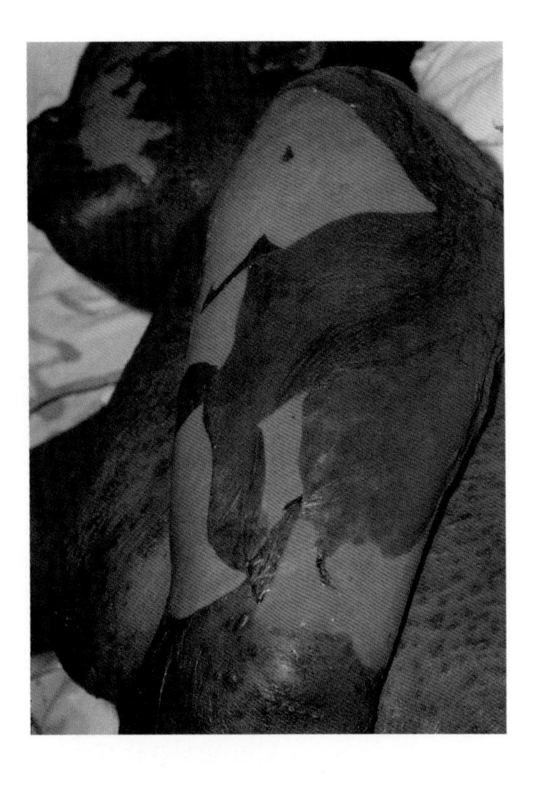

**Figure 193** This is a rare but serious drug reaction. Necrosis of the lower half of the epidermis causes the skin to slide off in sheets. It is most commonly due to thiacetazone and sulphonamides. It often occurs in those who are HIV positive.

*Treatment:* Good nursing care, fluid replacement and prevention of secondary bacterial infection.

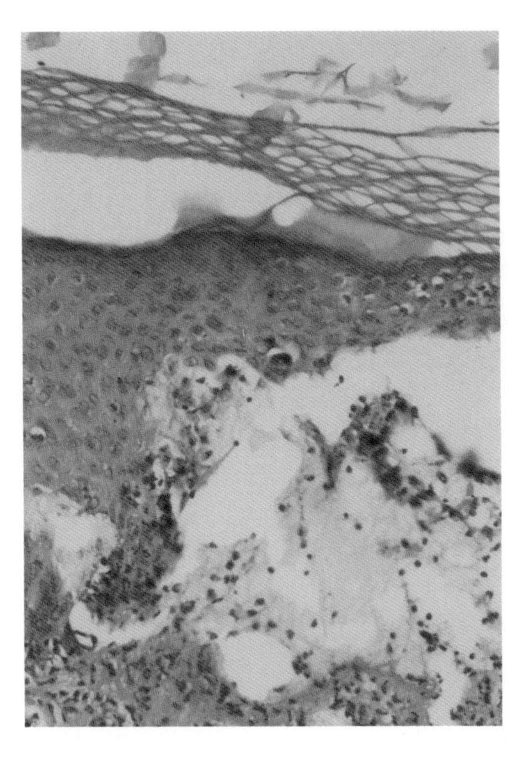

**Figure 194** Histology of TEN. Necrosis of the lower half of the epidermis. If you cut off the blister roof it will contain keratin and several layers of epidermal cells. Compare this with the histology of staphylococcal scalded skin syndrome where the blister roof is only keratin (*see* Figure 590).

## ECTHYMA

**Figure 195** Round punched out ulcer with a crust on top due to infection of the full thickness of the epidermis with *Staphylococcus aureus* (*see* Figure 309) or *Streptococcus pyogenes* (*see* Figure 124). Usually secondary to an insect bite, scabies or eczema.

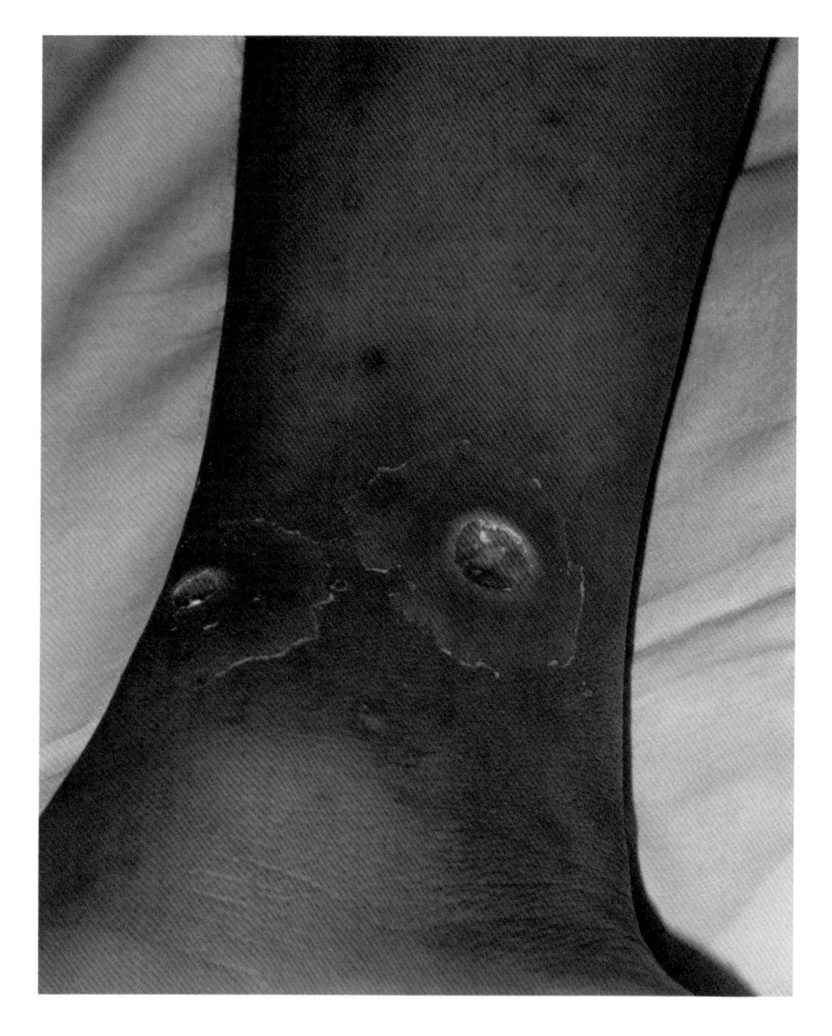

*Treatment:* Oral cloxacillin (if due to staphylococcus) or phenoxymethylpenicillin (if due to streptococcus). The ulcer will take at least 4 weeks to heal.

# ECZEMA OR DERMATITIS

**Figure 196** The word 'eczema' comes from a Greek word meaning to 'bubble through'. The word 'dermatitis' means 'inflammation in the skin'. The two words, eczema and dermatitis, are used interchangeably for a condition in the skin in which fluid accumulates in and between the prickle cells of the epidermis. Clinically the picture varies from overt blistering to slight scaling or lichenification.

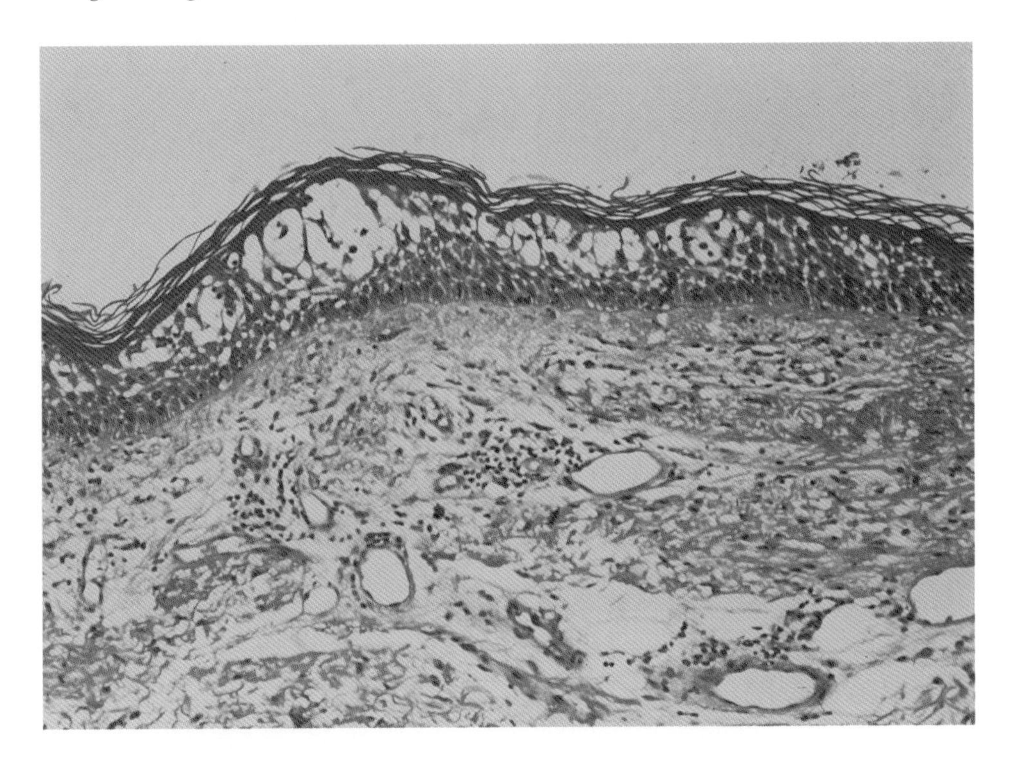

## Classification of eczema

### Endogenous eczema (coming from the inside)

- Atopic eczema.
- Seborrhoeic eczema.
- Discoid (nummular) eczema.
- Unclassifiable eczema (symmetrical eczema which does not fit into one of the categories above).

### Exogenous eczema (coming from the outside)

- Primary irritant eczema.
- Allergic contact eczema.

## Atopic eczema

**Figures 197, 198** Atopic means an inherited predisposition to eczema, asthma and hay fever. The individual, and other members of the family, may have one, two or all three manifestations of the disease. The eczema most commonly begins in infancy (after 3 months of age) on the face and scalp, although it can begin later.

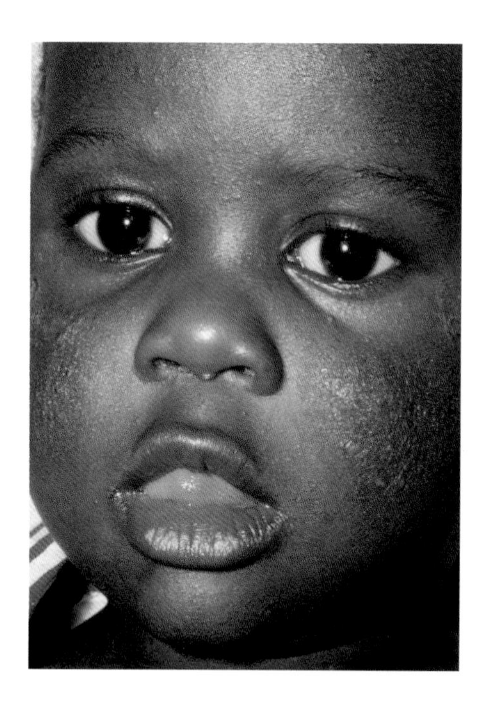

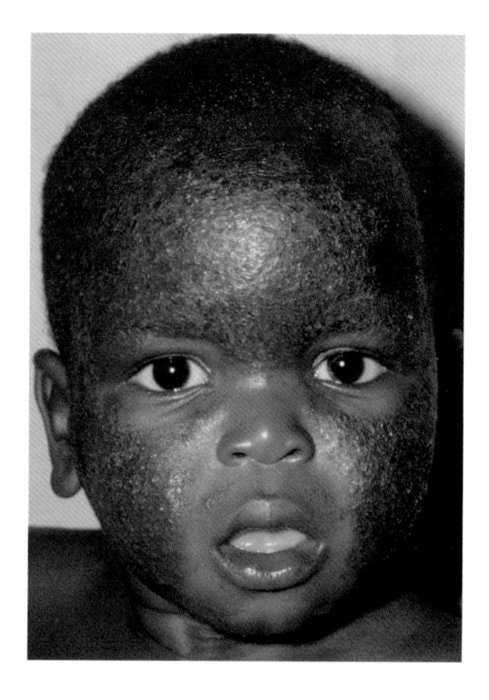

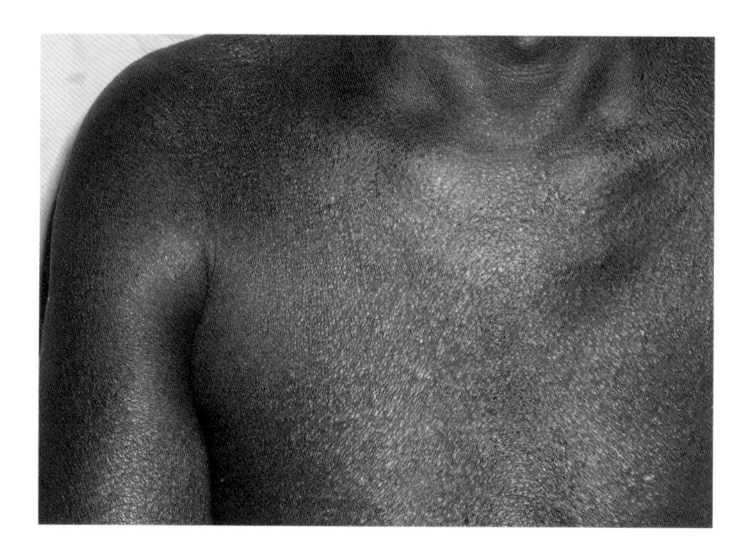

**Figure 199** It may then spread to the rest of the body as a poorly defined scaly rash.

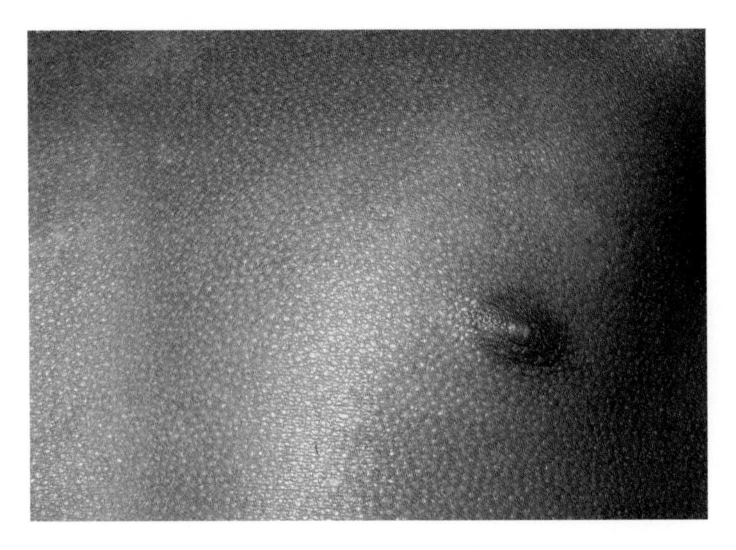

**Figure 200** This pattern of tiny papules on the trunk is a common pattern in children.

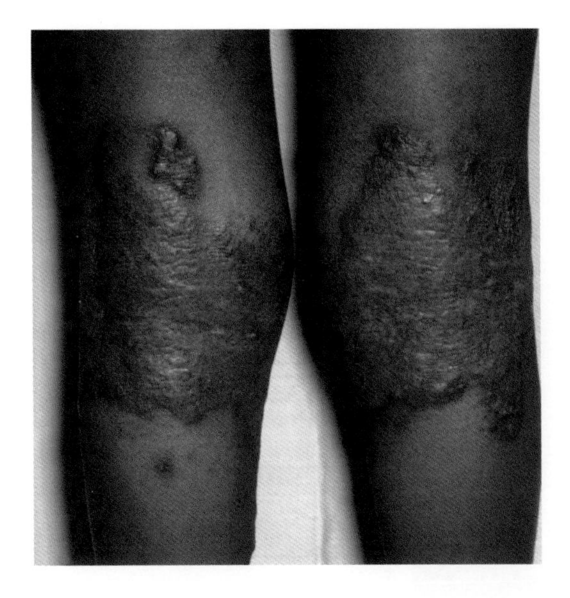

**Figure 201** As the child gets older the rash may localise in the flexures. In adults the eczema may start in the flexures.

*Treatment:* Topical steroid ointment not cream. Start with 0.5% or 1% hydrocortisone ointment applied bd. Use a slightly stronger topical steroid ointment if there is lichenification or the hydrocortisone does not work. For secondary infection add a systemic antibiotic (cloxacillin) not a topical antibiotic.

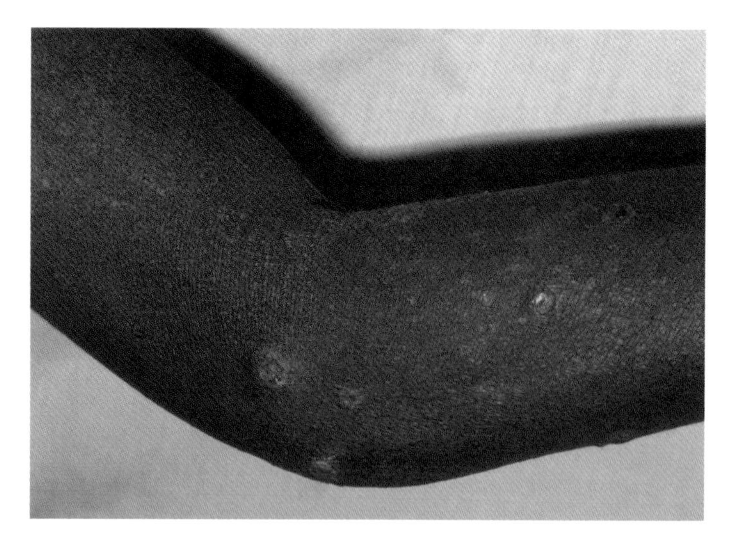

**Figure 202** Atopic eczema is a very itchy rash. Scratching produces excoriations.

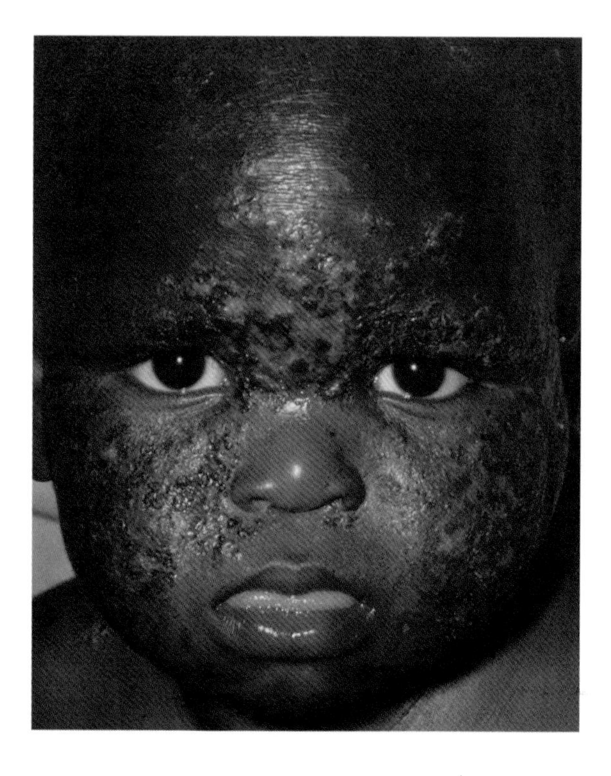

**Figure 203** Scratching can also lead to secondary infection, usually with *Staphylococcus aureus* (same child as in Figure 198).

**Figures 204, 205** Rubbing, rather than scratching with the nails, produces lichenification (thickening of the epidermis and increased skin lines).

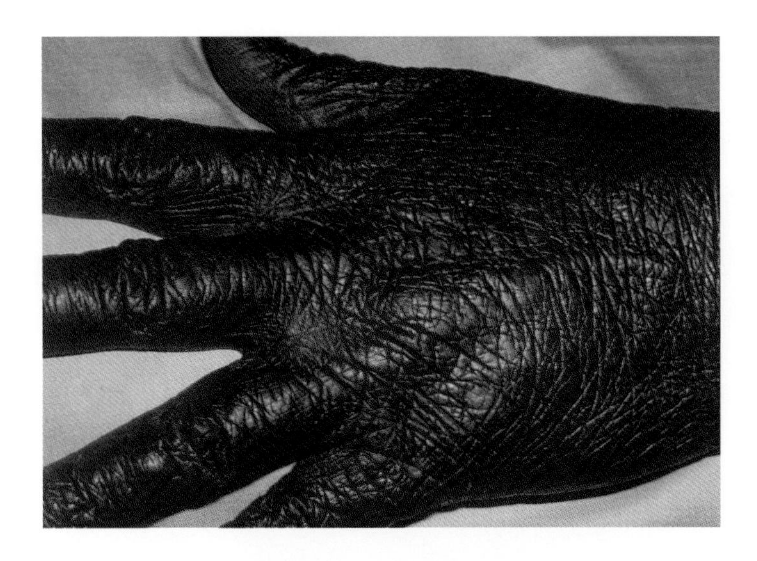

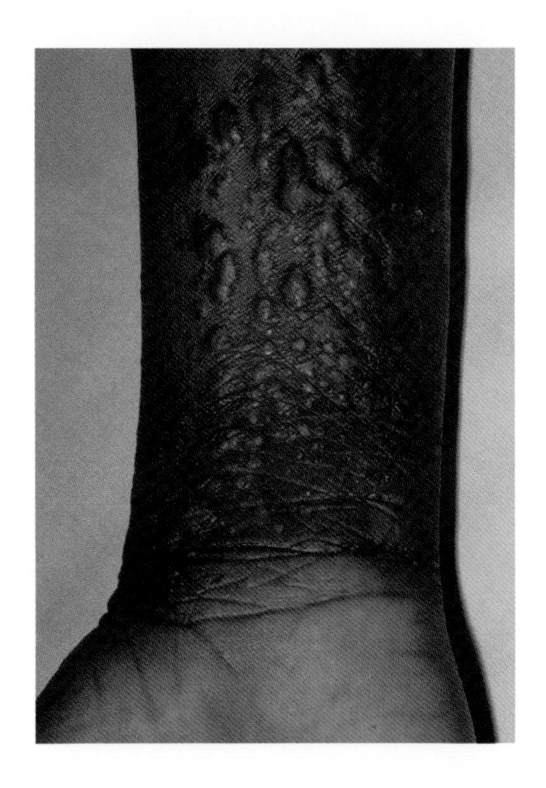

**Figure 206** Shiny nails. As well as lichenification of the skin (*see* Figures 204–5) constant rubbing of itchy skin causes the nails to become polished (shiny).

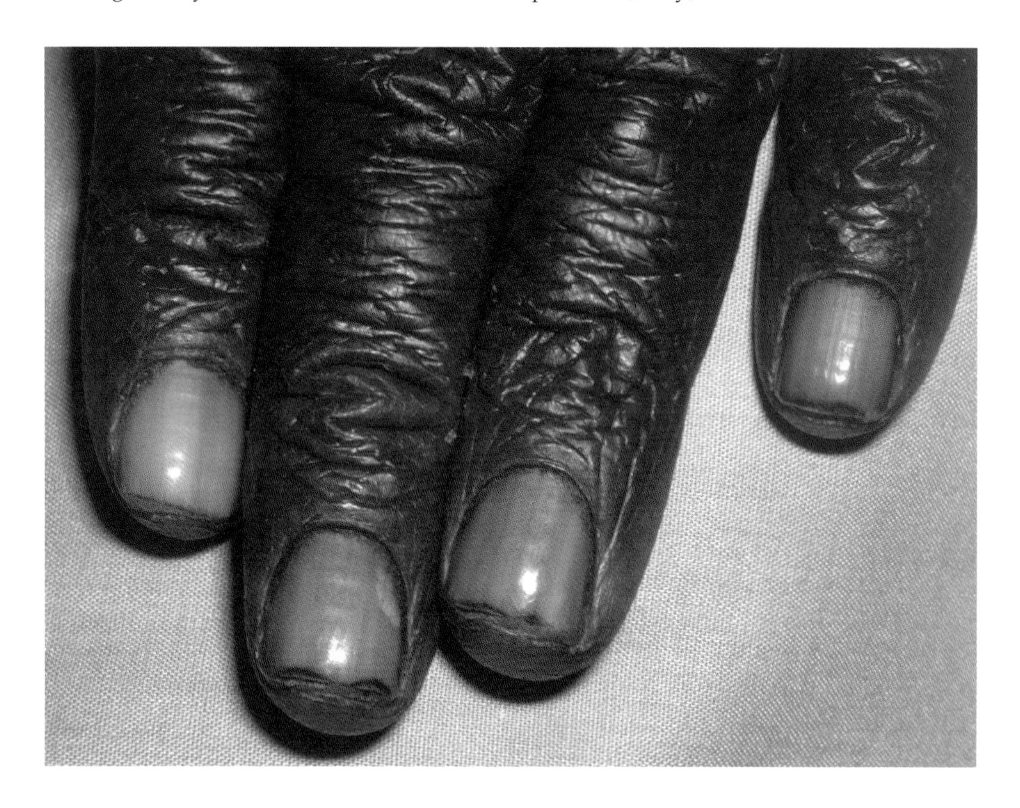

## Seborrhoeic eczema

**Figures 207, 208** The diagnosis of seborrhoeic eczema is made on the distribution of the rash. It occurs on the scalp (dandruff), eyebrows, eyelashes, nasolabial folds, external ear (otitis externa), the centre of the back and centre of the chest. Rarely, the flexures (axillae and groins) are involved. It is a disease of adults; it does not occur before puberty. It tends to come and go, especially at times of stress.

*Treatment:* 1% hydrocortisone cream or ointment applied bd or a topical imidazole cream applied bd when the rash is there. Leave it off when the rash is not present.

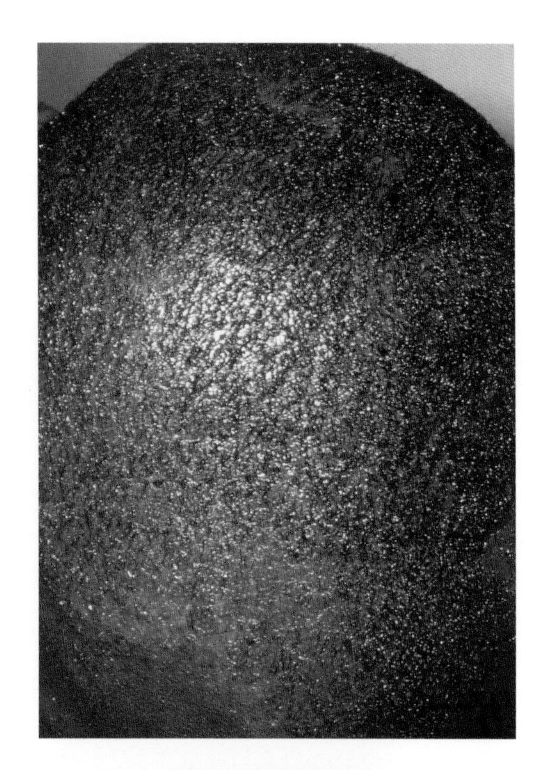

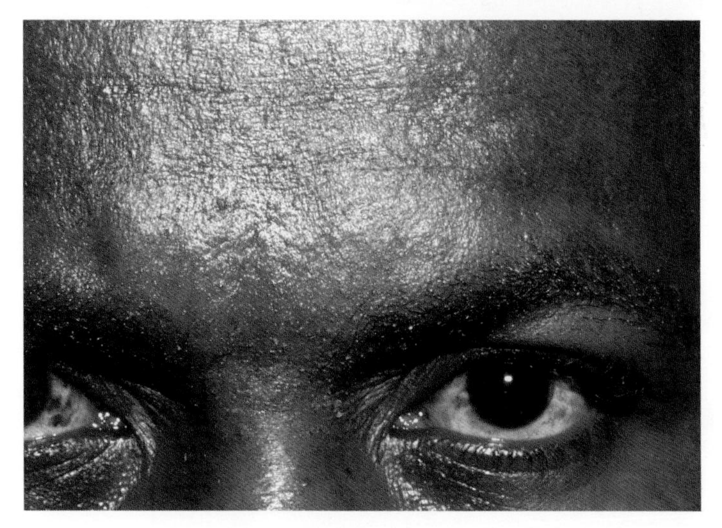

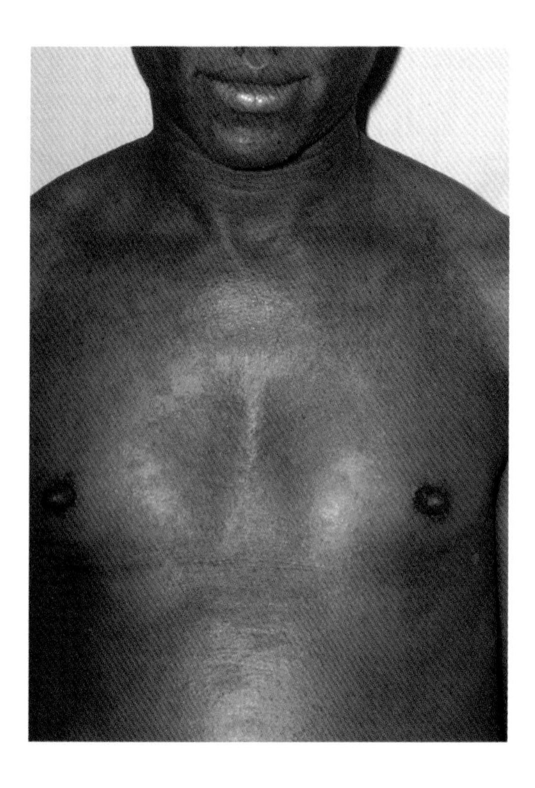

**Figure 209** Seborrhoeic eczema involving the centre of the chest.

## Infantile seborrhoeic eczema

**Figure 210** Unusual type of eczema occurring in early infancy (usually 2–6 weeks after birth). It begins with 'cradle cap' (scaly scalp) and then spreads to the face, nappy area, axillae and elsewhere. It differs from infantile atopic eczema by its early age of onset (before 12 weeks), the fact that it is not itchy and that it gets better after a few weeks and does not recur. It has nothing to do with the ordinary adult type of seborrhoeic eczema.

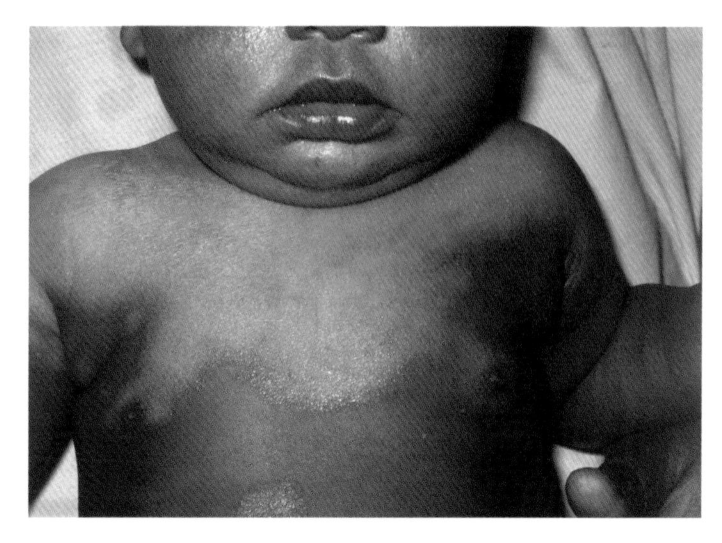

*Treatment:* Usually none is needed because it is not itchy. Explain to the parents that it will get better on its own after a few weeks.

## Discoid eczema

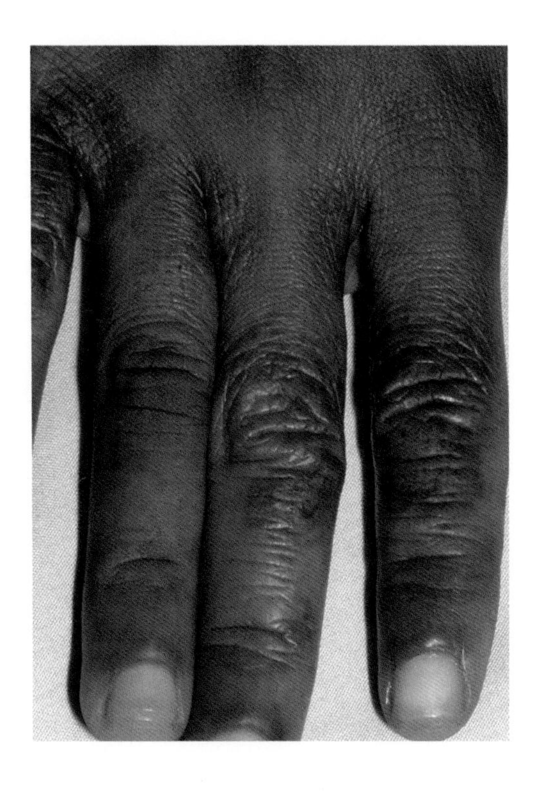

**Figure 211** Round or oval discs of eczema on the backs of the hands of young adults or on the lower legs of the middle aged and elderly.

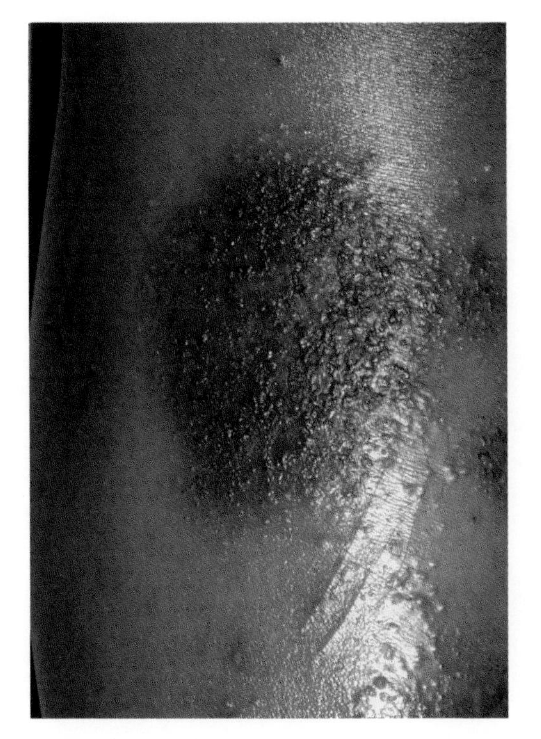

**Figure 212** Often vesicles and crusts rather than just scaling.

*Treatment:* Responds better to topical tar than to topical steroids. 3% crude coal tar in Vaseline or Lassar's paste applied bd.

## Primary irritant eczema

**Figure 213** A primary irritant eczema is due to weak acids or weak alkalis being in contact with the skin. Anyone can get it if they have enough contact with these substances. In nappy rash the bacteria in the stool break down the urea in the urine to ammonia which is alkaline. It is caused by the baby being in a wet, soiled nappy.

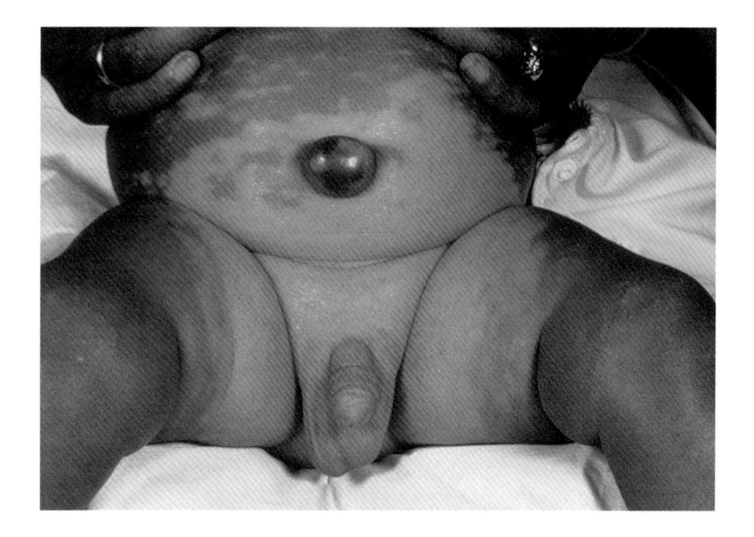

*Treatment:* Change the nappies frequently.

**Figure 214** Primary irritant eczema due to the frequent application of benzyl benzoate for scabies. The emulsion has been used twice a day for 14 days rather than applied only twice.

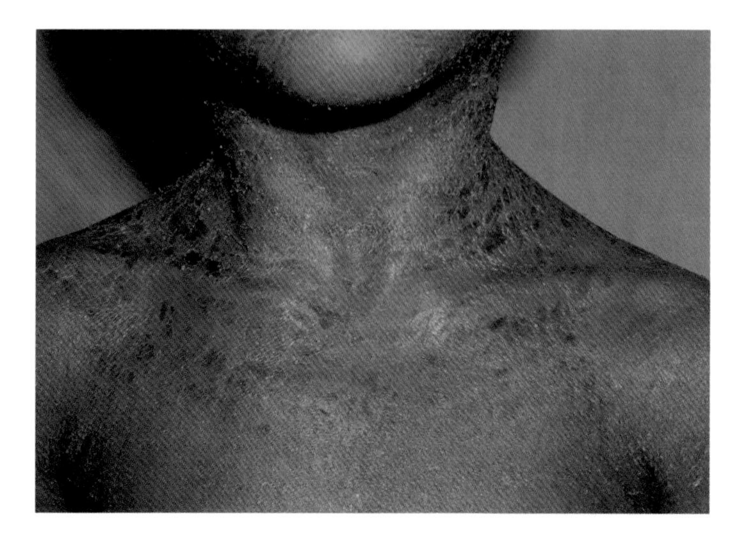

*Treatment:* Stop the benzyl benzoate and apply a weak topical steroid ointment, e.g. 1% hydrocortisone ointment bd, until it is better.

## Allergic contact eczema

An allergic contact eczema is a Type IV allergic reaction (delayed hypersensitivity) to an allergen in contact with the skin. The rash, usually an acute (blistering) eczema at the site of contact, occurs 48–96 hours after that contact. Once sensitised, an individual will get a rash whenever he is in contact with the allergen for the rest of his life, but always after a delay of 48–96 hours.

**Figures 215, 216** Allergic contact eczema due to mercaptobenzothiazole in the rubber of these sandals. Note that the rash is exactly where the sandals are in contact with the skin.

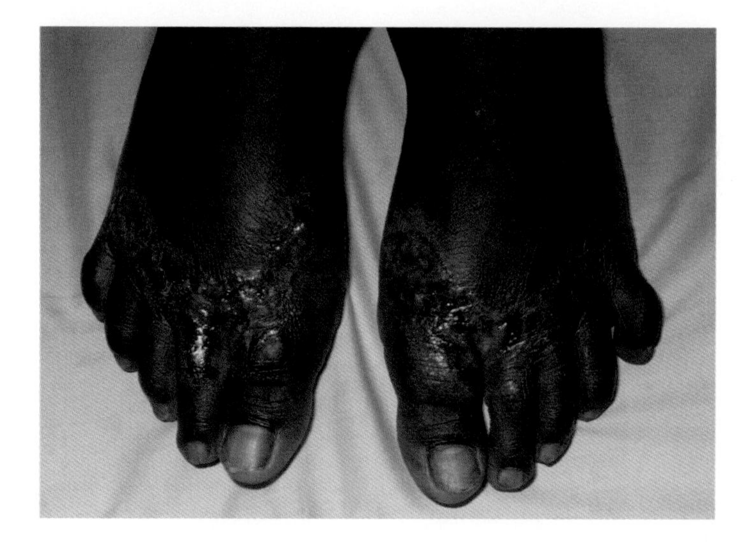

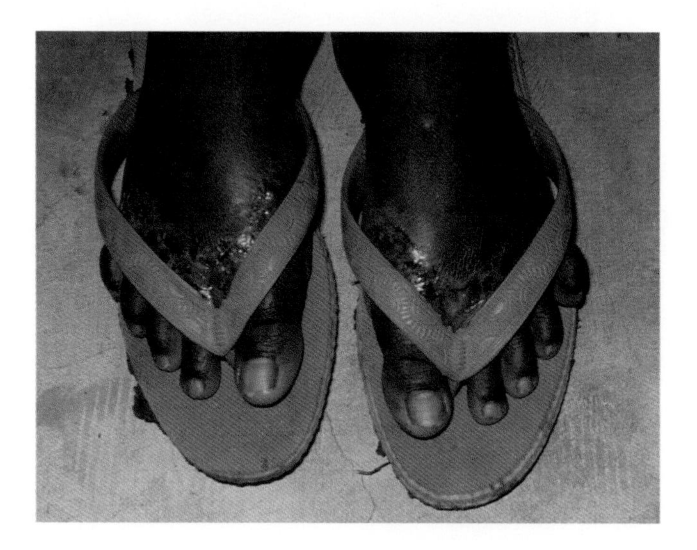

**Figures 217, 218** Allergic contact eczema from nickel in watch buckle and bra clips.

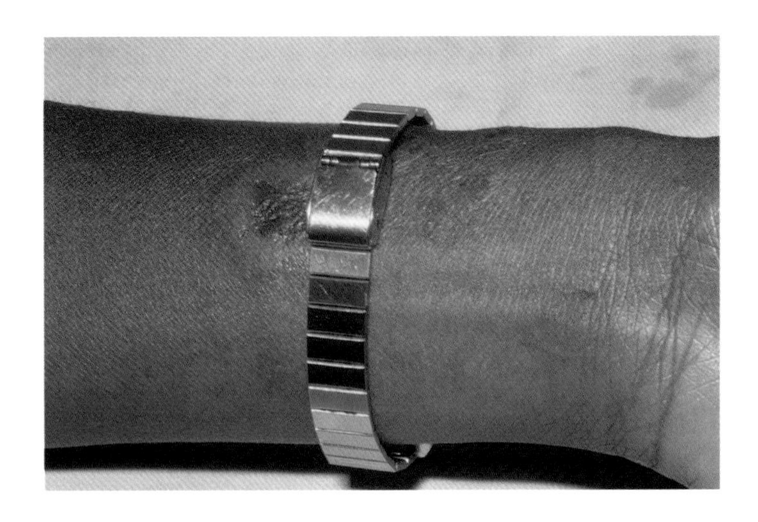

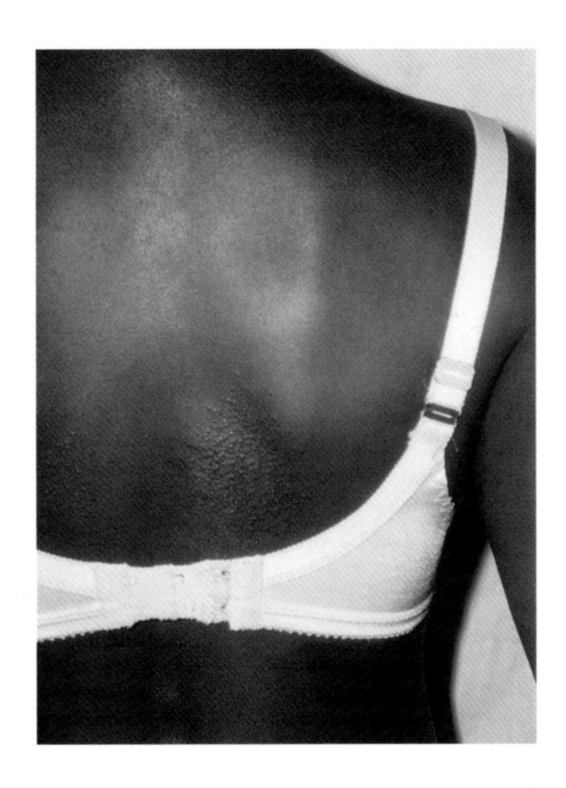

**Figure 219** Allergic contact eczema due to nickel in the buckle of a belt.

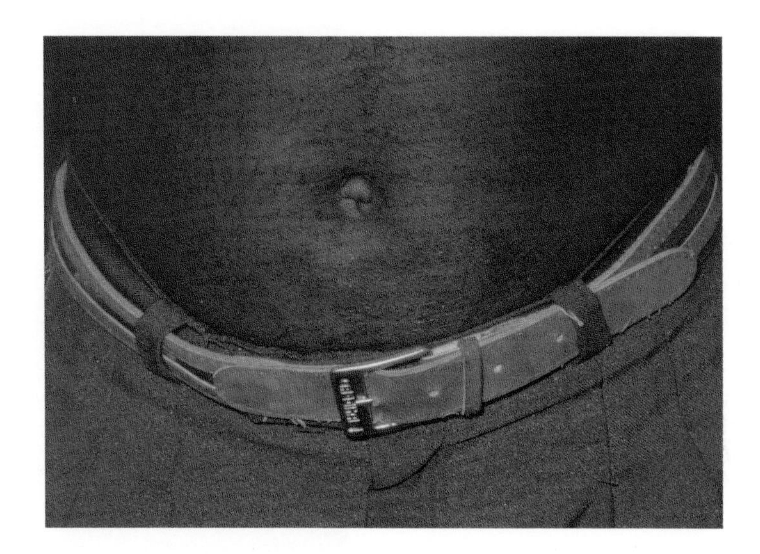

**Figure 220** Allergic contact eczema due to potassium dichromate in cement dust. The rash is usually on the backs of the hands and the face (i.e. the exposed parts of the skin).

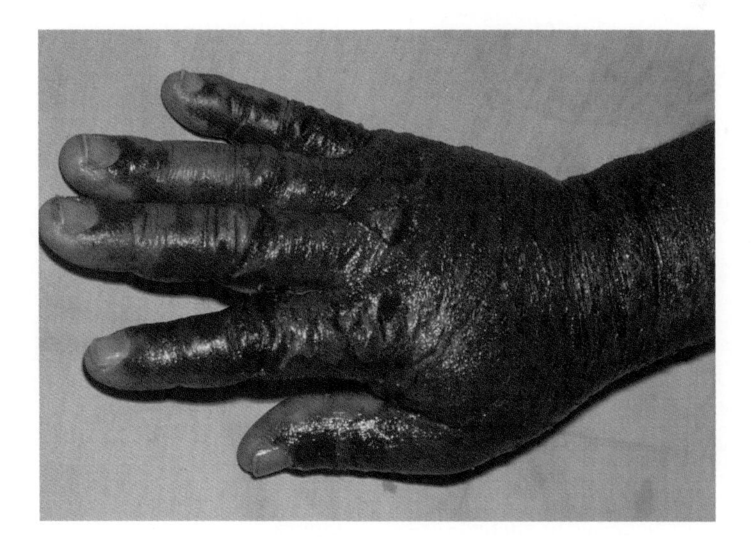

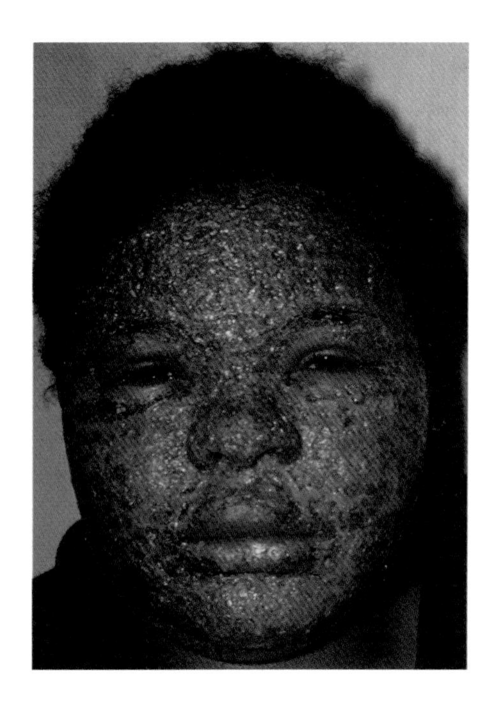

**Figure 221** Allergic contact eczema due to a topical medicine applied to the face. Note the blistering and crusting from an acute eczema.

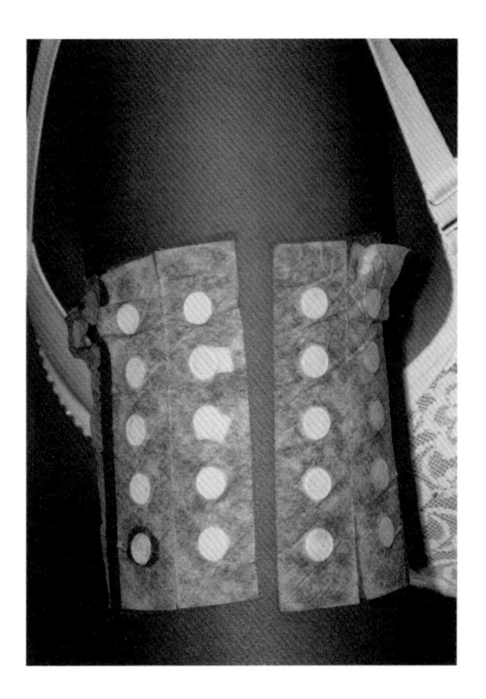

**Figure 222** The diagnosis of allergic contact eczema can be confirmed by patch tests. The allergen is applied to the skin and left in place for 96 hours.

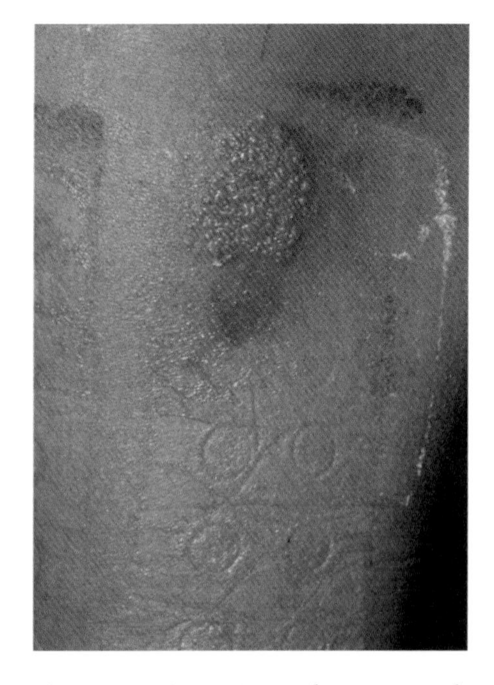

**Figure 223** A positive patch test is a patch of eczema (erythema and vesicles) at the site of the test after 96 hours.

## EHLERS-DANLOS SYNDROME

**Figure 224** A group of inherited disorders in which there is defective collagen in the skin +/– the bowel, cartilage and bone. Minor injuries leave gaping wounds which heal slowly leaving scars.

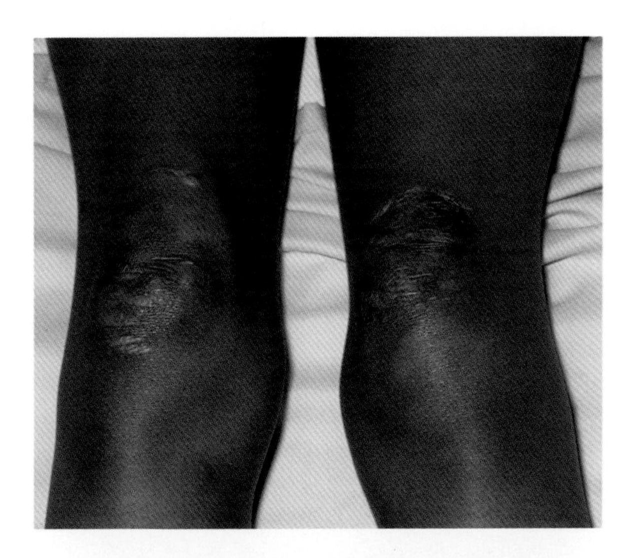

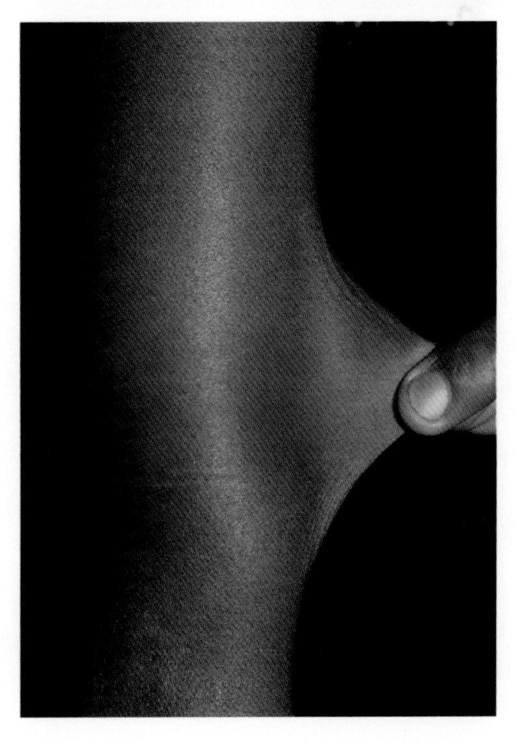

**Figure 225** The skin is hyperextensible as are the joints.

## EPIDERMODYSPLASIA VERRUCIFORMIS OF LEWANDOWSKY AND LUTZ

**Figure 226** A genetic condition, inherited as an autosomal recessive trait (*see* Figure 18), in which there is an abnormal response to wart viruses. Patients develop extensive warts which may become almost confluent. Here the warts are plane warts. These patients are at risk of developing skin cancer in one or more of their warts.

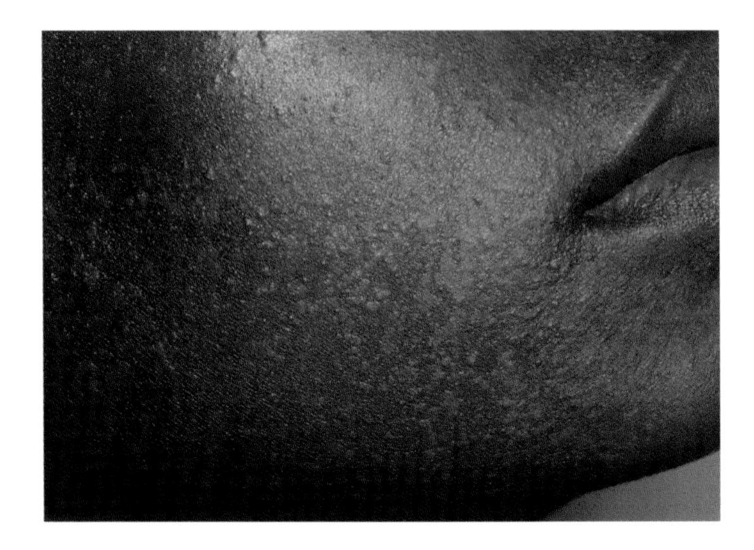

*Treatment:* Genetic counselling and advice to see a doctor immediately if tumours develop.

**Figure 227** Squamous cell carcinoma in the groin of a patient with epidermodysplasia verruciformis. The tumours in these patients contain wart virus (particularly HPV5).

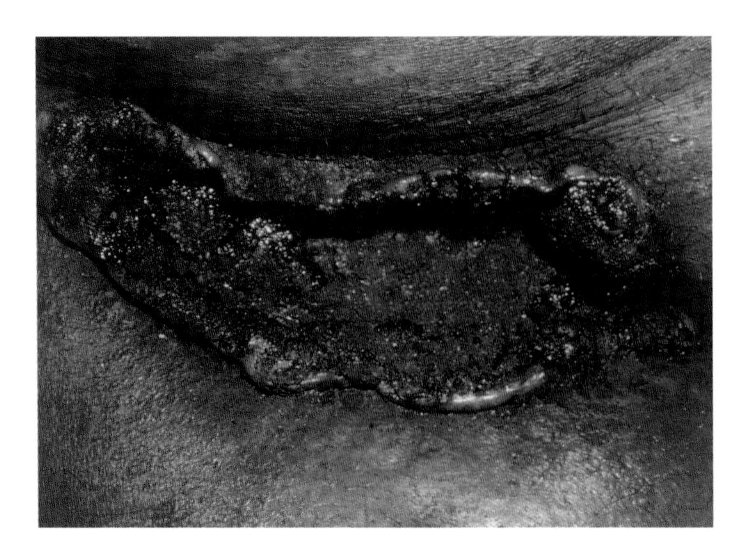

## EPIDERMOLYSIS BULLOSA

This term encompasses a number of different genetically determined diseases in which blisters appear on the skin in response to trauma. There are three main types depending on where the split in the skin is:

- Simplex.
- Junctional (usually lethal in the first 2 years of life).
- Dystrophic (autosomal dominant and recessive types).

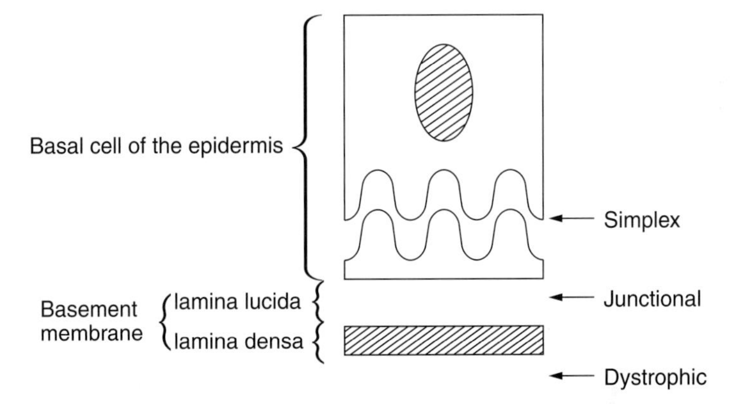


**Figure 228** Classification of epidermolysis bullosa according to the site of the blisters on electron microscopy.

**Figures 229, 230** Dystrophic epidermolysis bullosa. Blisters and erosions present from birth. There are less severe types of epidermolysis bullosa in which blisters only occur when the patient wears a new pair of shoes which rub.

*Treatment:* Genetic counselling to the parents. Protection from injury. Potassium permanganate soaks to blisters and erosions.

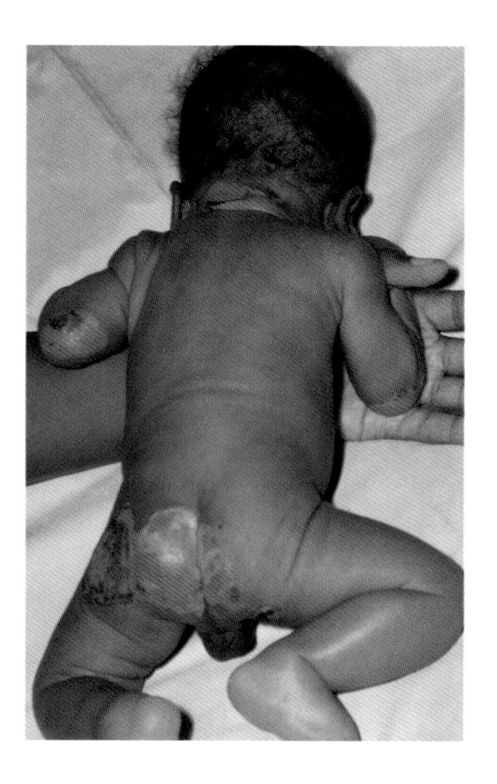

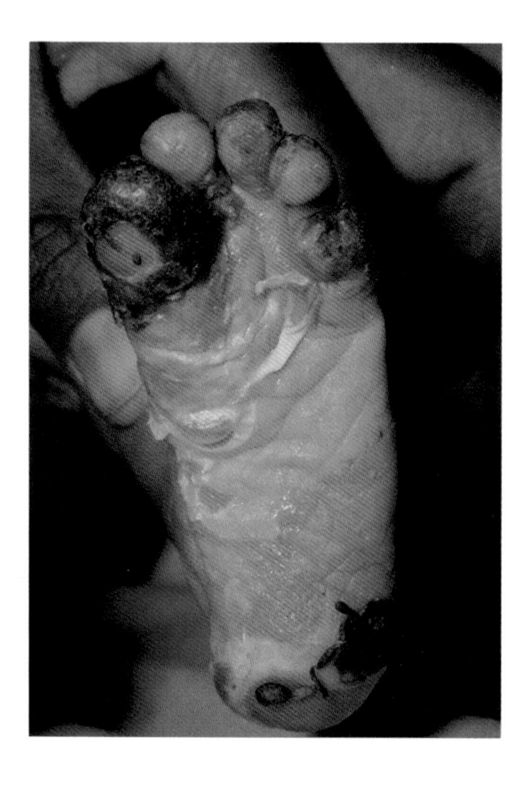

## ERYSIPELAS

**Figure 231** Infection of the upper dermis with *Streptococcus pyogenes* (*see* Figure 124). The patient is unwell with fever, rigors and general malaise. The rash is erythematous, well demarcated and may or may not contain large blisters in the centre. There is no associated lymphangitis or lymphadenopathy, and usually no obvious portal of entry.

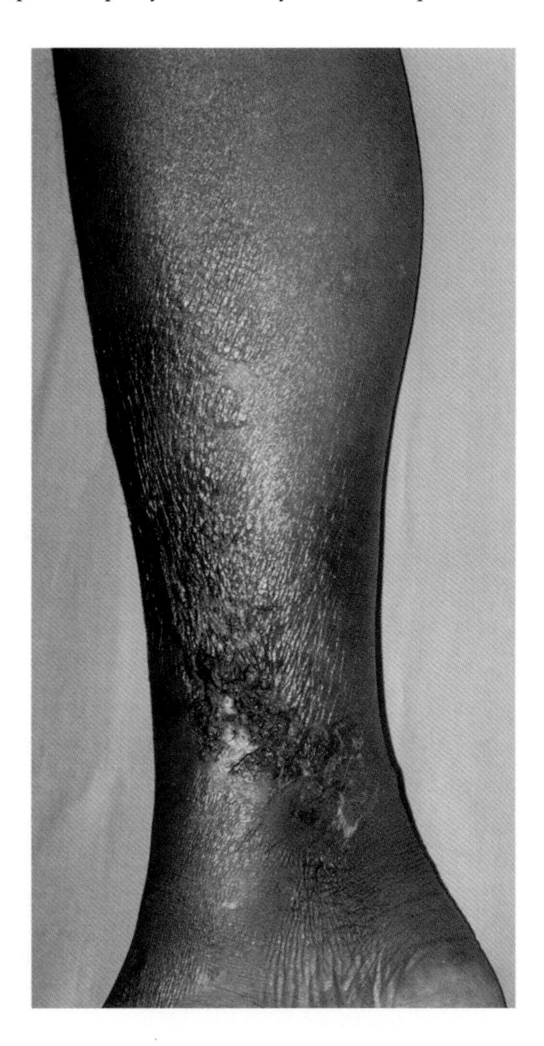

*Treatment:* Benzyl penicillin 1 mega-unit 6 hourly by intravenous or intramuscular injection for 7 days. The temperature should settle within 24 hours.

## ERYTHEMA ANNULARE CENTRIFUGUM

**Figure 232** Gradually enlarging plaque(s) with a scaly edge. By marking the edge it is possible to see it extend from day to day. Differs from a fungal infection in that it extends more rapidly and no fungus is found on microscopy. Occurs at any age and no cause can usually be found.

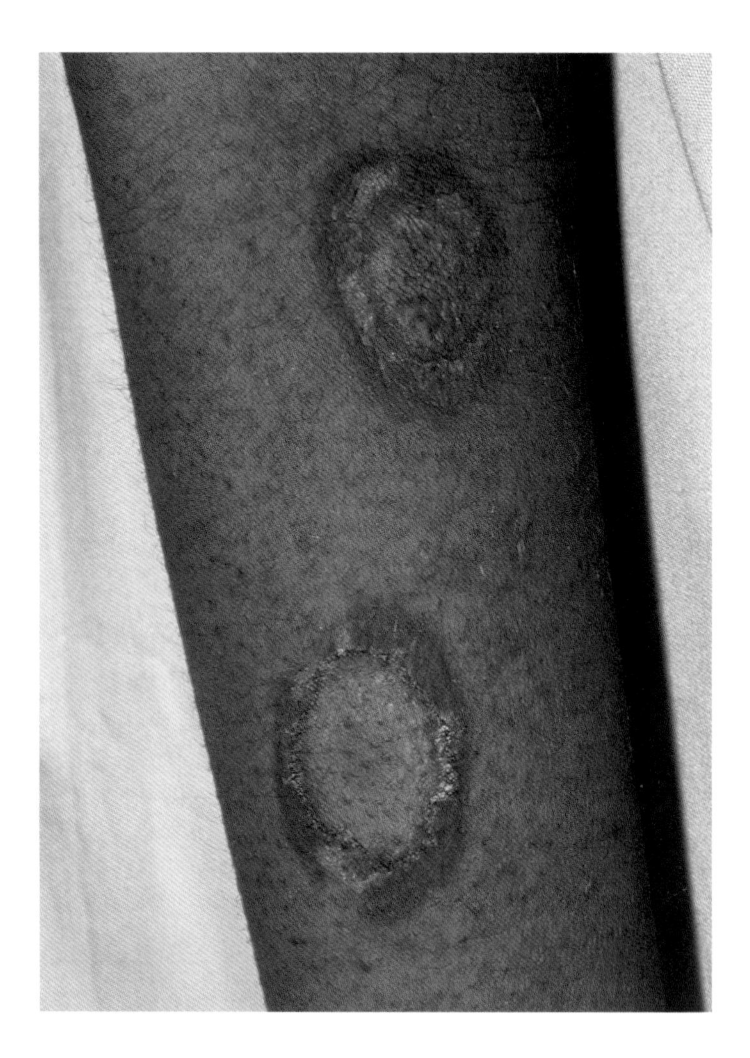

*Treatment:* Reassure the patient that it will get better spontaneously.

## ERYTHEMA NODOSUM

**Figures 233, 234** Crops of tender erythematous nodules on the lower legs, especially the front of the shins which continue to erupt for 6–12 weeks. Individual nodules heal in 7–10 days. The cause can be a streptococcal sore throat, tuberculosis or some other infection.

*Treatment:* Look for an underlying cause and treat that if necessary (e.g. tuberculosis). Give analgesics for the pain.

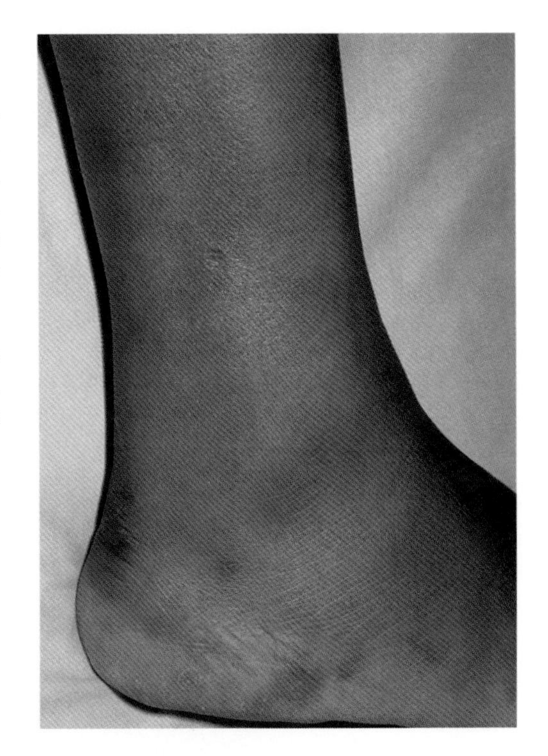

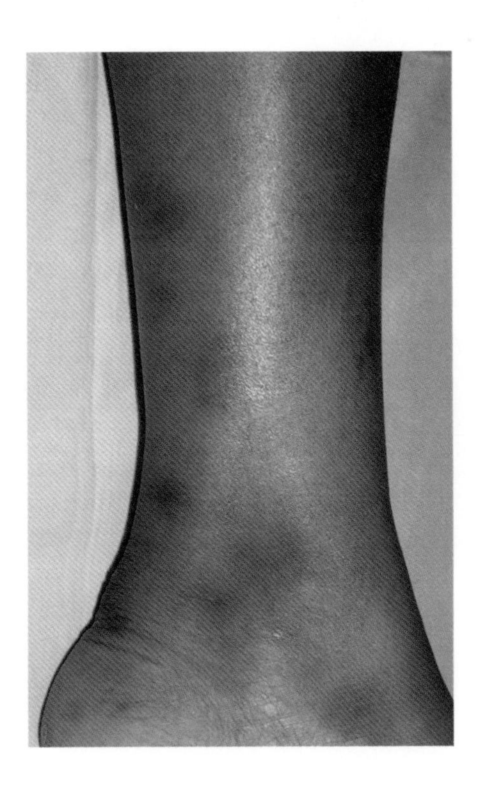

## ERYTHRASMA

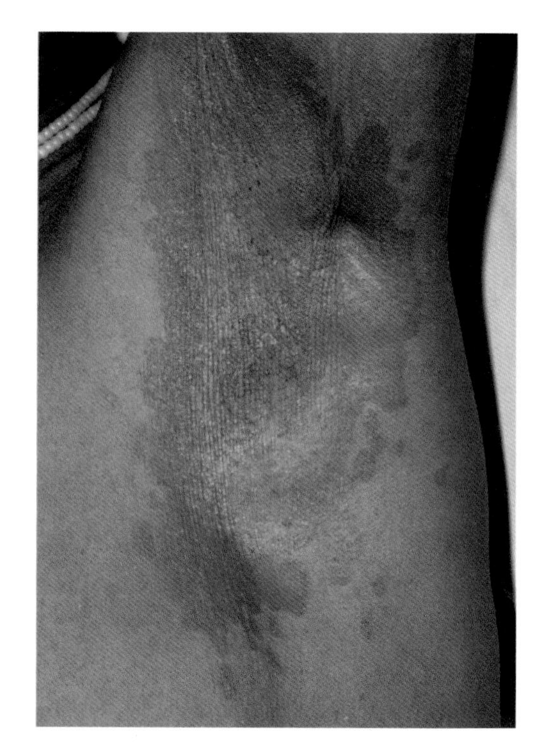

**Figures 235, 236** This is an infection of the stratum corneum with the Gram positive bacteria, *Corynebacterium minutissimum*. It causes a well defined, uniformly scaly, slightly hyperpigmented rash in the flexures (axillae, groins, submammary area and toe webs). The rash extends across the flexure and it fluoresces bright pink under a Wood's light.

*Treatment:* Erythromycin 250mg qds for 2 weeks.

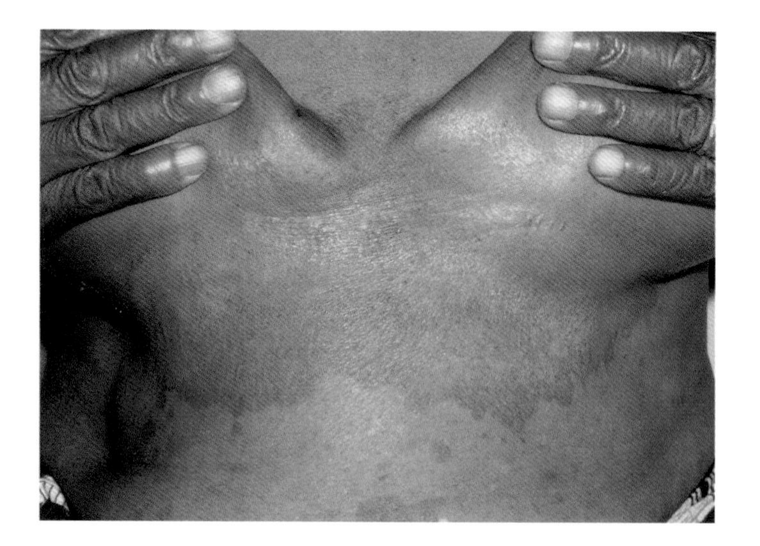

## ERYTHRODERMA (Exfoliative dermatitis)

Erythroderma is the term used when more than 90% of the body is red and scaly. The same rash is also called exfoliative dermatitis and the two terms are used interchangeably. The common causes are eczema, psoriasis, drug rashes and lymphomas.

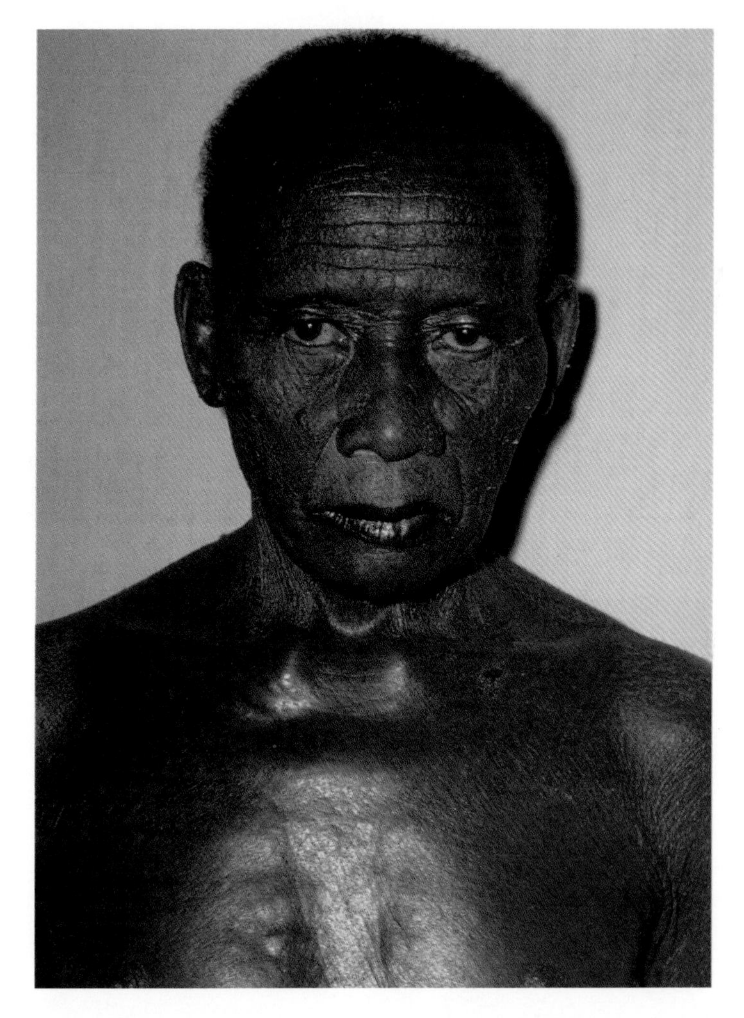

**Figure 237** Erythroderma due to eczema. The skin is hyperpigmented rather than red. Note the lichenification on the forehead.

*Treatment:* Topical steroid ointment bd. If no improvement consider systemic steroids or azathioprine.

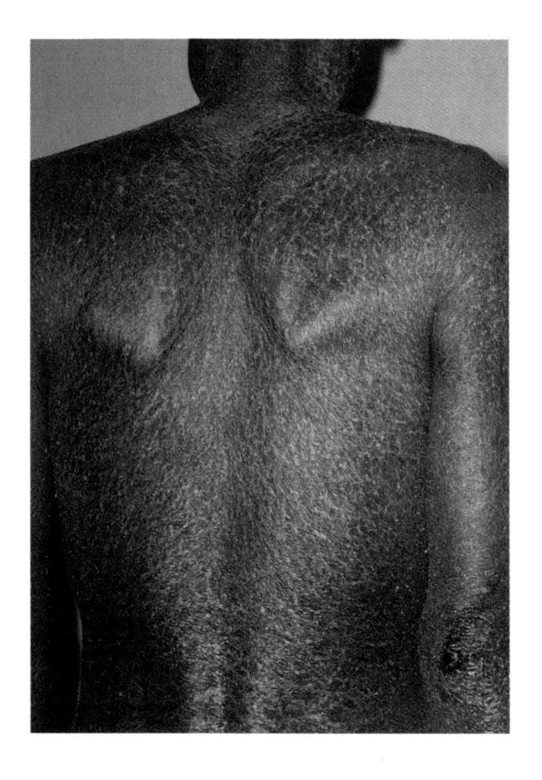

**Figure 238** Erythroderma due to psoriasis (*see also* Figure 544).

*Treatment:* Apply bland greasy ointments, e.g. Vaseline, frequently until it settles. Do not use tar, dithranol or topical steroids. If bland ointments do not work consider oral or intramuscular methotrexate once a week.

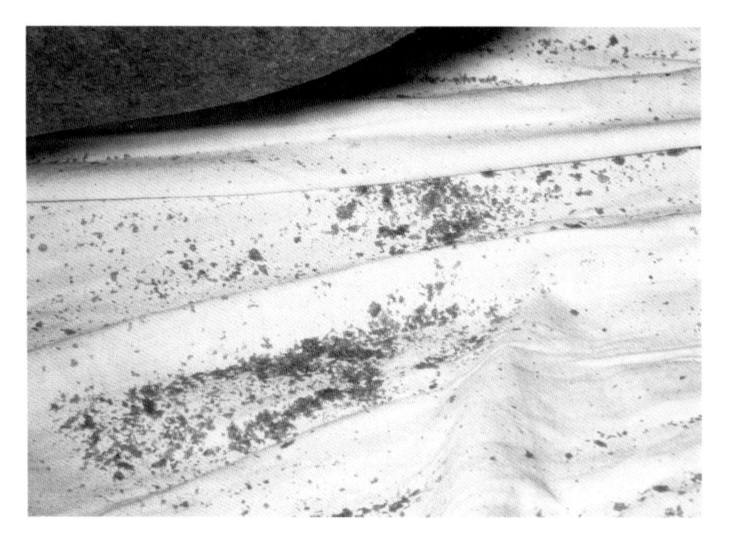

**Figure 239** In erythroderma due to psoriasis the skin shows some erythema and there is a lot of scaling. If the bed and the floor are full of scales, it is likely that the diagnosis is psoriasis.

## FILARIASIS

Lymphatic filariasis is due to the nematode worm, *Wuchereria bancrofti*. The disease is transmitted by mosquitos which bite infected humans thus picking up the microfilaria in the blood stream. Inside the mosquito the microfilaria develop into larvae which migrate to the mouth-parts ready for inoculation into the mosquito's next victim. In the host these larvae develop into adult worms which lodge in the lymphatics and lymph nodes and produce microfilaria for the next 2–4 years. Infection may be asymptomatic or it may cause elephantiasis of the legs or genitalia.

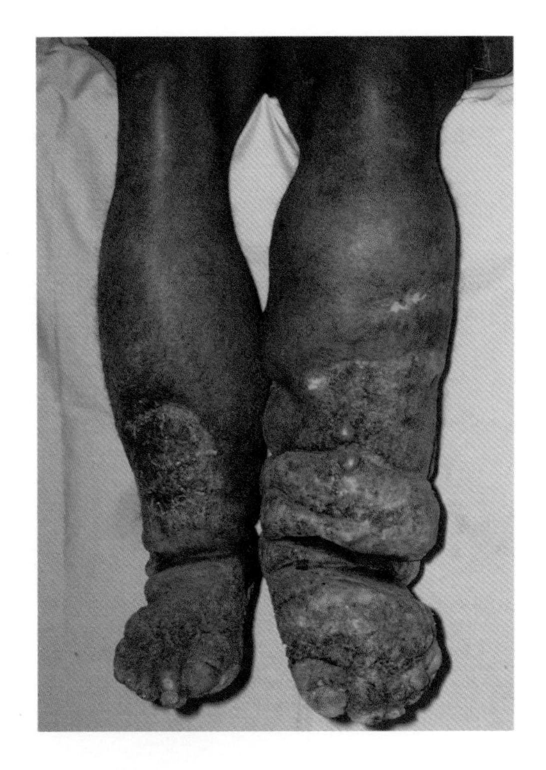

**Figure 240** Elephantiasis of the legs.

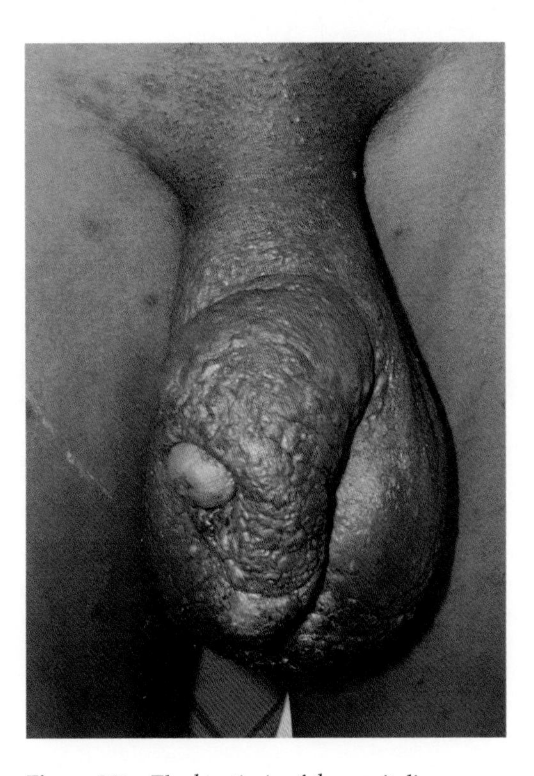

**Figure 241** Elephantiasis of the genitalia.

**Figures 242, 243** Histology of lymph node showing microfilaria (H&E stain).

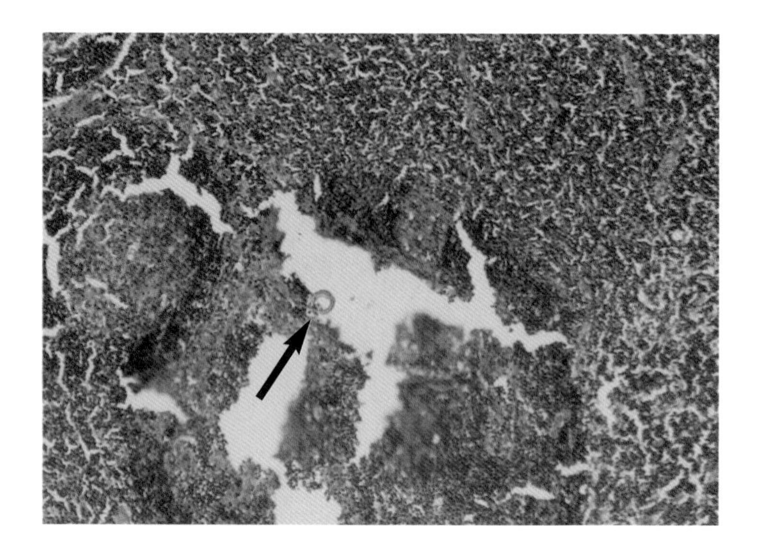

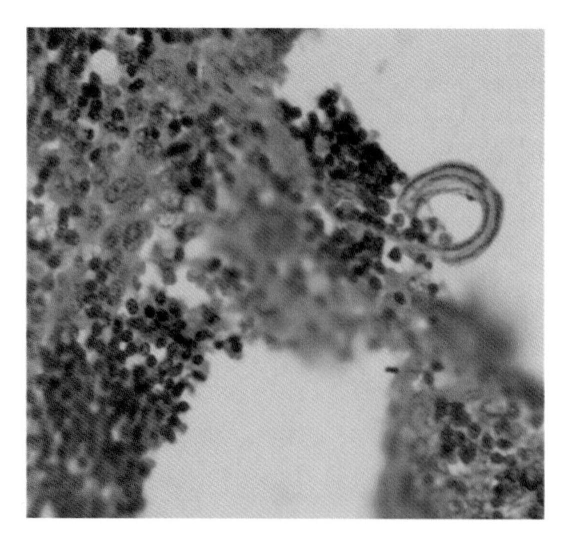

*Diagnosis:* The simplest method of diagnosis is to use the ICT filariasis test, a rapid card test which detects circulating *W. bancrofti* antigens.

*Treatment:* Whole communities in endemic areas should be treated with a single dose of two drugs once a year for 4–6 years. Albendazole 600mg together with ivermectin 400μg/kg body weight or diethylcarbamazine (DEC) 6mg/kg body weight. Simple hygiene measures such as washing with soap and water and moisturising the skin can prevent recurrent bacterial infection in an area of lymphoedema. Other ways of reducing lymphoedema include deep breathing for 10 minutes (before getting out of bed in the morning) to empty the lymphatics of the thorax and abdomen, moving the limb and sitting with the legs raised when resting.

## FOLLICULAR MUCINOSIS (Alopecia mucinosa)

**Figure 244** Boggy plaques on the skin and/or scalp with loss of hair. The diagnosis can be confirmed by histology which shows mucinous degeneration of the external root sheath of the hair follicle and sebaceous glands. In some patients it is a manifestation of mycosis fungoides (*see* Figures 414–15).

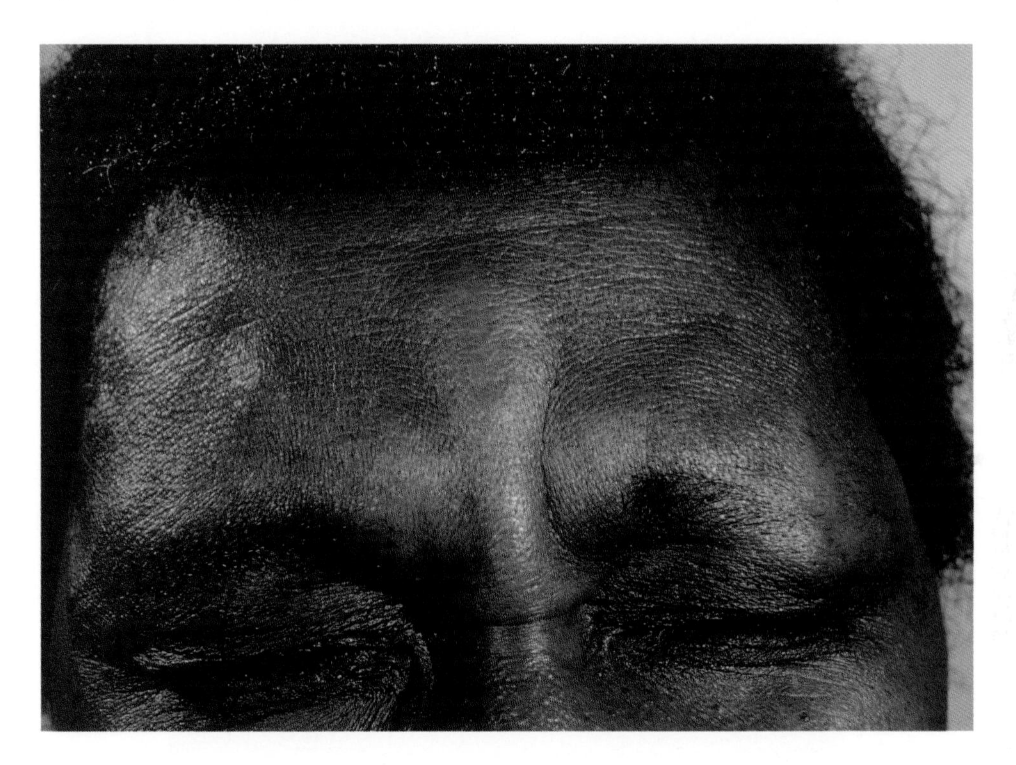

*Treatment:* Apply a potent topical steroid such as 0.1% betamethasone 17-valerate ointment bd.

## FOLLICULITIS

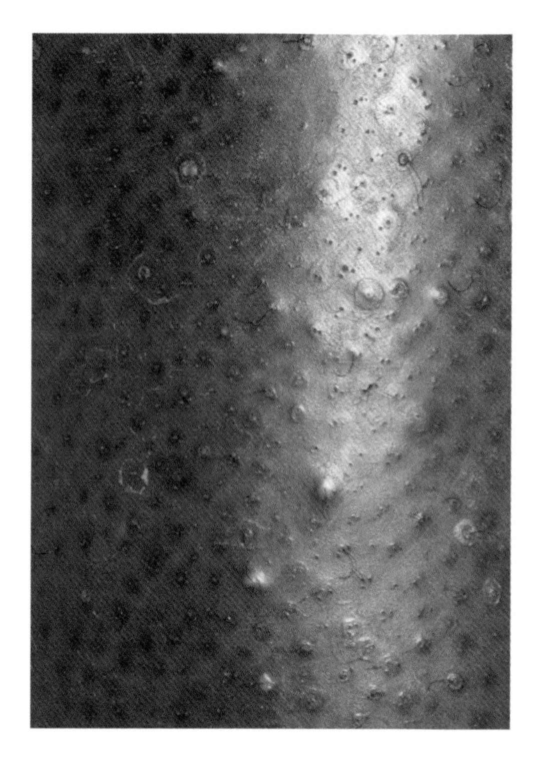

**Figure 245** Bacterial infection of the mouth of a hair follicle with *Staphylococcus aureus* (*see* Figure 309). Each pustule has a hair emerging from the centre. It is often caused by applying Vaseline or other greasy ointments to the skin.

*Treatment:* Stop applying greasy ointments. May need oral cloxacillin 500mg qds for 7 days in addition.

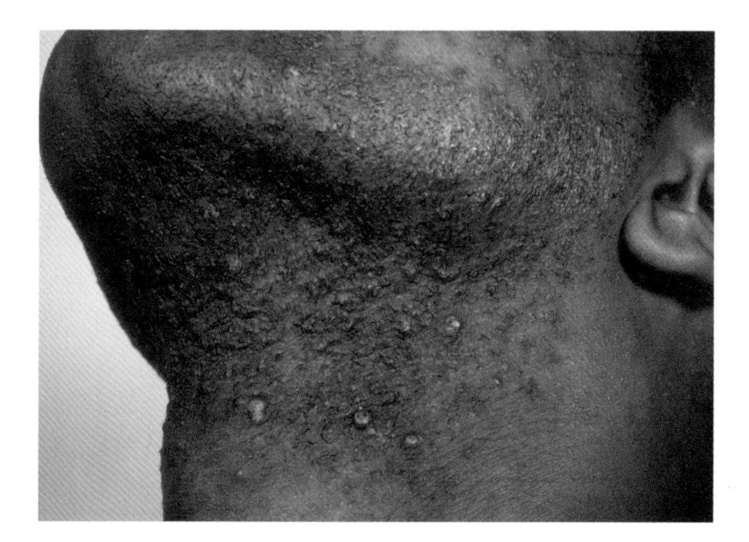

**Figure 246** Folliculitis of the beard area is called sycosis barbae. A condition which looks similar due to ingrowing beard hairs is called pseudosycosis barbae or pili incarnati.

*Treatment of sycosis barbae:* Stop any greasy ointments being applied to the face +/– oral cloxacillin 500mg qds for 7 days.

*Treatment of pseudosycosis barbae:* Grow a beard; this will cause the hairs to uncurl.

## FORDYCE SPOTS

**Figure 247** Yellow papules on the lips or buccal mucosa due to sebaceous gland hyperplasia.

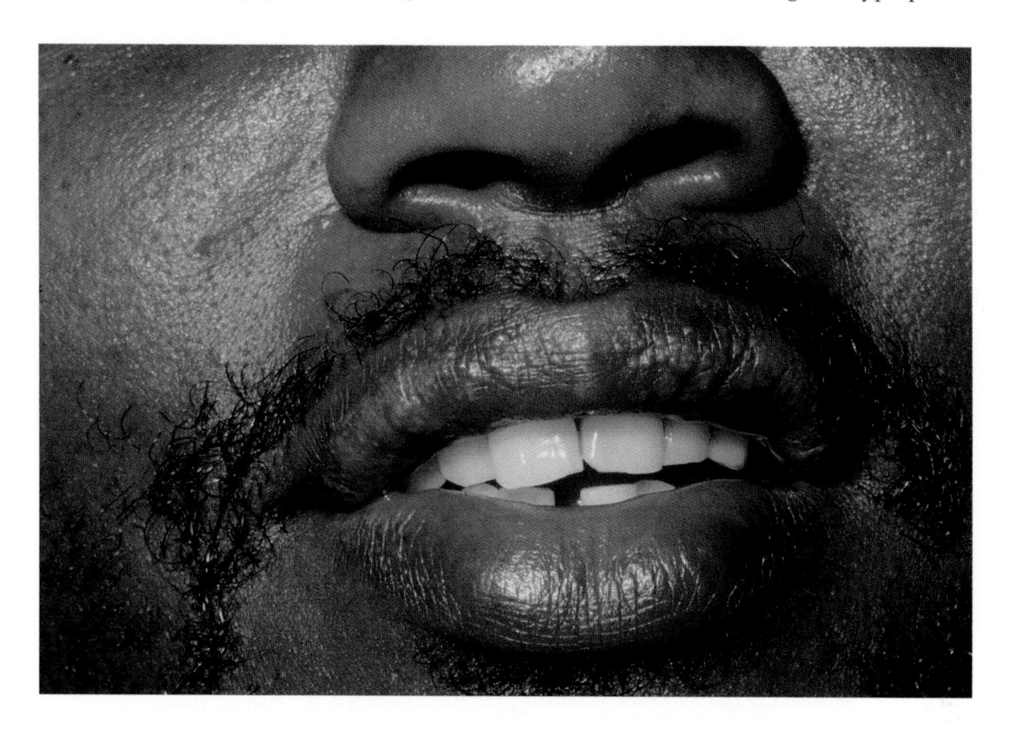

*Treatment:* This is a common normal finding and needs no treatment other than reassurance.

## FOX FORDYCE DISEASE

**Figure 248** Itchy rash in the axillae due to blockage of the apocrine ducts.

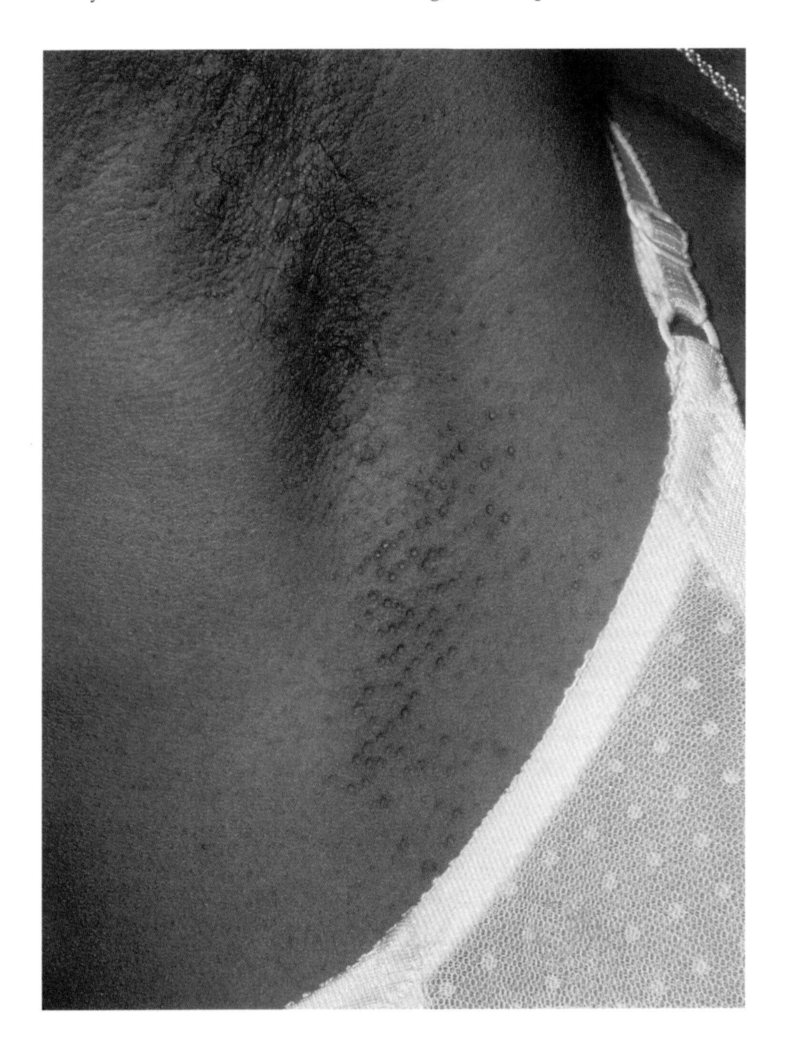

*Treatment:* Unsatisfactory. Sometimes topical steroids help. If the itching is intolerable the sweat bearing skin of the axillae can be excised.

## GANGRENE

**Figure 249** Gangrene is the death of tissue due to lack of arterial blood supply.

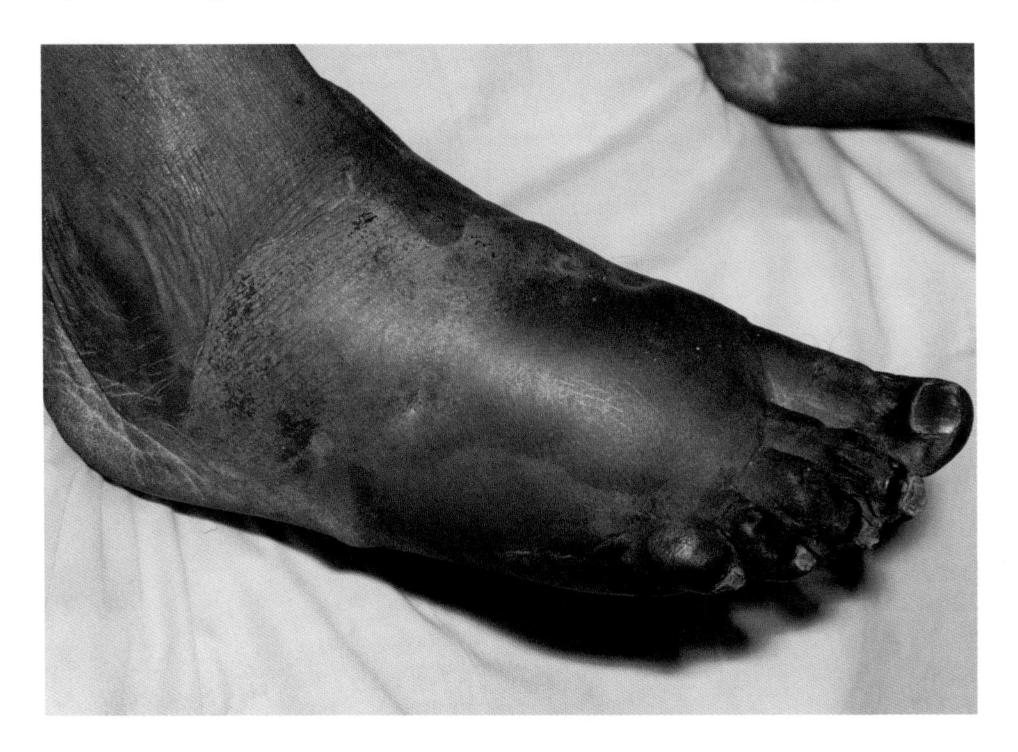

*Treatment:* Amputation to remove all the dead tissue.

## GIANOTTI CROSTI SYNDROME (Papular acrodermatitis of childhood)

**Figures 250, 251** Disease of pre-school children which is a response to a viral infection such as hepatitis B (but can be any). Small, firm, discrete papules on buttocks and extremities. The child is not usually unwell and the rash gets better spontaneously after 3–4 weeks.

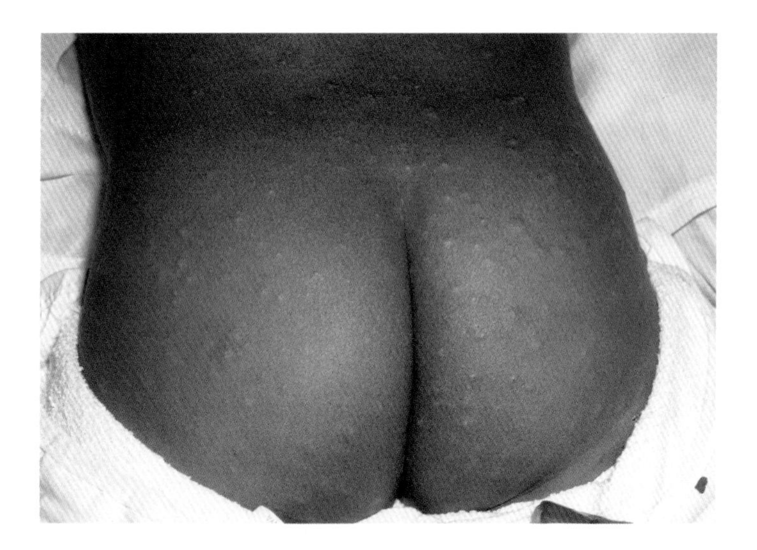

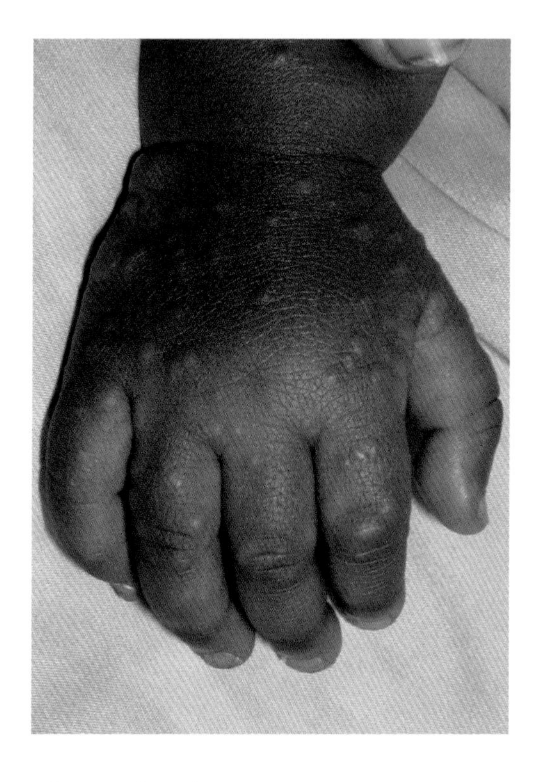

*Treatment:* Reassurance that it will get better on its own.

## GIANT CELL EPULIS

**Figure 252** Firm reddish-purple nodule or plaque in the mouth. Often occurs during pregnancy. Not to be confused with Kaposi's sarcoma in the mouth (*see* Figure 324).

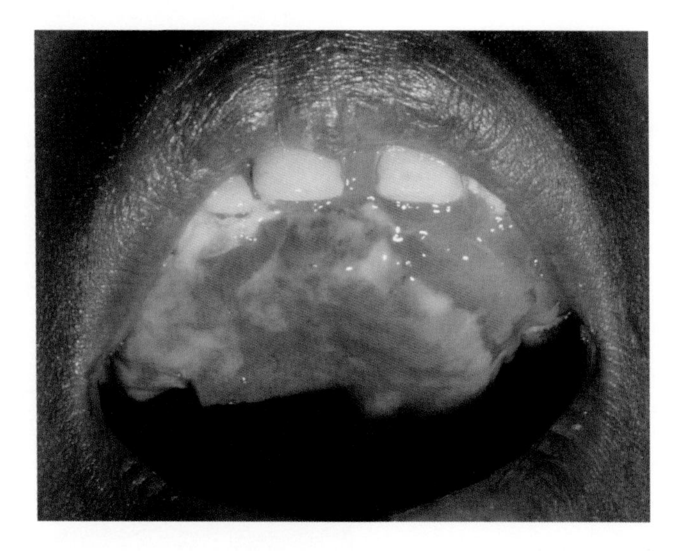

*Treatment:* Surgical excision if it is a nuisance.

**Figure 253** The histological picture is characteristic with numerous multinucleated giant cells in a vascular stroma.

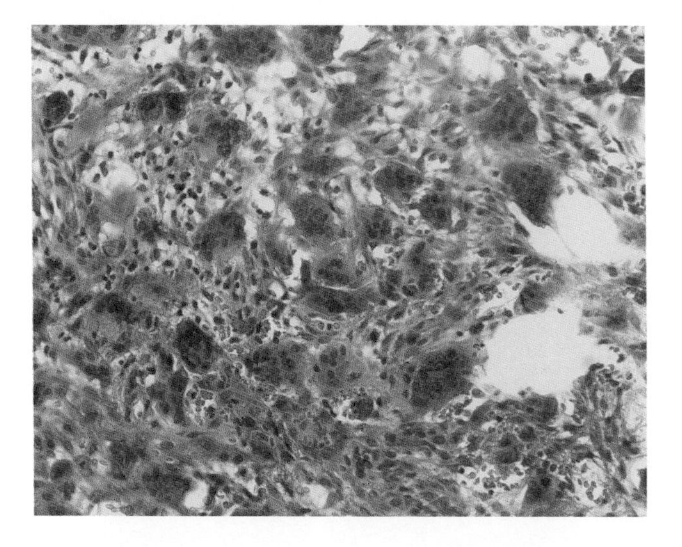

## GOLTZ SYNDROME (Focal dermal hypoplasia)

**Figures 254, 255** Rare syndrome inherited as an X-linked dominant trait which is lethal in males, so it is only seen in females. From birth there are linear atrophic, telangiectatic, hypo- and hyperpigmented plaques arranged along Blaschko's lines down the limbs and around the trunk.

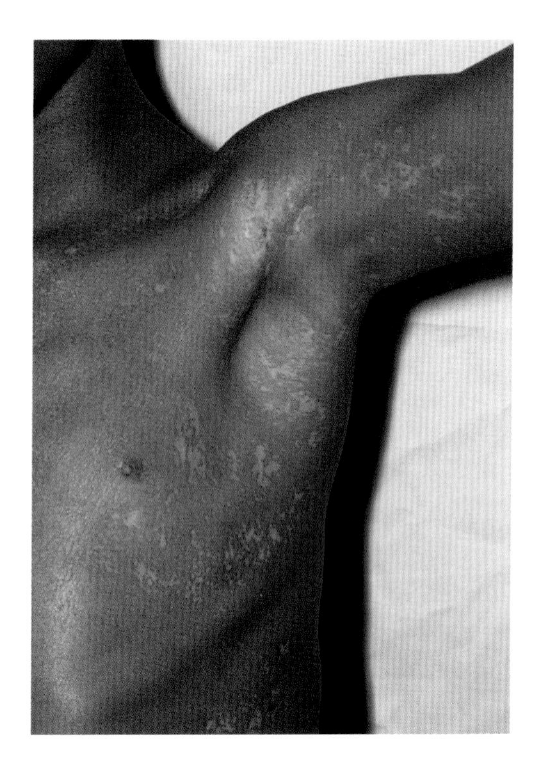

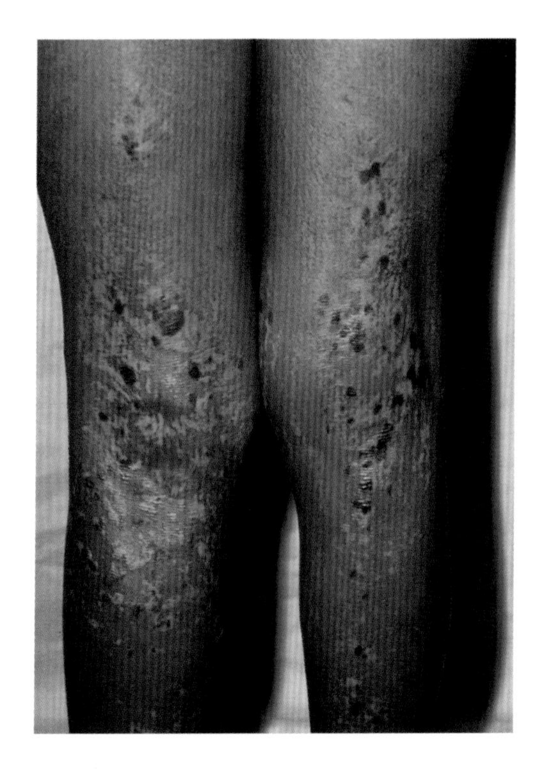

**Figure 256** Multiple papillomas on the lips. These are present from birth.

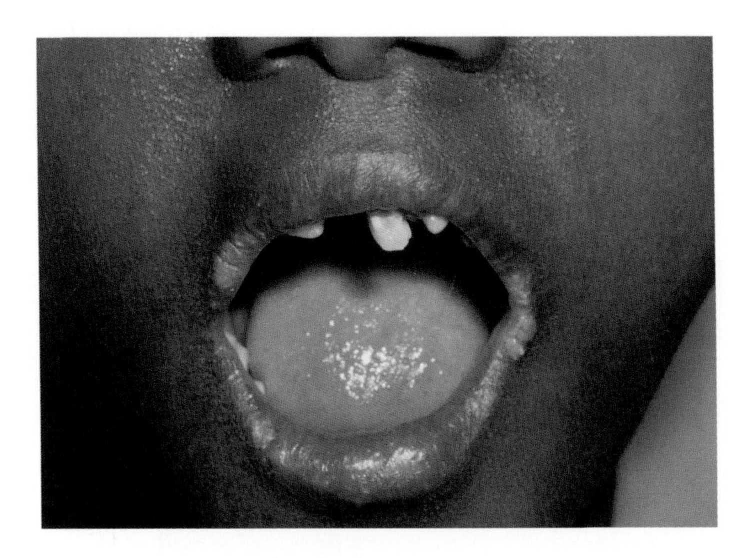

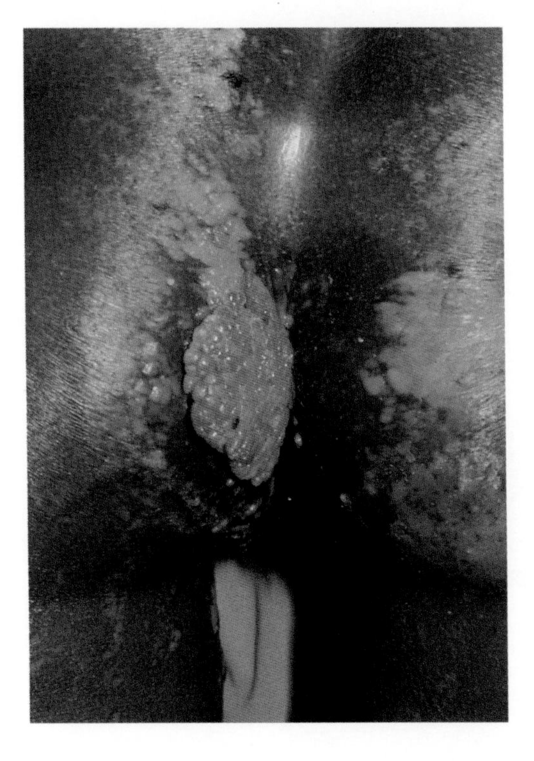

**Figure 257** Raspberry tumours around the anus. In addition the child is short, has sparse, brittle hair, dystrophic nails, syndactyly or polydactyly, other skeletal defects and eye problems such as microphthalmia or squint.

*Treatment:* There is nothing that can be done for this condition.

## GONORRHOEA

**Figure 258** Sexually transmitted disease caused by *Neisseria gonorrhoeae*. In males it causes a purulent urethral discharge 2–5 days after infection followed by dysuria. The discharge is often profuse. In females infection is often asymptomatic but later it causes salpingitis which leads to infertility, ectopic pregnancy and chronic pelvic pain. Rarely, the infection can become disseminated causing a monoarthritis of one of the large joints together with a few pustules or haemorrhagic pustules on the skin.

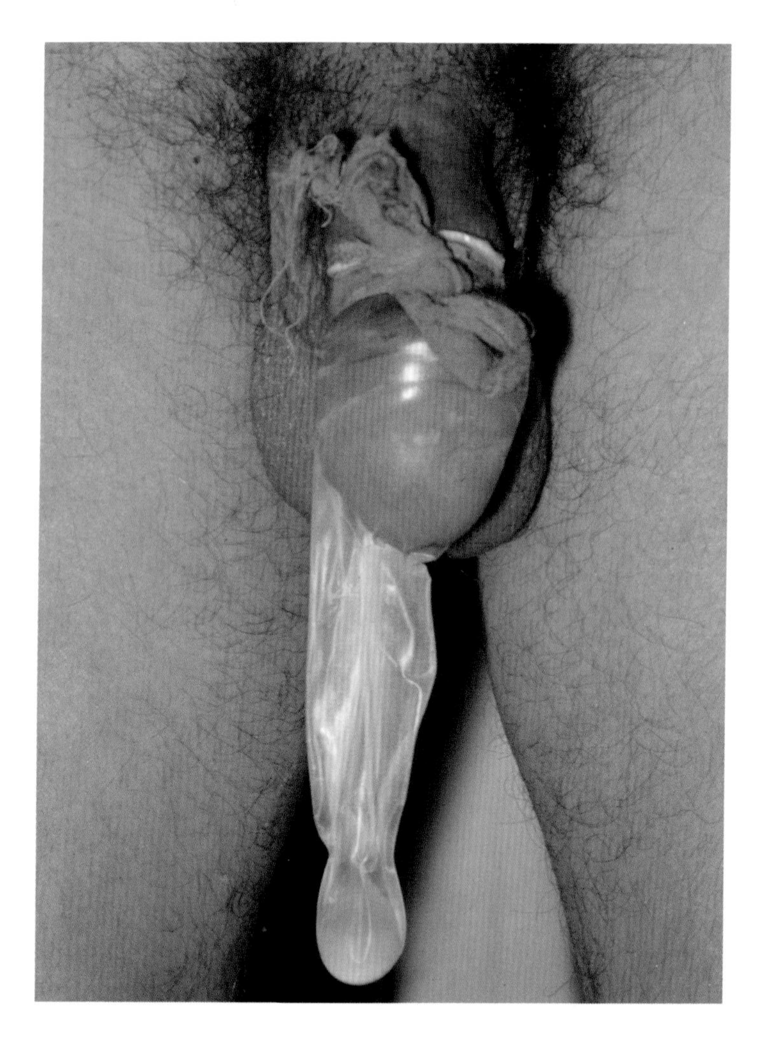

*Treatment:* Antibiotics to patient and all sexual partners depending on the local sensitivities of the organism. Almost all gonococci are now resistant to penicillin.

**Figure 259** Gram stain of smears taken from the urethra, endocervix or rectum will show the *Neisseria gonorrhoeae* as a Gram negative (stained red) diplococcus found within polymorphonuclear leukocytes. Culture on modified Thayer-Martin medium is even more specific.

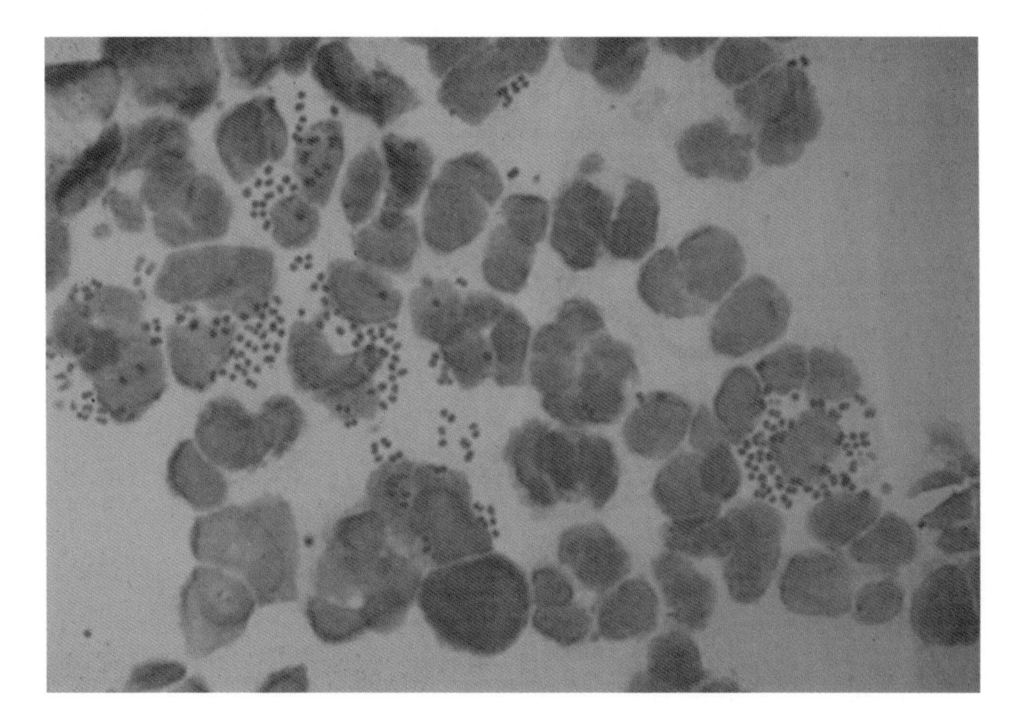

**Figure 260** In babies gonorrhoea can cause ophthalmia neonatorum. This is a serious infection which can lead to blindness because the gonococcus produces a toxin which dissolves the cornea. Babies develop a purulent discharge from the eyes within the first 4 weeks of life. Ophthalmia neonatorum can also be due to *Chlamydia trachomatis, Staphylococcus aureus* or *Streptococcus pneumoniae* infection.

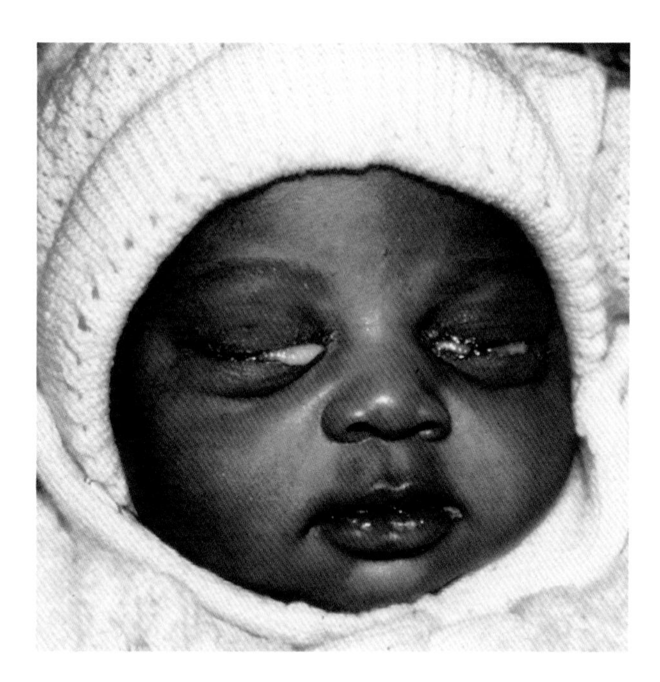

*Prevention:* Wipe the eyelids clean with cotton wool soaked in normal saline and instil 2–3 drops of 2.5% povidone iodine solution into the eyes of all babies immediately after birth. An alternative would be to use 1% tetracycline eye ointment instead of the povidone iodine.

*Treatment:* Apply 1% tetracycline eye ointment every minute for 5 minutes, every 5 minutes for 1 hour, then hourly until all symptoms subside.

## GOUTY TOPHI

**Figure 261** Deposits of uric acid crystals in the dermis in patients with gout. The antihelix of the ear is a common site.

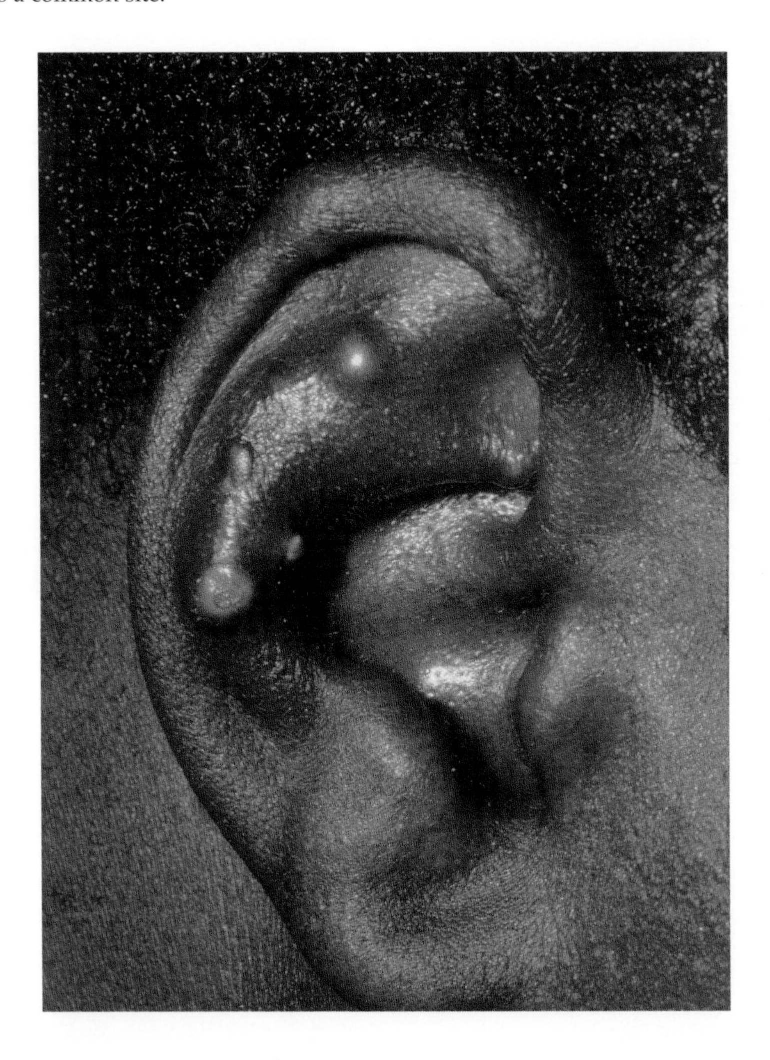

*Treatment:* Allopurinol 100–200mg/day orally.

## GRANULOMA ANNULARE

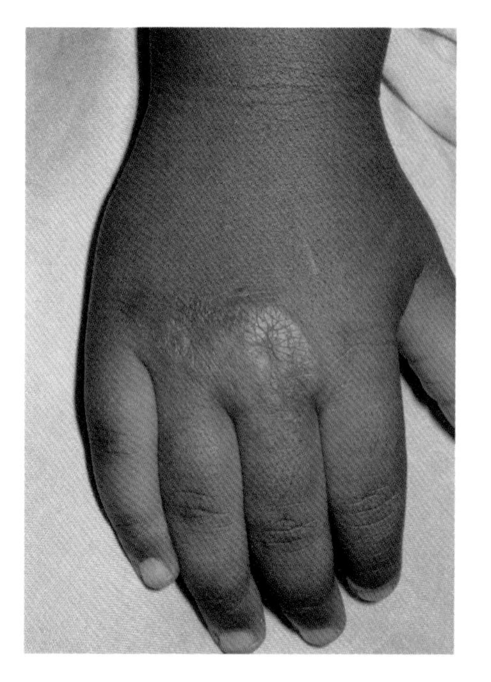

**Figure 262** Small skin-coloured papules in rings on the dorsum of the hands or fingers. They are usually asymptomatic but can be painful if knocked. The cause is unknown.

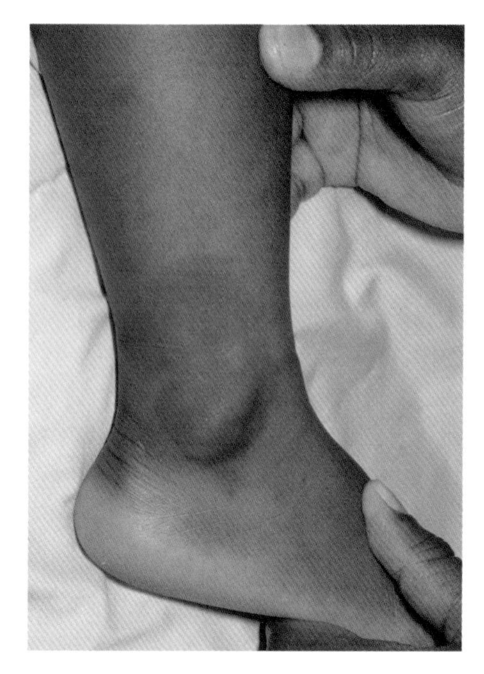

**Figure 263** It can present as a patch or plaque rather than small papules.

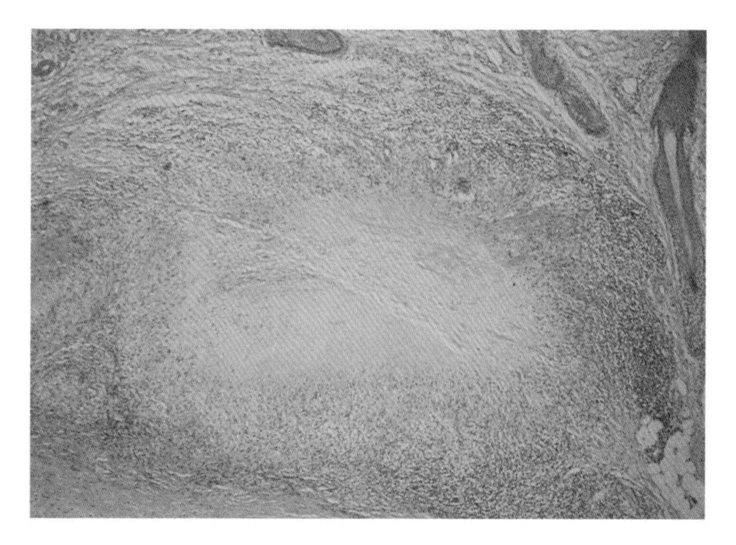

**Figure 264** The diagnosis can be confirmed by biopsy which shows a palisading granuloma with no organisms inside.

*Treatment:* It gets better on its own and needs no treatment other than reassurance.

## GRANULOMA INGUINALE (Donovanosis)

**Figure 265** Sexually transmitted disease caused by *Calymmatobacterium granulomatis*. After an incubation period of 14–60 days (average 21 days) multiple painless nodules appear on the genitalia. These have well defined borders and adjacent nodules coalesce to form large plaques. If left untreated they may become large deep-seated ulcers which can cause lymphatic obstruction and elephantiasis of the genitalia.

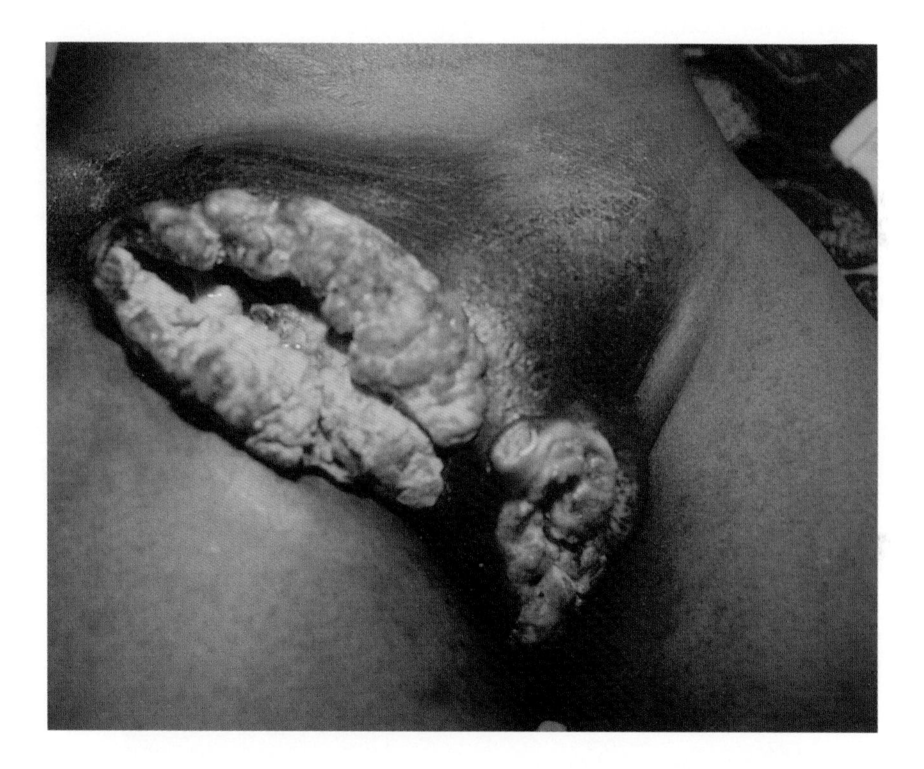

*Diagnosis:* Take multiple punch biopsies from the edge of the lesion and crush them between two glass slides. Stain with Wright's stain or Giemsa stain and see the Gram negative rods within macrophages. Always send one of the specimens for histology to rule out a squamous cell carcinoma which is the main differential diagnosis.

*Treatment:* Azithromycin 500mg bd for 7 days. Check for other sexually transmitted diseases and HIV infection.

## HAILEY-HAILEY DISEASE (Chronic benign familial pemphigus)

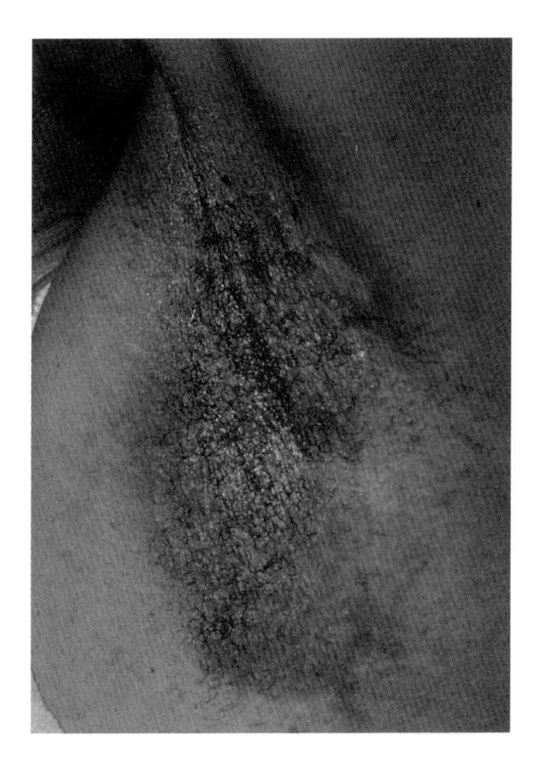

**Figure 266** Genetic condition inherited as an autosomal dominant trait (*see* Figure 295). Does not become apparent until after puberty when it causes a rash in the flexures (neck, axillae and groins). Small flaccid blisters quickly rupture to leave erosions and fissures.

*Treatment:* It is often helped by the application of moderately potent or potent topical steroids. Treat any secondary infection with antibiotics or antifungals as necessary. If it is very severe, methotrexate orally once a week can be helpful.

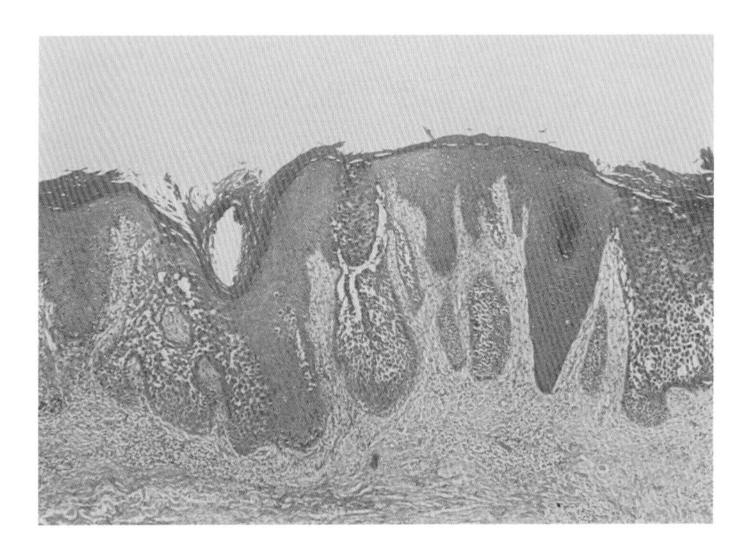

**Figure 267** A biopsy shows acantholysis with a suprabasal split in the epidermis similar to that seen in pemphigus vulgaris (*see* Figure 500), but the cells remain partially in contact with one another giving what is often described as a 'dilapidated brick wall' appearance.

## HERPES GESTATIONIS

**Figure 268** Rare, very itchy rash occurring in pregnancy. Begins at any time after the end of the first trimester and usually occurs earlier in each successive pregnancy. Begins with an erythema multiforme-like rash (*see* Figure 186) which then blisters. Immunofluorescence of a skin biopsy shows deposition of $C_3$ along the basement membrane and the serum shows a $C_3$ binding factor (HG factor). Rarely, the rash is present in the newborn infant presumably due to passive transfer of the HG factor across the placenta.

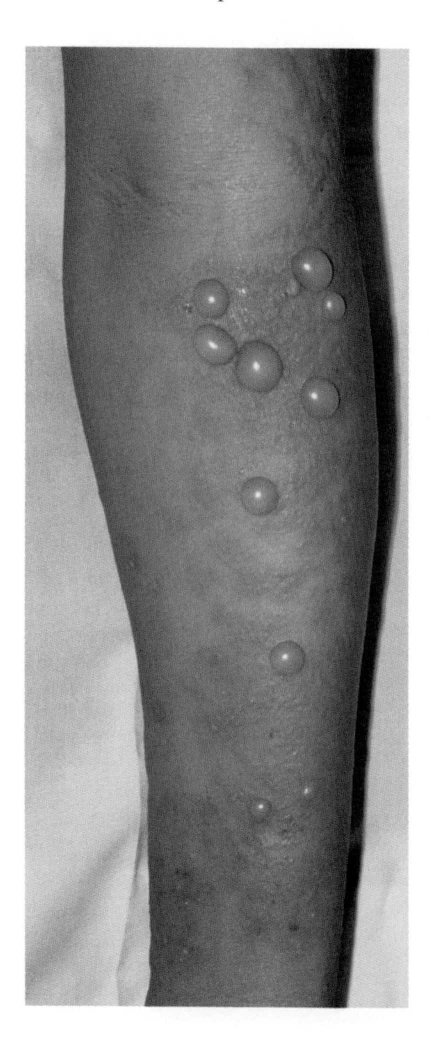

*Treatment:* Ice applied to the skin is often helpful for the itching. If the itching is intolerable use systemic steroids (60mg prednisolone daily, gradually reducing).

# HERPES SIMPLEX

The herpes simplex virus, *Herpesvirus hominis* (HSV), belongs to the alpha subgroup of herpes viruses. There are two antigenic types of HSV, type 1 and type 2.

## Herpes simplex type 1

Most primary infections with *Herpesvirus hominis* type 1 occur in the mouth in early childhood and are asymptomatic. Occasionally, they may cause an acute gingivostomatitis with fever and general malaise. After the primary infection the virus remains latent in the sensory nerve ganglia (or the peripheral nerve ganglia) for the rest of the patient's life. Recurrent episodes can then occur and are precipitated by fever, menstruation or stress.

**Figure 269** Recurrent herpes simplex usually affects the lips if the primary site was in the mouth, or the same site as the primary infection if it was on the skin. It is usually preceded by a prodromal sensation of itching, burning or tingling for a few hours before grouped vesicles appear. These break, crust and heal in 7–10 days.

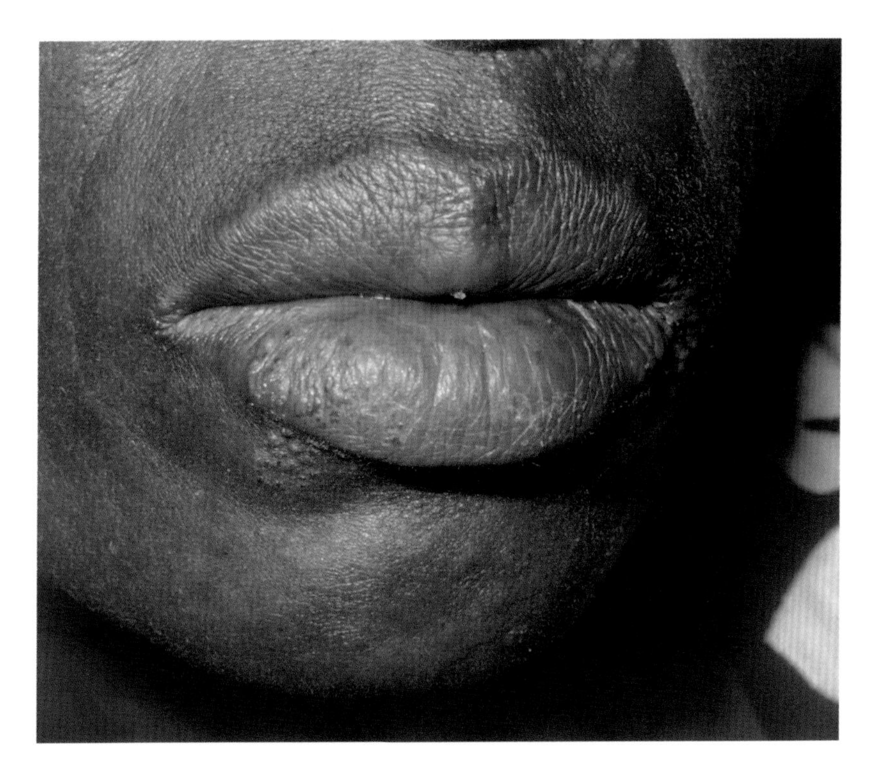

*Treatment:* Usually none is necessary as it gets better spontaneously.

**Figure 270** Crusted herpes simplex in a patient with HIV infection.

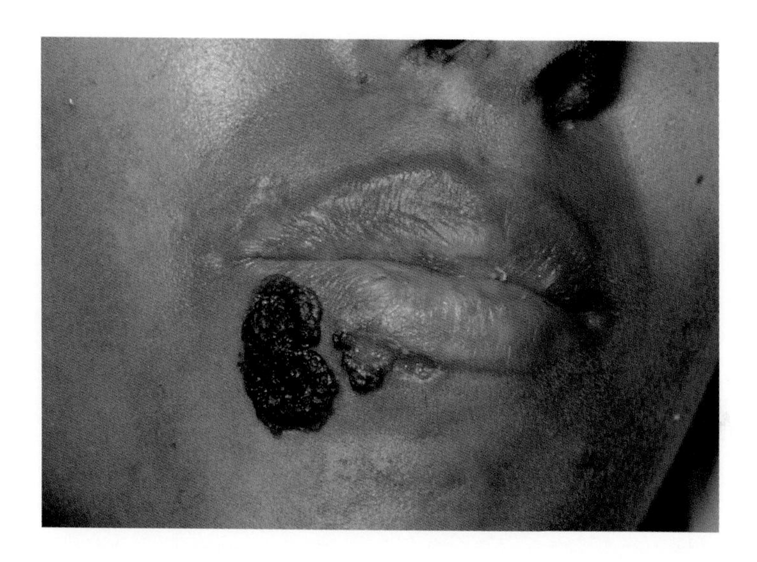

**Figure 271** Chronic crusting and ulceration caused by herpes simplex in a patient with HIV infection. This kind of picture can last weeks or months.

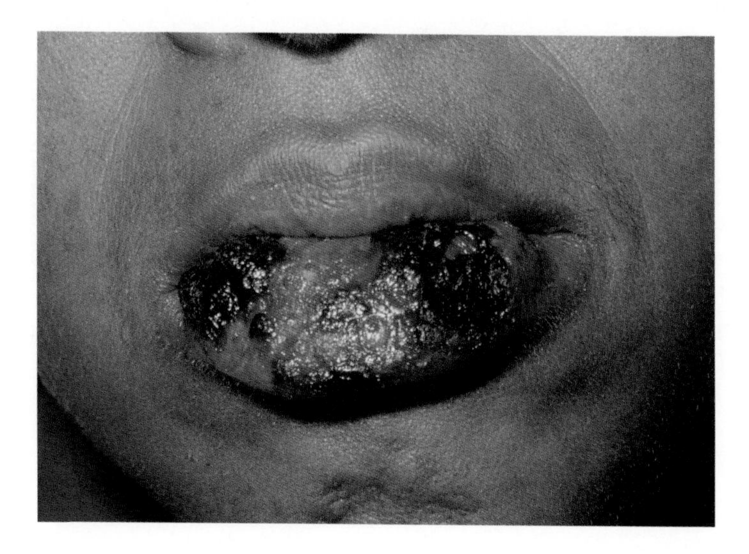

**Figure 272** Disseminated herpes simplex in a patient with HIV infection (same patient as in Figure 270).

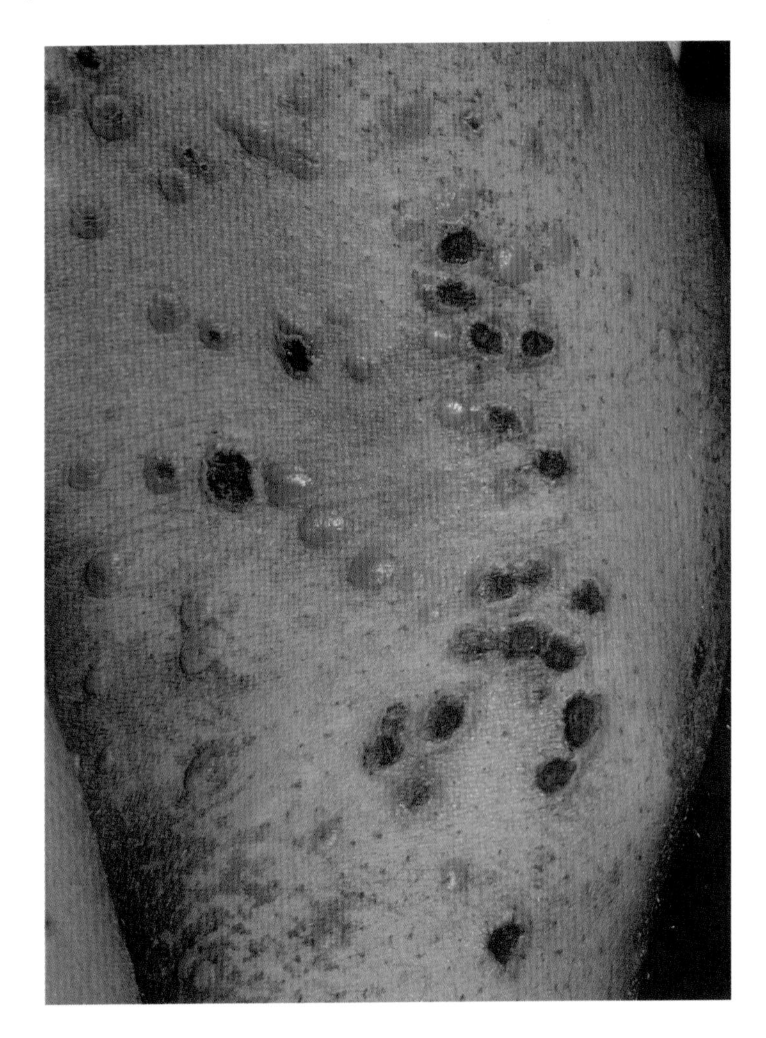

*Treatment:* Extensive herpes simplex can be treated with oral acyclovir 200mg five times daily for 7 days. This only works if it is started within 48 hours of the first symptoms (because the drug has to be phosphorylated by the actively multiplying virus to work).

**Figures 273, 274** Primary herpes simplex infection in a patient with atopic eczema can be very extensive; it is called eczema herpeticum. This pattern can also be seen in patients with pemphigus vulgaris, pemphigus foliaceus and Darier's disease, when it is known as Kaposi's varicelliform eruption.

*Treatment of eczema herpeticum/Kaposi's varicelliform eruption:* If it is available, oral acyclovir 200mg five times daily for 7 days.

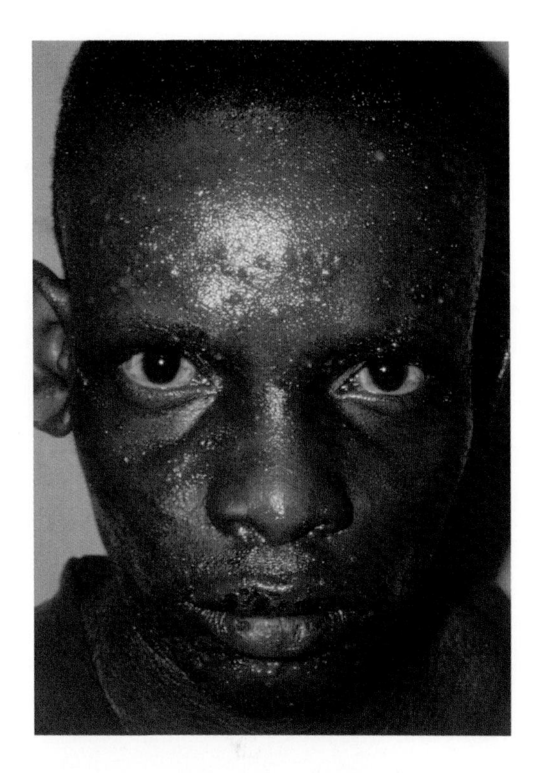

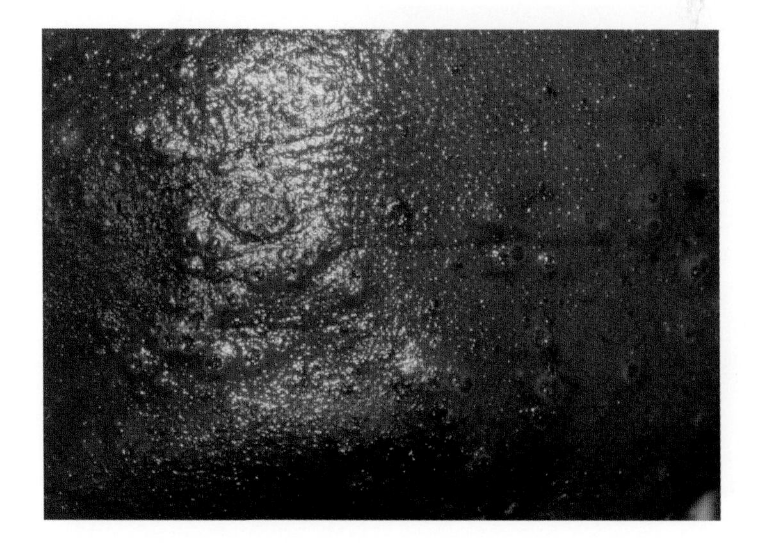

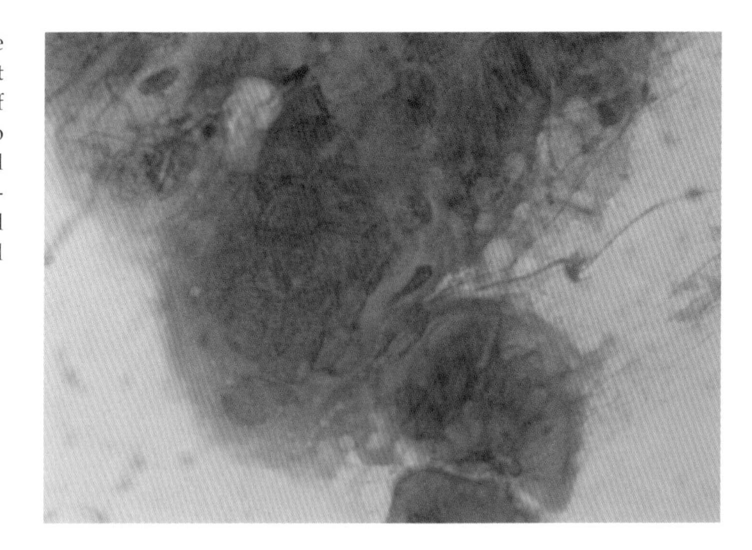

**Figure 275** If there is any doubt about the diagnosis of herpes simplex, do a Tzank smear and stain with Papanicalou stain; you will see multinucleated giant cells.

## Herpes simplex type 2 (herpes genitalis)

**Figure 276** This is the most common cause of recurrent genital ulceration.

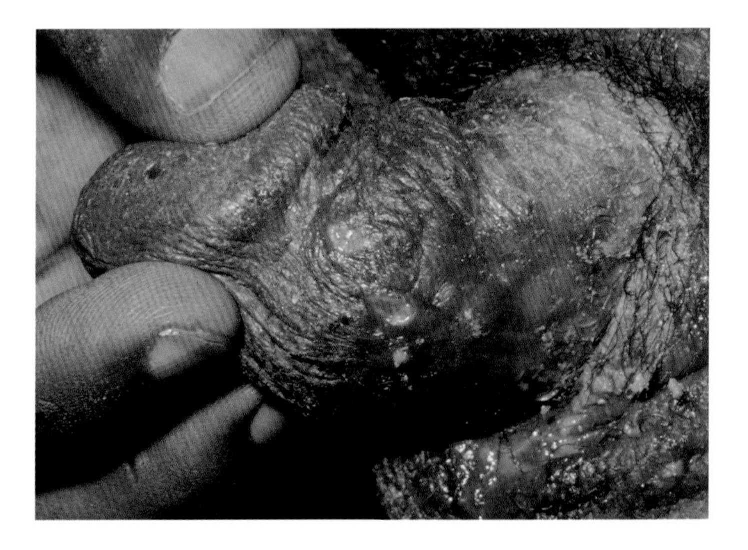

**Figure 277** The primary infection with *Herpesvirus hominis* type 2 begins with painful grouped vesicles which rapidly break down to form erosions. The lesions heal in 7–10 days. Recurrent episodes are common but the symptoms are usually less severe than in the primary infection.

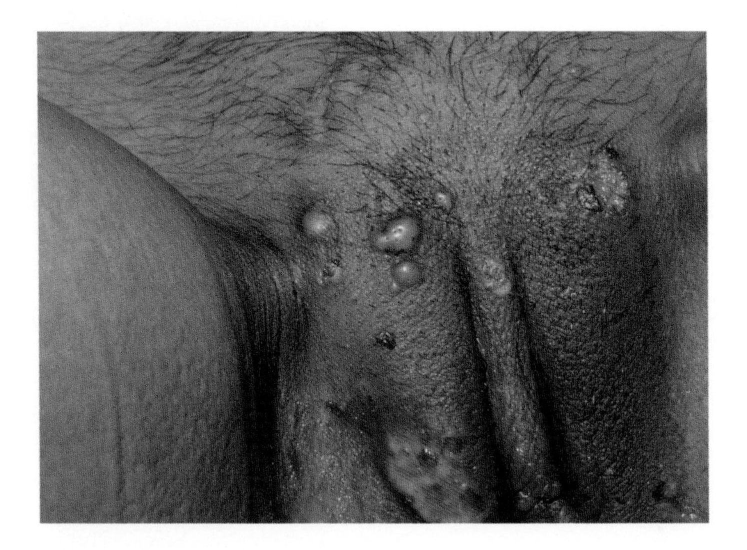

*Treatment:* Saline soaks (1 tablespoon of salt in a pint of water) for 10 minutes bd may be soothing. If the pain is severe use oral acyclovir 200mg five times daily for 5 days, but only if the patient is seen within the first 24 hours after the vesicles appear.

**Figure 278** In patients who are HIV positive, herpes genitalis is often extensive and may take months to heal. These two ulcers have been present for 4 months.

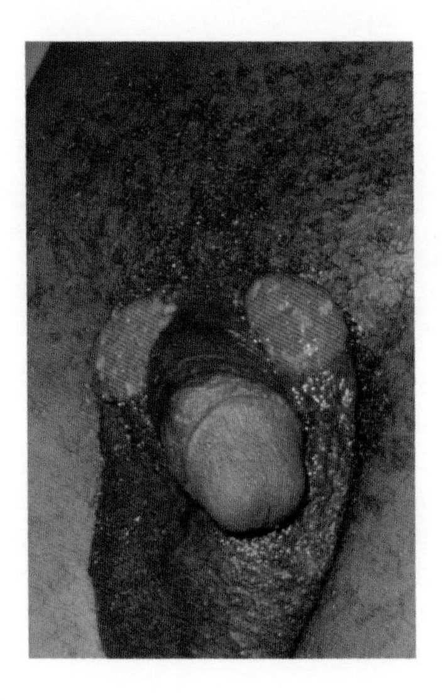

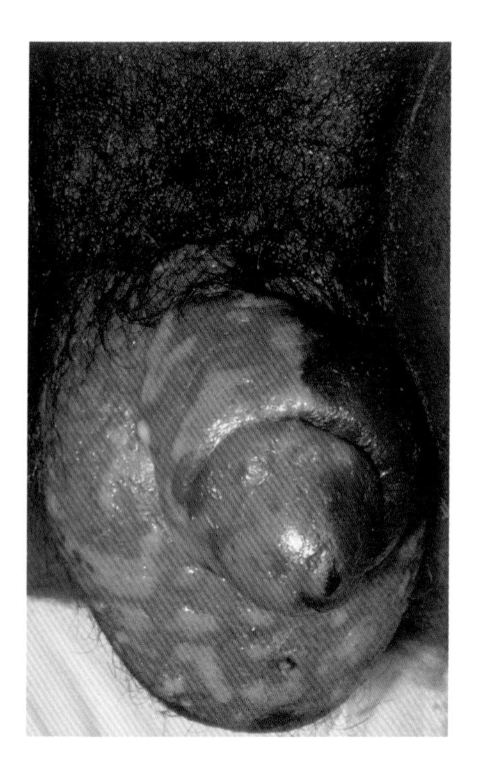

**Figure 279** Extensive ulceration of the genitalia due to herpes simplex type 2 in a patient with HIV infection.

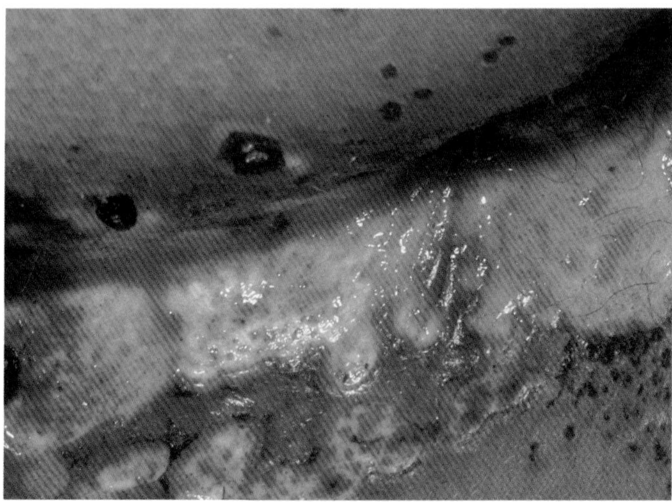

**Figure 280** Extensive perianal herpes simplex type 2 in a patient with HIV infection.

*Treatment of genital herpes associated with HIV infection:* Oral acyclovir 200mg five times daily for 7 days is very helpful if the patient is seen early (within 24–48 hours of the onset). Very frequent recurrences can be treated with prophylactic acyclovir 400mg bd. It is, however, a very expensive drug.

## HERPES ZOSTER

Herpes zoster is the reactivation of the *Herpes varicella zoster* virus. After chicken pox, the virus lies dormant in the posterior root ganglion and later travels down the cutaneous nerves to infect the epidermal cells in the skin. This usually occurs when the immune response is decreased, in old age or in younger patients with HIV infection. Almost everyone with herpes zoster less than 10 years of age and in the 20–50-year age group is HIV positive.

**Figure 281** Herpes zoster of the left $T_4$ dermatome in an 80-year-old man. This is a painful rash made up of grouped vesicles along the course of the dermatome. The rash stops abruptly at the midline. The pain may begin several days before the rash appears.

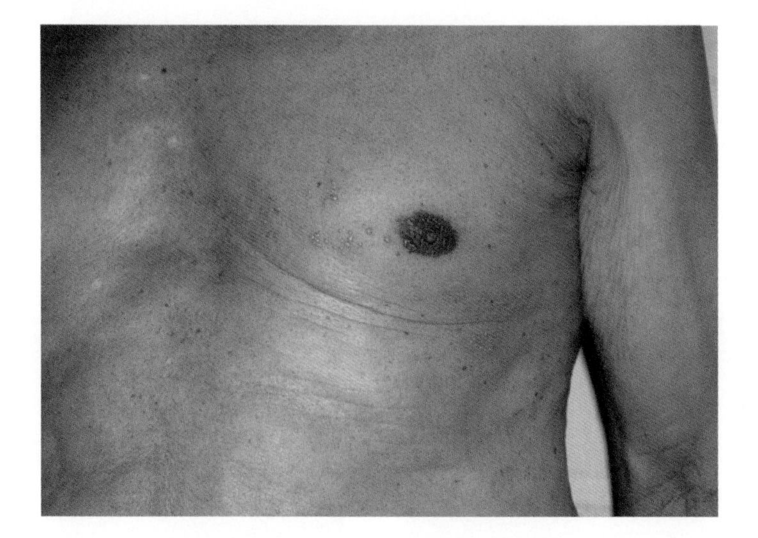

**Figure 282** Herpes zoster of the left $T_3$ dermatome. The vesicles have now become confluent.

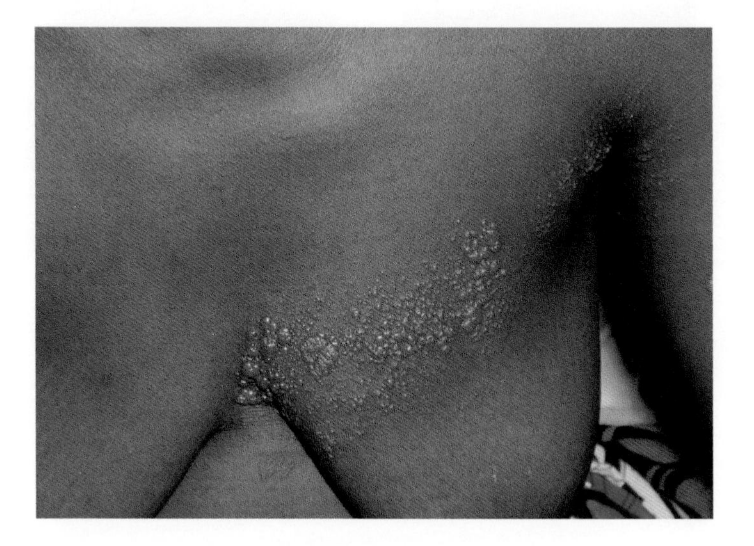

**Figure 283** The vesicles then break leaving erosions and crusts. Without treatment the rash will heal in 3–4 weeks.

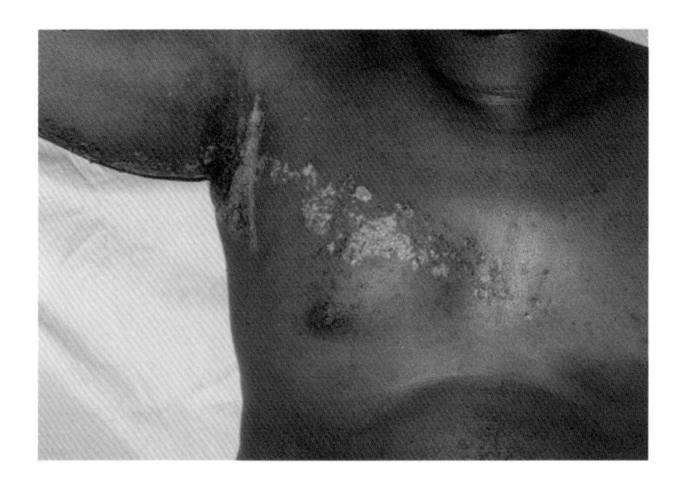

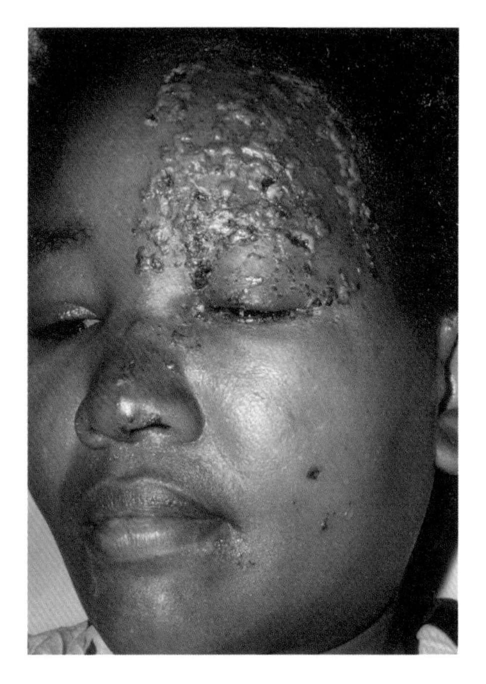

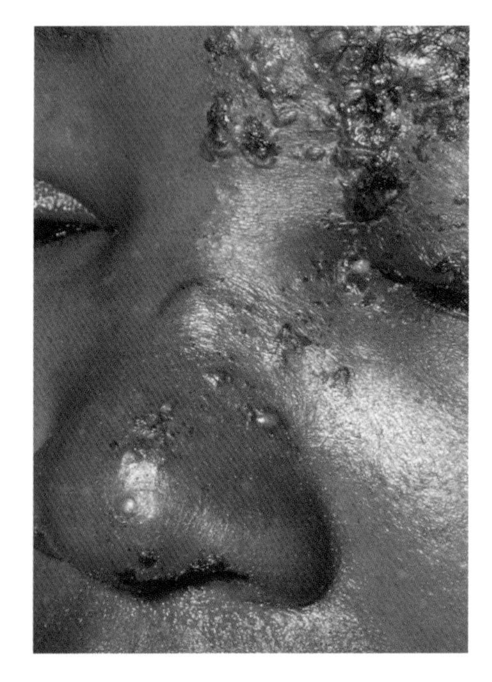

**Figures 284, 285** Ophthalmic herpes zoster. Involvement of the nasociliary branch of the nerve, with vesicles going down the side of the nose, means that the eye will also be involved.

**Figures 286, 287** Herpes zoster of the mandibular branch of the 5th cranial nerve; the anterior ⅔ of the tongue is involved as well as the skin of the chin and side of the cheek.

*Treatment:* Regular analgesics for the pain. Topical Gentian Violet (0.5%) once the vesicles have burst to prevent secondary bacterial infection. If the patient is seen within 48 hours of the onset, oral acyclovir 800mg five times daily for 7 days will shorten the course of the disease, but this drug is very expensive.

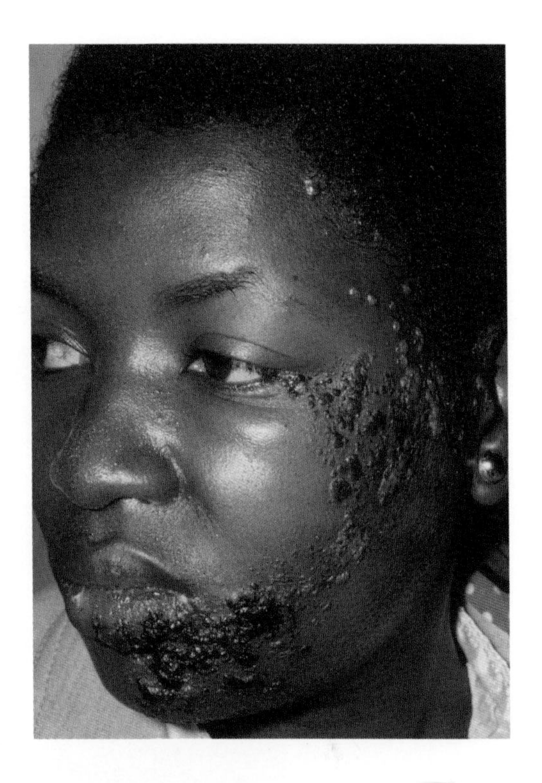

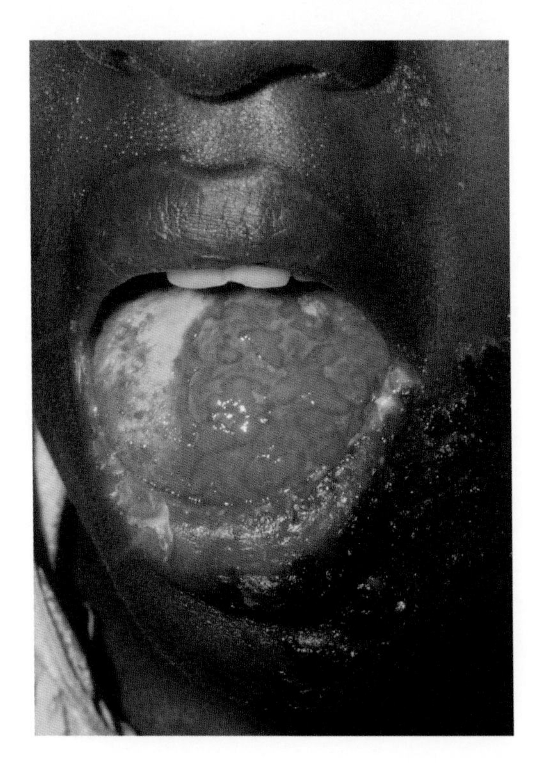

## HIRSUTISM

**Figure 288** Hairy chin in a 27-year-old lady. Hirsutism is male pattern hair in a female.

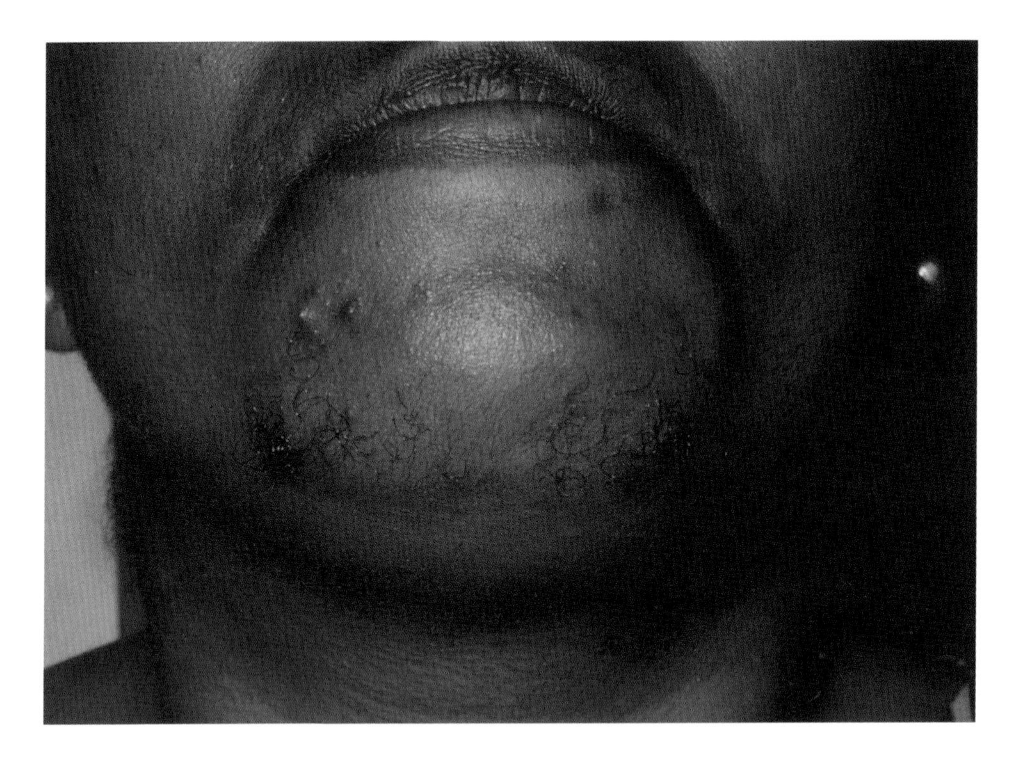

*Treatment:* If normal menstruation, reassure the patient that it is not serious. If abnormal menstruation look for androgen producing tumour. If the hirsutism is not too noticeable it can be left alone. If the patient does not like it, bleach the hairs with lemon juice or hydrogen peroxide, or remove them with depilatory creams or by shaving.

## HISTIOCYTOMA (Dermatofibroma)

**Figure 289** Small firm hyperpigmented papule at the site of a previous insect bite or other trauma.

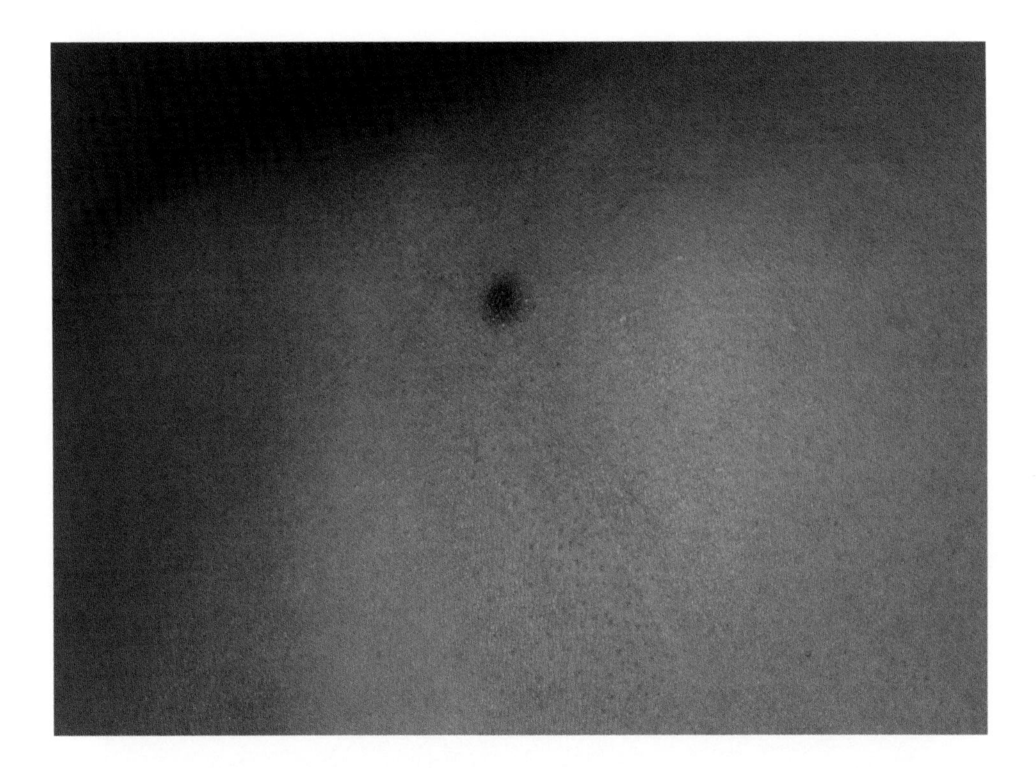

*Treatment:* It is quite harmless and needs no treatment.

## HISTOPLASMOSIS

**Figure 290** Infection due to *Histoplasma capsulatum* var *duboisii.* Umbilicated papules and nodules which may ulcerate appear on the skin and sometimes enlarge to form large vegetating plaques. It is most commonly seen in patients who are HIV positive.

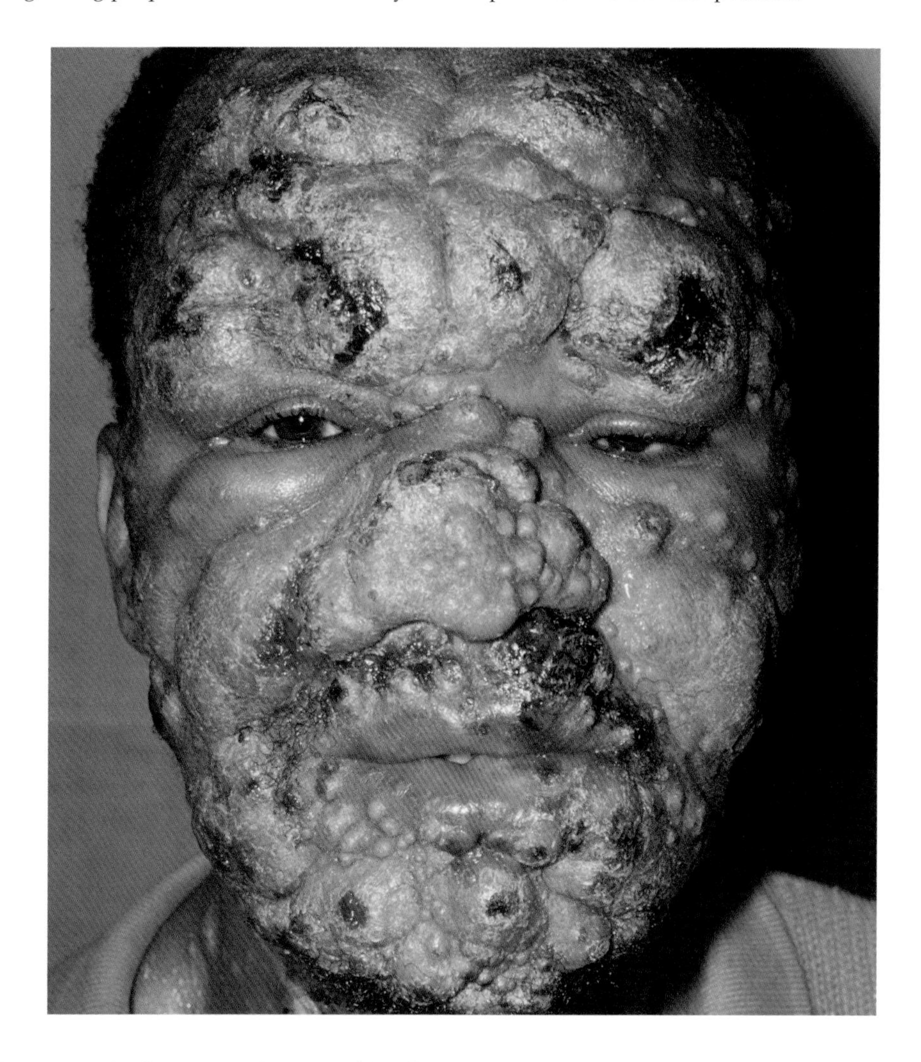

*Treatment:* Oral itraconazole 200mg/day for 6–8 weeks. Repeat if it recurs.

**Figures 291, 292** The diagnosis can be confirmed by biopsy. The organism is seen within macrophages in the dermis on H&E and PAS stains. The organism can also be cultured on Sabouraud's dextrose agar, without antibiotics, but it takes 2 months to grow.

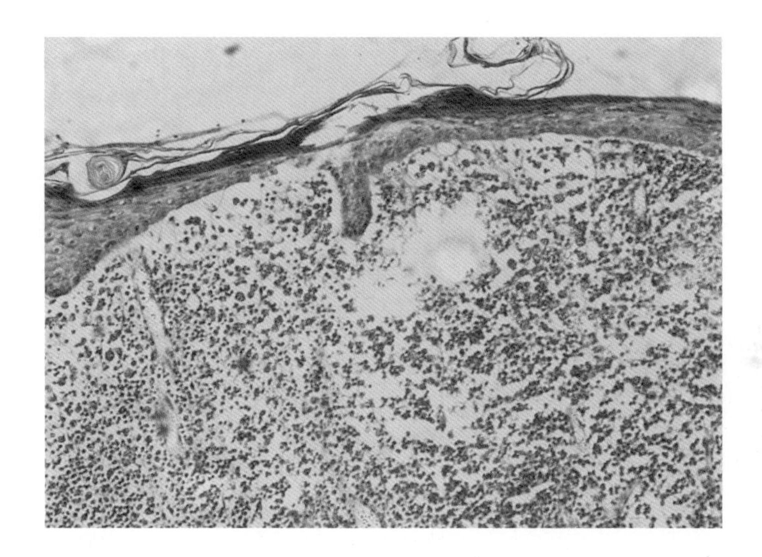

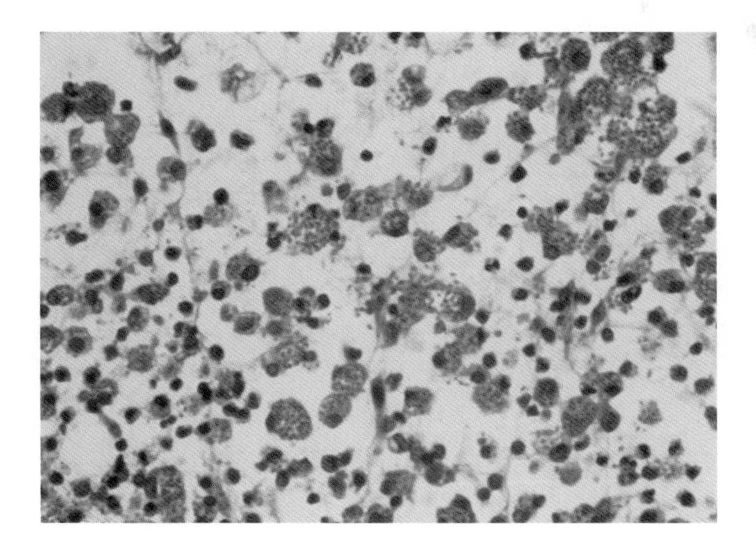

## HYPERHIDROSIS

**Figure 293** Excessive production of sweat most commonly affects the axillae, hands and feet.

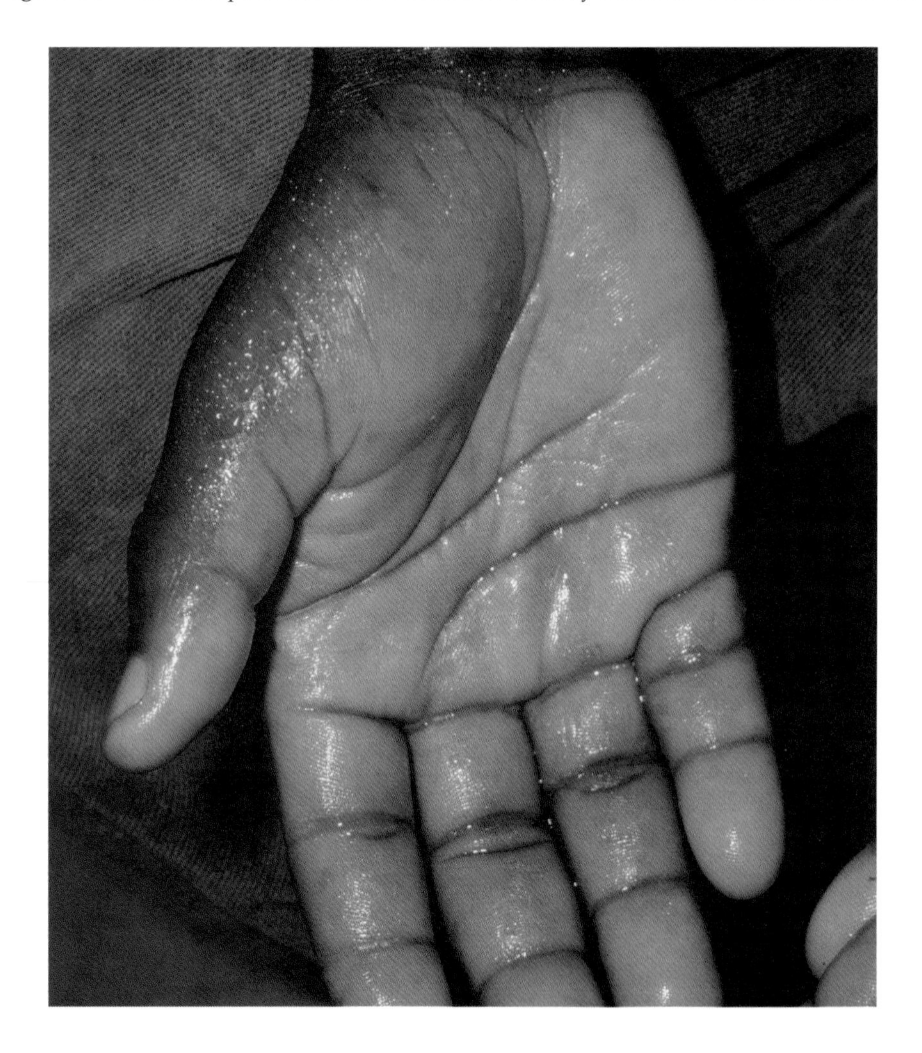

*Treatment:* For the axilla, apply 20% aluminium chloride hexahydrate in absolute alcohol once or twice a week, or excise the central axillary skin (axillary vault). For hands and feet, soak in 5% formalin. If this does not help the patient may need a sympathectomy.

## HYPERTRICHOSIS

**Figure 294** Foetal hair is not replaced by vellus and terminal hair but remains present throughout life. The child is not noticed to be particularly hairy at birth, but by early childhood the whole skin, apart from the palms and soles, is covered by silky hair up to 10cm long.

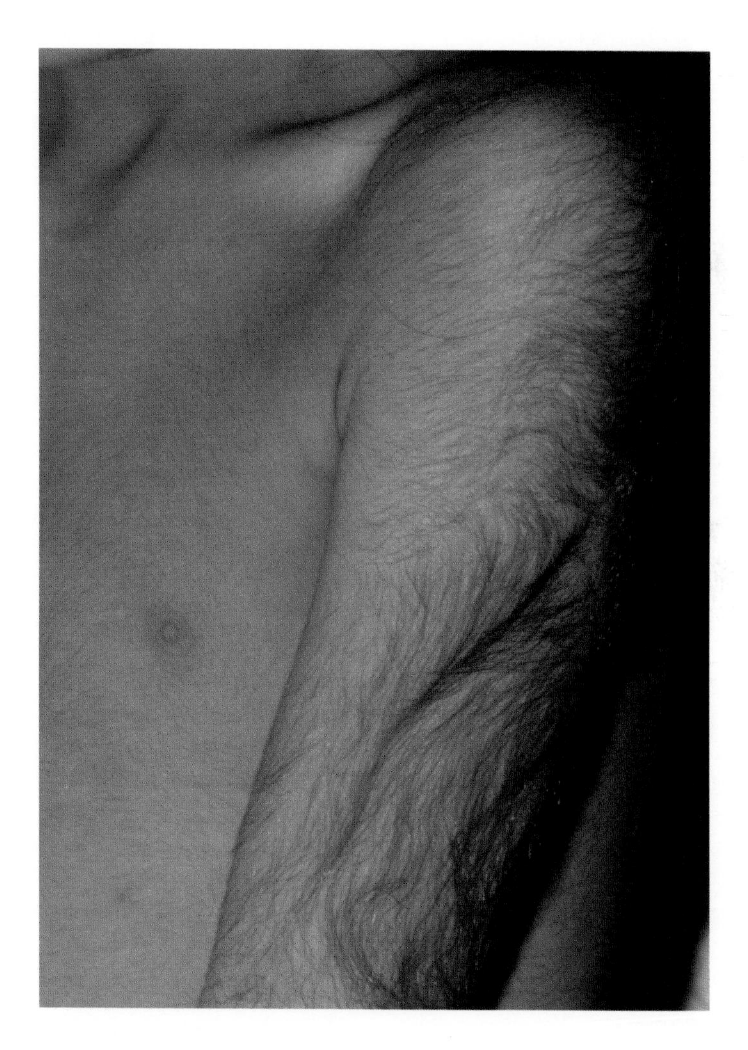

*Treatment:* Nothing can be done for this.

# ICHTHYOSIS

The word 'ichthyosis' comes from the Greek *ichthys*, meaning fish. It is applied to a group of diseases which are characterised by a dry scaly skin. Most of them are genetically determined and are present from birth.

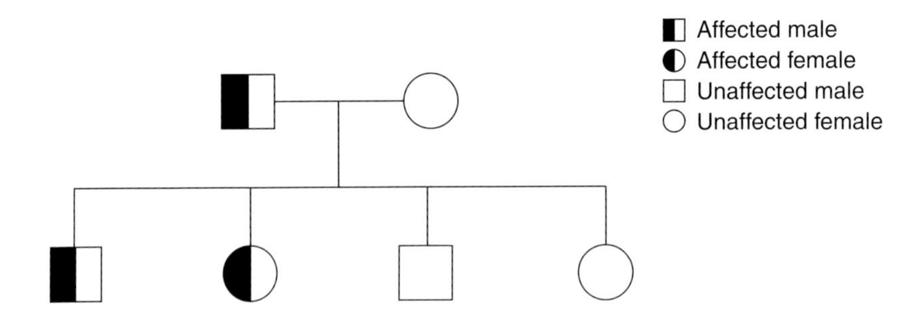


**Figure 295** Autosomal dominant inheritance. The condition is present in the heterozygous state, so affected individuals will pass it on to half their children, regardless of sex. Unaffected individuals do not have the abnormal gene and cannot therefore pass it on to their children.

The types of ichthyosis inherited in this way are:

- Ichthyosis vulgaris.
- Bullous ichthyosiform erythroderma.

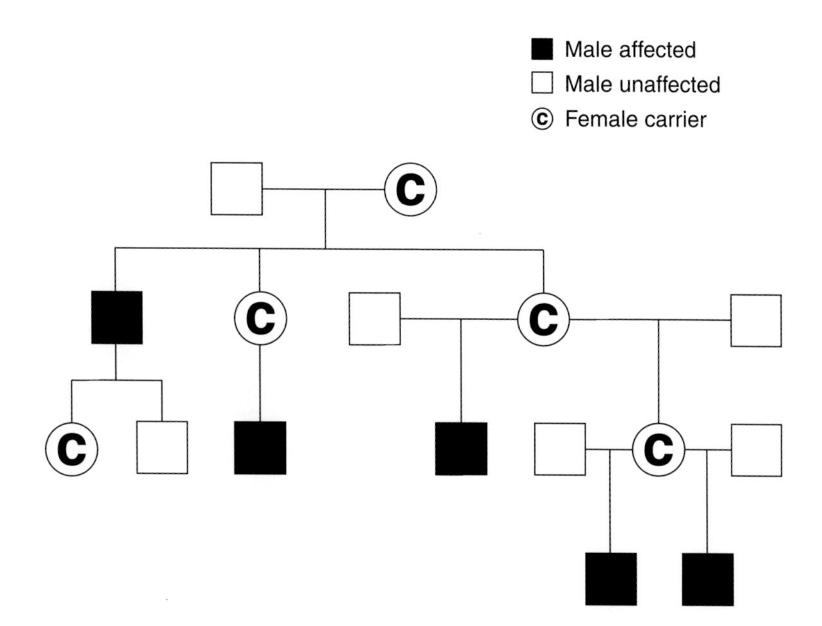


**Figure 296** X-linked recessive inheritance. The abnormal gene is on the X chromosome. Females have two X chromosomes and do not show the disease, but they are carriers and can pass it on to half their sons. Males only have one X chromosome. If it is abnormal they will show the disease. They cannot pass the disease on to their sons but will pass the abnormal gene on to all their daughters who will be carriers. The type of ichthyosis inherited in this way is:

- Sex-linked ichthyosis.

Autosomal recessive inheritance (*see* Figure 18).

The types of ichthyosis inherited in this way are:

- Non-bullous ichthyosiform erythroderma.
- Lamellar ichthyosis.
- Harlequin foetus.

When ichthyosis occurs later in life it is called acquired ichthyosis and can be due to malnutrition, lepromatous leprosy or a lymphoma.

## Ichthyosis vulgaris

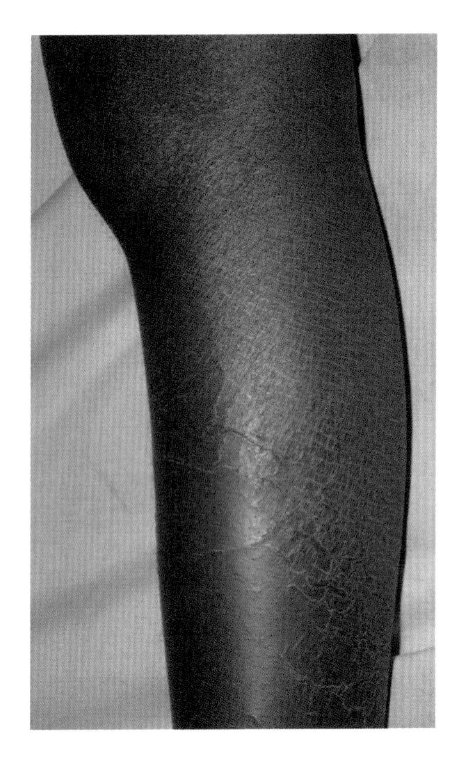

**Figure 297** The whole skin apart from the antecubital and popliteal fossae is dry and scaly.

*Treatment:* Application of moisturisers as and when necessary, e.g. Vaseline, animal fat, coconut oil, cocoa butter or whatever is available locally.

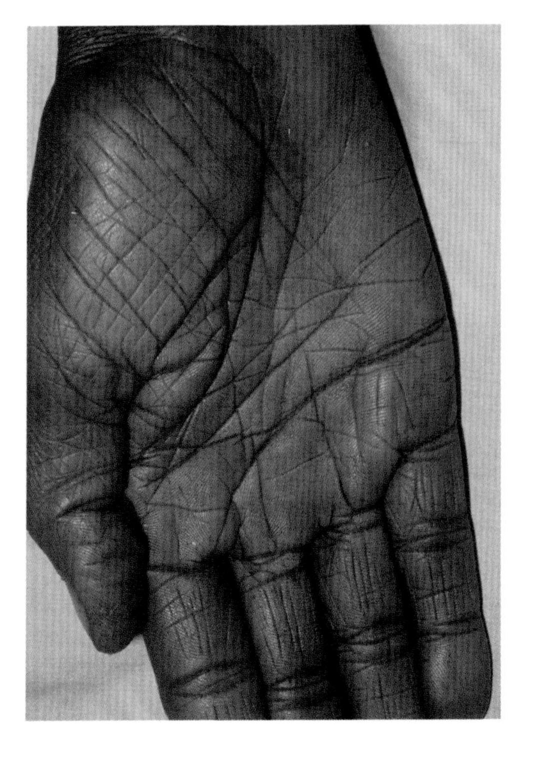

**Figure 298** The palms and soles show increased skin markings.

## Sex-linked ichthyosis

**Figure 299** This is an X-linked recessive condition which is seen only in males, although it is transmitted through females (*see* Figure 296). The scales are large and hyperpigmented. They are particularly noticeable in the flexures, and remain throughout life.

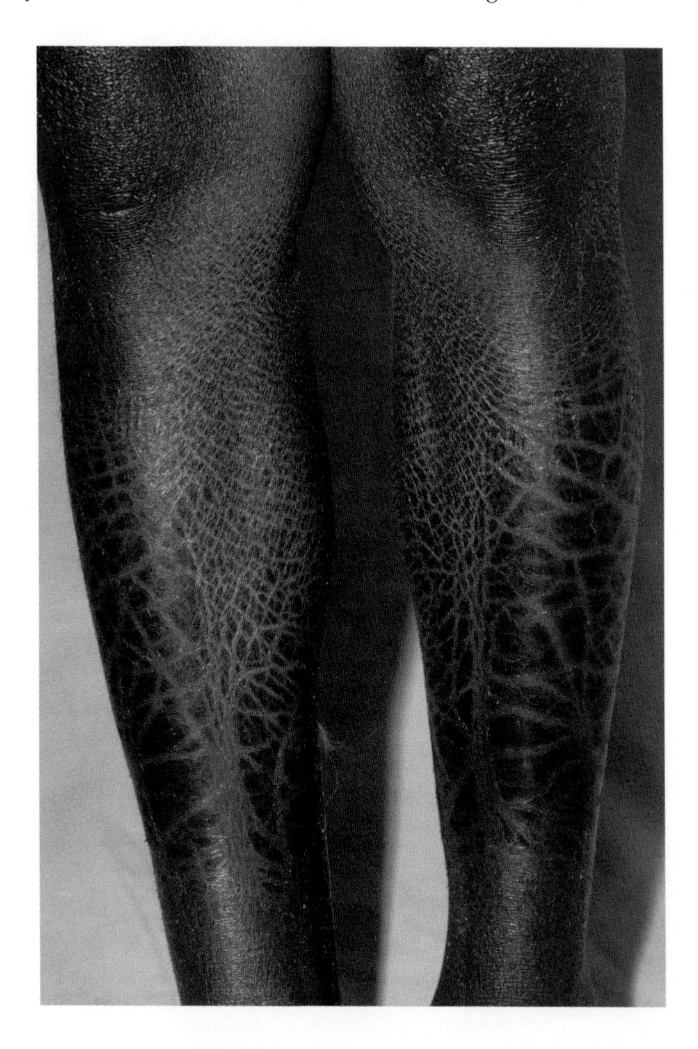

*Treatment:* Application of moisturisers as and when necessary, e.g. Vaseline, animal fat, coconut oil, cocoa butter or whatever is available locally.

## Bullous ichthyosiform erythroderma

**Figures 300, 301** At birth the baby is red and scaly, and blisters and erosions are prominent at sites of trauma. By the end of the first year of life the most obvious feature is warty hyperkeratosis forming ridges. The face, palms and soles are spared.

*Treatment:* Application of greasy ointments is helpful, e.g. Vaseline, animal fat, coconut oil, cocoa butter or whatever is available locally. Oral retinoids (acetretin 0.5mg/kg body weight/day) can be very helpful but the long-term risks have to be weighed against the benefits. Oral retinoids are very expensive.

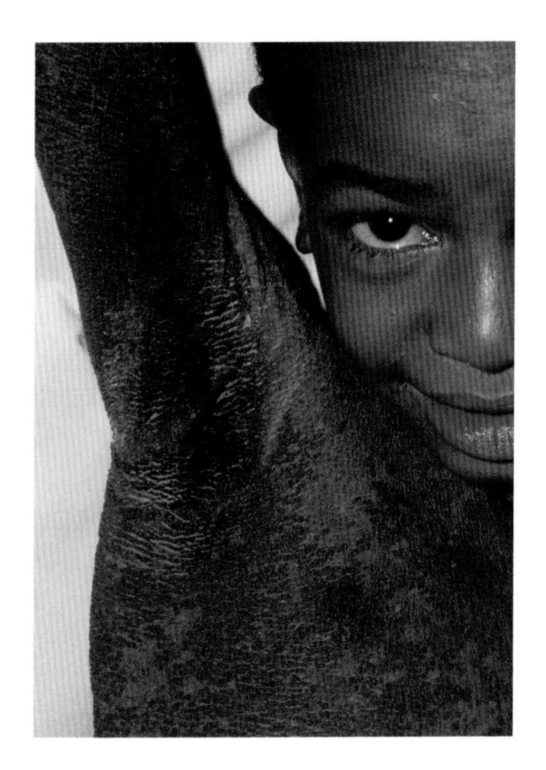

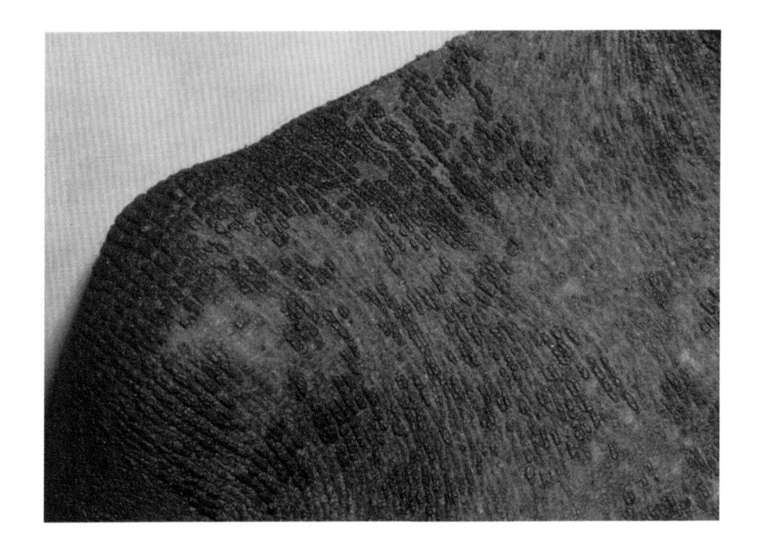

## Non-bullous ichthyosiform erythroderma

**Figures 302, 303** The baby may be born encased in a thick membrane ('Collodion baby'). When the 'collodion' comes off the skin is red and scaly all over, and it remains like this throughout life.

*Treatment:* Application of greasy ointments is helpful, e.g. Vaseline, animal fat, coconut oil, cocoa butter or whatever is available locally. Oral retinoids (acetretin 0.5mg/kg body weight/day) can be very helpful but the long-term risks have to be weighed against the benefits. Oral retinoids are very expensive.

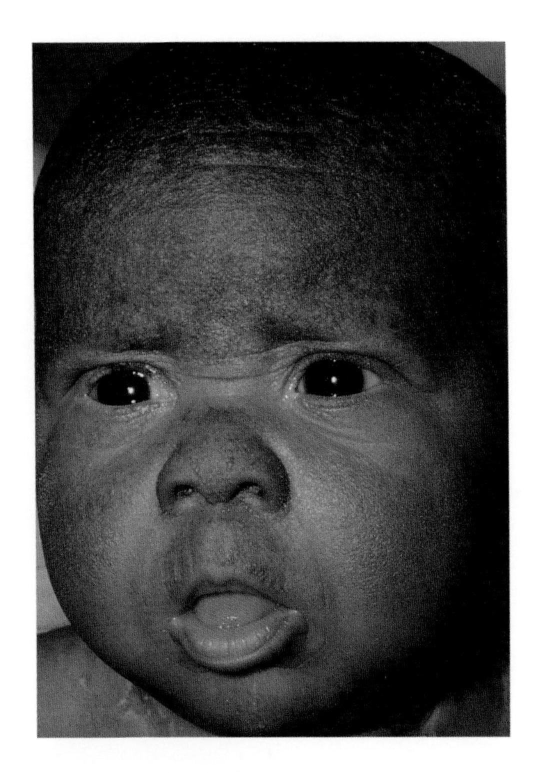

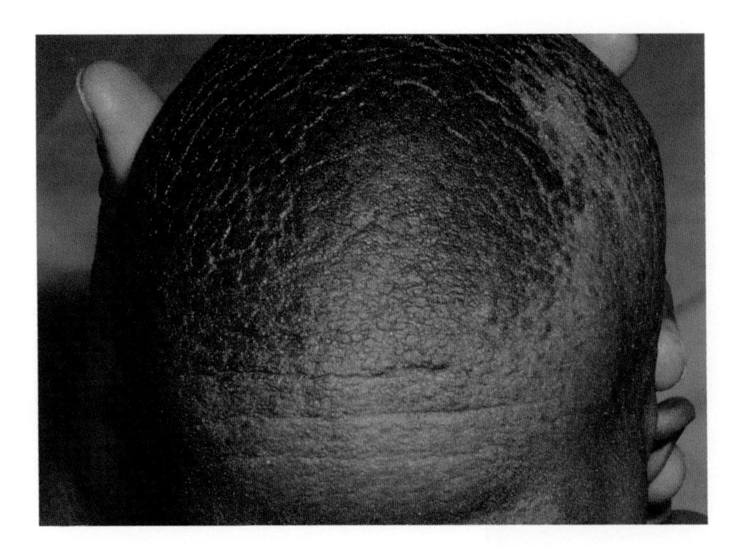

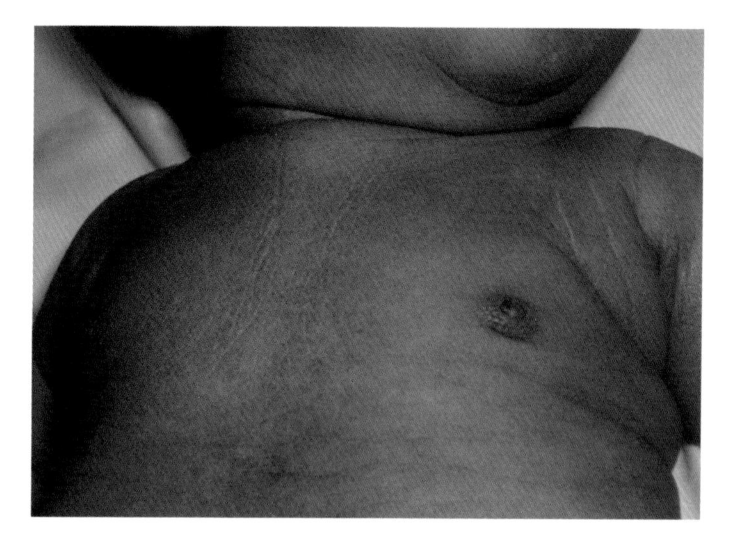

**Figure 304** Non-bullous ichthyosiform erythroderma – the skin is red and scaly all over.

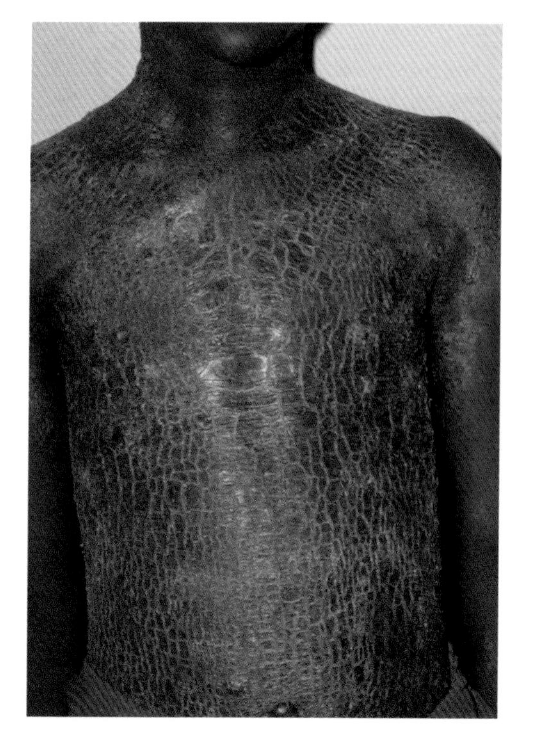

## Lamellar ichthyosis

**Figure 305** Most babies with this condition are born encased in a thick membrane ('Collodion baby'). When the 'collodion' comes off the baby is covered with large, hyperpigmented scales.

*Treatment:* As for bullous and non-bullous ichthyosiform erythroderma (*see* Figures 300–4).

**Figure 306** In lamellar ichthyosis the palms and soles are spared.

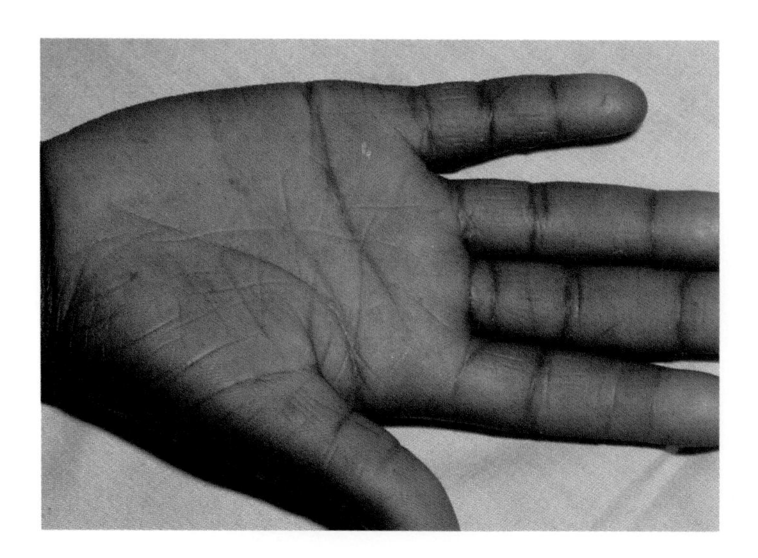

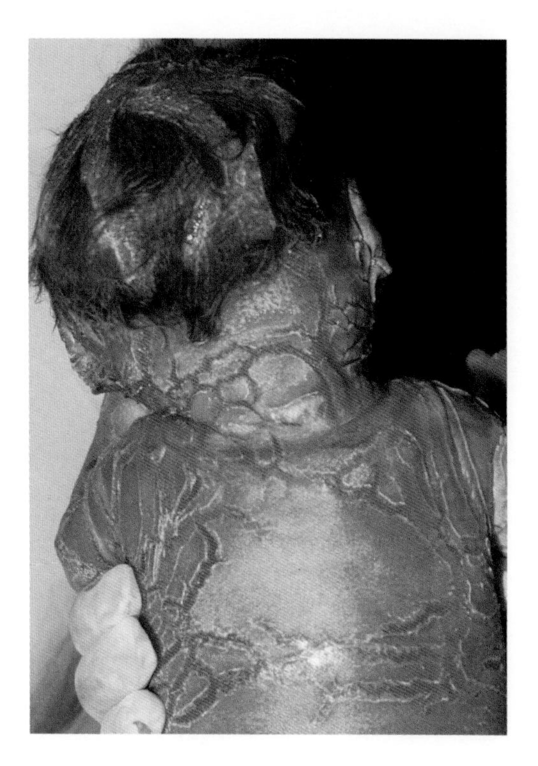

## Harlequin foetus

**Figure 307** The child is born with thick hyperkeratosis over the whole body. This splits in diamond shaped fissures resembling a harlequin costume. Most of these babies die in the first few days or weeks of life.

*Treatment:* Oral acetretin may be life saving if it is available (0.5mg/kg body weight/day), but it is very expensive and will have to be continued throughout life.

## IDIOPATHIC GUTTATE HYPOMELANOSIS

**Figure 308** Small white macules on the arms and legs are a common and normal finding.

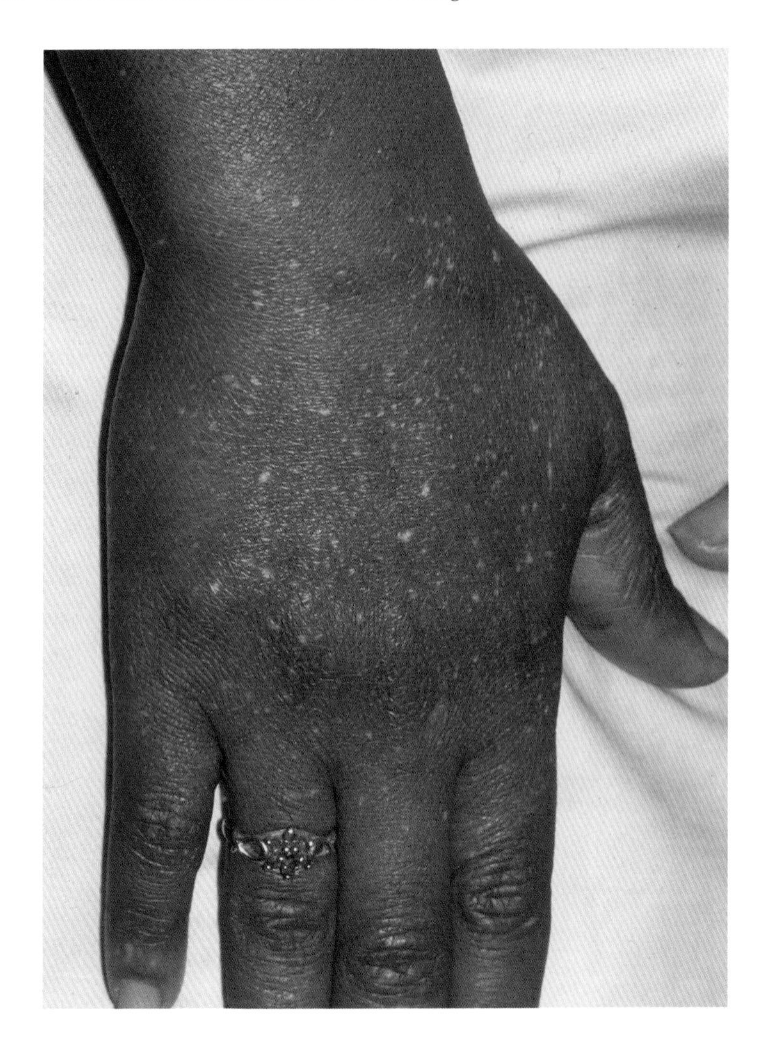

*Treatment:* It needs no treatment other than reassurance.

## IMPETIGO

**Figure 309** Diagram to show sites of infection with *Staphylococcus aureus*. Impetigo is a very superficial infection of the epidermis (just under the stratum corneum) with *Staphylococcus aureus* or *Streptococcus pyogenes* (*see* Figure 124) or a mixture of both.

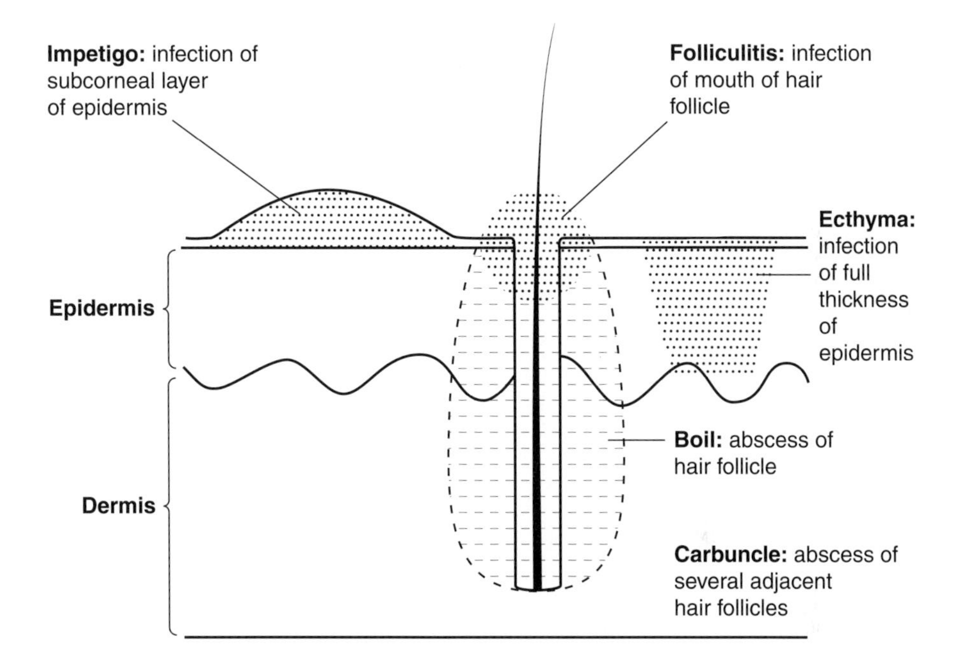


**Figure 310** Small vesicles rapidly rupture to give honey-coloured crusts.

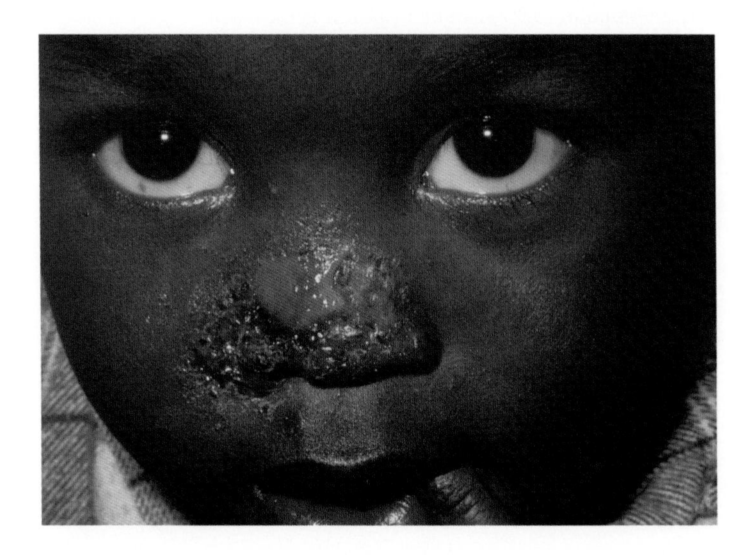

*Treatment:* Remove crusts by soaking them in soapy water or oil, then apply 0.5% Gentian Violet paint bd for 3 days. If it is streptococcal rather than staphylococcal add oral phenoxymethylpenicillin (Penicillin V) to prevent subsequent acute glomerulonephritis.

## Bullous impetigo

**Figure 311** In infants, especially in the newborn, impetigo due to *Staphylococcus aureus* is often bullous. The subcorneal blisters remain intact instead of bursting and a fluid level of pus is often seen.

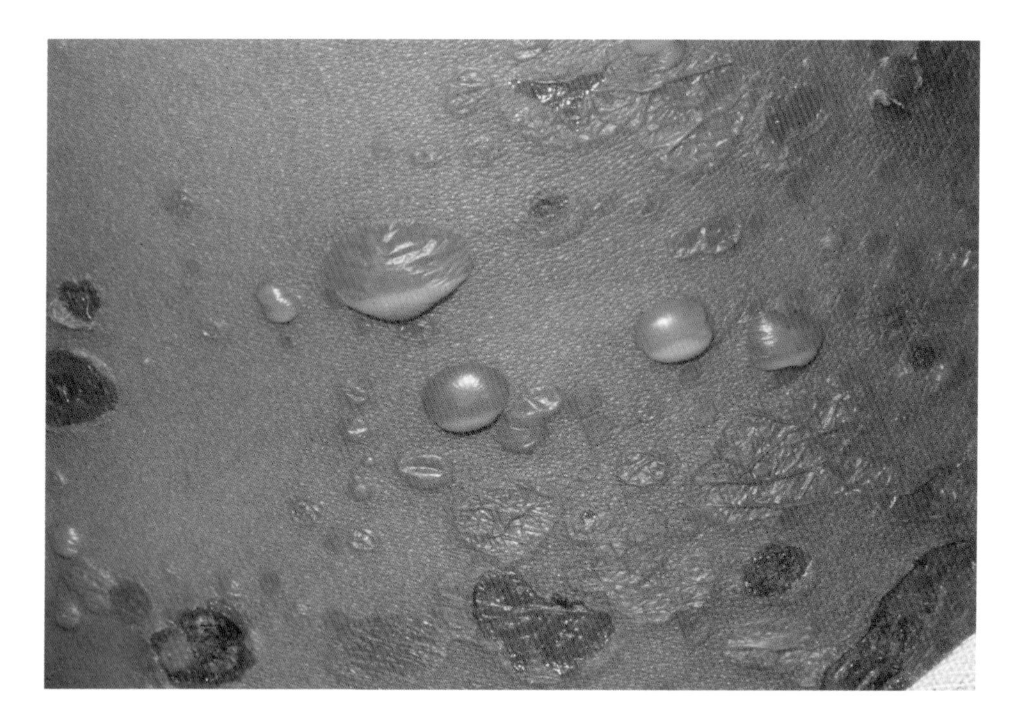

*Treatment:* If it is widespread give oral antibiotics; cloxacillin elixir 62.5mg qds for 7 days. Topical Gentian Violet paint (0.5%) can be used if it is localised.

## INCONTINENTIA PIGMENTI

**Figure 312** Rare genetic disorder inherited as an X-linked dominant trait which is fatal in males, so it is only seen in females. At birth there is erythema and linear vesiculation on the trunk and limbs. After 2 weeks or so the vesicles are replaced by linear warty plaques.

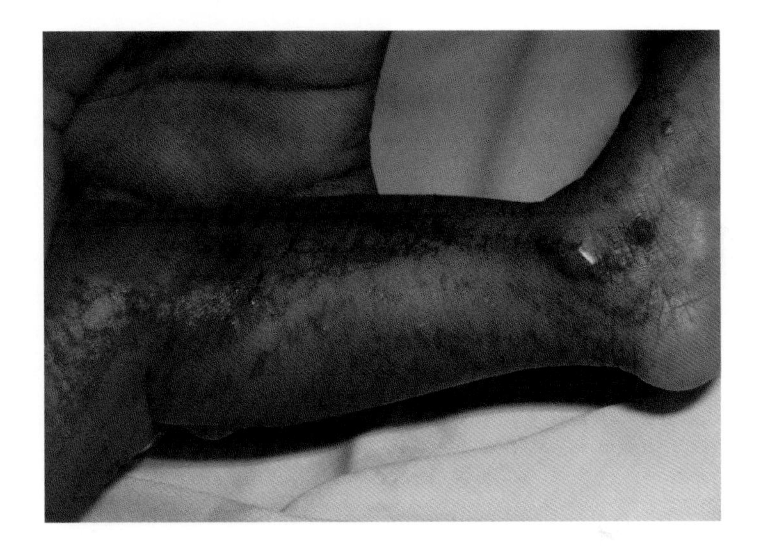

**Figure 313** After about 6 months hyperpigmented streaks and whorls appear in the groins or following Blaschko's lines on the trunk. These disappear by the early–mid-teens. It is a multisystem disorder with abnormalities also in the central nervous system (mental retardation and convulsions), eyes (squint, cataracts, blindness) and teeth (partial or complete absence of teeth or conical teeth).

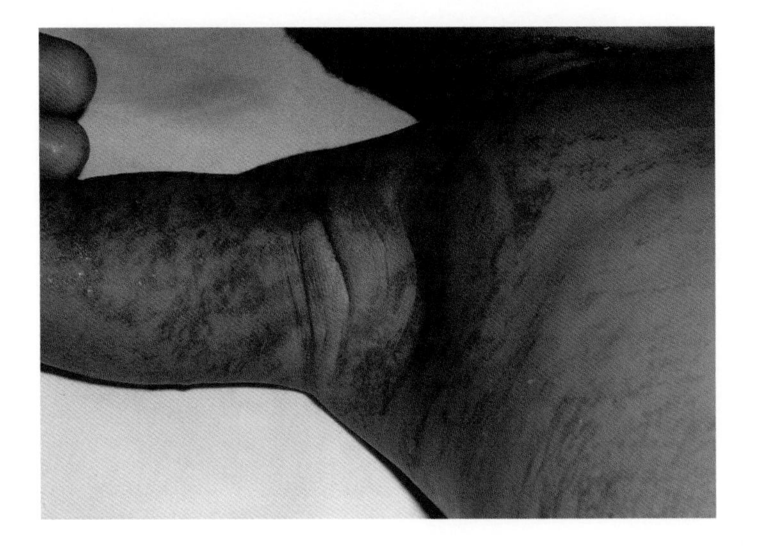

## INCONTINENTIA PIGMENTI ACHROMIANS (Hypomelanosis of Ito)

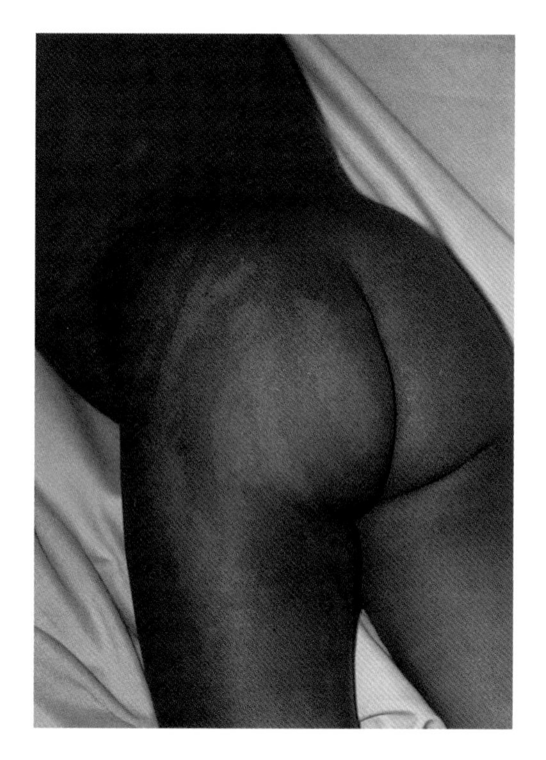

**Figures 314, 315** Hypopigmented streaks and whorls on the skin which look like those of incontinentia pigmenti but are hypo- rather than hyperpigmented. No preceding blistering or warty hyperkeratosis but associated abnormalities of the CNS, eyes and teeth as in incontinentia pigmenti. It appears to be due to a variety of chromosomal abnormalities (the more common ones are mosaic trisomy 18, diploidy/triploidy, mosaicism for sex chromosome aneuploidy, and tetrasomy 12p).

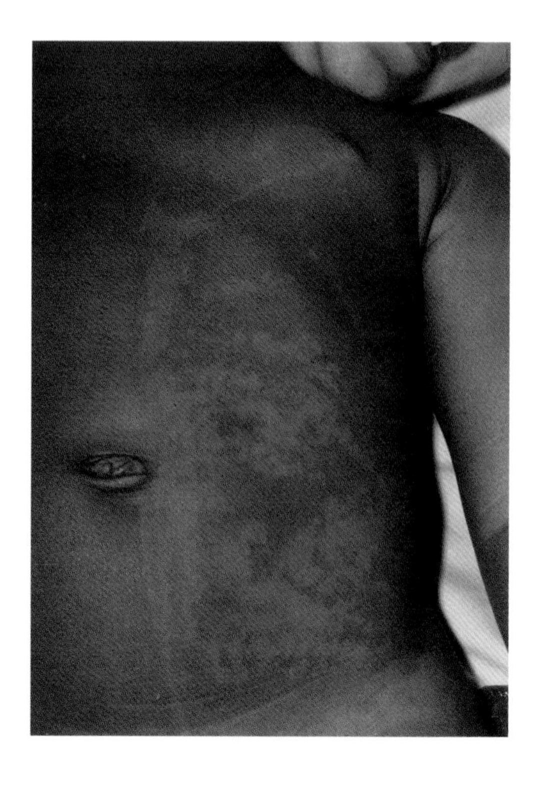

## INTERTRIGO

**Figure 316** Inflammation of the skin due to two moist surfaces rubbing together. Occurs on the upper thighs, in the submammary area and in the belly folds of people who are too fat.

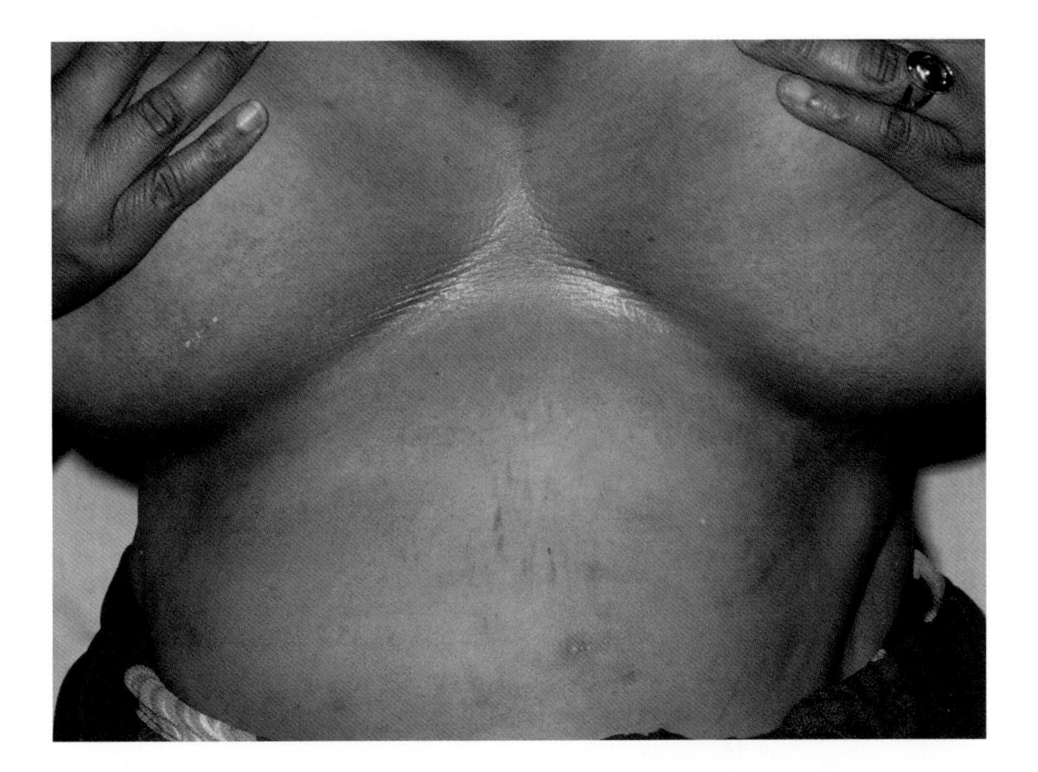

*Treatment:* The patient needs to lose weight.

## KAPOSI'S SARCOMA

Kaposi's sarcoma (KS) is one of the cancers found in AIDS. It is due to infection with human herpes virus-8 (HHV-8). 90% of individuals with KS have AIDS (epidemic KS), the other 10% have endemic KS (*see* Figures 330–1).

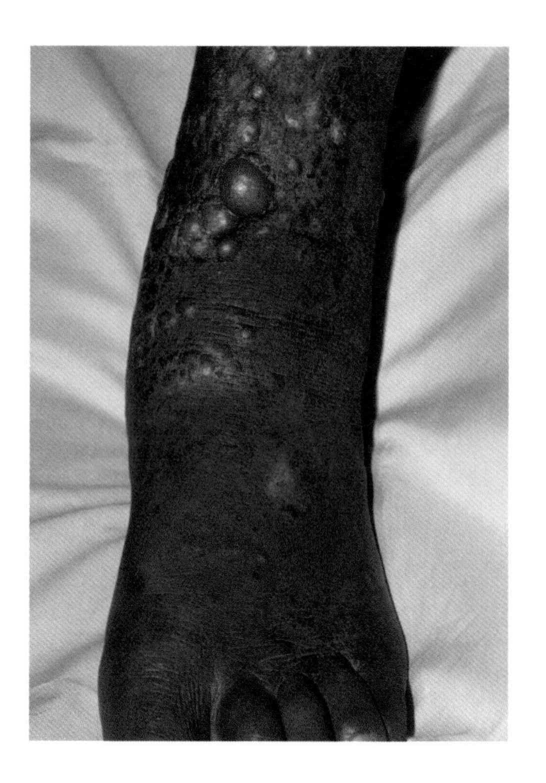

### Epidemic Kaposi's sarcoma

**Figure 317** Often begins on the legs and feet with hyperpigmented papules, nodules or plaques. The whole lower leg may be sclerotic and woody hard, and there may be associated lymphoedema.

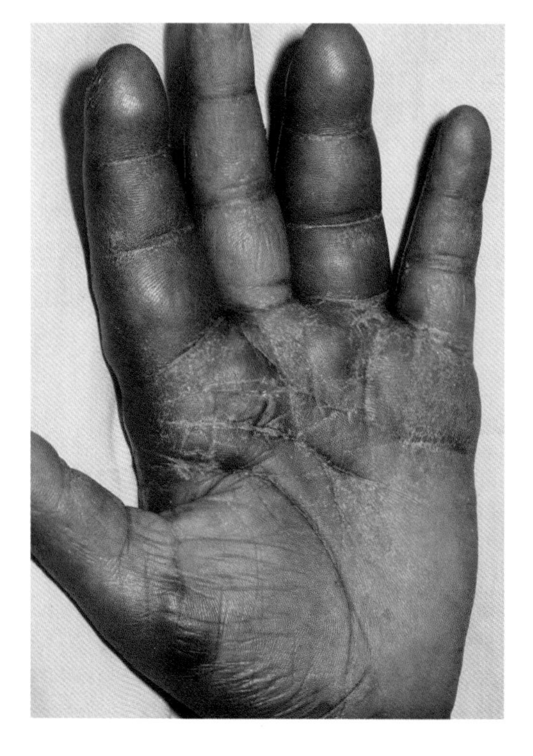

**Figure 318** On the lighter skin of the palms and soles the typical dark reddish-purple colour of the lesions can be seen.

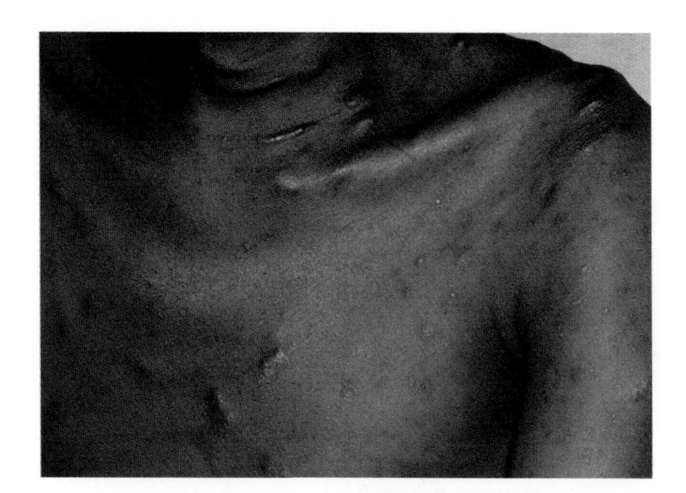

**Figure 319** Widespread skin lesions can be linear in shape.

**Figures 320, 321** Lesions on the face are often unsightly.

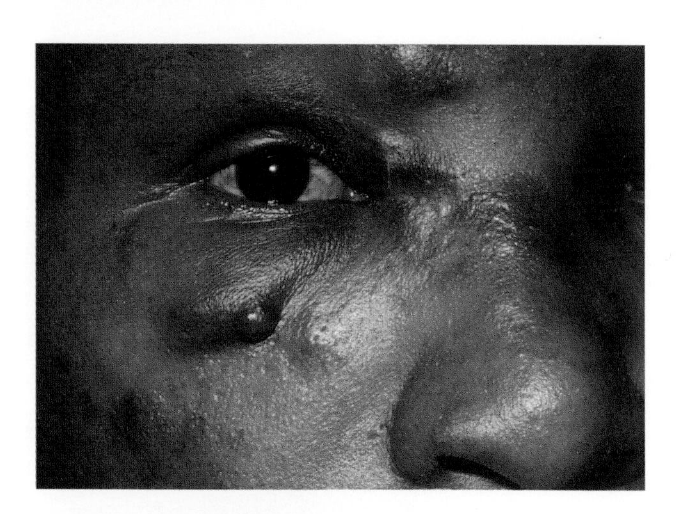

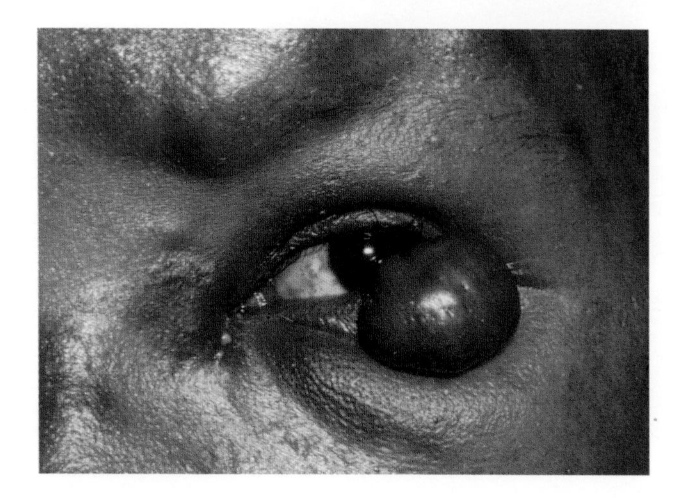

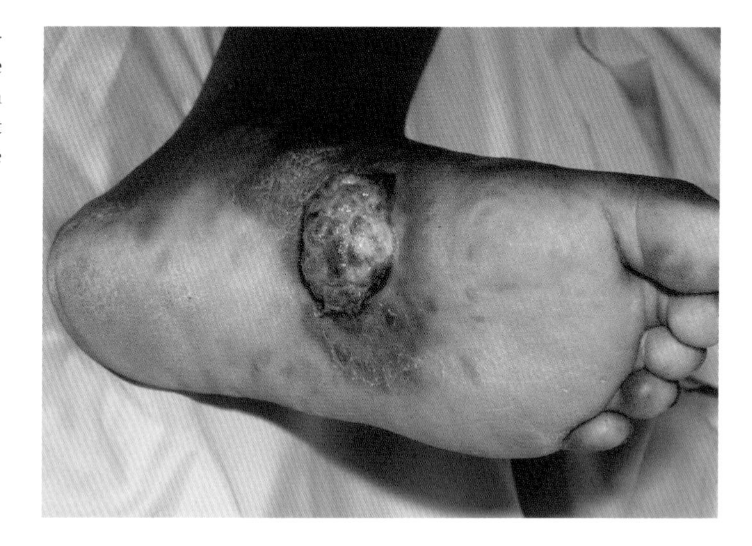

**Figure 322** A nodular lesion of KS on the sole may resemble an amelanotic malignant melanoma (*see* Figure 121).

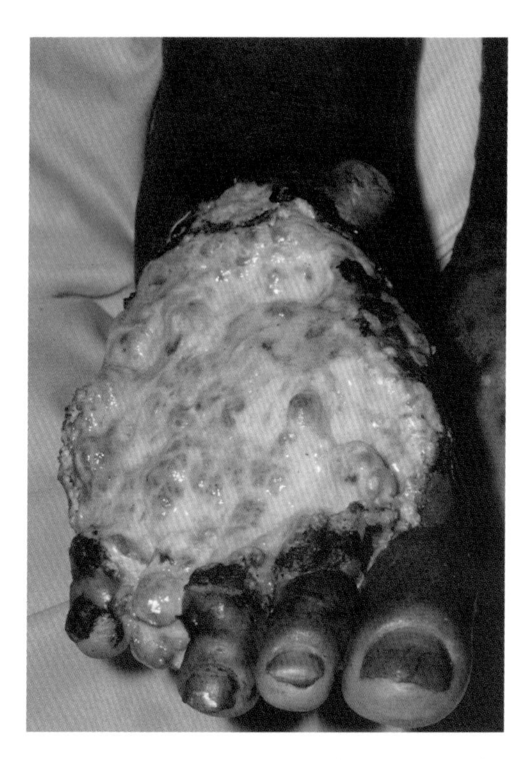

**Figure 323** Fungating KS on the dorsum of the foot.

**Figure 324** Mucous membrane involvement with KS is common. Lesions in the mouth are dark red in colour, not brown (*see also* Figures 632–3). The palate is the most common site for mucous membrane involvement. Here the gum and buccal mucosa are also involved.

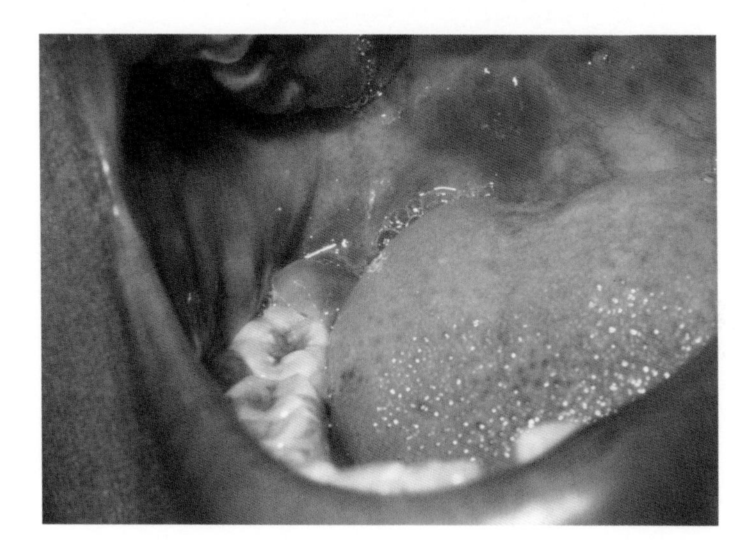

**Figure 325** Kaposi's sarcoma of the gum.

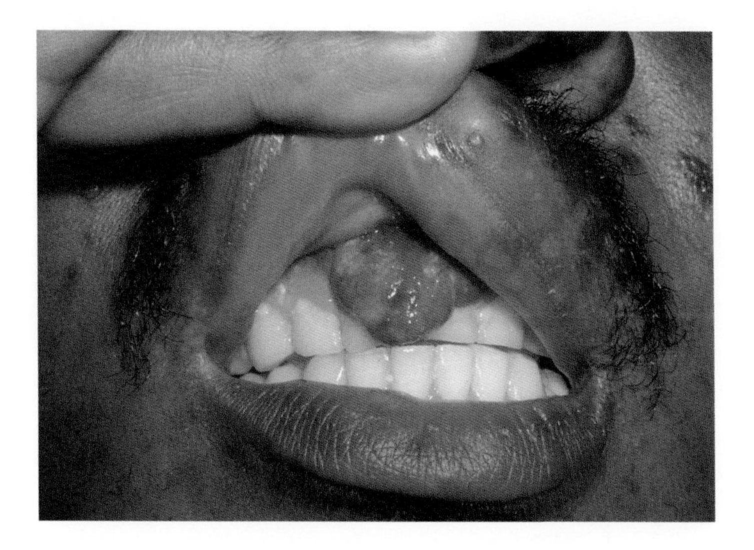

**Figures 326, 327** Kaposi's sarcoma of the tongue.

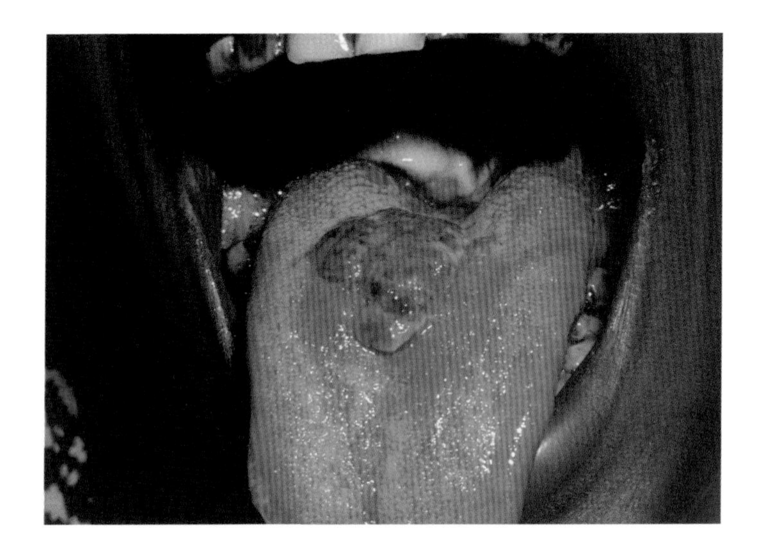

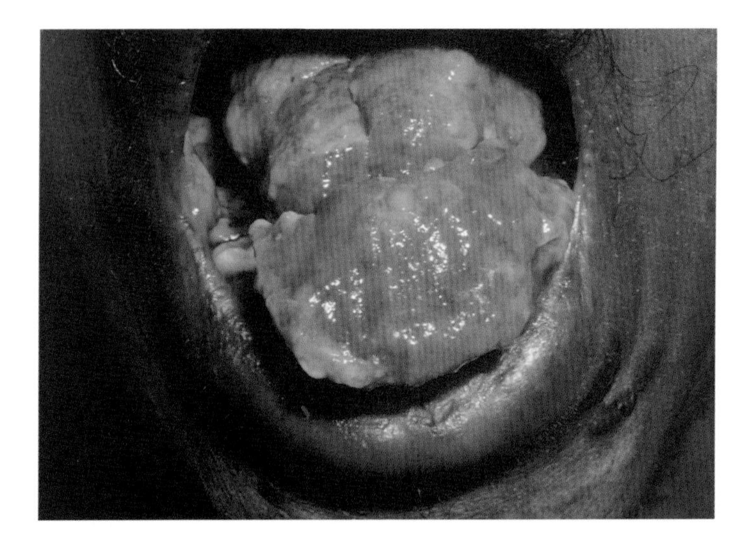

**Figure 328** Kaposi's sarcoma of the conjunctiva.

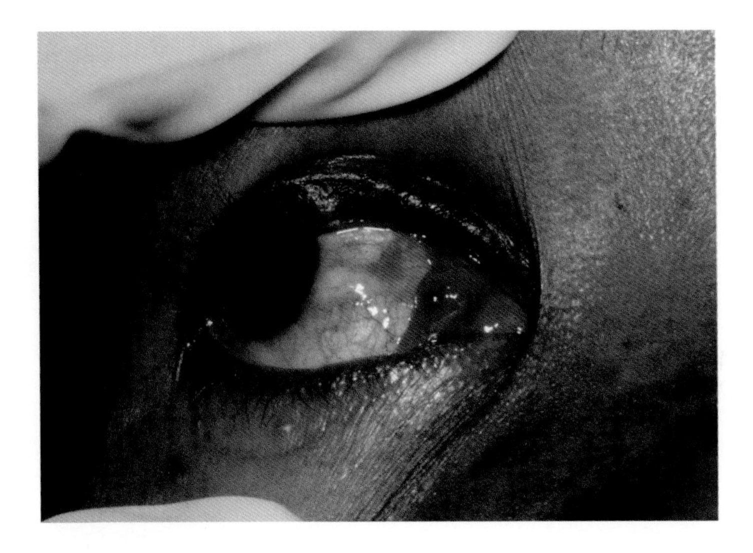

**Figure 329** The diagnosis is usually obvious clinically. If in doubt a biopsy will show proliferation of dermal capillaries which have a single layer of plump endothelial cells, vascular slits, extravasation of red blood cells and a proliferation of spindle cells. It should not be confused with giant cell epulis in the mouth (*see* Figures 252–3).

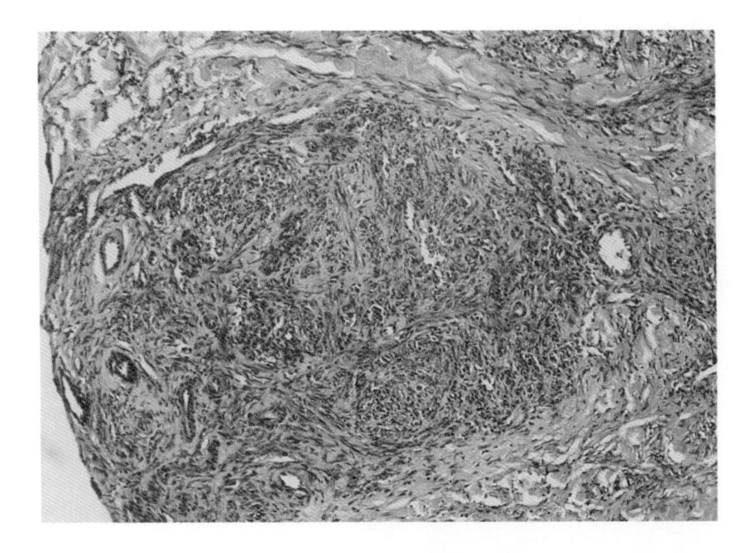

*Treatment of epidemic Kaposi's sarcoma:* Only treat if symptomatic (painful or unsightly). Chemotherapy with vincristine, doxorubicin and bleomycin gives good palliation for a time but these drugs are extremely expensive. If the disease is localised to a limb, radiotherapy may be helpful.

## Endemic Kaposi's sarcoma

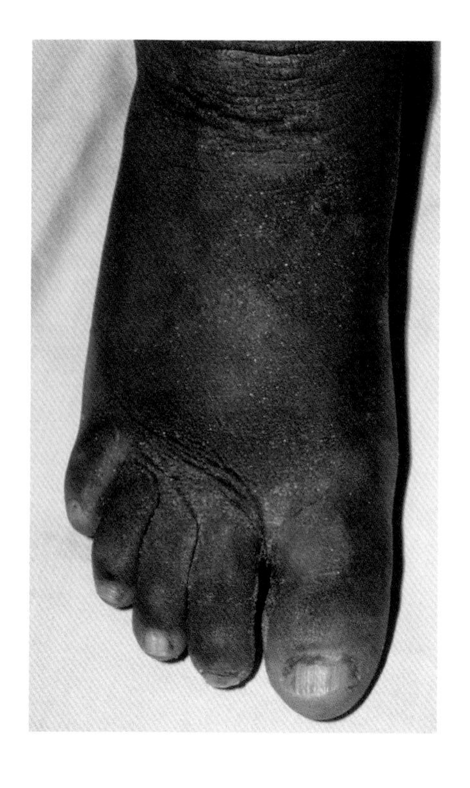

**Figure 330** Endemic Kaposi's sarcoma most commonly affects elderly men on the extremities. These lesions contain the same human herpes virus-8 as the lesions in patients with AIDS. Diffuse KS on the foot and lower leg in an elderly man.

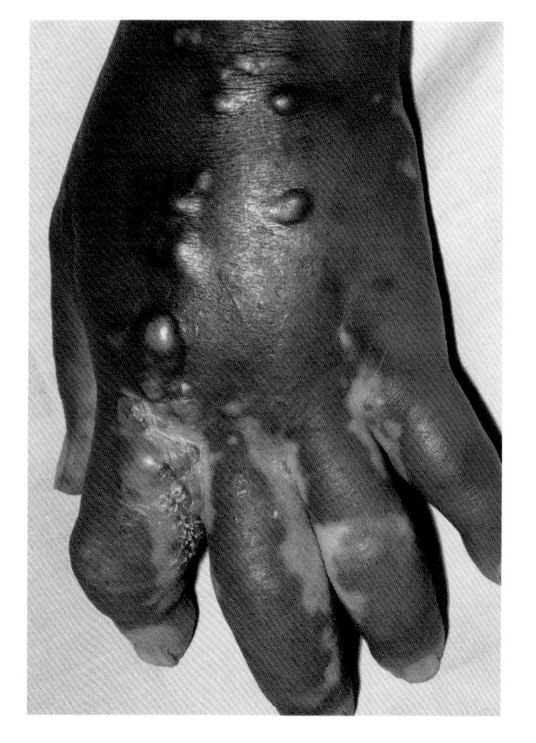

**Figure 331** Kaposi's sarcoma on the hand of a 75-year-old man.

*Treatment:* Radiotherapy works well for endemic KS if it is available.

## KELOID SCAR

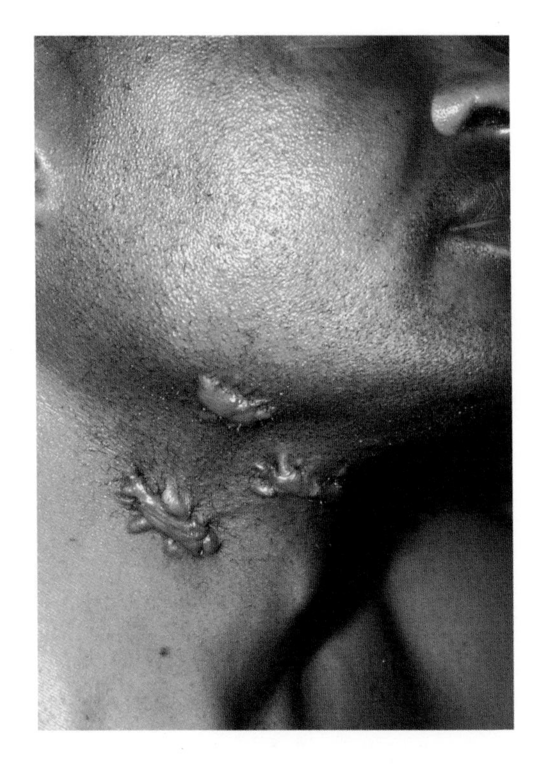

**Figure 332** A keloid scar is a scar which extends beyond the original site of injury. A hypertrophic scar is similar but confined to the site of injury.

*Treatment:* Small scars can be left alone or injected with triamcinolone (10mg/ml) monthly until they are flat. Larger scars can be excised and treated with radiotherapy within 24 hours of the surgery. Excision alone is likely to result in a recurrence.

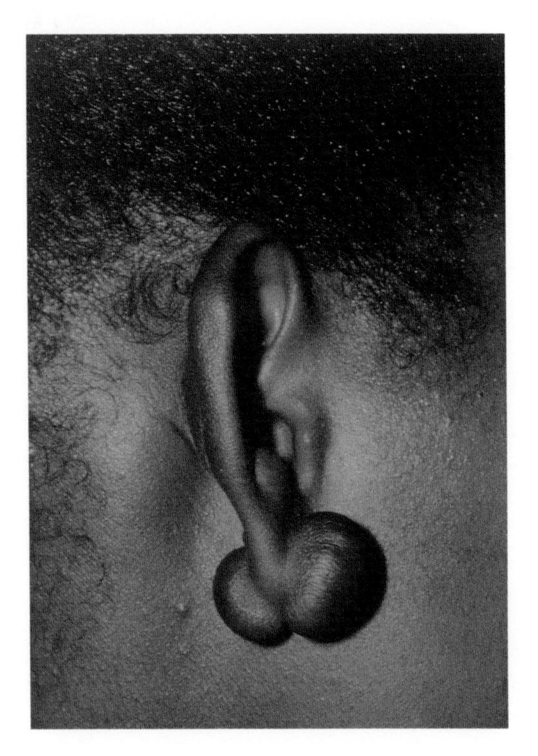

**Figure 333** Keloid scar on the ear lobe following ear piercing.

## KERATODERMA PALMARIS ET PLANTARIS

**Figures 334, 335, 336** This is a heterogeneous group of genetic disorders, which are characterised by abnormal keratinisation of the palms and soles. This variety is called diffuse palmoplantar keratoderma and is inherited as an autosomal dominant trait (*see* Figure 295).

*Treatment:* Topical salicylic acid (3% gradually increasing to up to 20%) applied bd.

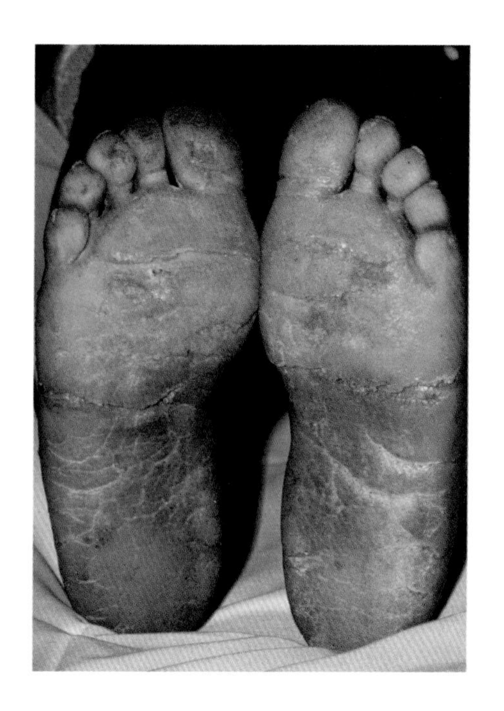

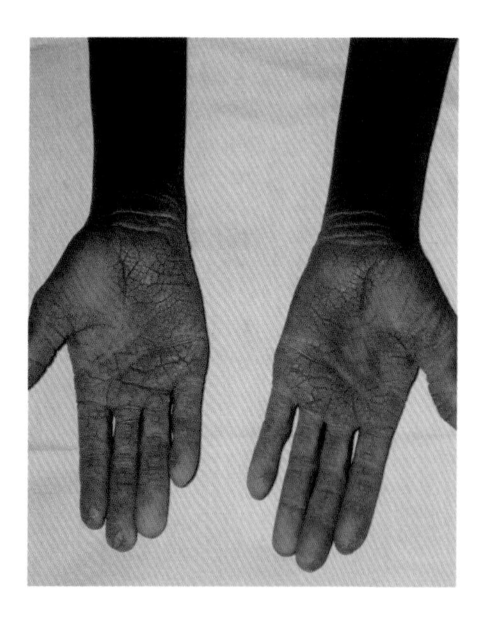

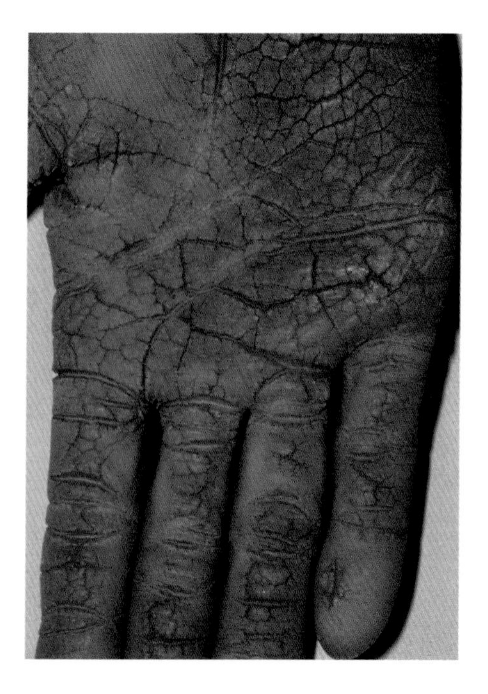

**Figure 337** Marginal keratoderma in a 9-year-old girl.

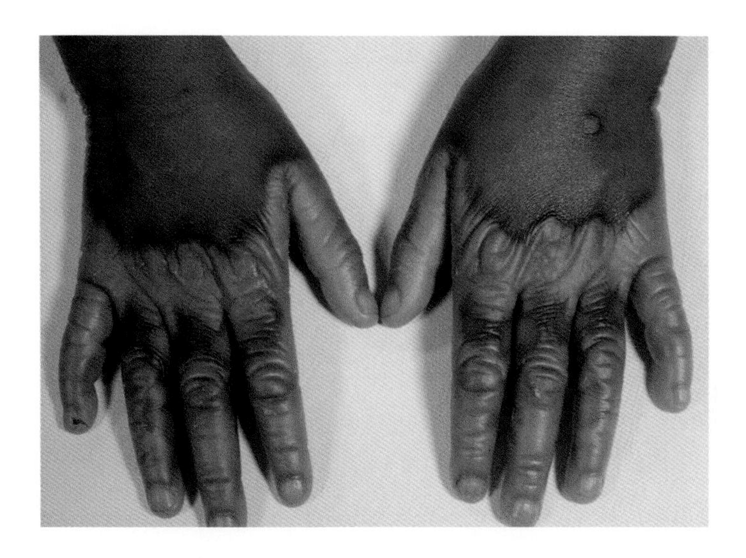

*Treatment:* Topical salicylic acid (3% gradually increasing to up to 20%) applied bd.

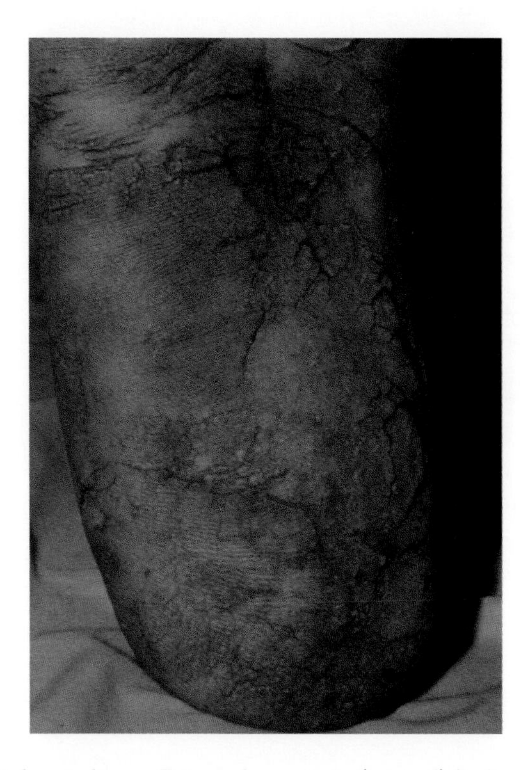

**Figure 338** Climatic keratoderma. Extremely common (normal) finding in people who walk around bare footed. The keratin thickens in response to constant trauma and the thick keratin splits causing fissures (which may be painful).

*Treatment:* Wear shoes (and socks).

## KERATOLYSIS EXFOLIATIVA

**Figure 339** Recurrent peeling of the skin of the palms. It is not really a disease but a normal variant.

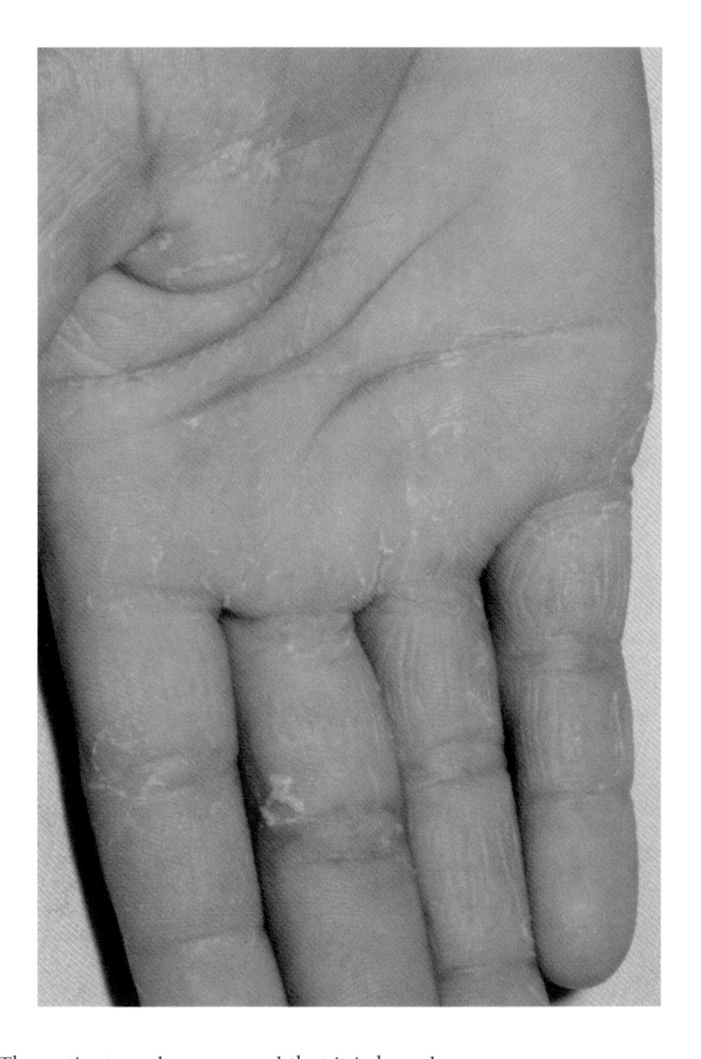

*Treatment:* The patient can be reassured that it is harmless.

## KERATOLYSIS – PITTED

**Figure 340** Infection of the stratum corneum with corynebacteria in individuals with sweaty feet. Small round holes appear in the keratin on the ball of the foot, the undersurface of the toes or the heel.

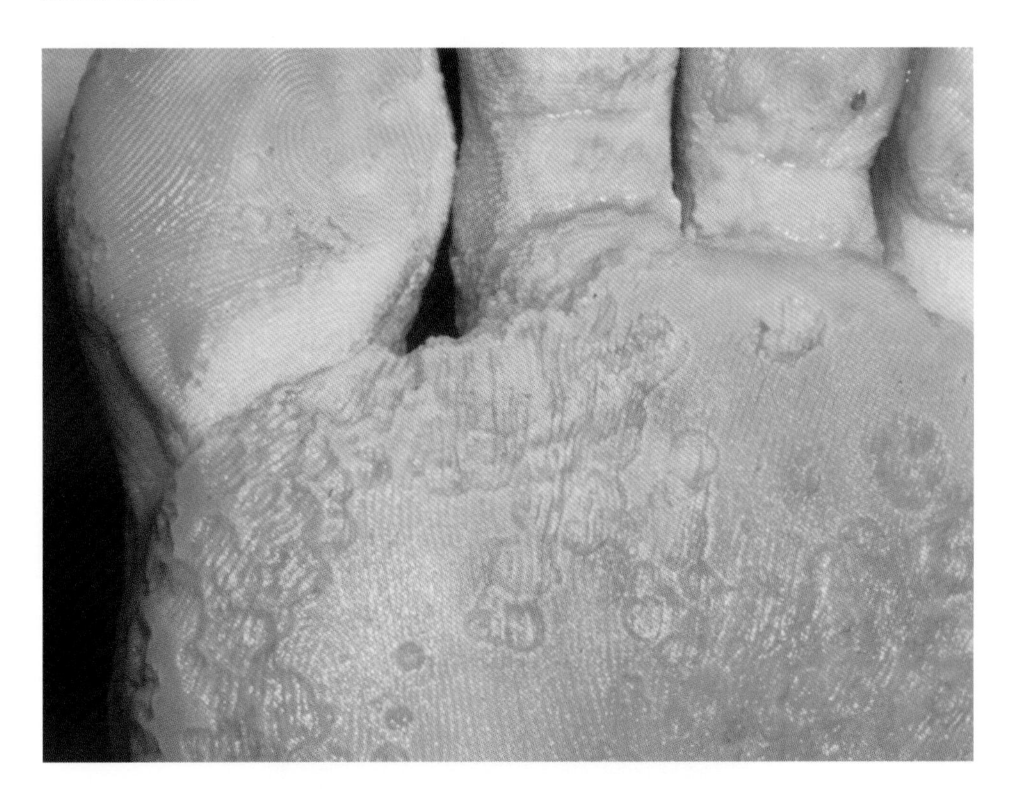

*Treatment:* Stop the sweating by soaking the feet in 5% formaldehyde for 10 minutes daily, or apply topical antibiotics (fusidic acid, erythromycin or mupiracin) bd.

## KERATOSIS PILARIS

**Figures 341, 342** Small follicular papules on the upper arms and thighs which feel rough to the touch. It is a common (normal) finding in children, and even more common in those with atopic eczema.

*Treatment:* Usually none is needed other than reassurance. If any treatment is wanted apply 10% urea cream or 3% salicylic acid ointment prn.

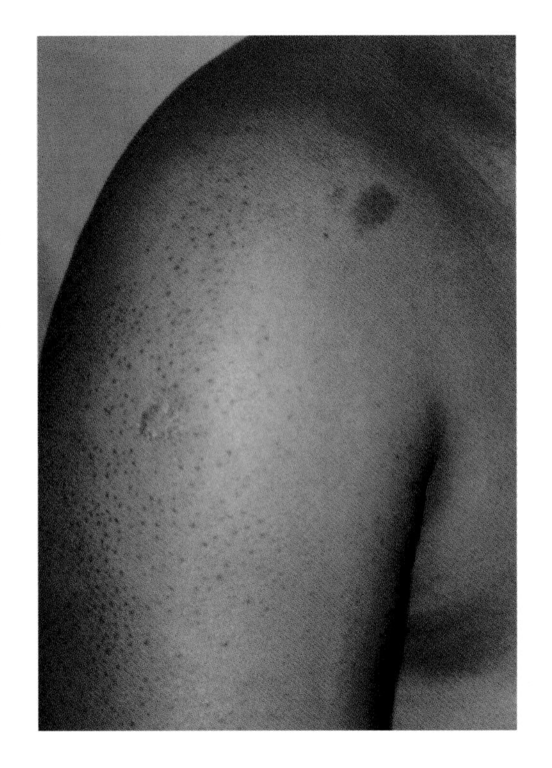

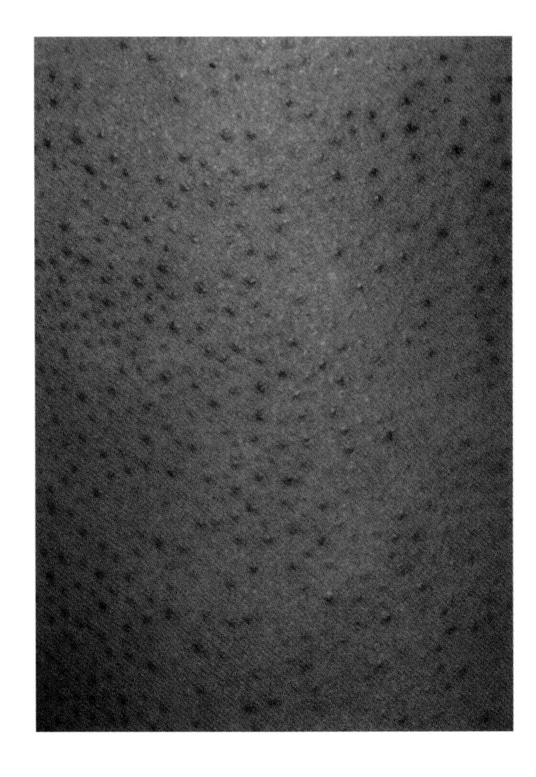

## KNUCKLE PADS

**Figure 343** Well circumscribed thickening of the epidermis over the joints of the fingers. Inherited as an autosomal dominant trait (*see* Figure 295), but not usually apparent until after puberty.

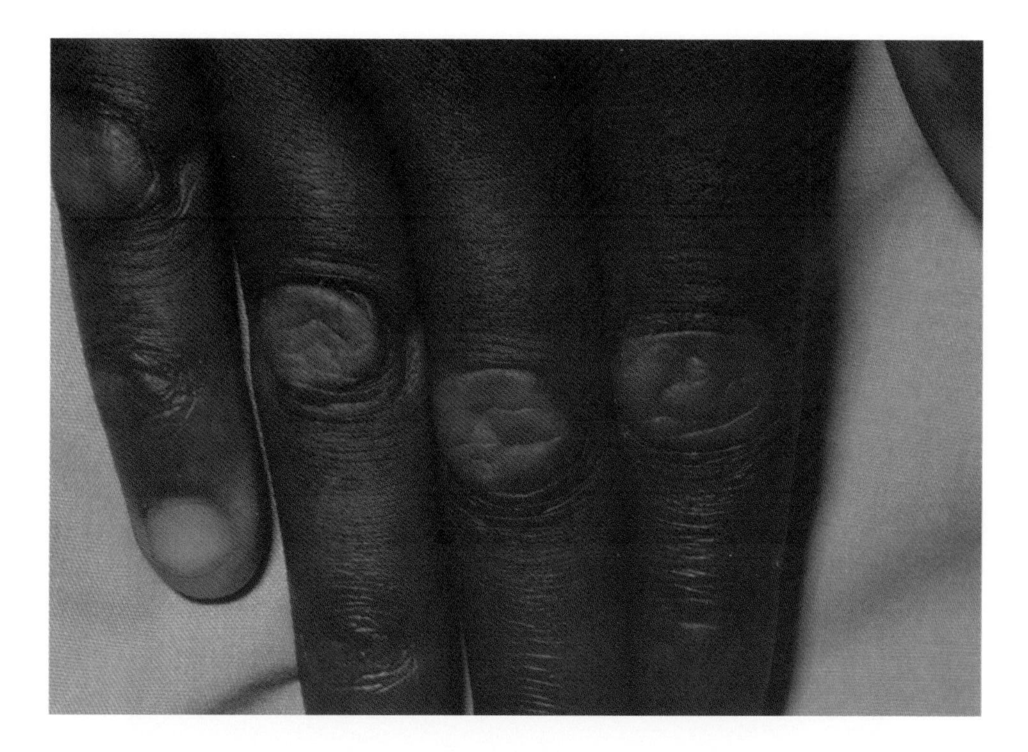

*Treatment:* None is needed other than reassurance that they are harmless.

## KOEBNER PHENOMENON

**Figure 344** Rash occurring at the site of an injury such as a scratch or cut. It occurs typically in psoriasis, lichen planus or plane warts. This picture shows numerous plane warts on the back of the hand and a single line of warts at the site of a scratch.

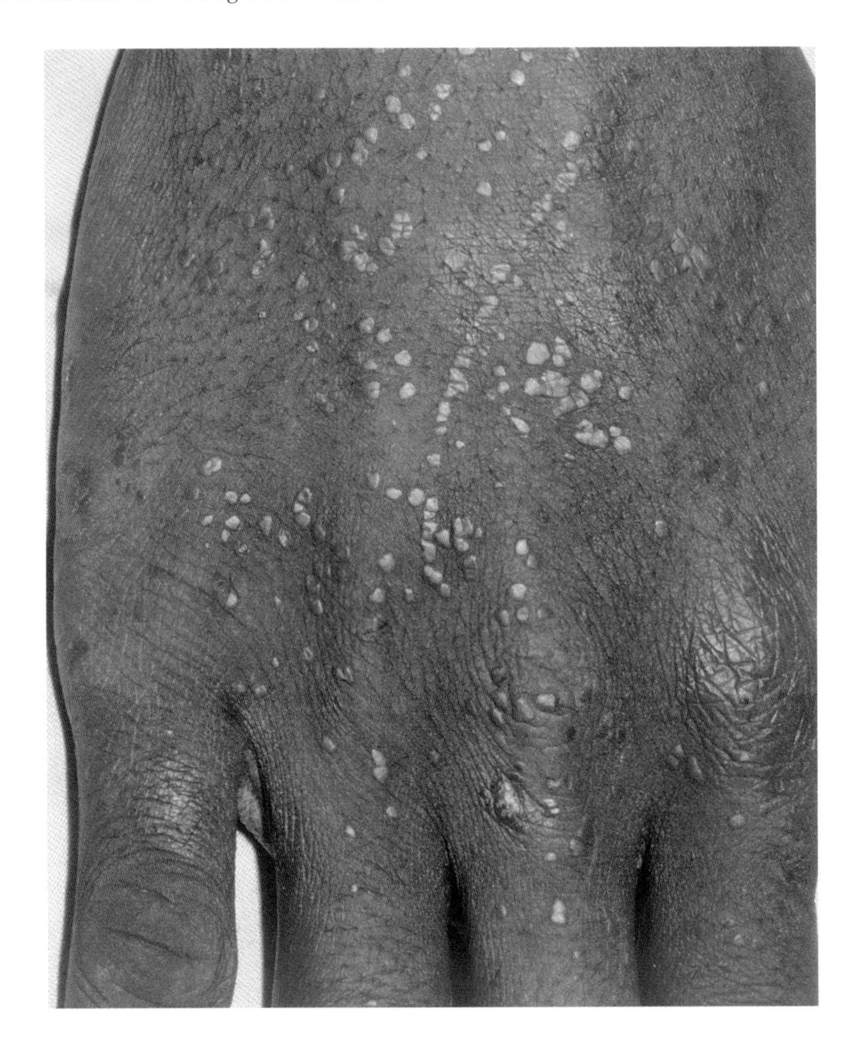

## KWASHIORKOR

**Figures 345, 346** Protein malnutrition which typically occurs in young children after measles. Clinically the skin of the legs looks like paint peeling off, there is marked oedema and the hair is sparse and looks as if it has had henna applied to it (reddish colour).

*Treatment:* Increase the protein in the diet and advise the mother about good eating habits for the future.

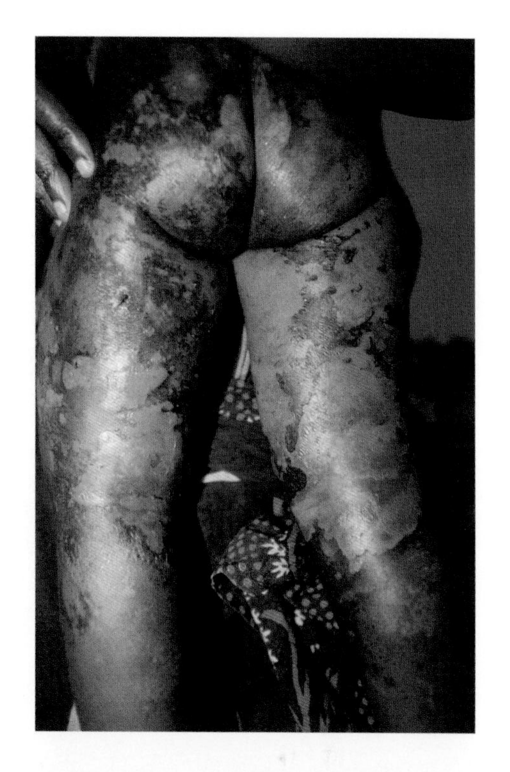

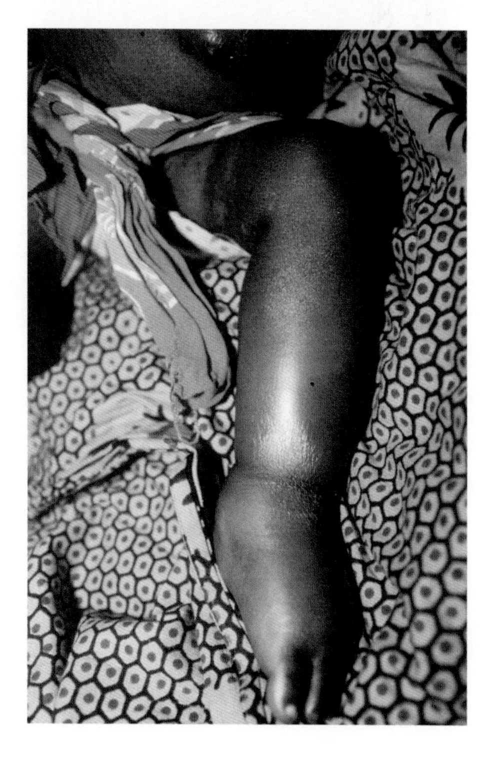

## LARVA MIGRANS

**Figure 347** Due to the dog or cat hookworm, *Ankylostoma braziliense*. The hookworm ova are excreted in the animal's faeces. In the soil the ova hatch into larvae after about 7 days. These can survive in the soil for several weeks. If children play in the soil the larvae can enter the skin and produce a 'creeping' eruption. This is a thin reddish line which moves each day in a serpiginous pattern. It is most commonly seen in children who have been playing in dirt where dog and cat faeces are found, but it is also often seen in foreign visitors to African beaches.

*Treatment:* 10% thiabendazole ointment applied topically qds for 1 week, or a single oral dose of ivermectin 200μg/kg body weight.

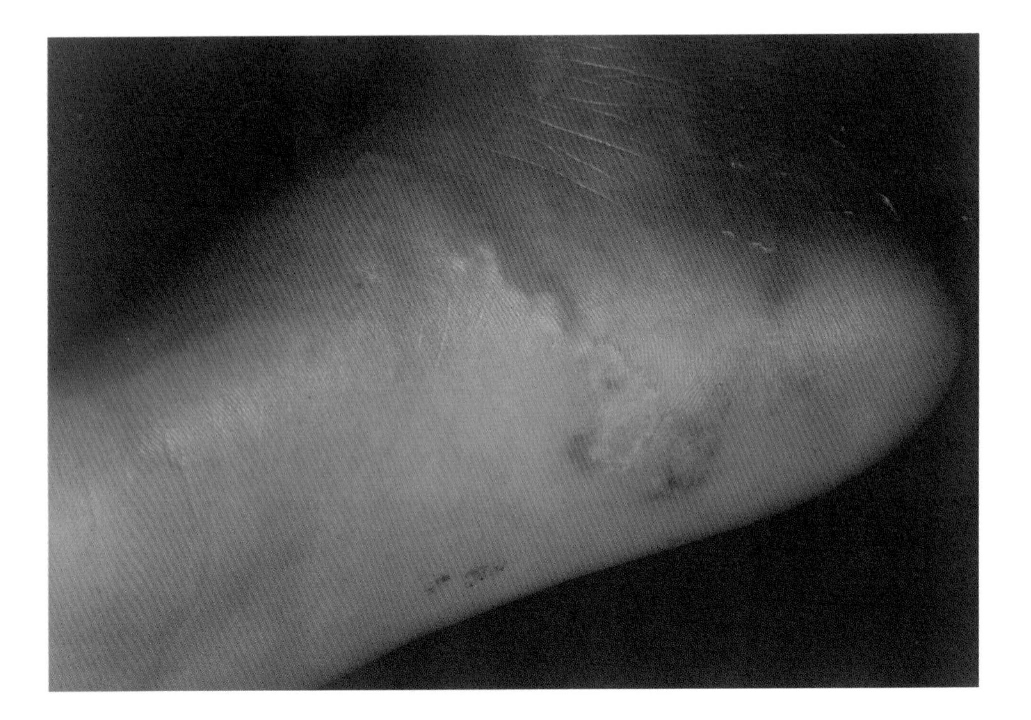

# LEISHMANIASIS

**Figure 348** Due to the protozoa, *Leishmania tropica*, and transmitted by the bite of a sandfly.

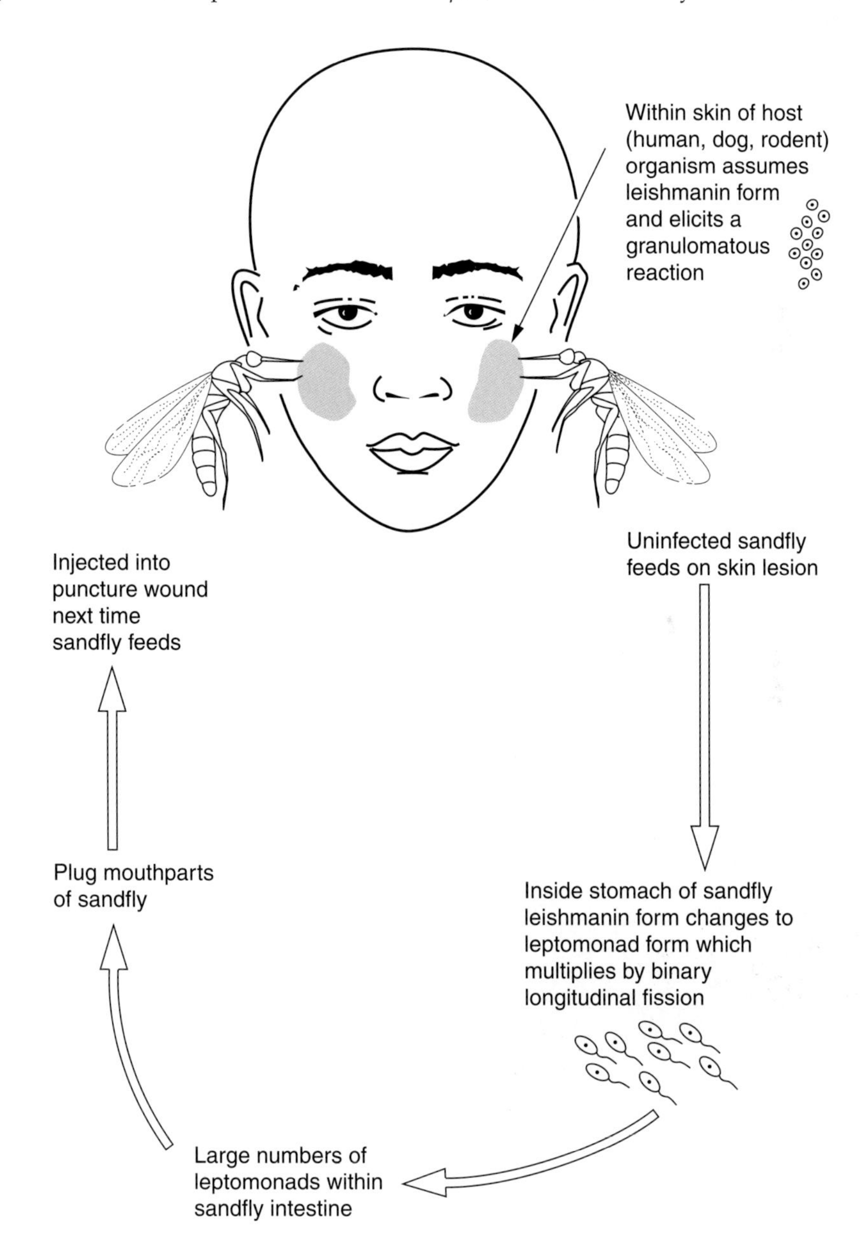

## Cutaneous leishmaniasis

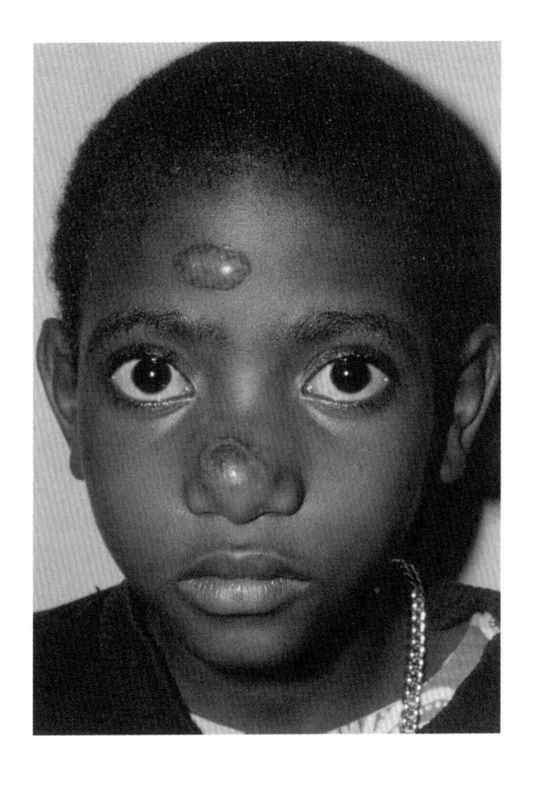

**Figure 349** An erythematous nodule develops at the site of the sandfly bite, in this case two nodules.

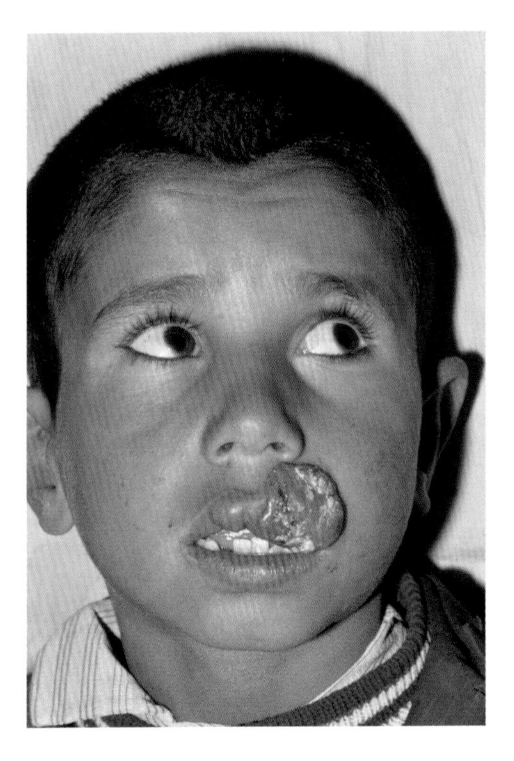

**Figure 350** The nodule flattens off to become a plaque.

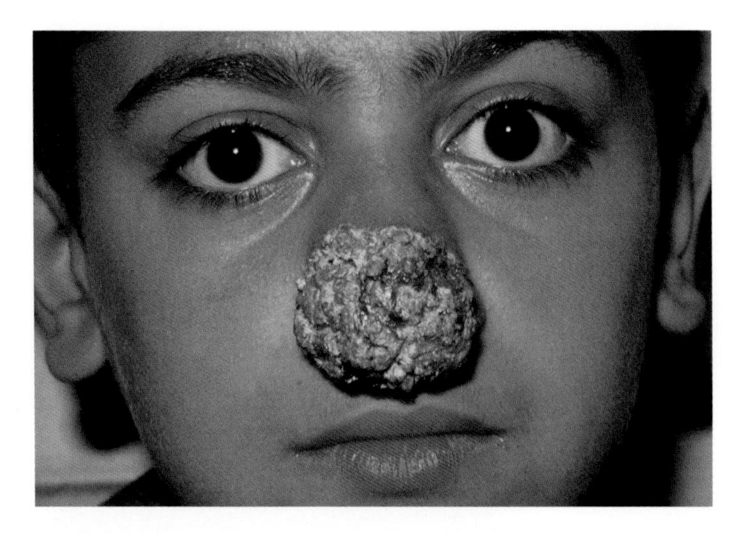

**Figure 351** The plaque may ulcerate and crust.

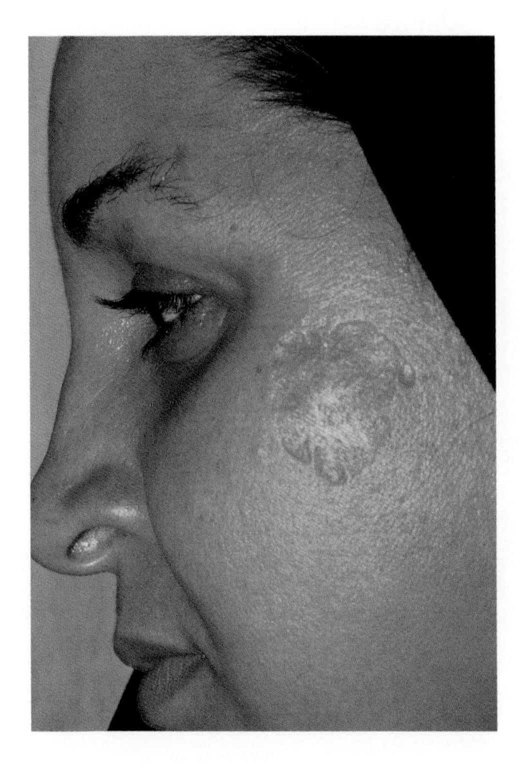

**Figure 352** After about 12 months it heals spontaneously leaving a depressed cribriform scar.

## Lupoid leishmaniasis

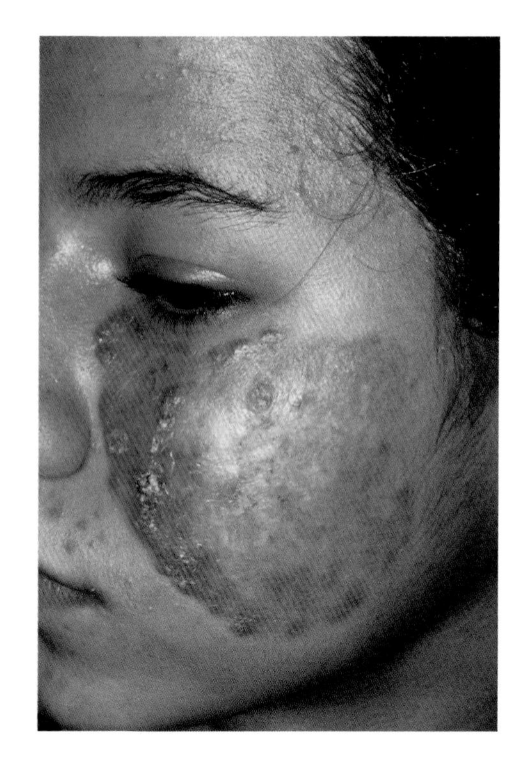

**Figure 353** In a patient who has previously had cutaneous leishmaniasis, new granulomatous papules occur around the edge of the scar. These do not heal spontaneously.

*Treatment:* Intramuscular injections of sodium stibogluconate 10mg/kg body weight daily until healing occurs.

## Diffuse cutaneous leishmaniasis

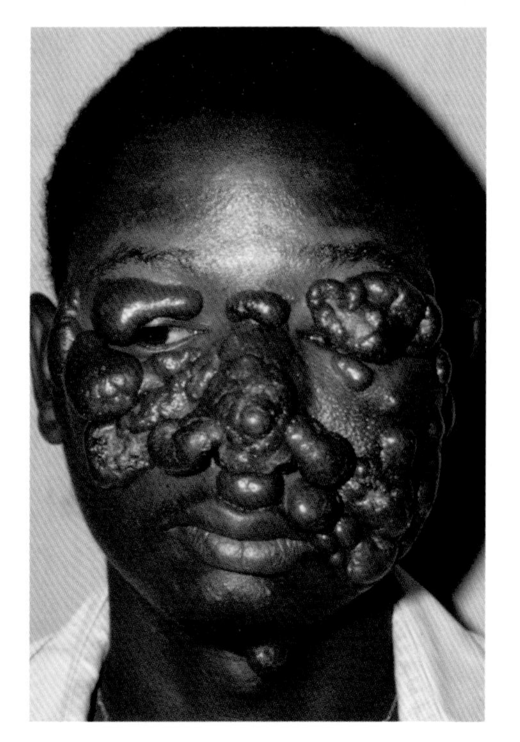

**Figure 354** This is leishmaniasis in an individual with no immunity to the organism (equivalent to lepromatous leprosy – *see* Figure 367). Extensive skin nodules which are full of organisms.

*Treatment:* Intramuscular injections of sodium stibogluconate 10mg/kg body weight daily until healing occurs.

## LEPROSY

Leprosy is a chronic bacterial infection due to *Mycobacterium leprae*. It is spread by droplet infection and has a long incubation period (anything from 2 months to 40 years). It principally affects the peripheral nerves and the skin. The cardinal features are palpably enlarged peripheral nerves, anaesthetic skin patches and the demonstration of acid fast bacilli (AFB) in the skin.

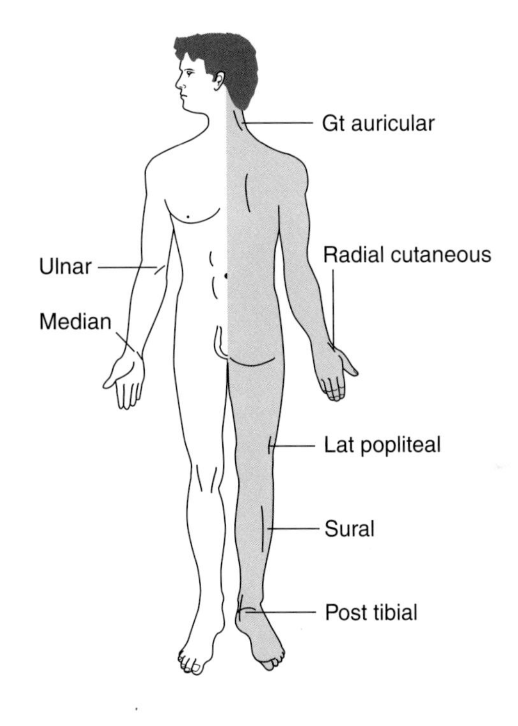


**Figure 355** The peripheral nerves which are enlarged are those that are near the skin's surface.

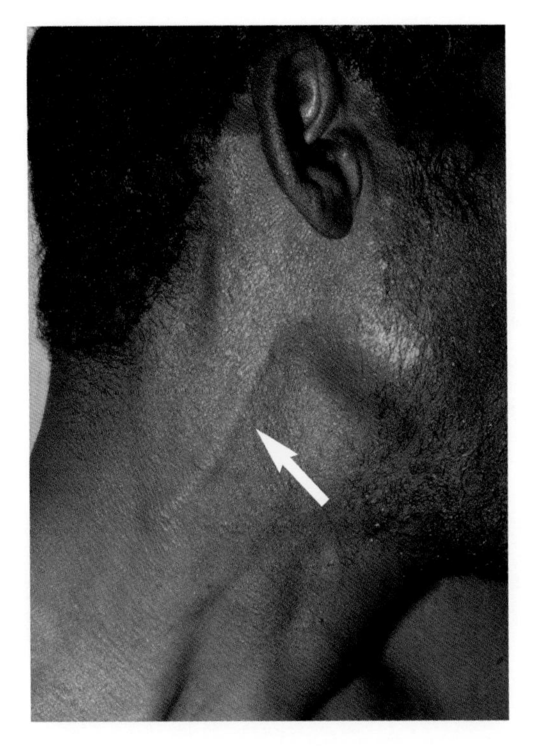

**Figure 356** The greater auricular nerve can sometimes be seen as well as felt.

## Diagnosis and classification of leprosy

**Figure 357** The clinical findings are very variable depending on the patient's cell mediated immunity to the leprosy bacillus.

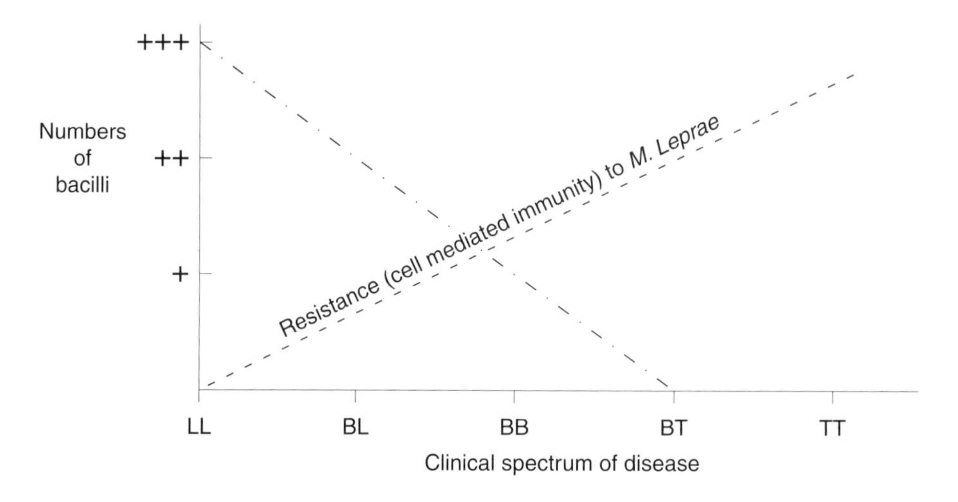


The diagnosis can be confirmed by doing slit skin smears and staining with a modified Ziehl-Neelson stain (Fite stain). Two things are measured on slit skin smears:

- *The bacterial index* (BI) is the density of leprosy bacilli and includes both living and dead bacilli.

  BI 1+ = 1–10 bacilli in 100 oil immersion fields

  2+ = 1–10 bacilli in 10 oil immersion fields

  3+ = 1–10 bacilli in 1 oil immersion field

  4+ = 10–100 bacilli in an average oil immersion field

  5+ = 100–1000 bacilli in an average oil immersion field

  6+ = >1000 bacilli (many globi) in an average oil immersion field

- *The morphological index* (MI) is the percentage of living bacilli in relation to the total number in the smear. It is given as a percentage.

A BI of 0 or 1+ is classified as paucibacillary leprosy.

A BI of 2+ or more is classified as multibacillary leprosy.

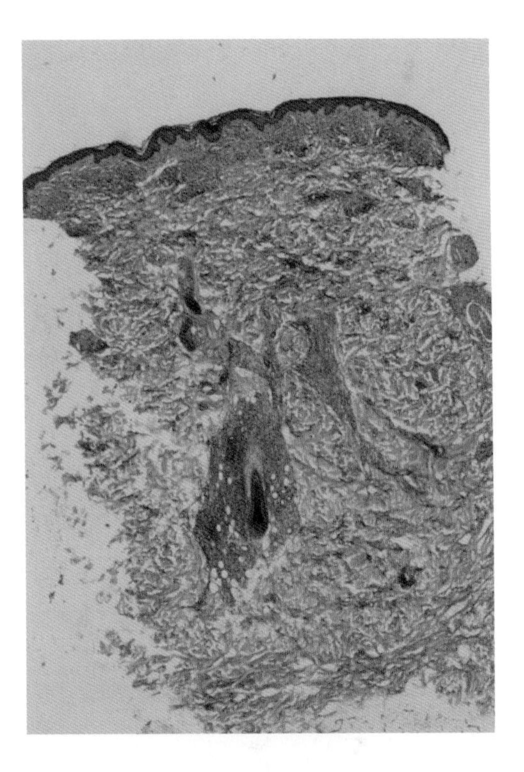

**Figures 358, 359** The diagnosis can also be confirmed by doing a biopsy of one of the skin lesions. In tuberculoid leprosy there are non-caseating granulomas in the upper dermis which extend right up to the dermo–epidermal junction. In addition, there is a granulomatous reaction in a cutaneous nerve.

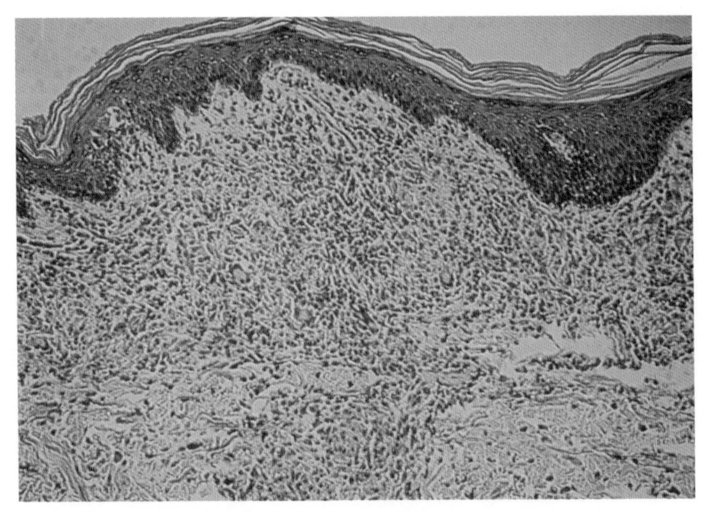

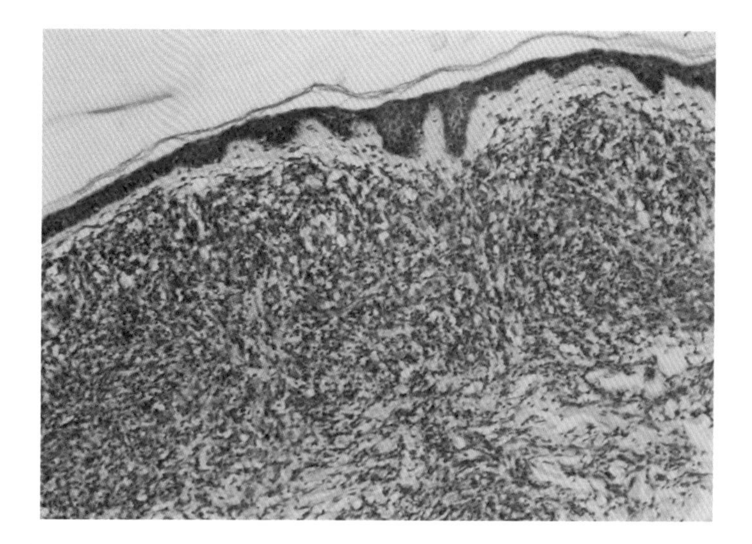

**Figure 360** Biopsy from lepromatous leprosy (Fite stain). There are foamy histiocytes in the dermis and a clear grenz zone between the dermis and the epidermis.

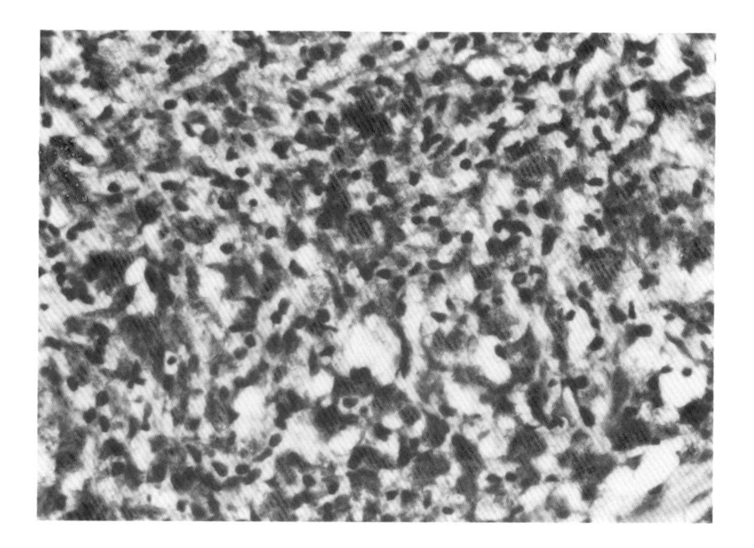

**Figure 361** Biopsy from lepromatous leprosy (same patient and same specimen as in Figure 360). Very numerous AFB (BI of 6+) seen staining red with Fite stain.

## Clinical features

**Figure 362** Indeterminate leprosy. Single or multiple hypopigmented, ill-defined macule(s) with normal sensation. One-third will disappear spontaneously, one-third will remain indeterminate, and one-third will develop into one of the clinical patterns of the disease.

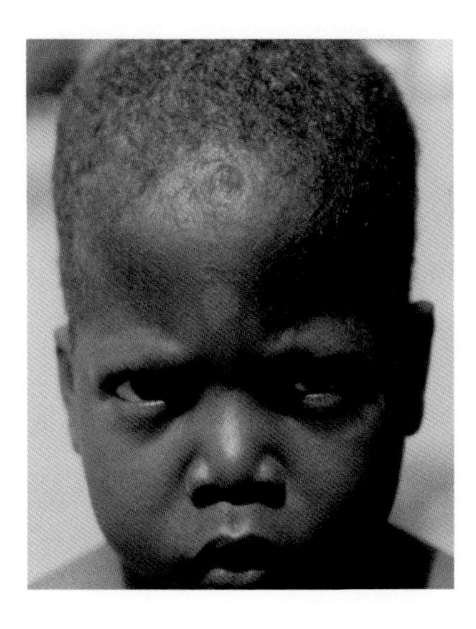

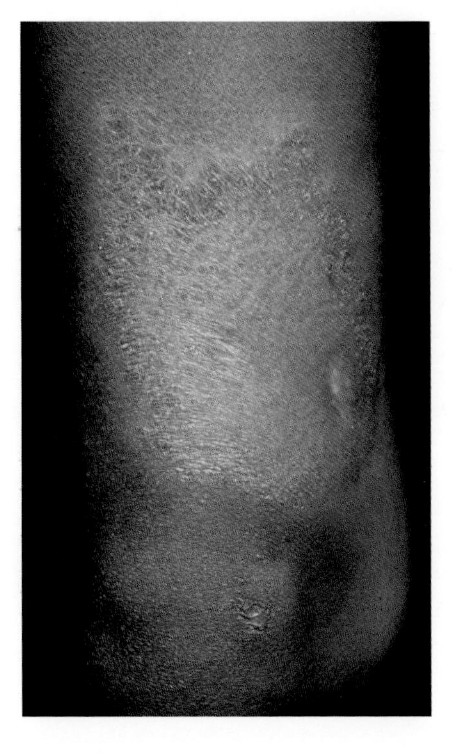

**Figure 363** Tuberculoid leprosy (TT leprosy) or paucibacillary leprosy. These patients have good cell mediated immunity and, on the skin, a single or few (2–5) anaesthetic plaque(s) with a raised border. Often there will be a single enlarged cutaneous nerve nearby.

**Figures 364, 365** Borderline tuberculoid leprosy (BT leprosy). Few, asymmetrical patches and/or plaques. Lesions may be coppery coloured or hypopigmented. This group of patients is particularly at risk of developing Type I reactions when started on treatment (BT stands for 'big trouble' – *see* Figures 376–7).

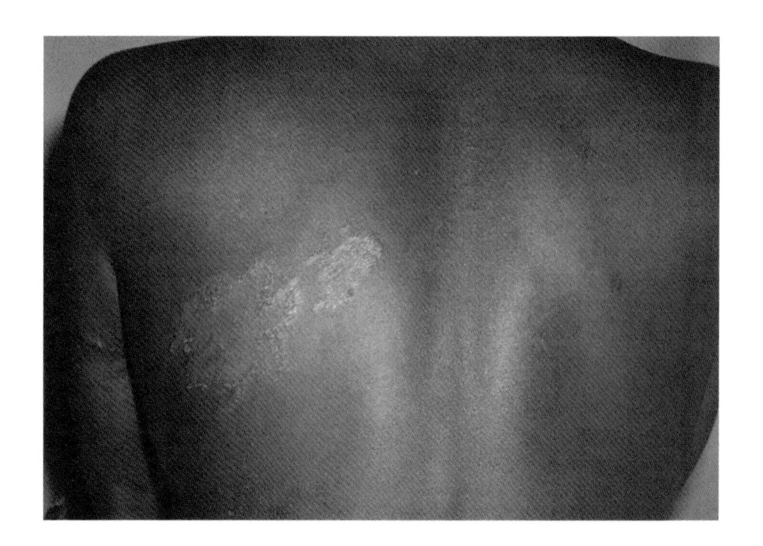

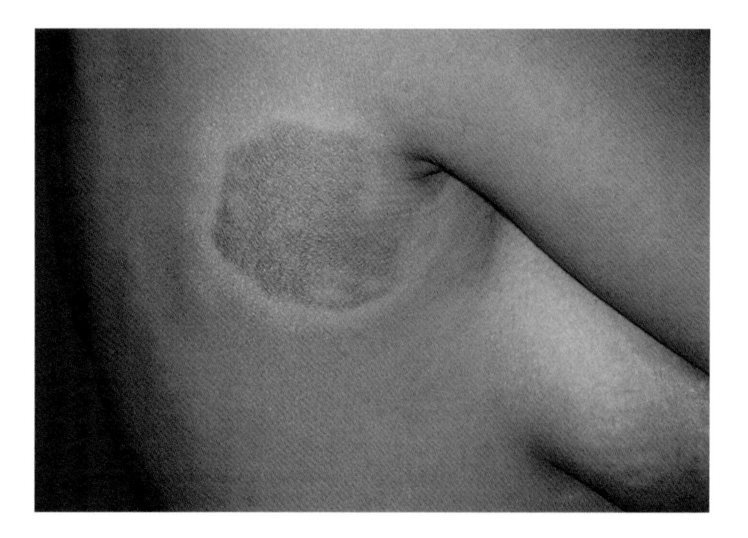

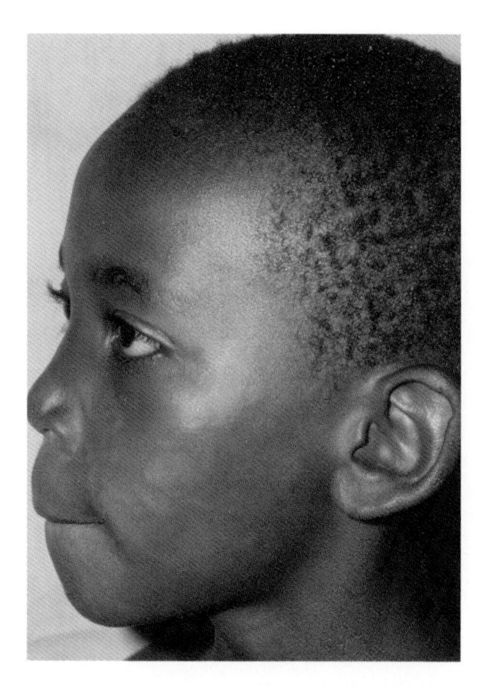

**Figure 366** Borderline lepromatous leprosy (BL leprosy). Multiple asymmetrical patches, nodules and plaques which are not anaesthetic.

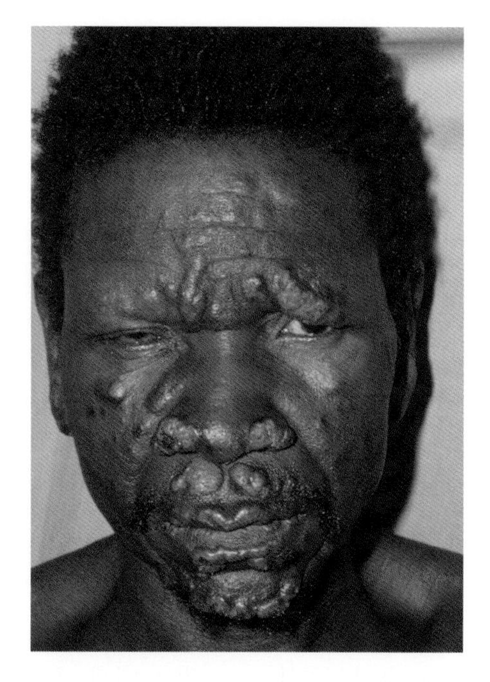

**Figure 367** Lepromatous leprosy (LL leprosy). Widespread symmetrical papules and nodules with loss of eyebrows (madurosis).

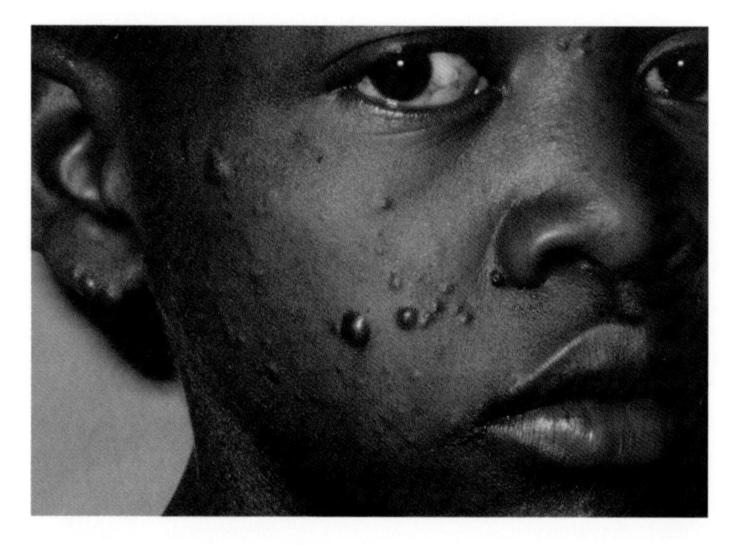

**Figure 368** LL leprosy. Shiny papules on the cheek and ear lobe. The ear is commonly involved.

**Figure 369** LL leprosy. Widespread non-anaesthetic plaques on the back.

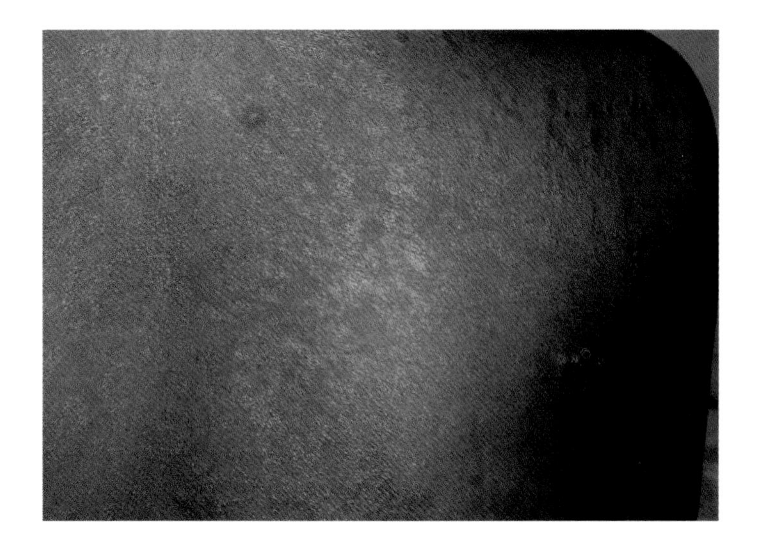

*Treatment of paucibacillary leprosy* (TT and BT): Rifampicin 600mg orally once a month, supervised, plus dapsone 100mg daily. Treatment is given for 6 months.

*Treatment of multibacillary leprosy* (BB, BL and LL): Rifampicin 600mg orally once a month, supervised, plus clofazamine 300mg orally once a month, supervised, plus clofazamine 50mg daily, plus dapsone 100mg daily. Treatment is given for 2 years.

## Disability in leprosy

Most of the disability in leprosy is due to sensory, motor or autonomic nerve damage. This can be due to invasion of the peripheral nerves with the leprosy bacilli (or the inflammatory reaction to those bacilli – *see* Figure 358), a leprosy reaction or secondary infection. Many patients present very late to the doctor with disability already present.

## WHO classification of disability

| | *Hands and feet* | *Eyes* |
|---|---|---|
| **Grade 0** | No anaesthesia<br>No visible deformity or nerve damage | No eye problems<br>No visual impairment |
| **Grade 1** | Anaesthesia present<br>No visible deformity or nerve damage | Eye problems present<br>Vision 6/60 (can count fingers at 6 metres) |
| **Grade 2** | Visible deformity | Severe visual impairment (<6/60) |

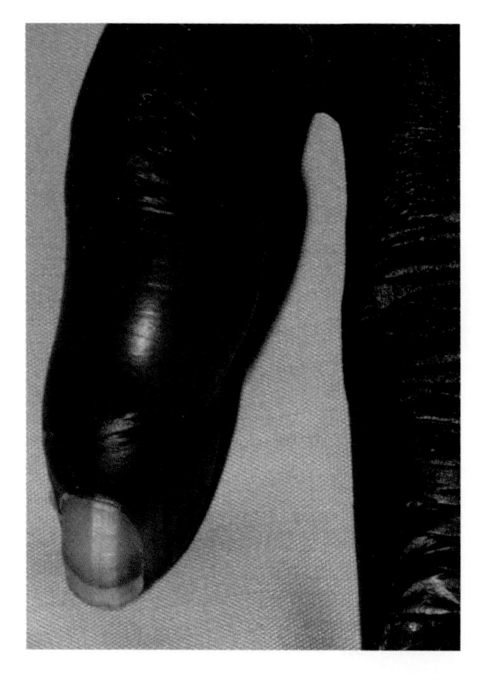

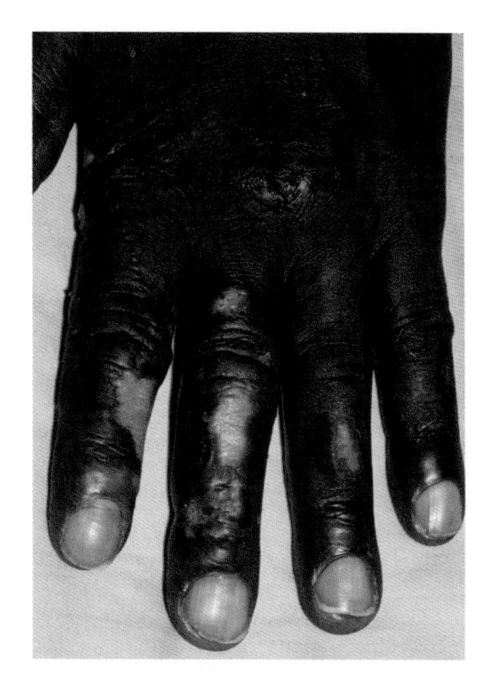

**Figures 370, 371** Widespread nerve damage with glove and stocking anaesthesia in patients with BL and LL leprosy. Patients develop blisters due to burns or other trauma, leading to scarring and loss of pigment.

**Figure 372** Ulceration on the sole in an anaesthetic foot is common following trauma.

*Treatment:* Soak the foot in warm, soapy water for half an hour, shave off all excess keratin from around the ulcer and use a moisturiser to keep the skin soft. Wear shoes with Plastazote insoles that fit well.

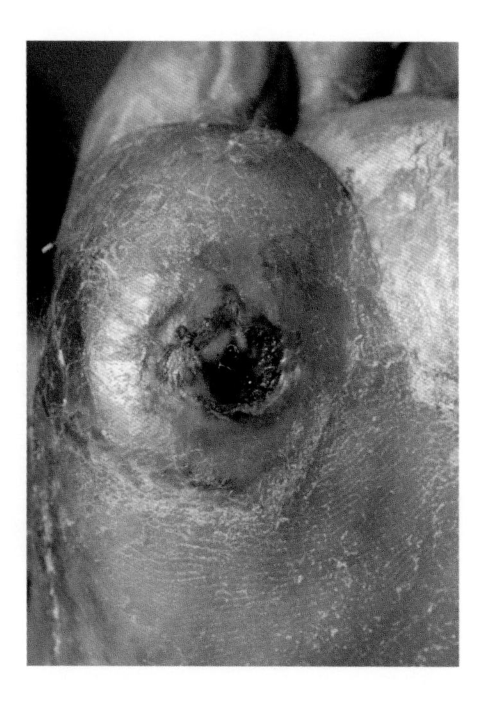

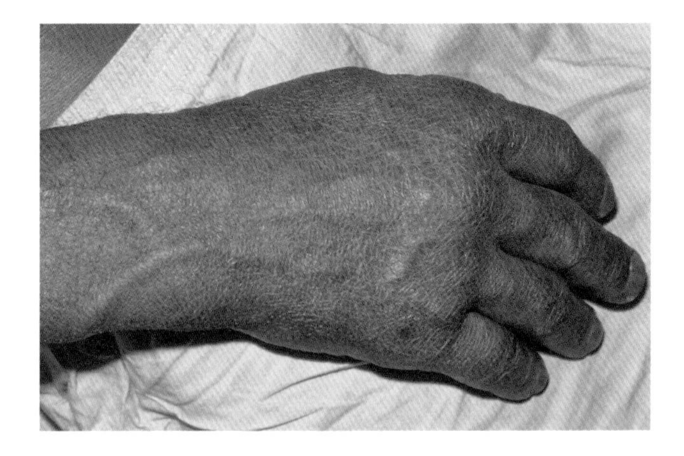

**Figure 373** Autonomic nerve damage leads to dryness of the skin, very noticeable when you shake the patient's hand.

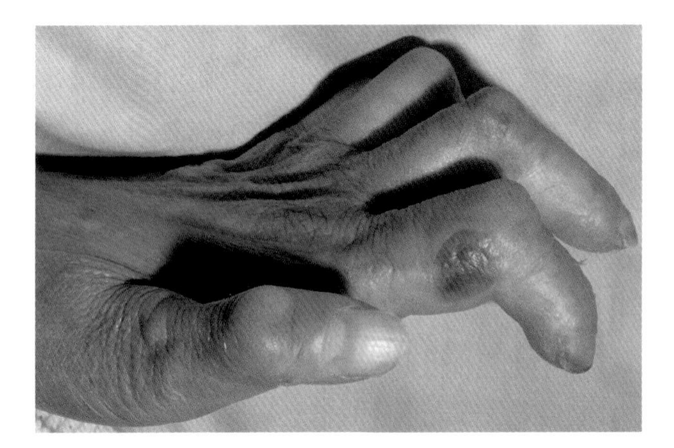

**Figure 374** Claw hand due to median and ulnar nerve damage.

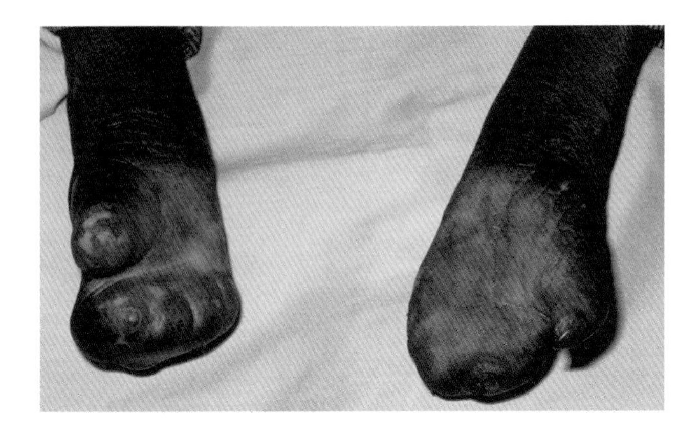

**Figure 375** Repeated trauma to anaesthetic limbs can cause resorption of the fingers and toes.

## Leprosy reactions

There are two types of leprosy reaction:

- *Type I reactions* are due to a change in cell mediated immunity (CMI). A reversal or upgrading reaction occurs where the CMI improves after starting treatment. A downgrading reaction occurs in patients receiving inadequate or irregular treatment; the CMI decreases and there is a shift towards the lepromatous end of the clinical spectrum.

- *Type II reaction* (erythema nodosum leprosum). This is an immune complex reaction (Type III allergic reaction) and is not associated with any change in CMI. It occurs in patients with BL and LL leprosy.

**Figure 376** Type I (reversal) reaction. This is a Type IV hypersensitivity reaction. Antigen from the dying bacilli reacts with T lymphocytes causing a rapid improvement in CMI. It is likely to occur in patients with borderline leprosy (mainly BT and BB) within the first 6 months of starting treatment. Acute swelling of skin lesions occurs.

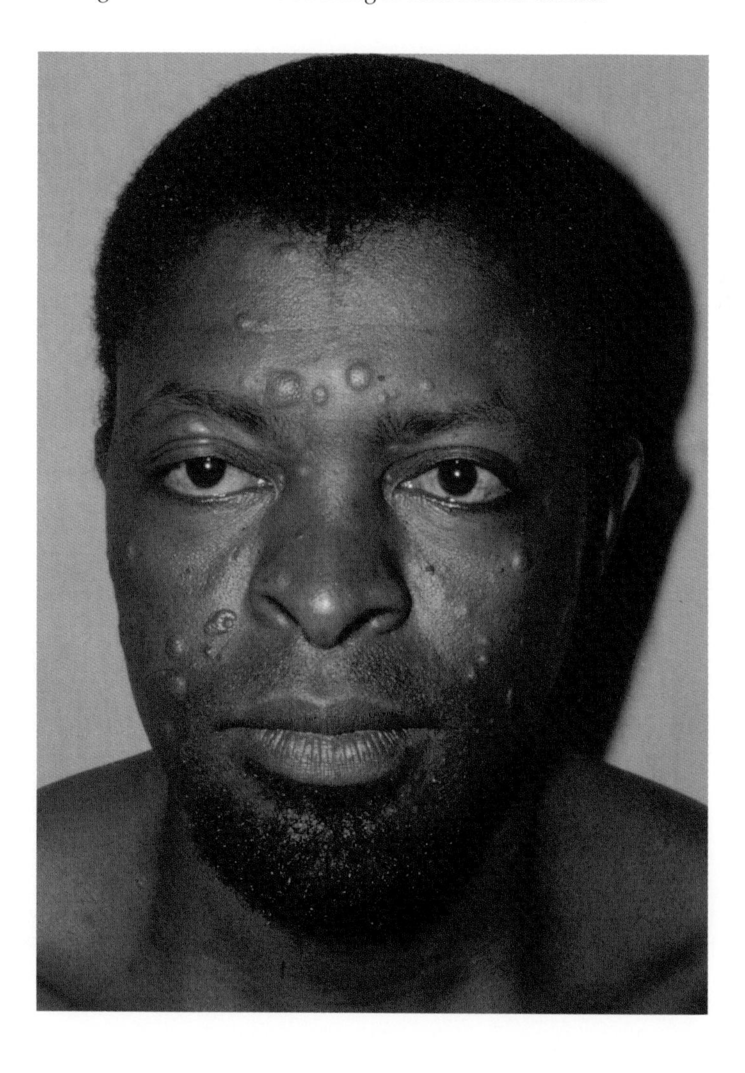

**Figure 377** Type I (reversal) reaction. Swelling of a hand or foot can occur. Also swelling and pain in cutaneous nerves can lead to wrist drop, drop foot or facial nerve palsy.

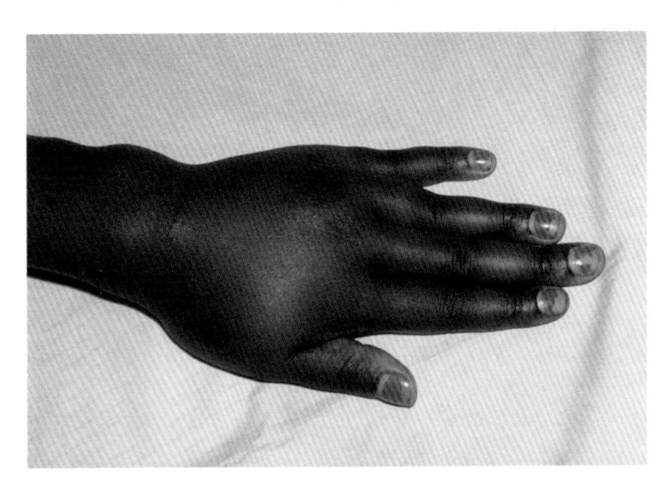

*Treatment:* Reversal reactions should be thought of as medical emergencies. Urgent treatment with high doses of systemic steroids (60mg of prednisolone daily) is required to prevent permanent nerve damage. The patient should stay on high doses of prednisolone until all symptoms subside. The dose is then gradually reduced over a period of 6 months.

**Figure 378** Type II reaction (erythema nodosum leprosum or ENL). Recurrent crops of tender red nodules occur symmetrically on the face, arms and legs. Some of them ulcerate. In addition, the patient may have orchitis, dactylitis, iridocyclitis and tender enlargement of peripheral nerves. ENL may become chronic and it can be very difficult to do much about it.

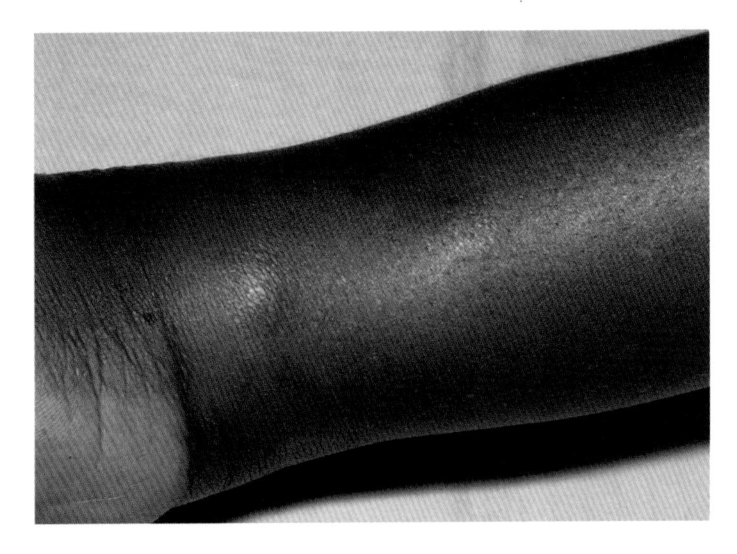

*Treatment:* Thalidomide is the drug of choice because it works within 48 hours. Start with 100mg tds, then taper it off over 3–4 weeks. Remember that this drug is teratogenic and must not be given to pregnant women. If thalidomide is not available, use prednisolone 60mg/day, but taper it down over a period of 2 weeks.

## LEUKAEMIA

**Figure 379** Acute myeloid leukaemia. Leukaemic cells in the skin may form nodules or plaques.

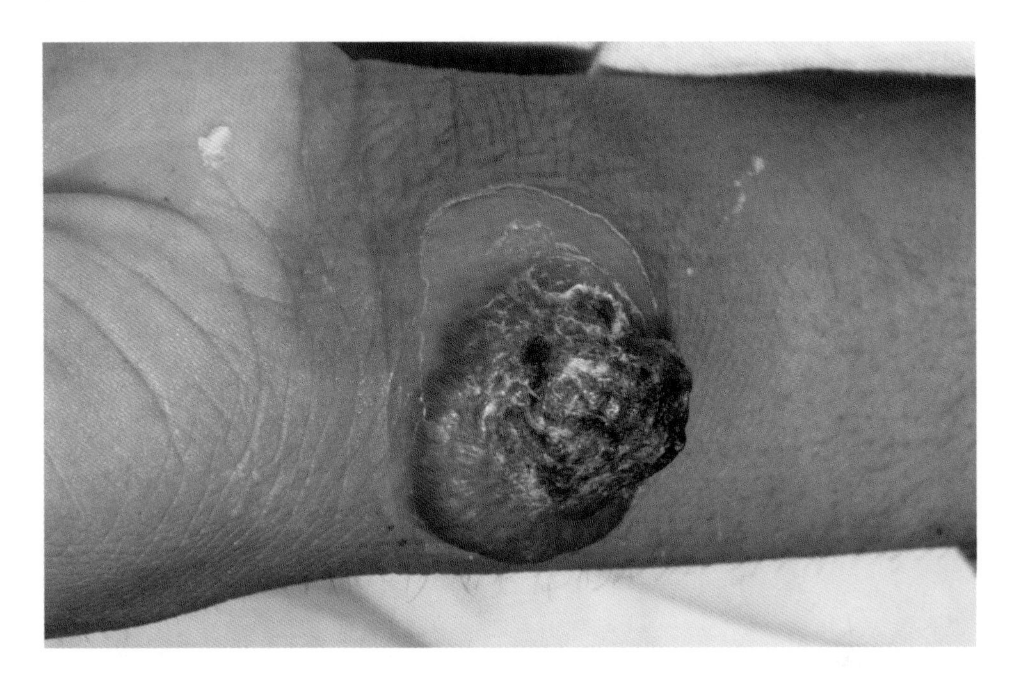

*Treatment:* Treat the leukaemia with cytotoxic drugs.

# LICE

Lice are wingless insects which pierce the skin to feed on human blood. There are three types: head lice, body lice and pubic (or crab) lice.

## Head lice

**Figure 380** The head louse (*Pediculus humanus capitis*) is about 3mm long and the female lays 7–10 eggs/day during a life span of one month. Infestation occurs by direct contact from head to head, mainly in children.

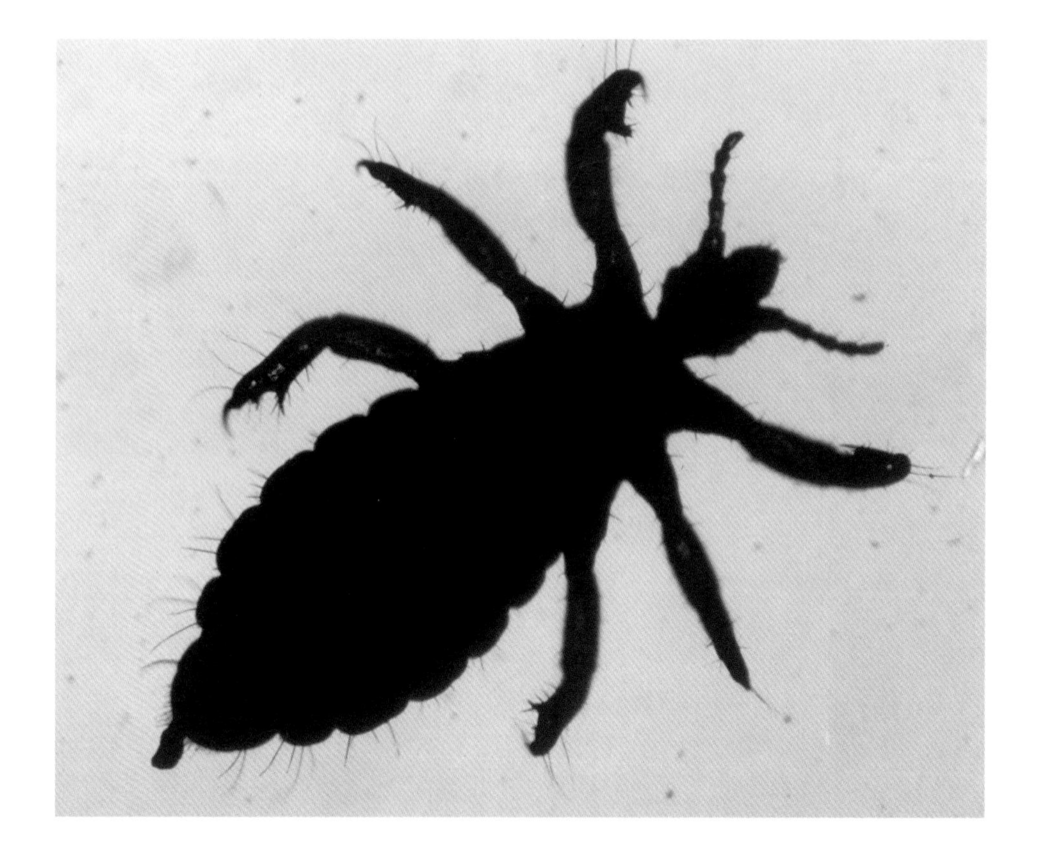

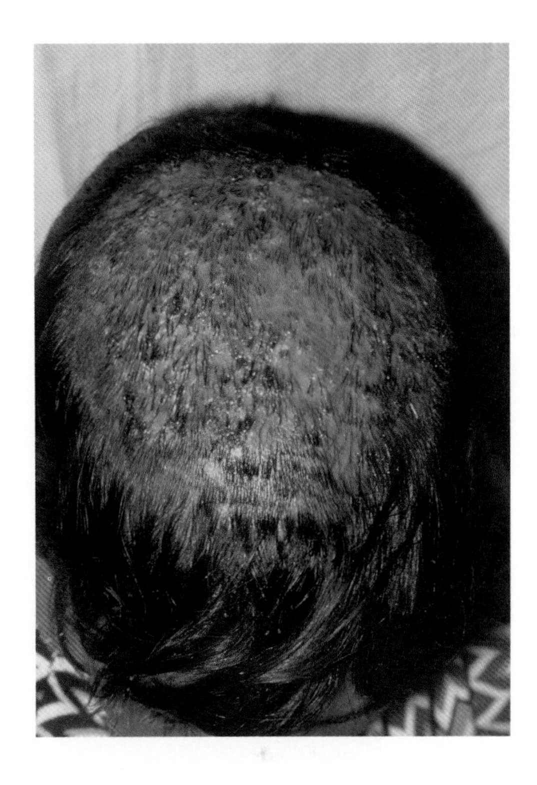

**Figure 381** Head lice are often asymptomatic, but if large numbers of lice are present there may be intolerable itching, with secondary bacterial infection and posterior cervical lymphadenopathy.

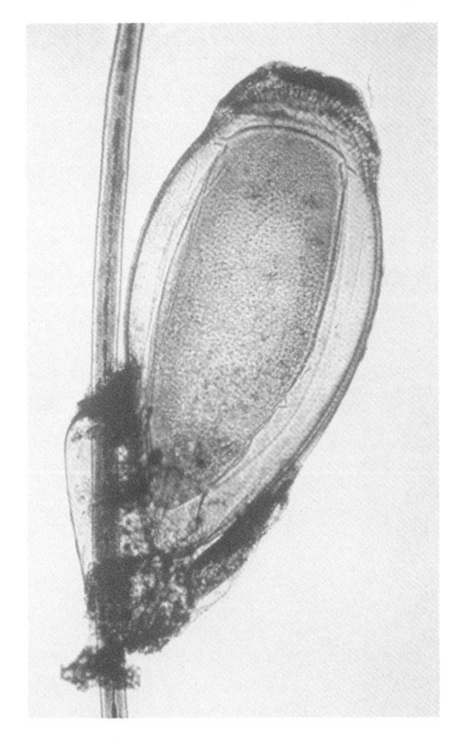

**Figure 382** The diagnosis is made by finding the nits (egg cases), which are white opalescent oval capsules firmly attached to the hairs.

*Treatment:* 0.5% Malathion or 0.5% Carbaryl in an alcoholic lotion applied to the scalp and left there for 12 hours. All children in the family should be treated at the same time. Alternatives would be to shave the head or to apply kerosene mixed with olive oil.

## Body lice

**Figure 383** The body louse (*Pediculus humanus corporis*) looks just like the head louse but it lives in the seams of clothing and lays its eggs there. It feeds on human blood, causing itching to the host.

*Treatment:* Wash and iron the clothes.

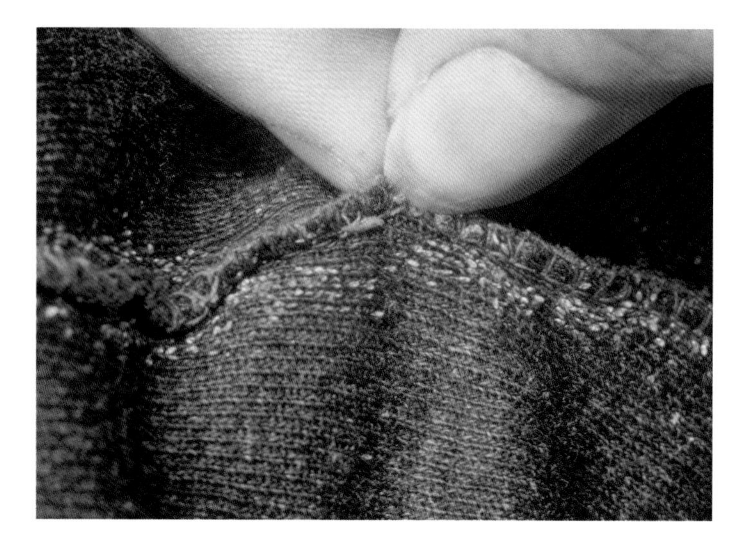

## Pubic (crab) lice

**Figure 384** Itching confined to the pubic area may be due to crab lice (*Pthirus pubis*). Look for the nits attached to the pubic hairs (they look just like the nits of head lice). The adult louse has large pincer-like legs (like those of a crab) with which it hangs on to adjacent pubic hairs whilst feeding. Crab lice are spread mainly by sexual intercourse.

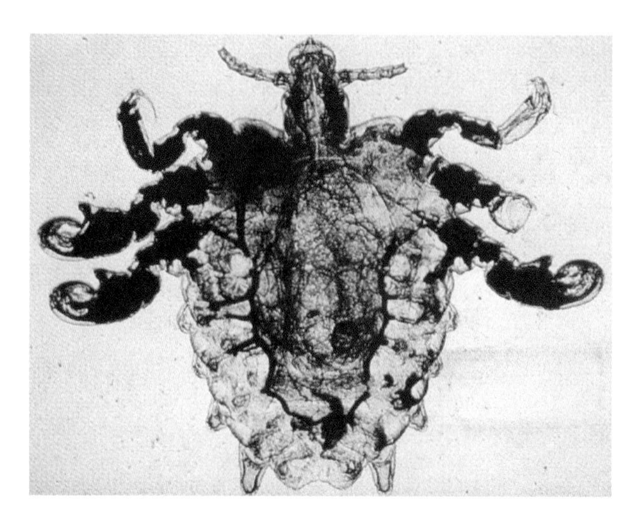

*Treatment:* Shaving the pubic hair is the simplest treatment. Alternatives are to apply 1% lindane cream or lotion, or 1% malathion lotion, and leave for 12 hours. For eyelashes, apply Vaseline and then pull off the lice and the egg cases.

**Figure 385** In individuals who are very hairy, the lice can move up through the body hair and be found in the axillae and even on the eyelashes.

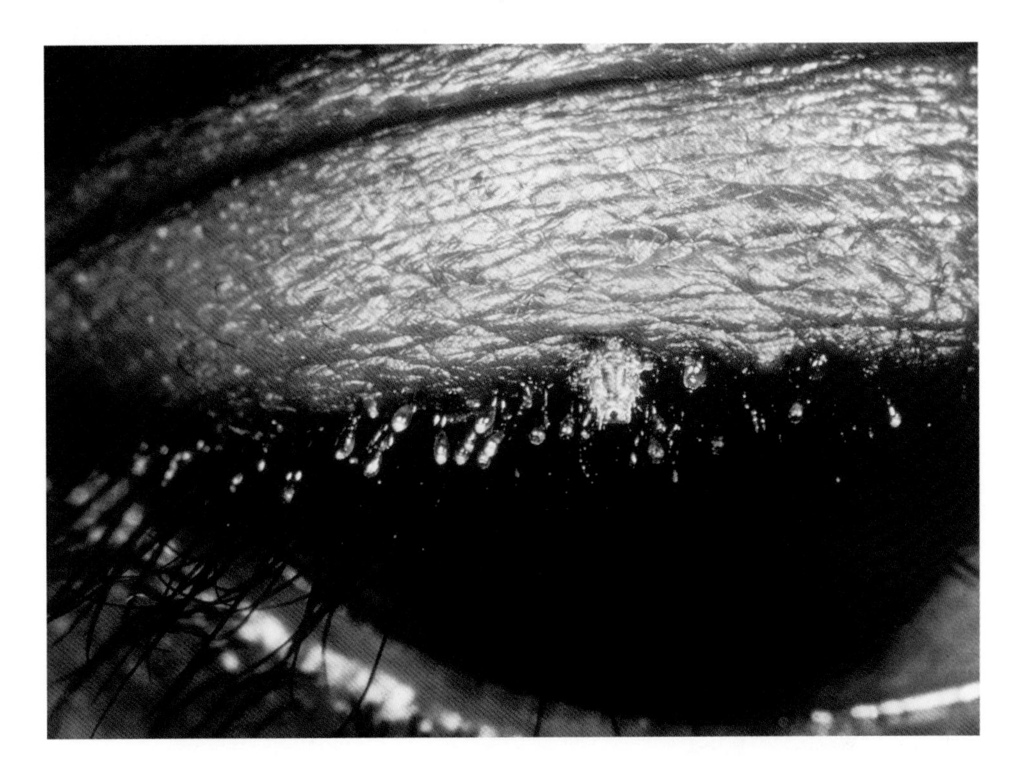

## LICHEN NITIDUS

**Figure 386** Disease of children or young adults. Non-itchy, tiny (pin head size), flat-topped shiny papules. They look like very small papules of lichen planus (*see* Figures 387–8) and can occur anywhere on the body. They may be grouped or generalised.

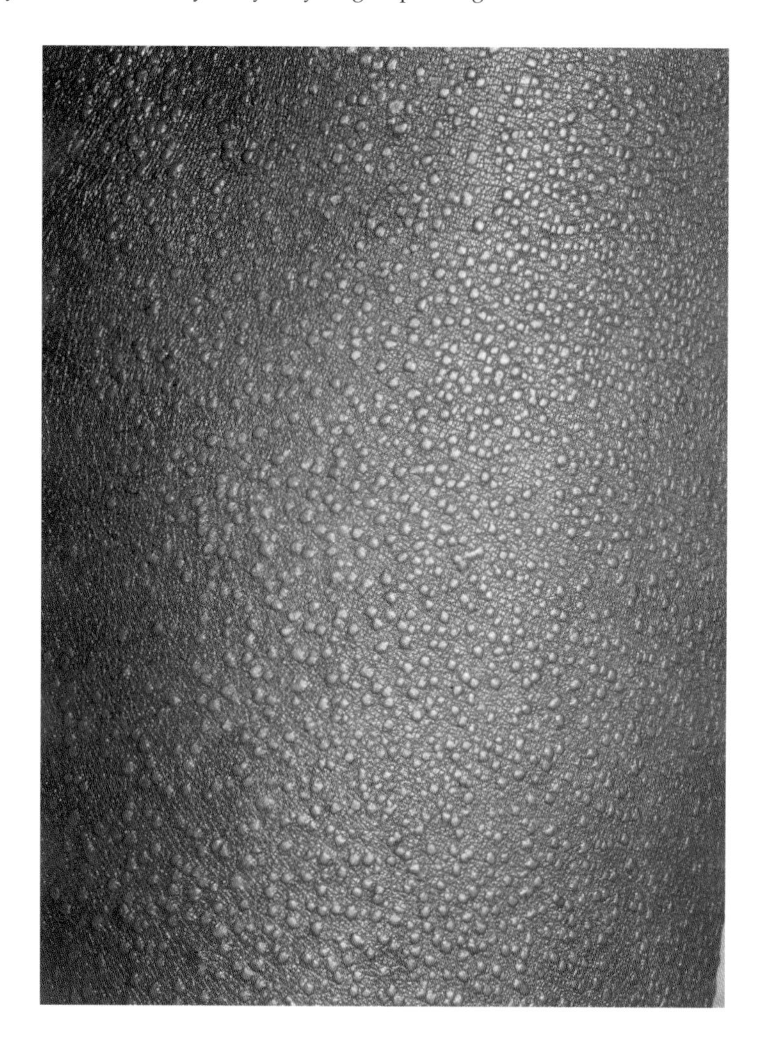

*Treatment:* Gets better spontaneously, so needs no treatment.

## LICHEN PLANUS

**Figures 387, 388** Mauve, flat-topped, shiny papules on the trunk and/or limbs. It is a very itchy rash which lasts 9–18 months. It mainly affects adults and is rare in children. It may cause the Koebner phenomenon (*see* Figure 344).

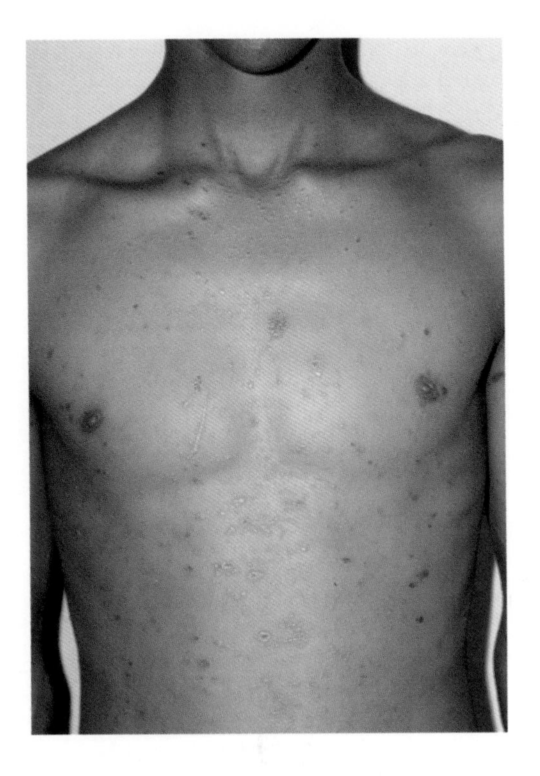

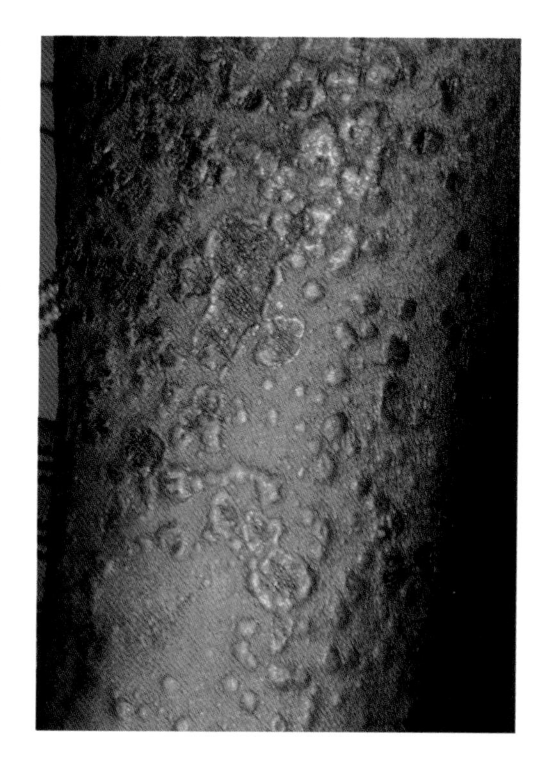

**Figure 389** Lichen planus may be very hyperpigmented with a characteristic bluish-black colour. Wickham's striae and white lacy lines in the mouth as described in Europeans are hardly ever seen.

*Treatment:* Moderately potent topical steroid (e.g. 0.025% betamethasone 17-valerate) ointment applied bd will help the itching; it will not make the rash go away until it has run its course.

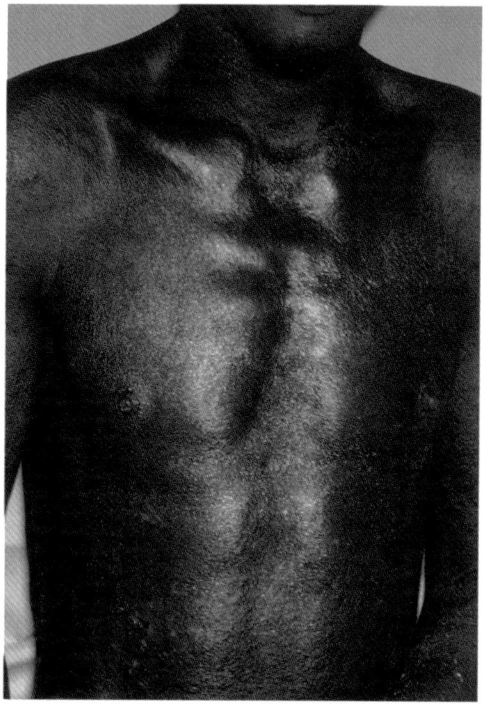

## Lichen planus-like drug eruption

**Figure 390** Bluish-black papules and plaques which are the colour of lichen planus, but more confluent, may be a lichenoid drug eruption. This one was due to ethambutol being taken for pulmonary TB in a patient who was HIV positive. Unusual drug eruptions should always make you think of HIV infection.

*Treatment:* Stop taking the offending drug.

## Lichen planus subtropicus

**Figure 391** This is a variant of lichen planus where the lesions are found on sun-exposed skin. It may sometimes be a manifestation of HIV infection.

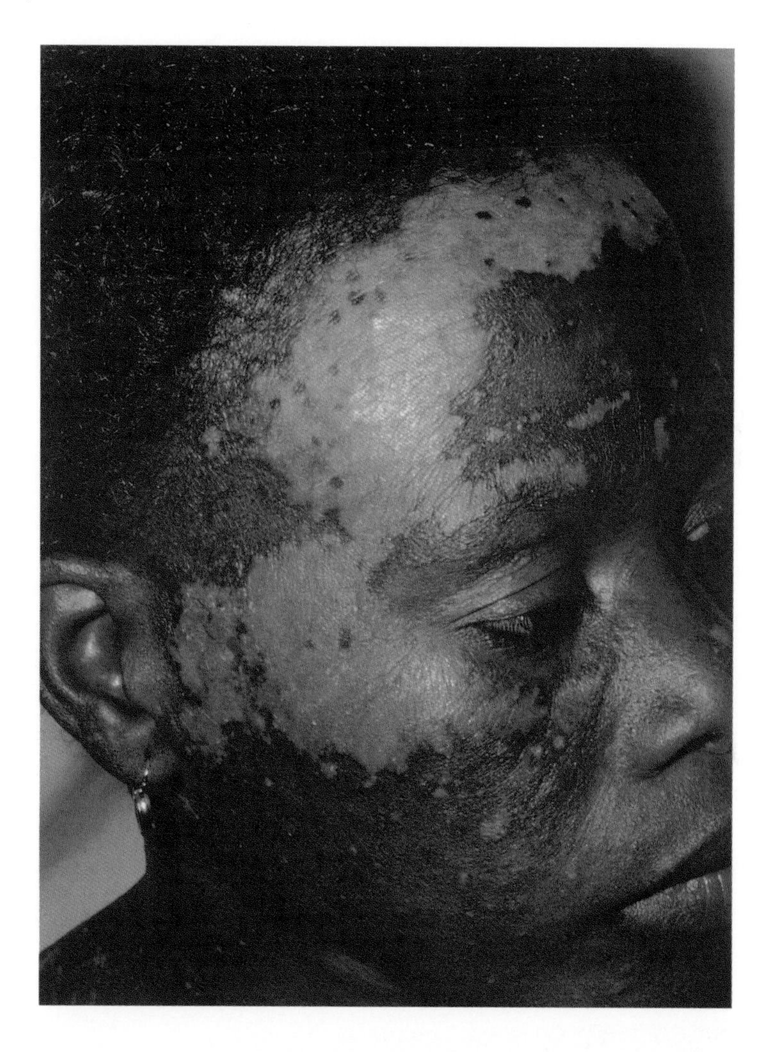

*Treatment:* Symptomatic with a topical steroid (e.g. 0.01% betamethasone 17-valerate) ointment bd.

## LICHEN SCLEROSIS ET ATROPHICUS

**Figure 392** Very itchy rash composed of white atrophic papules and plaques on the vulva and perianal skin in young girls and middle-aged women. There may be follicular plugging and haemorrhagic blisters. Occasionally similar lesions may appear on other parts of the body. It can be confused with vitiligo on the vulva (*see* Figure 663), but in vitiligo there is only a colour change, a white patch, without atrophy, haemorrhage or follicular plugging, and vitiligo is not itchy. In males the condition is called balanitis xerotica obliterans (*see* Figure 51).

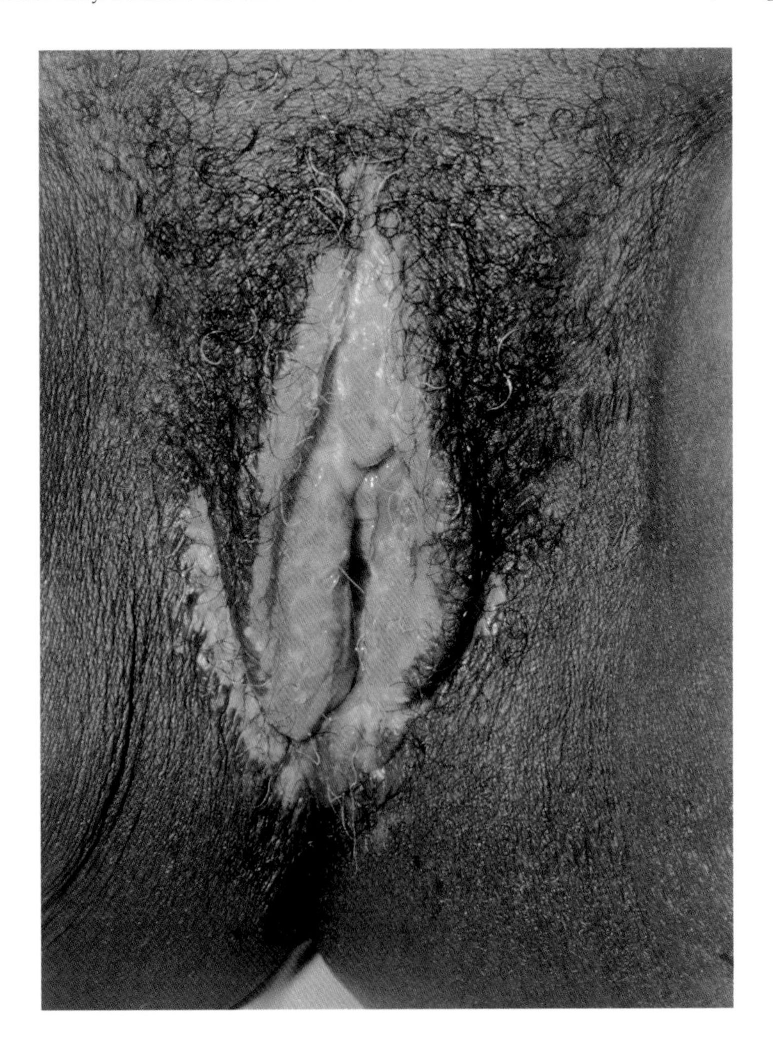

*Treatment:* In young children the condition usually gets better spontaneously at puberty. In older women it does not remit spontaneously. At all ages apply a potent topical steroid (e.g. 0.1% betamethasone 17-valerate) cream or ointment bd to alleviate the itching. Reduce the strength of the topical steroid once the itching has been controlled.

## LICHEN SIMPLEX

**Figure 393** A single well defined lichenified plaque produced by an individual continually rubbing and/or scratching the skin. The most common sites are the occiput, the ankle and the scrotum.

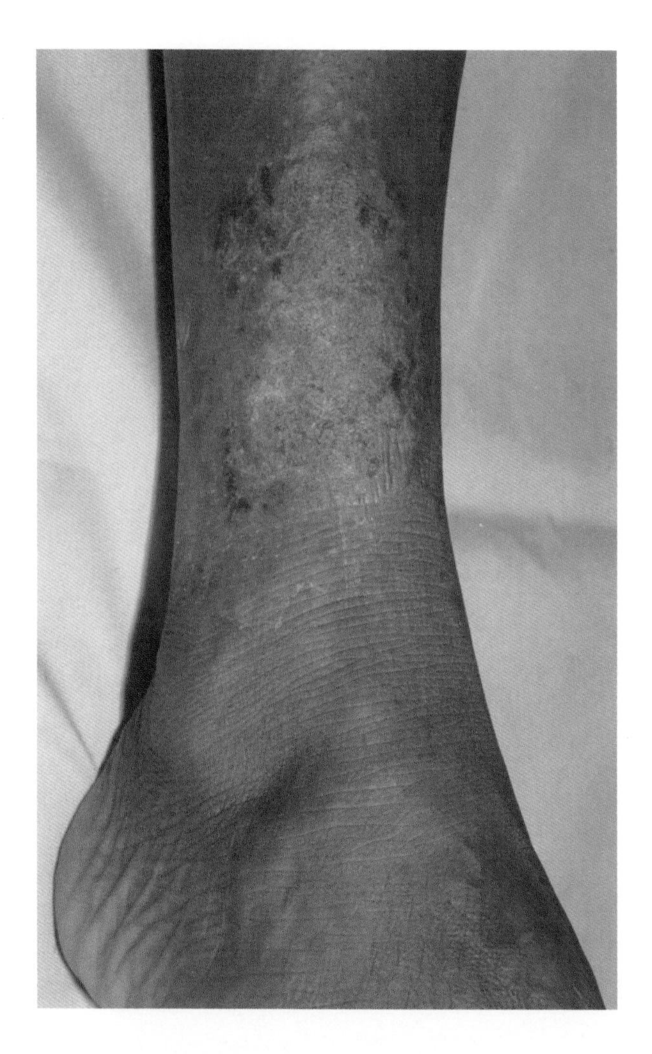

*Treatment:* It will get better if the patient stops scratching.

## LICHEN SPINULOSA

**Figures 394, 395** Common symmetrical rash in children in which there are minute perifollicular papules with a central horny spine. It gets better spontaneously after a few months.

*Treatment:* Reassurance that it will get better on its own.

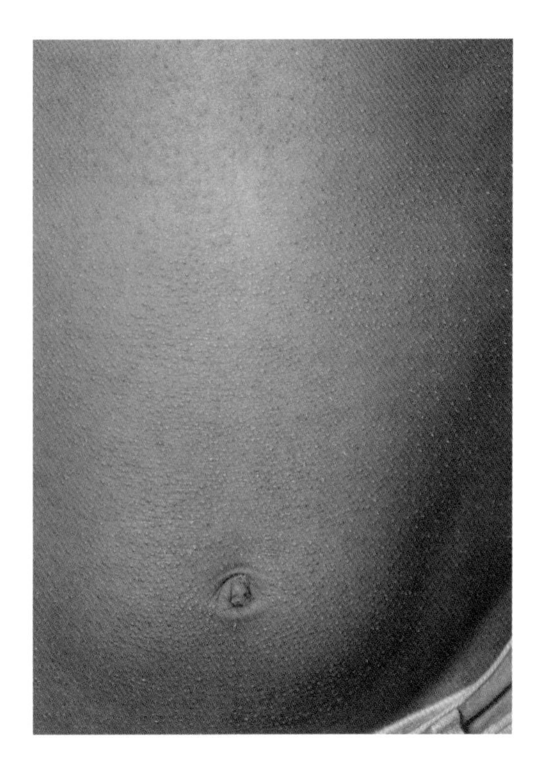

## LICHEN STRIATUS

**Figure 396** It looks like a line of lichen planus going down a limb, round the trunk or, in this case, along the angle of the jaw. More common in children than adults. Histologically it looks more like eczema than lichen planus. It lasts for 1–3 years and then gets better spontaneously.

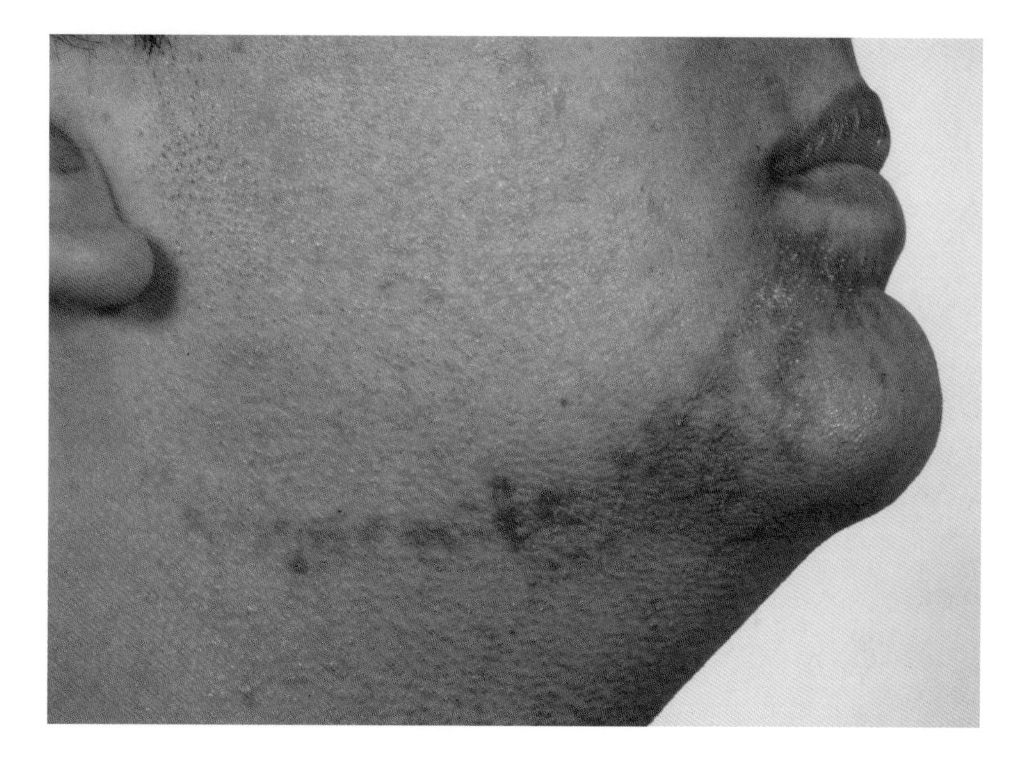

*Treatment:* Reassurance that it is harmless and will get better on its own.

## LINEAR IgA DISEASE

**Figure 397** Very itchy rash with annular grouped vesicles. Histology shows a subepidermal blister and immunofluorescence shows a linear band of IgA at the basement membrane.

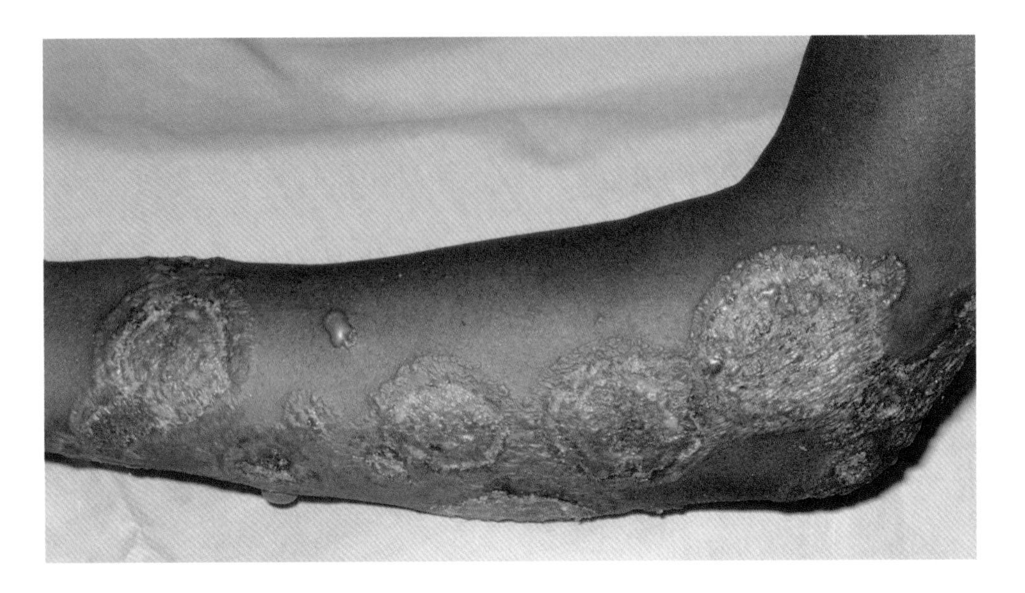

*Treatment:* Usually responds nicely to dapsone (diaminodiphenylsulphone) 50–100mg/day orally.

## LIP LICKING OR LIP SUCKING

**Figures 398, 399** Many children lick or suck their lips giving a hyperpigmented patch around the mouth which extends as far as the tongue can reach.

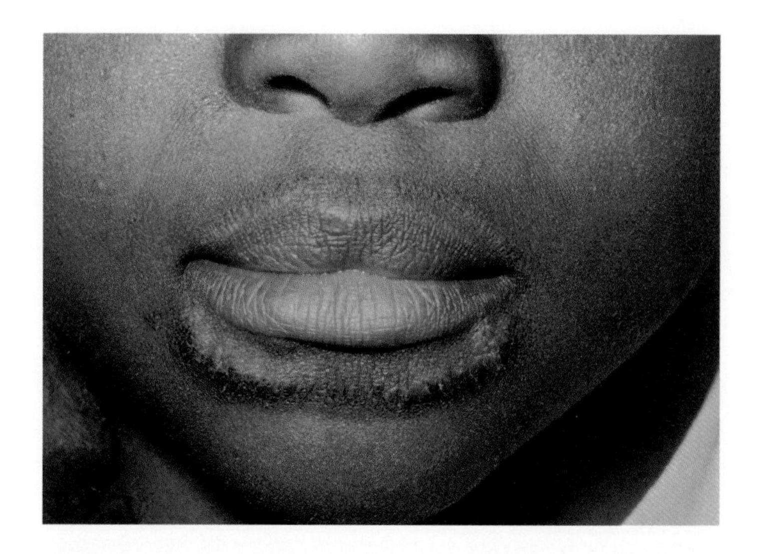

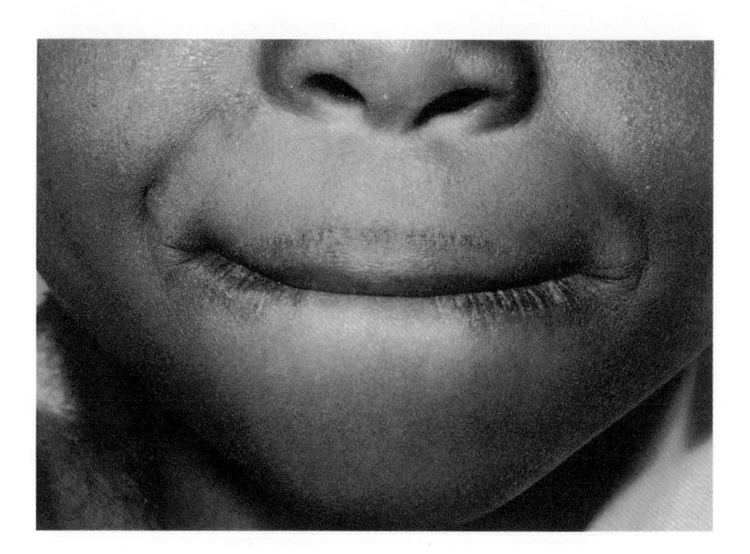

*Treatment:* Most children do not know they are doing it. Explain what is happening to the parents and get them to tell the child every time he or she does it. If this does not work, apply something that tastes nasty to the lips.

## LIPOMA

**Figure 400** Soft swelling in the skin. Can be single or multiple.

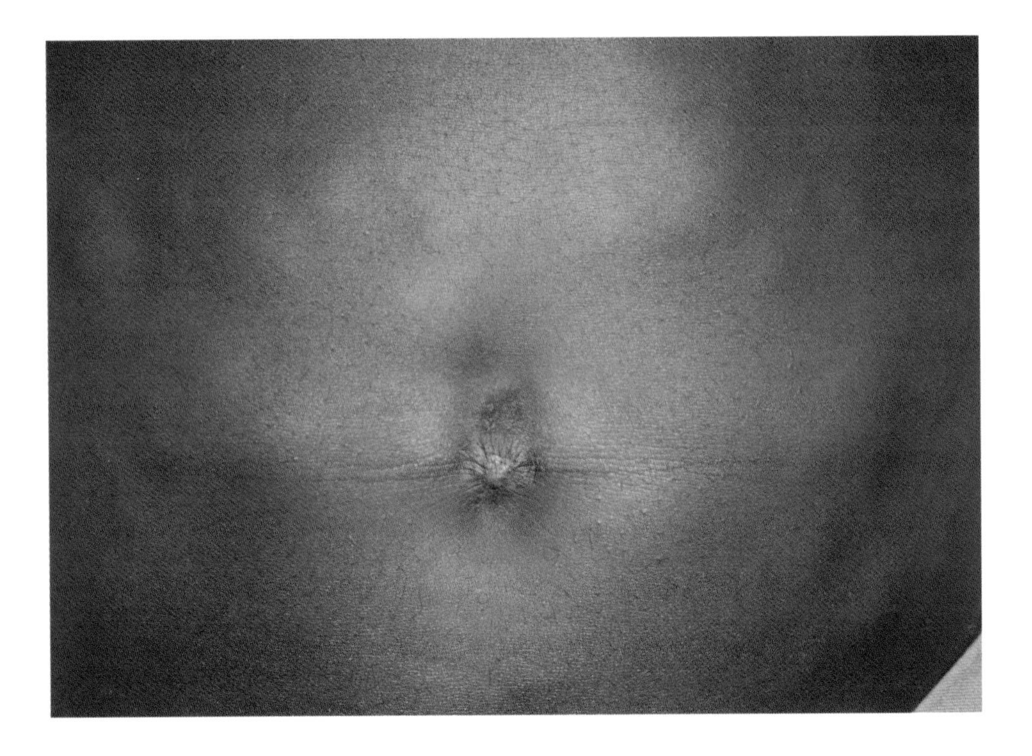

*Treatment:* Reassure the patient that it is harmless. Surgical excision only if it is unsightly.

## LOIASIS (Calabar swellings)

**Figure 401** Infestation with the filarial worm, *Loa loa,* which is transmitted by various species of mango fly (genus *Chrysops*). The female fly ingests circulating microfilaria when sucking human blood. Inside the fly infective larvae develop after about 10 days. These are then inoculated into a new host (human or baboon) when the fly takes its next blood meal. Adult worms develop after 1–4 years and discharge microfilaria into the blood stream. The adult worms migrate to the conjunctiva and skin where they can be seen. Calabar swellings are oedematous swellings, especially around the wrists and ankles, which are a hypersensitivity reaction to the presence of the worms.

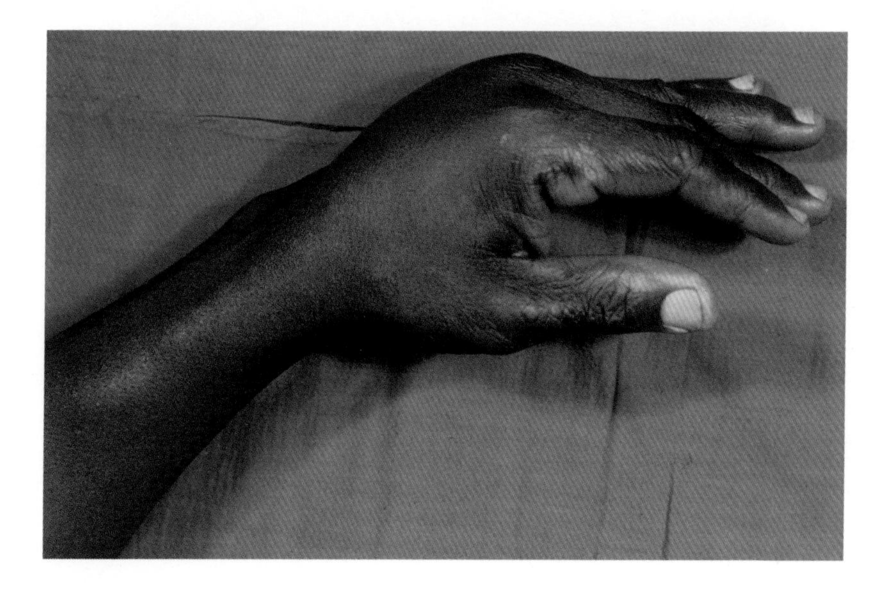

*Diagnosis:* The microfilaria can be seen on a thin blood film taken during the day.

*Treatment:* A single dose of ivermectin 400μg/kg body weight or a 3-week course of albendazole 400mg/kg body weight/bd. Do not use diethylcarbamazine as this can cause death as a result of a reaction to toxins from the rapid destruction of the microfilaria.

# LUPUS ERYTHEMATOSUS

## Discoid lupus erythematosus

**Figure 402** Unsightly rash on the face and scalp made up of well defined, red scaly plaques with follicular plugging. They heal leaving hypopigmentation and/or hyperpigmentation.

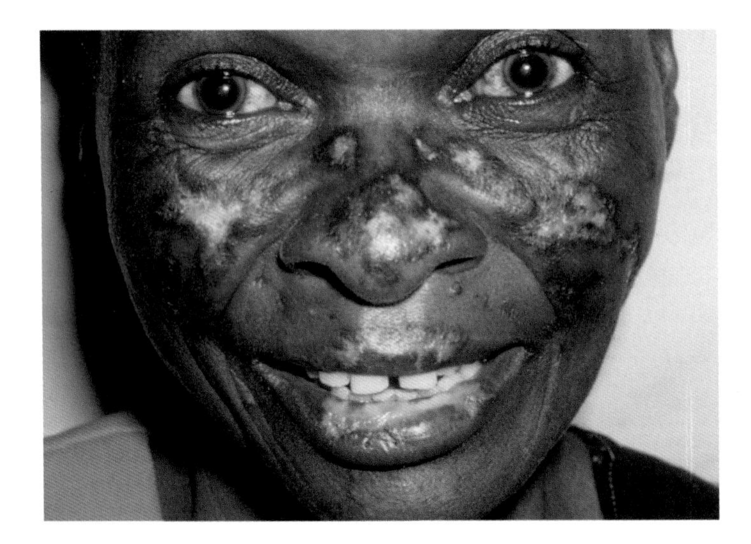

*Treatment:* If there are few lesions, apply a potent (e.g. 0.1% betamethasone 17-valerate) or very potent (e.g. 0.05% clobetasol propionate) topical steroid bd until the lesions are no longer red and scaly. If there are extensive lesions use oral chloroquine phosphate 200mg/day for at least 3 months. It may need to be continued longer if the disease is not fully controlled or recurs.

**Figure 403** On the scalp the lesions look similar while the disease is active. It causes a scarring alopecia which is permanent.

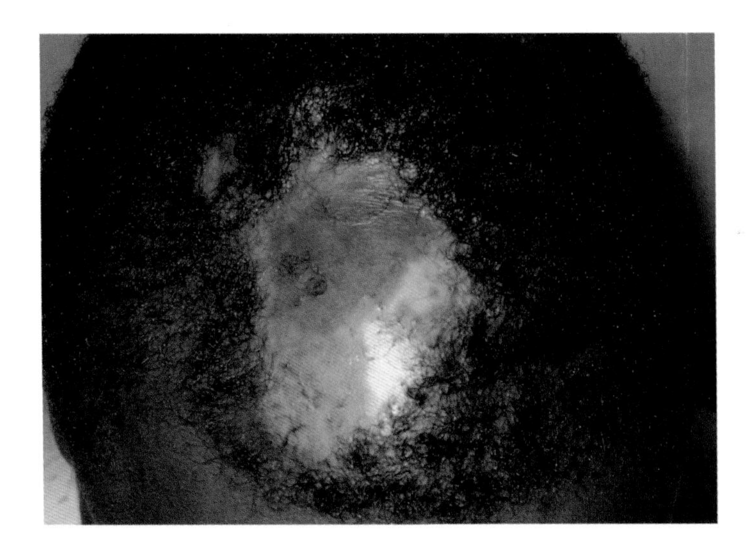

## Subacute cutaneous lupus erythematosus

**Figures 404, 405** This is a benign variant of systemic lupus erythematosus. There is an erythematous rash on sun-exposed skin which looks like discoid LE but without the scaling or follicular plugging. May be associated with arthritis, fever and general malaise but there are no serious systemic manifestations such as involvement of the central nervous system or kidneys.

*Treatment:* Chloroquine phosphate 200mg/day orally.

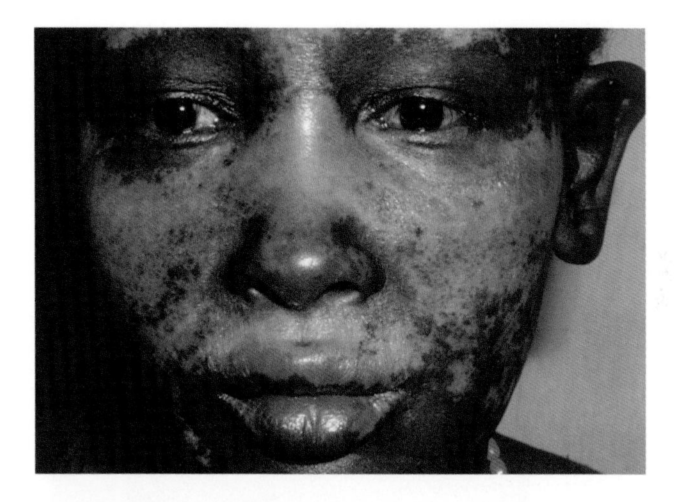

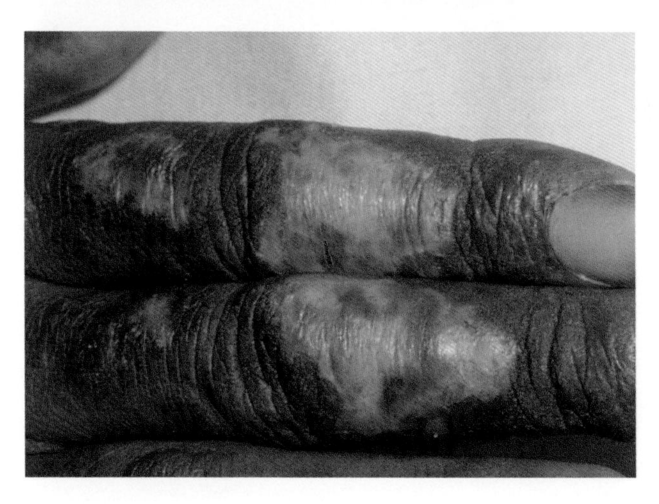

## Systemic lupus erythematosus

This is an autoimmune multi-system disorder mainly of females. On the skin there is a butterfly erythema (erythema on the cheeks and nose – *see* Figure 404), nail fold telangiectasia (*see* Figure 178) and diffuse non-scarring alopecia (*see* Figure 37). The systemic manifestations include fever, arthritis, nephritis, endocarditis, pericarditis, pulmonary fibrosis and CNS and psychiatric changes.

*Treatment:* Control the disease with high-dose systemic steroids (60mg prednisolone/day) and gradually reduce the dose to a maintenance dose of 5–10mg/day. Chloroquine or methotrexate may have to be added if the steroids do not control the disease or if it relapses when the dose is lowered.

## LYMPHOEDEMA

**Figure 406** Lymphoedema is an accumulation of lymph in the interstitial spaces caused by a problem with lymphatic drainage. It can be a congenital abnormality due to absence, or hypoplasia, of the lymphatics (primary lymphoedema), or be due to recurrent inflammation (after recurrent cellulitis) or blockage of the lymphatics and/or lymph nodes by cancer or filariasis (secondary lymphoedema).

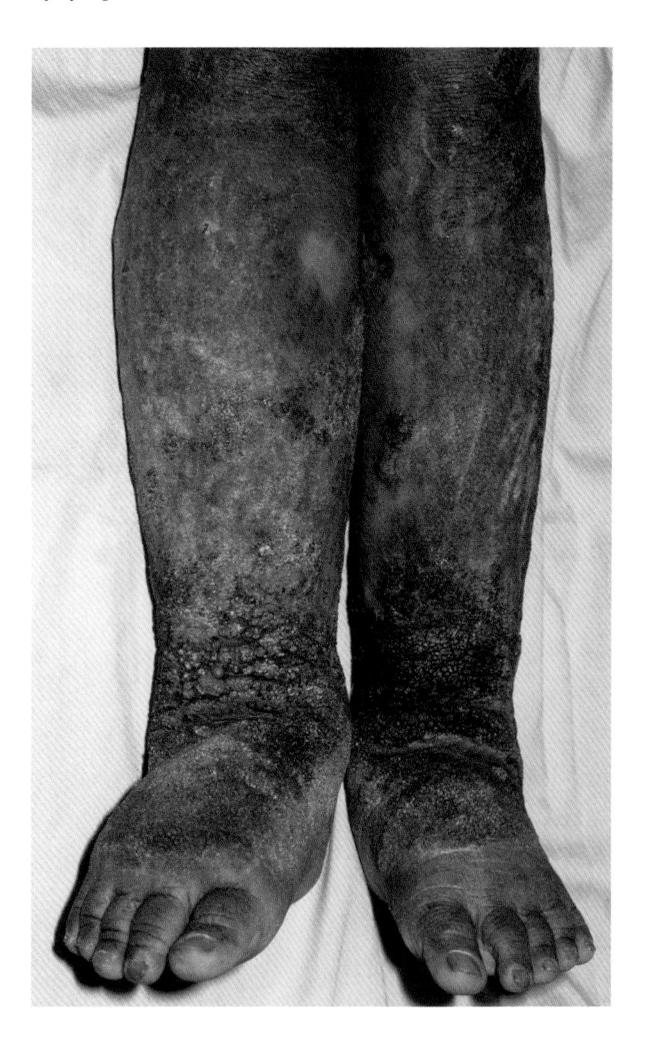

*Treatment:* Nothing can be done for primary lymphoedema. For secondary lymphoedema treat the underlying cause – long-term penicillin prophylaxis for recurrent cellulitis and yearly albendazole and ivermectin for filariasis. Prevent secondary bacterial infection of the swollen limb by frequent washing with soap and water (*see* Figures 240–1).

## LYMPHOGRANULOMA VENEREUM

Sexually transmitted disease due to *Chlamydia trachomatis,* mainly serotypes $L_{1,2,\&3}$. The incubation period is short in most cases (< 1 week) and there are two different clinical patterns:

- Primary lesion-inguinal adenitis syndrome.
- Ano-rectal-genital syndrome.

**Figure 407** Primary lesion inguinal adenitis syndrome. The primary lesion is often described by the patient as a 'pimple'. It is a small painless papule, vesicle or pustule on the genitalia which appears about 1 week after sexual contact. 2–3 weeks later the main problem begins with huge inguinal lymphadenopathy. Enlargement of the lymph nodes above and below the inguinal ligament gives rise to the characteristic 'groove' sign (a transverse line separating the two groups of glands).

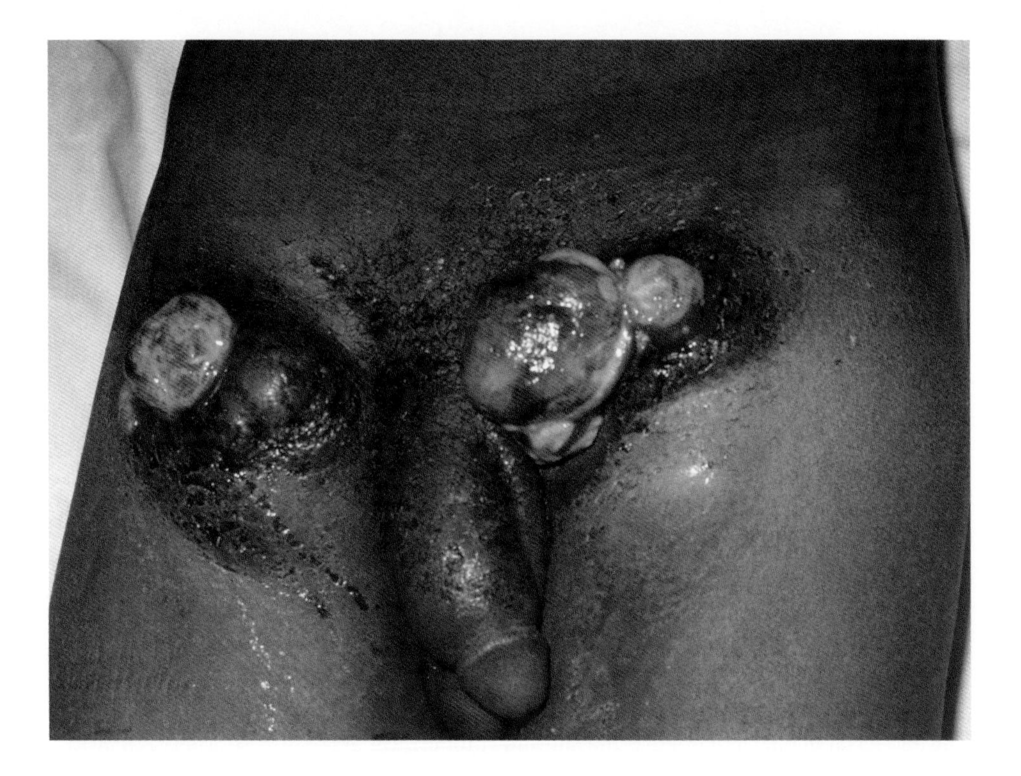

**Figure 408** The nodes are very tender and may suppurate forming multiple discharging sinuses (same patient as in Figure 407 but 3 weeks later).

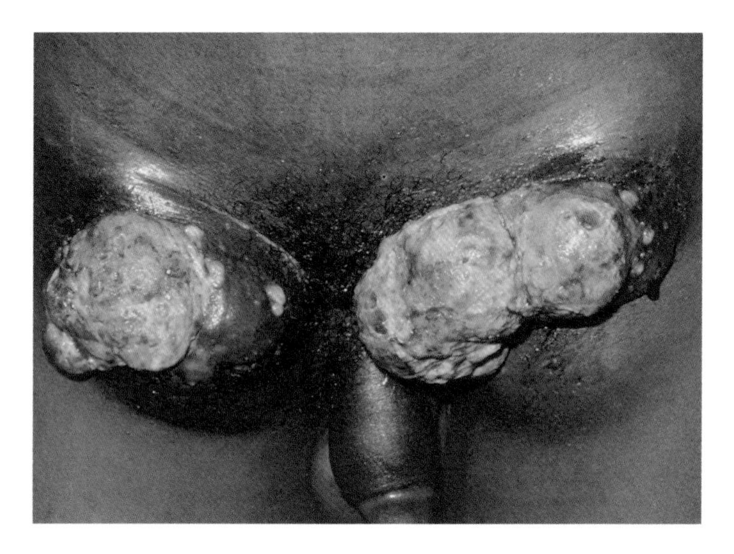

**Figure 409** Multiple discharging sinuses from LGV in a female.

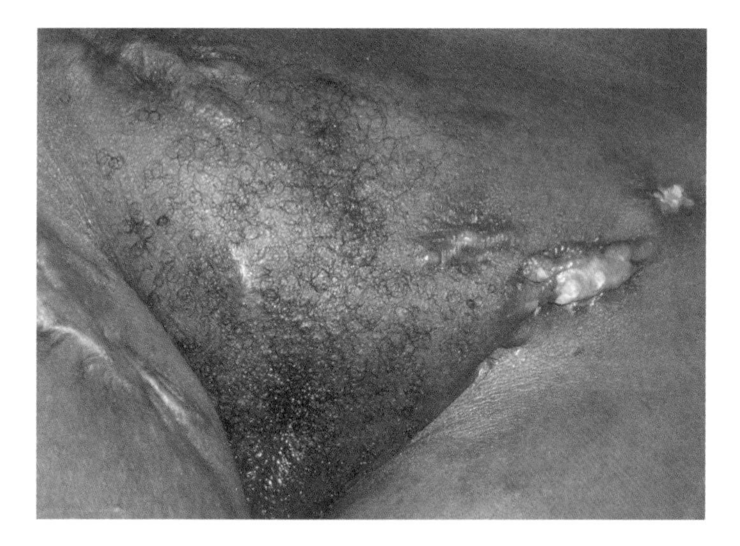

The ano-rectal-genital syndrome is the late and chronic form of the disease. There is a history of small blisters on the genitalia followed by inguinal adenitis. Then a proctitis occurs, starting with a muco-purulent bloody rectal discharge followed by a rectal stricture. There may also be perirectal abscesses, rectovesical or rectovaginal fistulae and genital elephantiasis.

*Diagnosis:* The diagnosis can be confirmed by culture in the yolk sac of a chick embryo or by a direct antibody fluorescent test on the patient's blood. LGV may give a biological false positive VDRL.

*Treatment:* Aspirate the glands using a large bore needle. Do not incise and drain or there will be chronic sinuses. Doxycycline 200mg bd or Septrin 960mg bd for 2–3 weeks. Check the RPR or VDRL for syphilis and check for HIV infection.

# LYMPHOMA

Lymphomas are a group of malignant neoplasms derived from B or T lymphocytes. They are subdivided into two broad categories:

- Hodgkin's disease.
- Non-Hodgkin's lymphoma, which includes tumours derived from B lymphocytes and mycosis fungoides derived from T lymphocytes.

## Hodgkin's disease

**Figure 410** This is a malignant lymphoma in which the Sternberg-Reed giant cell is the characteristic histological finding (a large, multinucleated cell with abundant cytoplasm). The patient usually presents with lymphadenopathy or generalised pruritis.

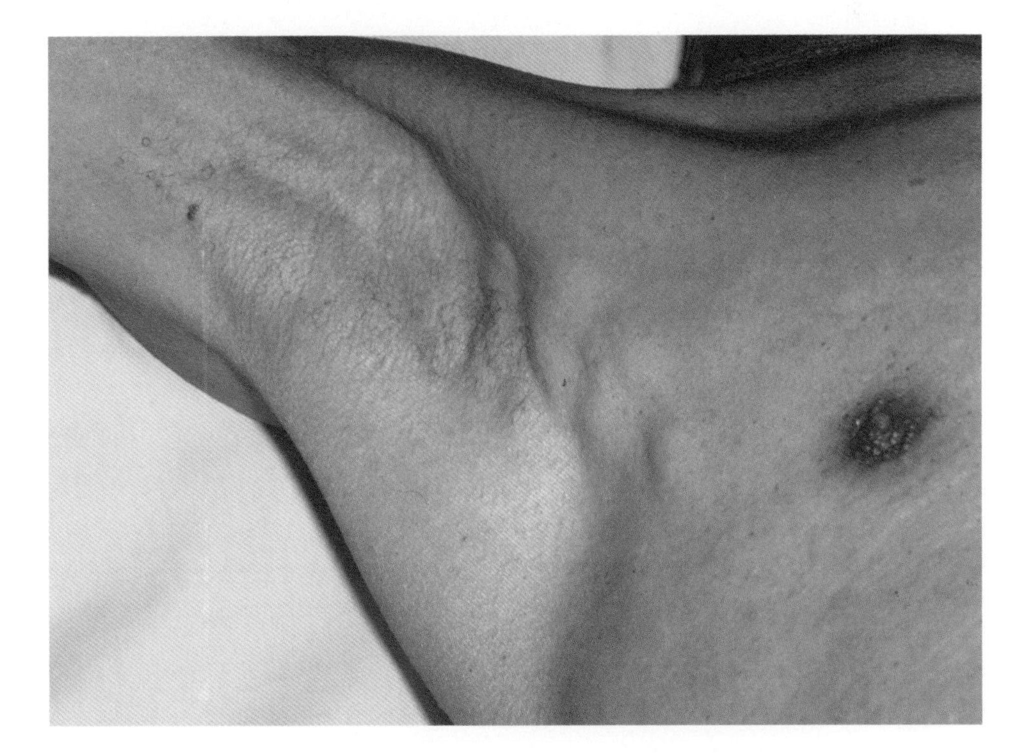

*Treatment:* Combination chemotherapy under the care of an oncologist.

## Non-Hodgkin's lymphoma

### Burkitt's lymphoma

**Figure 411** B-cell lymphoma due to infection with Epstein-Barr virus. The most common cancer seen in African children. Presents with swelling of face (especially jaws) or lymph nodes.

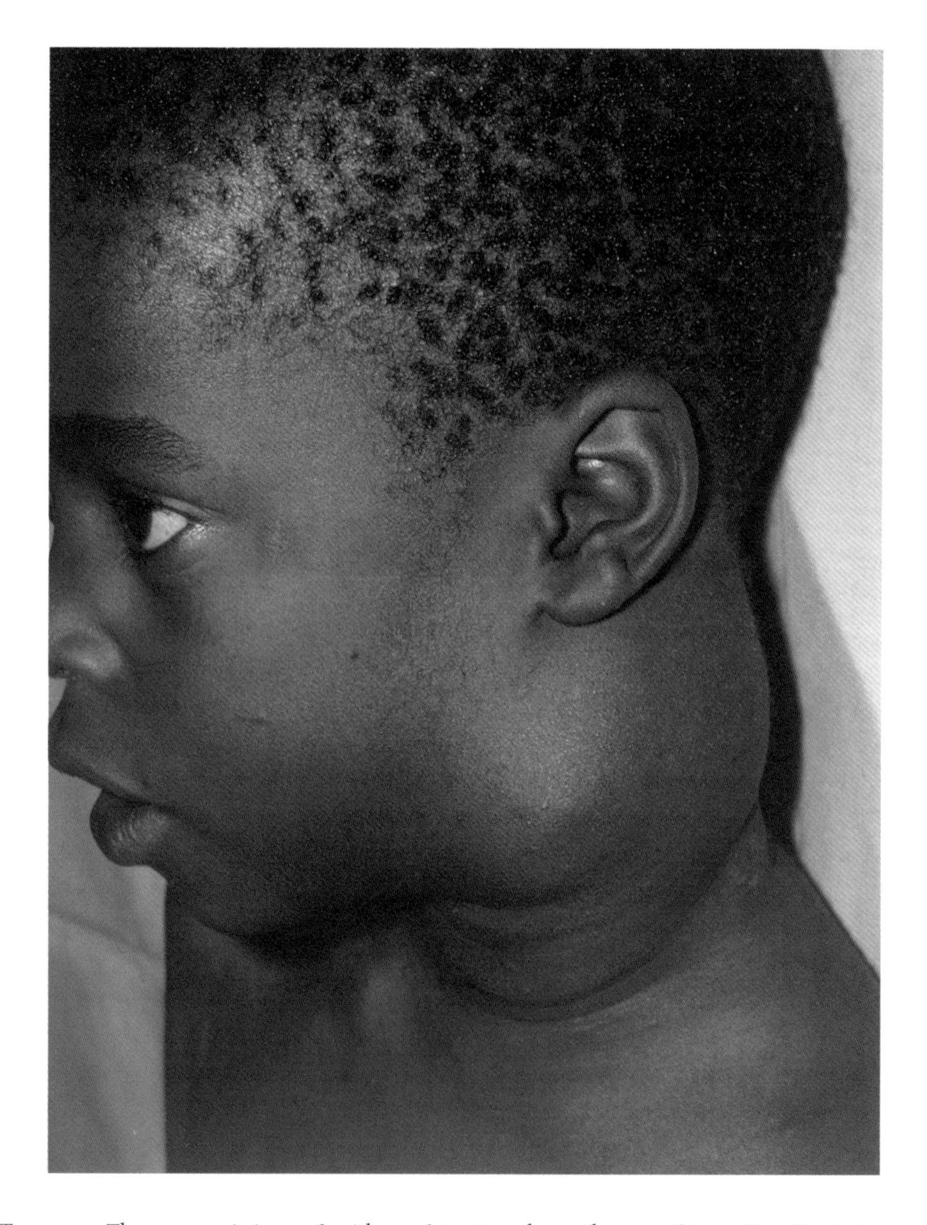

*Treatment:* The prognosis is good with combination chemotherapy if it can be afforded.

## Non-Hodgkin's lymphoma associated with HIV infection

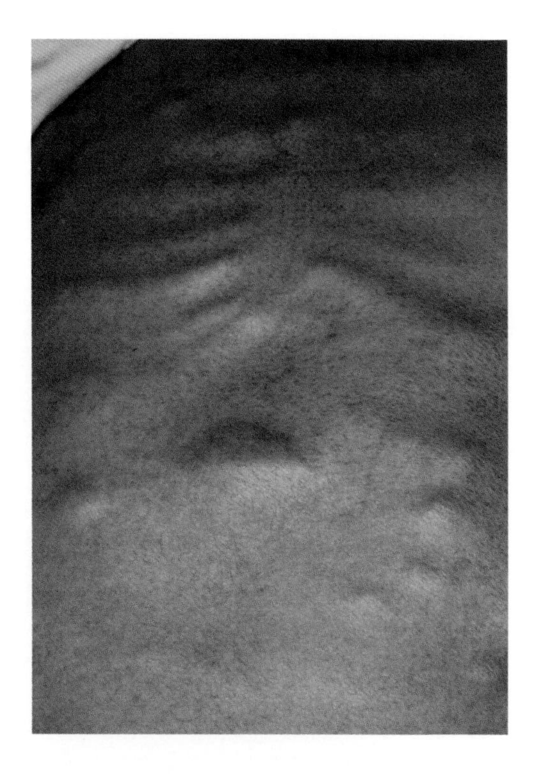

**Figure 412** Multiple skin-coloured nodules and plaques associated with widespread lymphadenopathy are seen in patients with HIV infection.

*Treatment:* The prognosis is poor because of the lymphoma itself and the risk of opportunistic infection. Combination chemotherapy can be tried but the drugs are very expensive.

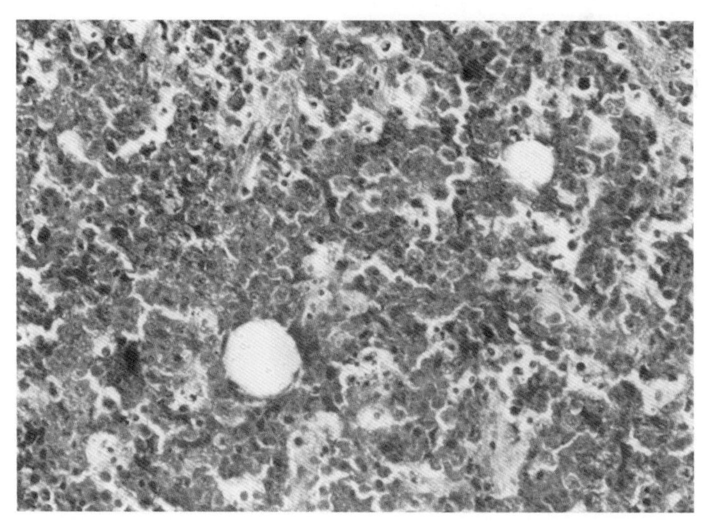

**Figure 413** Skin biopsy gives what is known as a 'starry sky' picture.

## Mycosis fungoides

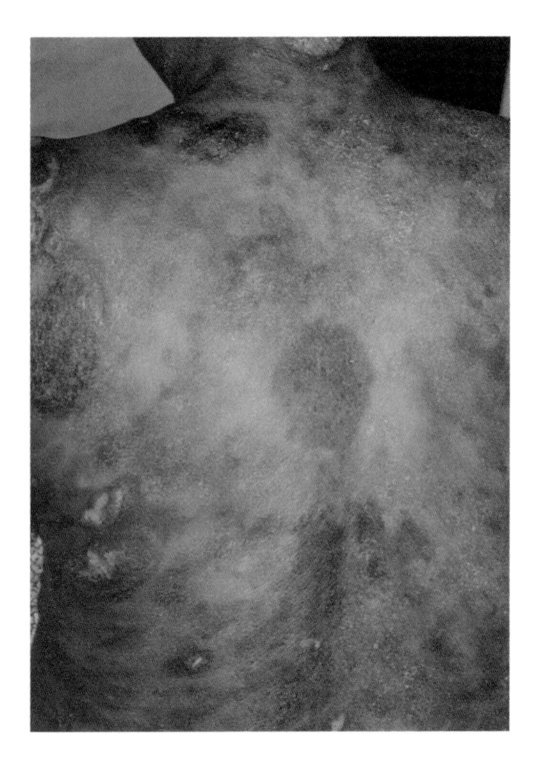

**Figure 414** This is a T-cell lymphoma which primarily involves the skin. The initial skin lesions are numerous scaly plaques of different colours. This stage of the disease can last 20 years or more.

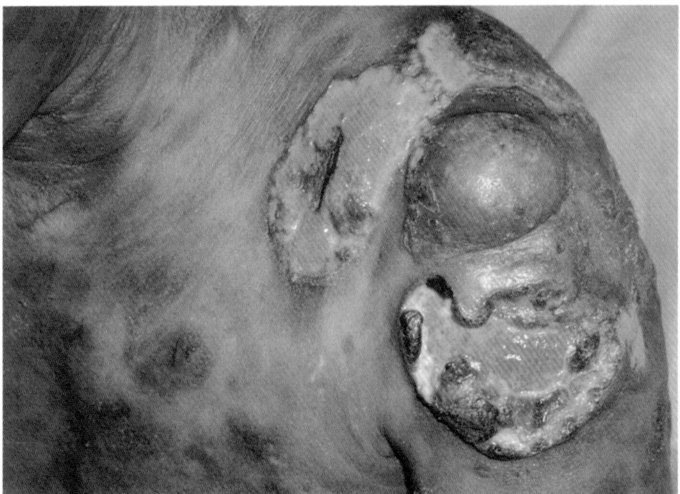

**Figure 415** Eventually tumours develop. At this stage the disease is often rapidly progressive with involvement of lymph nodes and internal organs leading to the patient's death.

**Figure 416** The diagnosis can be confirmed by biopsy. There is a lymphoid infiltrate in the dermis and groups of abnormal T-lymphocytes in the epidermis (Pautrier's microabscesses).

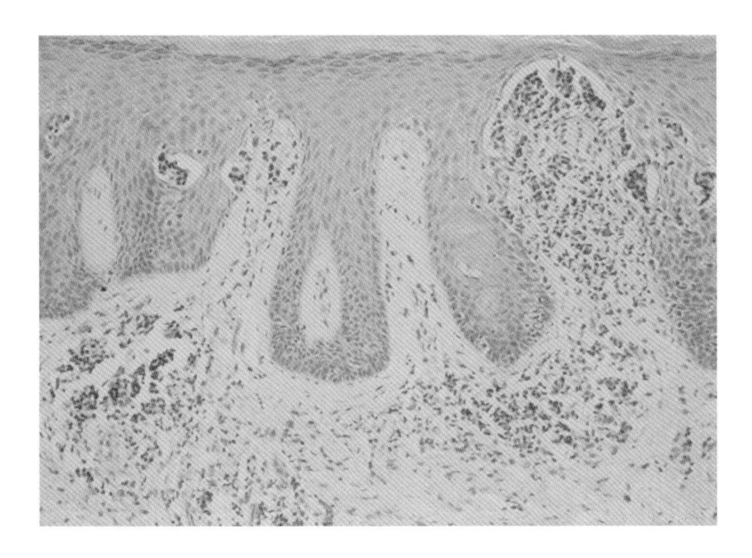

**Figure 417** Electron microscopy shows that the cells in the infiltrate and in the Pautrier's microabscesses have cribriform nuclei.

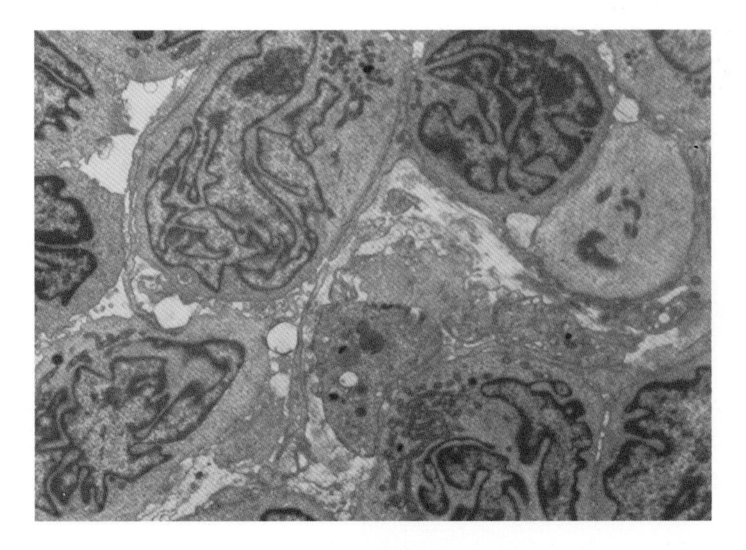

*Treatment:* In the early stages of the disease, topical steroids or PUVA (oral psoralens plus long-wave ultraviolet light). At the tumour stage, if the tumours are few, radiotherapy works nicely. If there are many tumours there is not much that can be done.

## Pagetoid reticulosis (Woringer-Kolopp disease)

**Figure 418** This is a rare pseudolymphoma which histologically can be confused with mycosis fungoides. It is a disease of young men. A single erythematous scaly or warty plaque occurs on a limb and extends slowly over many years; it never spreads systemically.

*Treatment:* Surgical excision or radiotherapy can be used.

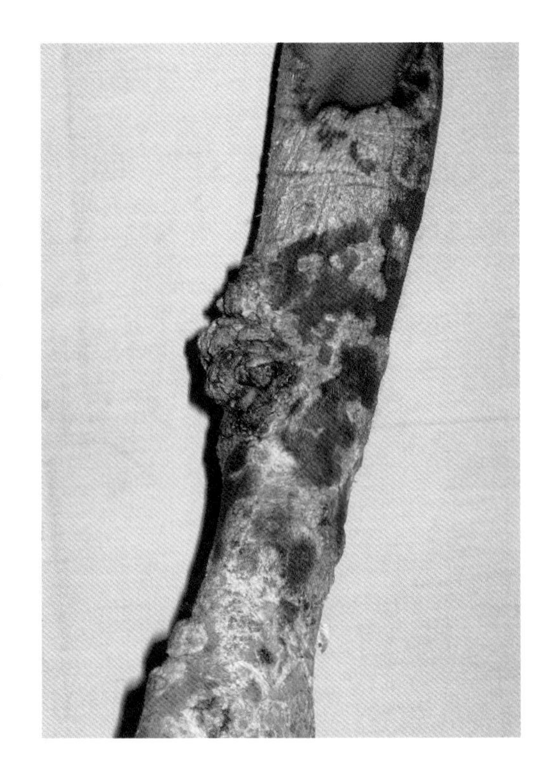

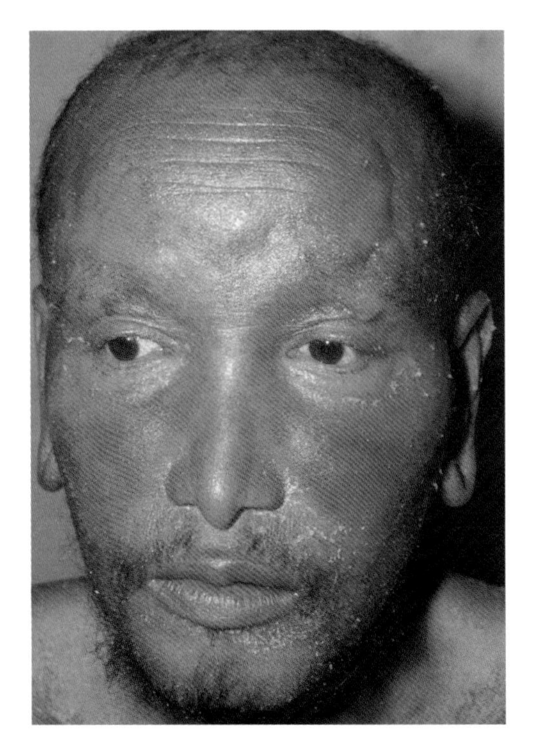

## Sezary syndrome

**Figure 419** This is the leukaemic phase of cutaneous T-cell lymphoma. The patient presents with erythroderma, alopecia and widespread lymphadenopathy. The normal skin pigment has entirely disappeared and the skin looks red. The diagnosis can be confirmed by skin biopsy (*see* Figure 416) and a blood film shows more than 20% atypical T-lymphocytes (Sezary cells – *see* Figure 417).

*Treatment:* Chlorambucil 4mg/day and prednisolone 30mg/day orally.

## MACULAR AMYLOID

**Figures 420, 421** Reticular hyperpigmentation on the back which is very itchy. It is easily missed or confused with other conditions such as eczema (*see* Figure 199).

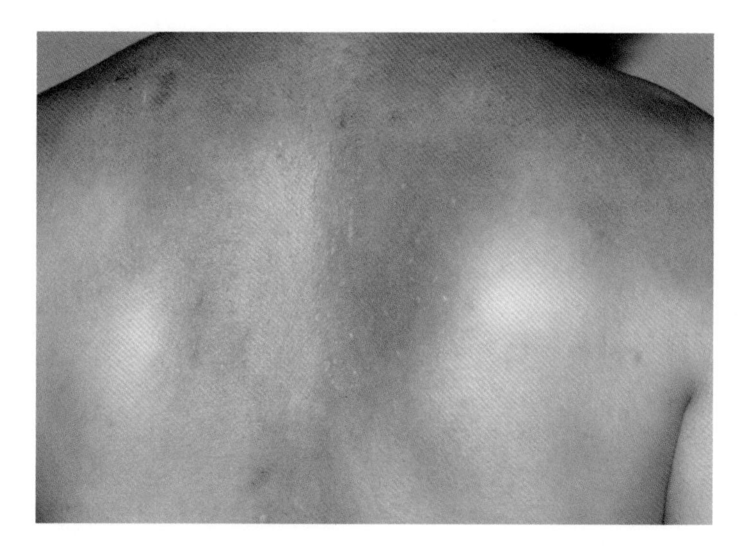

*Treatment:* Unsatisfactory. Topical steroids can be tried but are not usually very helpful.

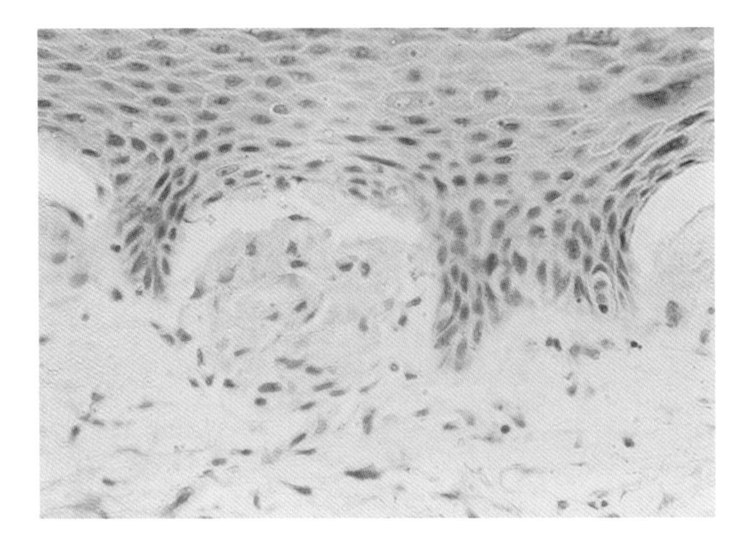

**Figure 422** The diagnosis can be confirmed by a skin biopsy; amyloid deposits stain red with a Congo Red stain.

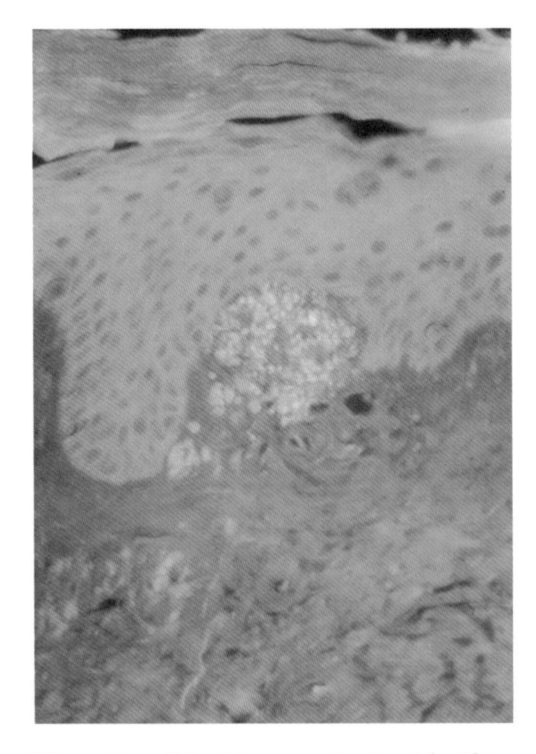

**Figure 423** Skin biopsy stained with Thioflavine T; the amyloid deposits stain green.

## MARASMUS

**Figure 424** An infant or child weighing less than 60% of their expected body weight for their age (this child is 2 years old). Failure of weight gain leads to emaciation. The subcutaneous fat disappears. There is no oedema as there is in kwashiorkor (*see* Figures 345–6). It is due to combined protein and calorie malnutrition and leads to death unless treated. It is seen commonly in young children with AIDS.

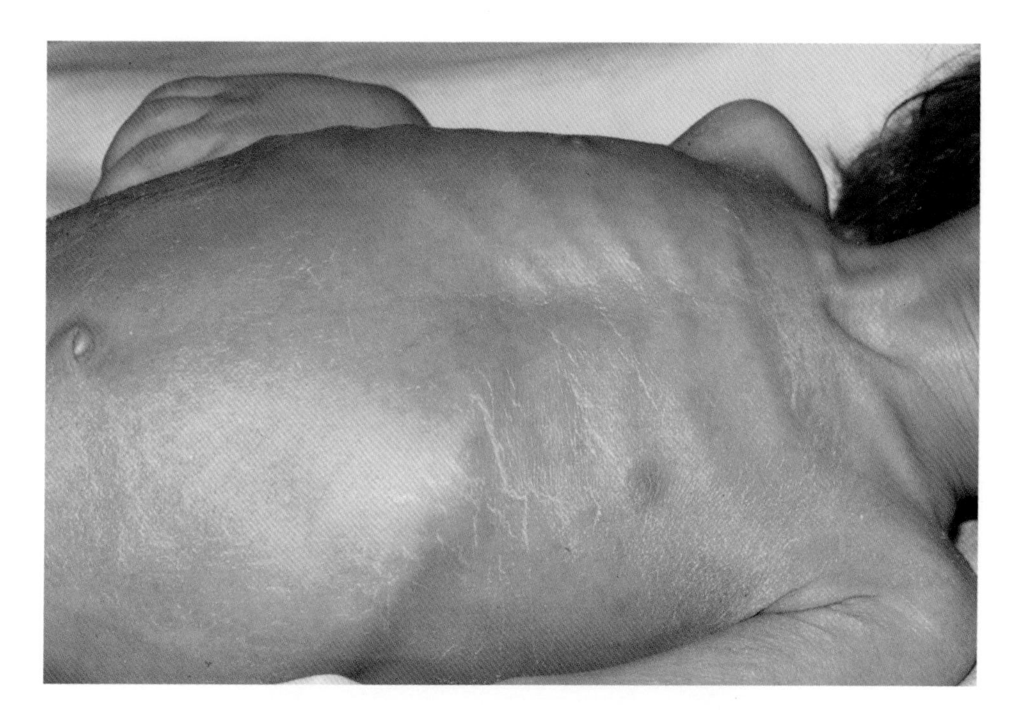

*Treatment:* The child should be given a high protein and high calorie diet.

## MEASLES

**Figures 425, 426** Viral infection due to a paramyxovirus. After an incubation period of 8–12 days the child develops a fever, runny nose, cough, photophobia and conjunctivitis. The rash starts behind the ears and spreads down the body to become generalised after 3 days. The initial reddish macules become confluent, then scaly and then peel off. The rash is not itchy. In the mouth Koplik's spots, which look like grains of salt, appear before the skin rash. Some children who are malnourished still die after measles.

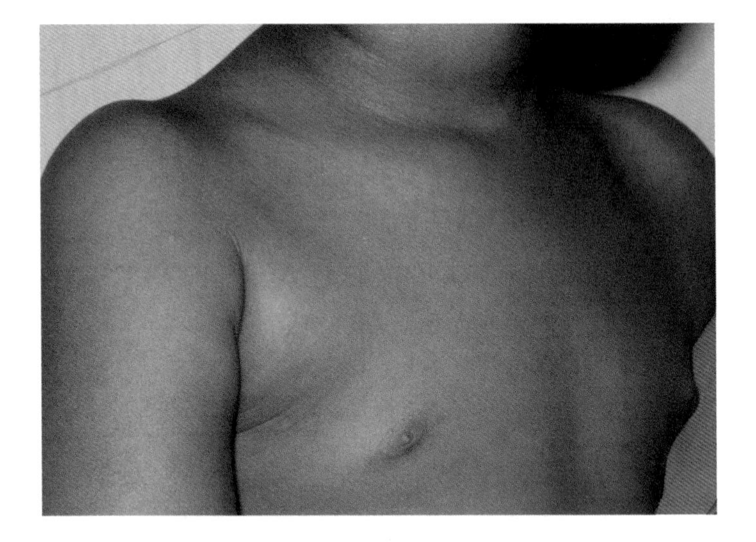

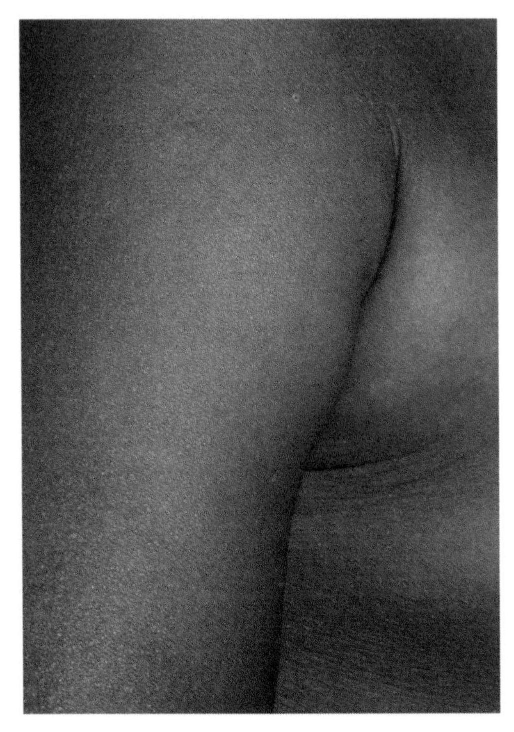

*Treatment:* All children with measles should be given vitamin A 100 000–200 000 IU on two successive days as soon as the diagnosis is made. This reduces the mortality considerably.

## MILIA

**Figure 427** These are tiny epidermoid cysts in the upper dermis. They are common on the cheeks in young adults and occur after blistering in all diseases with subepidermal blisters, e.g. bullous pemphigoid, epidermolysis bullosa and porphyria cutanea tarda.

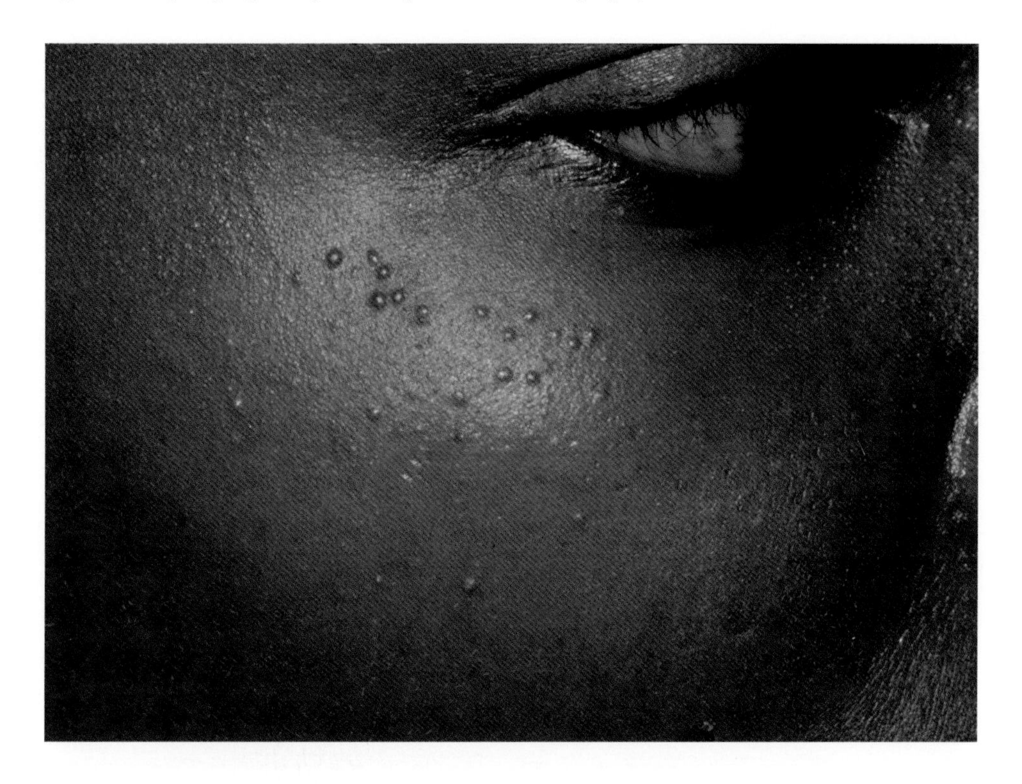

*Treatment:* They are quite harmless and no treatment is needed.

## MILIARIA

**Figure 428** Tiny vesicles due to the blockage of eccrine sweat ducts. Most commonly seen in the flexures (particularly around the neck) in the newborn who are covered with Vaseline or other greasy ointments, especially premature babies who are being kept in a hot room.

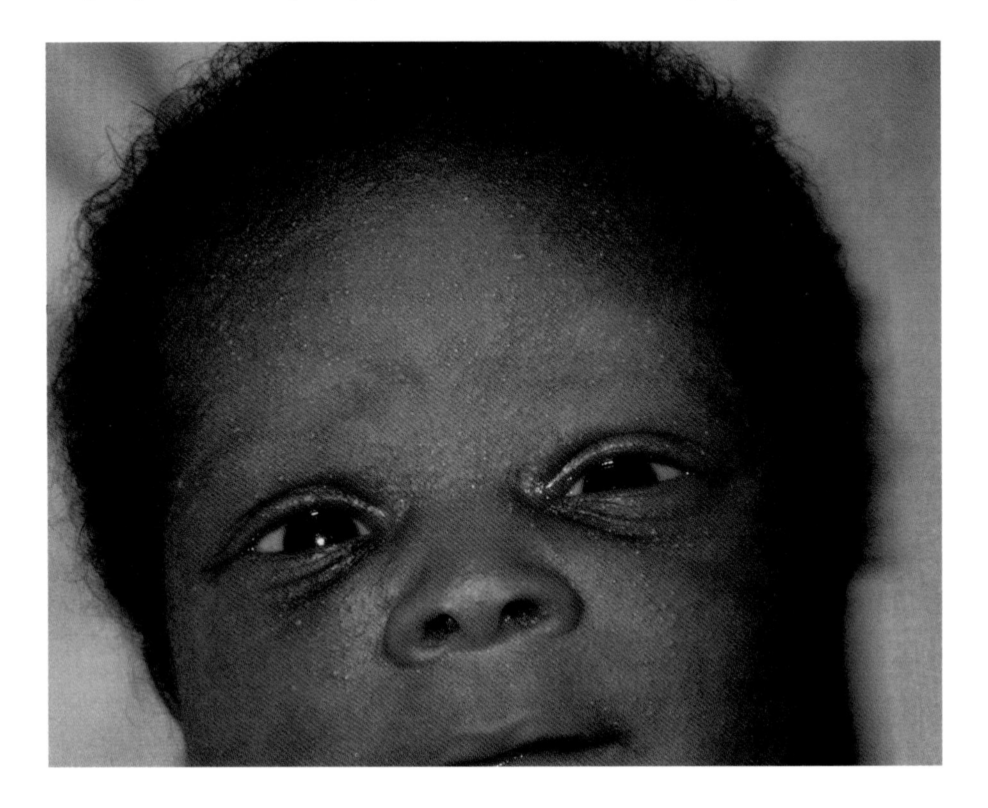

*Treatment:* Stop using greasy ointments. Remove excessive clothing.

## MILKER'S NODULE

**Figure 429** Parapoxvirus infection acquired from the teats of cows or the mouths of calves. Small papule/vesicle on the fingers of those involved in milking cows or taking care of the calves.

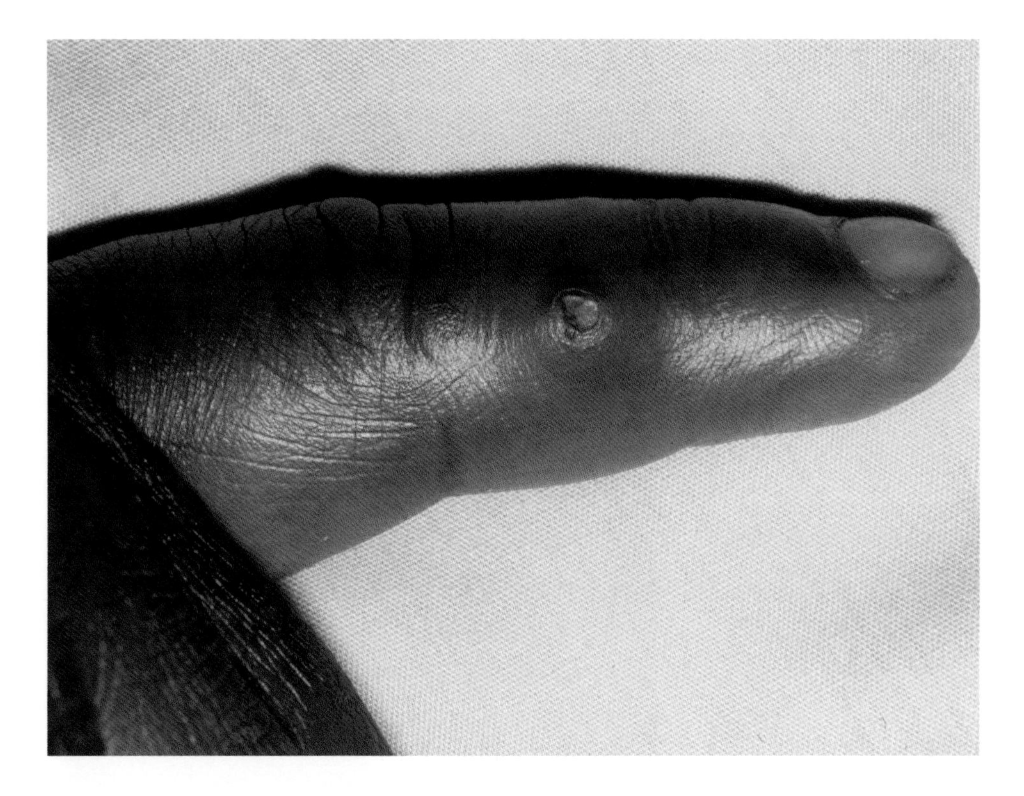

*Treatment:* None needed. It gets better spontaneously after 4–6 weeks. Lifelong immunity is acquired after infection, so it does not recur.

## MOLLUSCUM CONTAGIOSUM

**Figures 430, 431** Pox virus infection which is common in children. Transmitted from child to child by direct contact. Small translucent umbilicated papules (1–5mm in diameter) appear anywhere on the skin and usually last 6–9 months before disappearing spontaneously. When they occur in adults think of HIV infection.

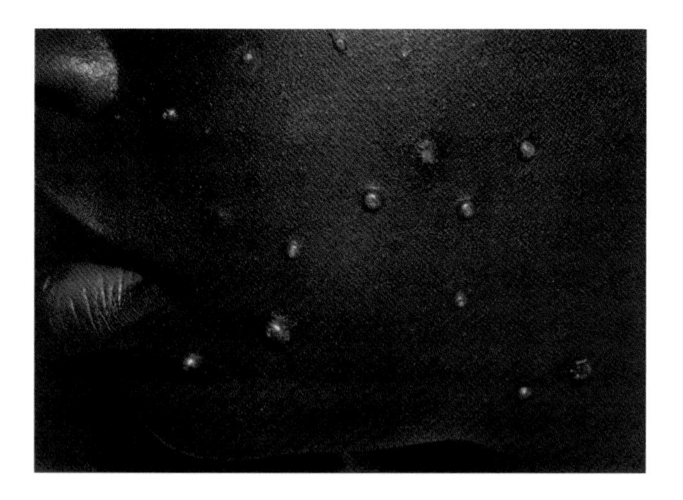

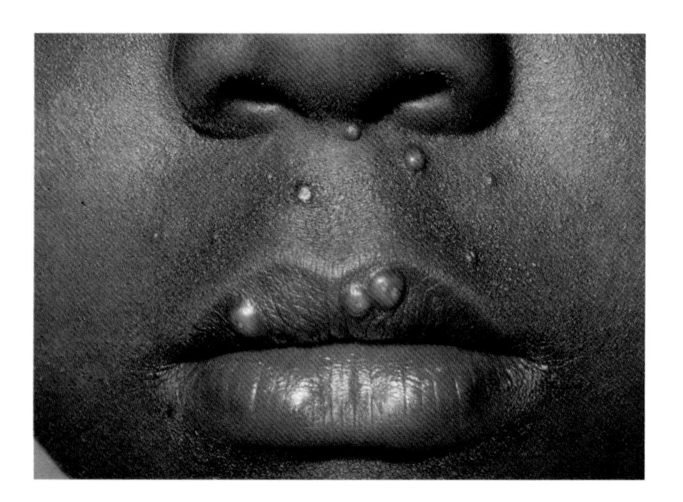

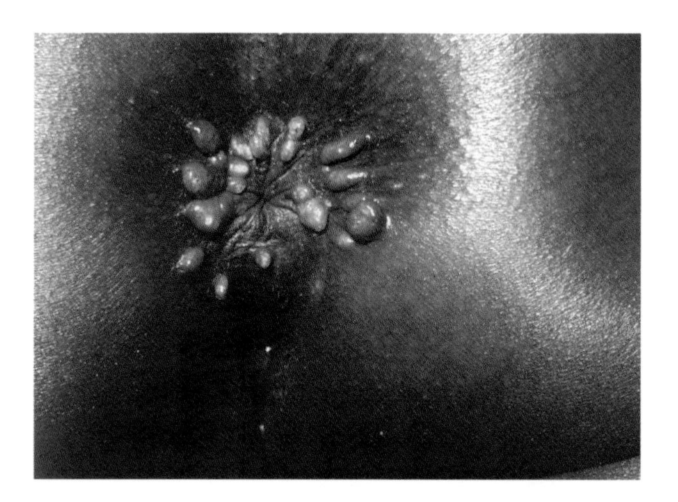

**Figure 432** If they occur around the anus in a child, suspect sexual abuse.

*Treatment:* Leave to resolve spontaneously.

## MORPHOEA (Localised scleroderma)

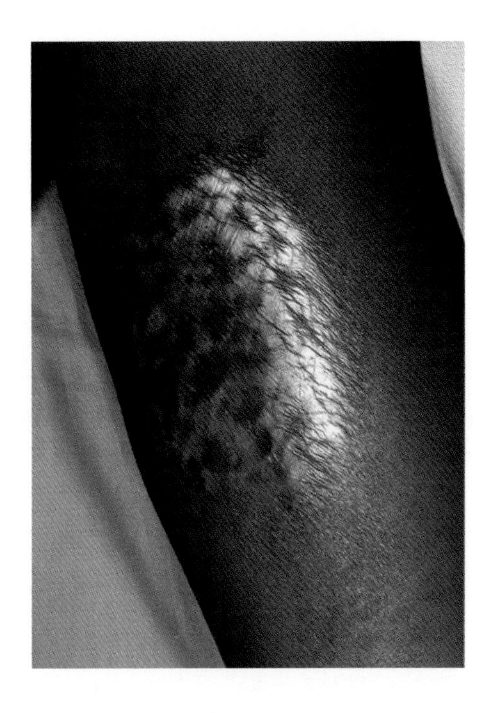

**Figure 433** Most commonly presents with a round or oval plaque which feels thicker than the surrounding skin. The edge may be raised and hyperpigmented.

*Treatment:* Reassure the patient that it usually resolves spontaneously.

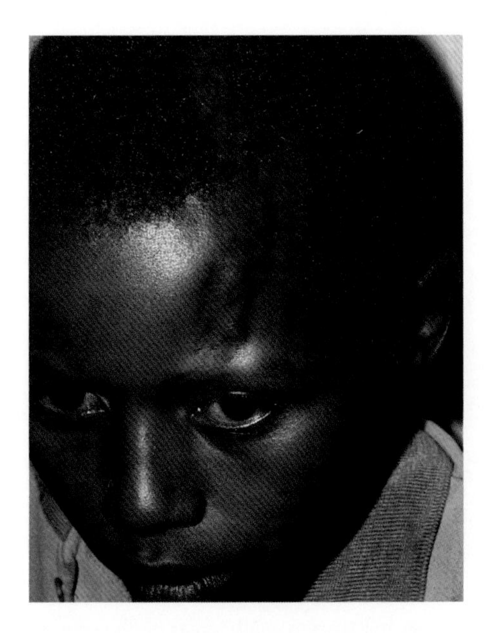

**Figure 434** Morphoea may be linear down a limb or on the forehead, when it is called 'en coup de sabre'. These lesions may resolve spontaneously or be permanent.

*Treatment:* There is no satisfactory treatment.

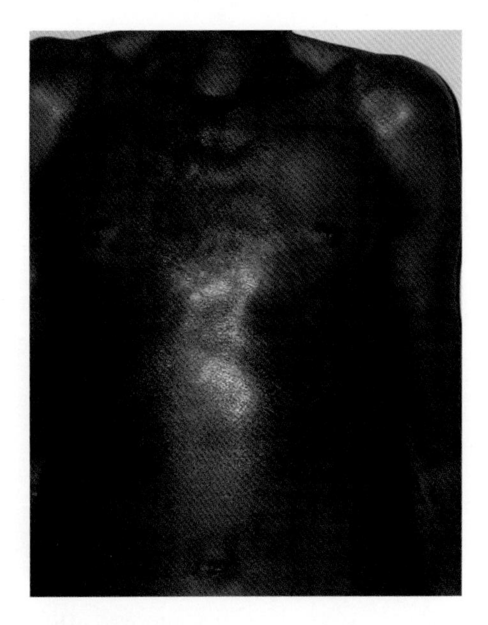

**Figure 435** Generalised morphoea. The skin of the trunk and/or limbs becomes tight and may make breathing difficult.

*Treatment:* There is no satisfactory treatment.

# MYIASIS

## Subcutaneous myiasis

**Figure 436** This is due to the larvae of *Cordylobia anthropophagia*, the tumbu fly or mango fly.

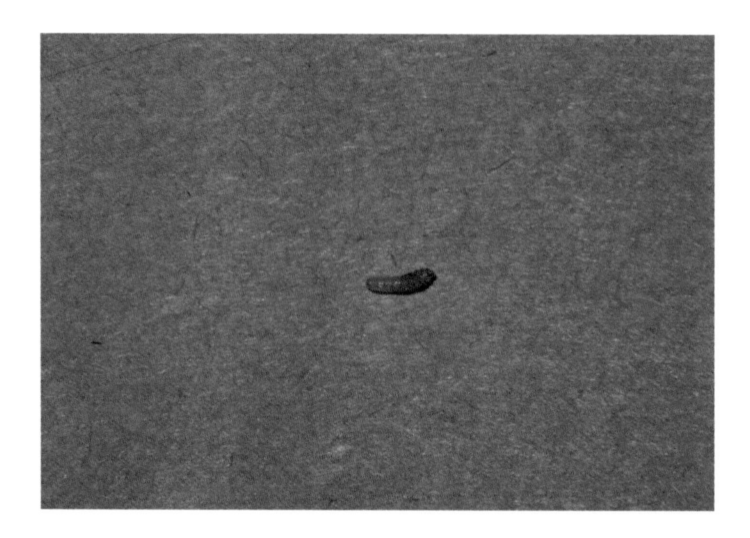

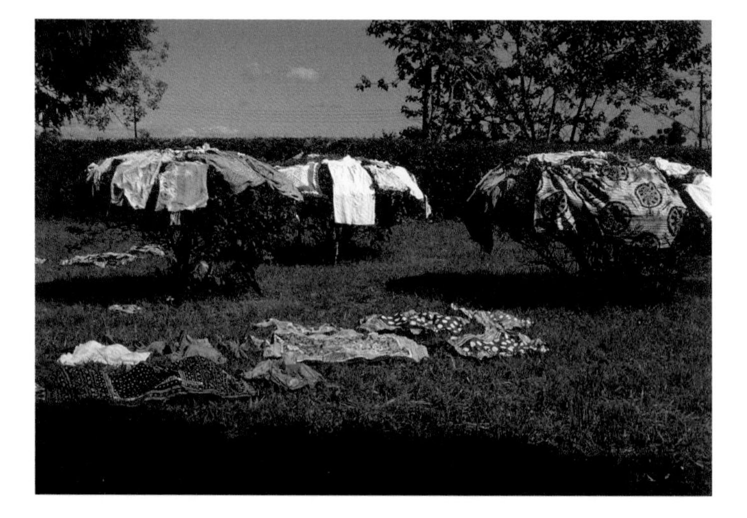

**Figure 437** The female fly lays her eggs in shady areas on the ground (especially ground contaminated with urine or faeces) or on clothes which are lying out to dry. She does not like bright sunshine and is only active between 7–9am and 4–6pm. Although the flies breed all the year round, most human infestations occur in the rainy season.

**Figure 438** Larvae hatch when the eggs are in contact with a warm body. The larvae penetrate (head down) through the host's unbroken skin into the subcutaneous fat. The burrowing is very quick (less than one minute) and is usually unnoticed by the patient. A small papule with a central pore develops which may be itchy or painful. The papule enlarges to look like a boil. There may be one or several 'boils', usually on parts of the body covered with clothes.

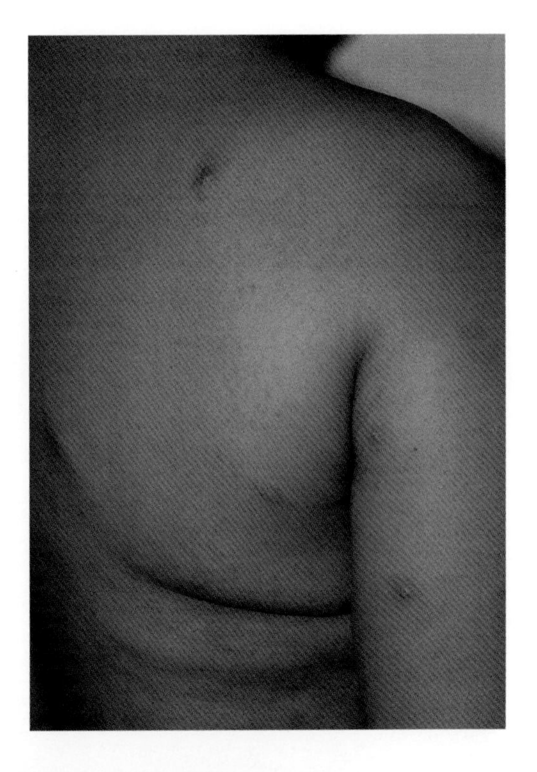

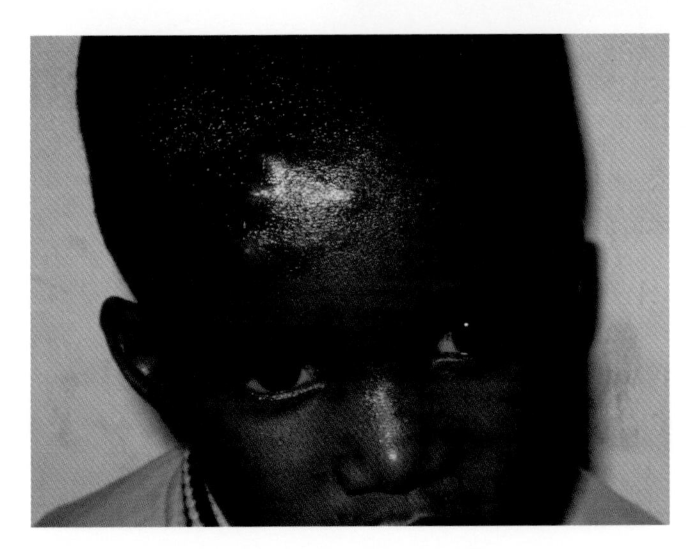

**Figure 439** They can appear on the face or scalp, from unironed pillow cases or sheets.

*Prevention:* Dry clothes in bright sunshine and iron before wearing them.

*Treatment:* Apply Vaseline or a piece of pork fat over the 'boil'. The larva will be unable to breath and will crawl out (*see* Figure 436).

## Wound myiasis

**Figure 440** Many different species of flies deposit their eggs in discharging wounds. The larvae hatch and feed on the necrotic tissue. It is a very good way of cleaning up dirty wounds.

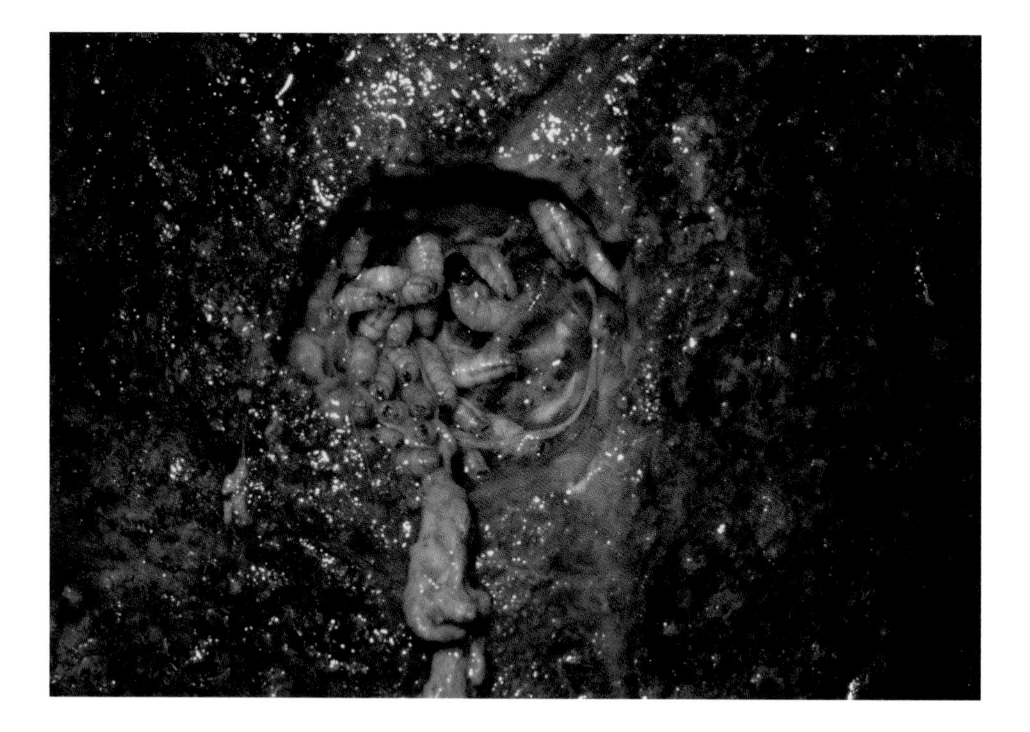

# NAIL ABNORMALITIES

**Figure 441** Anatomy of the nail apparatus.

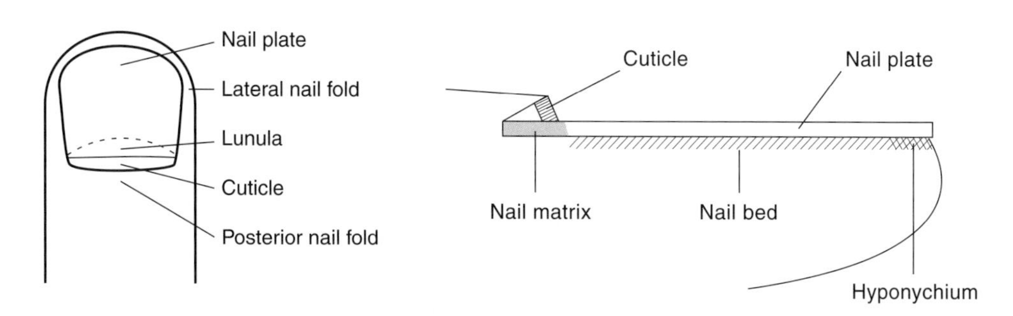


## Abnormalities of the nail matrix

**Figure 442** Longitudinal ridging. Lichen planus of the nails produces longitudinal ridges, as does Darier's disease (*see* Figure 153). A few longitudinal ridges are a normal finding.

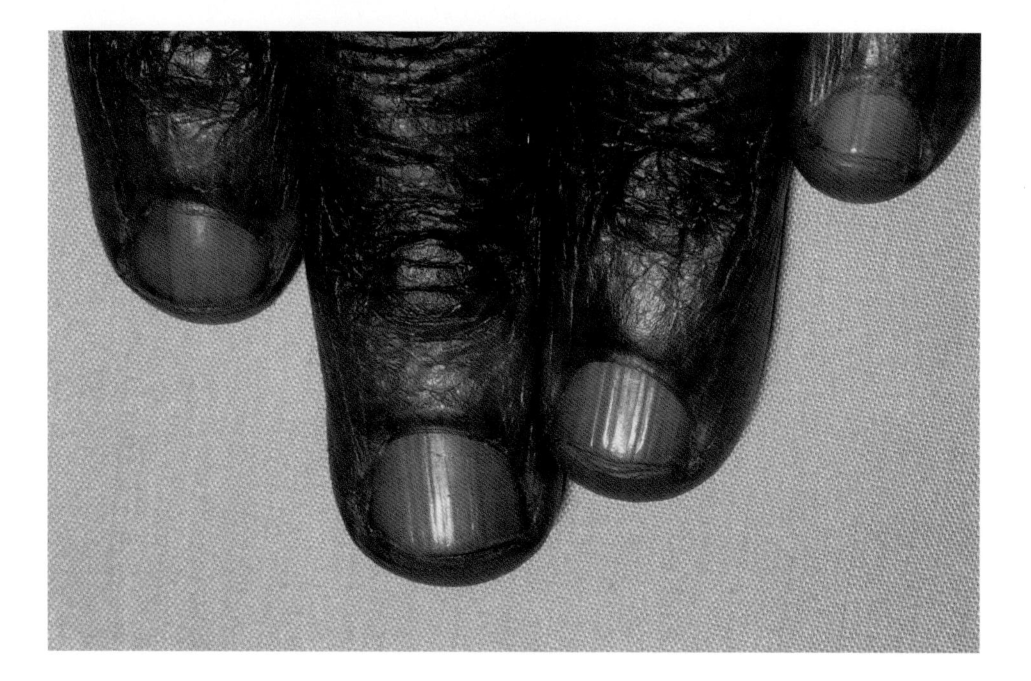

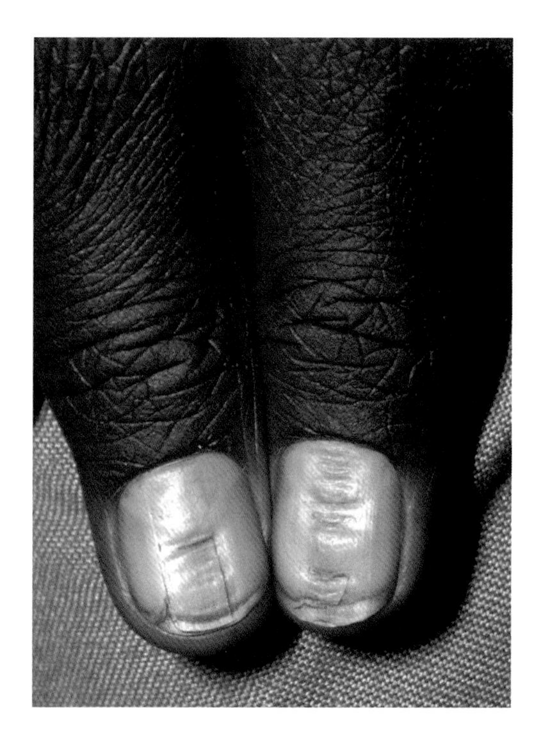

**Figure 443** Habit tic deformity. A depression down the centre of one or both thumb nails, due to constant picking of the cuticle or nail.

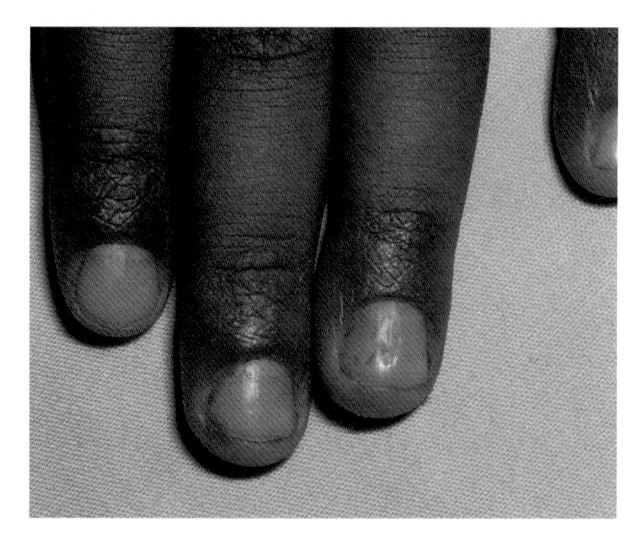

**Figure 444** Pitting. Occurs in eczema (as in this figure – note the eczema on the dorsum of the fingers over the distal phalanges), psoriasis (*see* Figure 540) and alopecia areata.

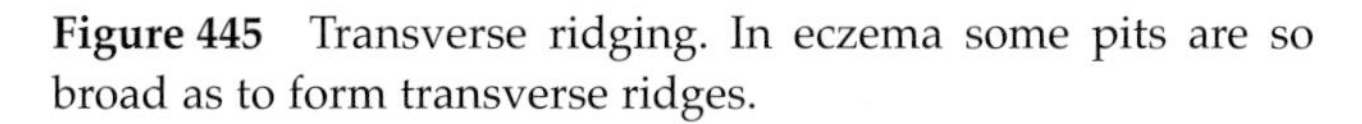

**Figure 445** Transverse ridging. In eczema some pits are so broad as to form transverse ridges.

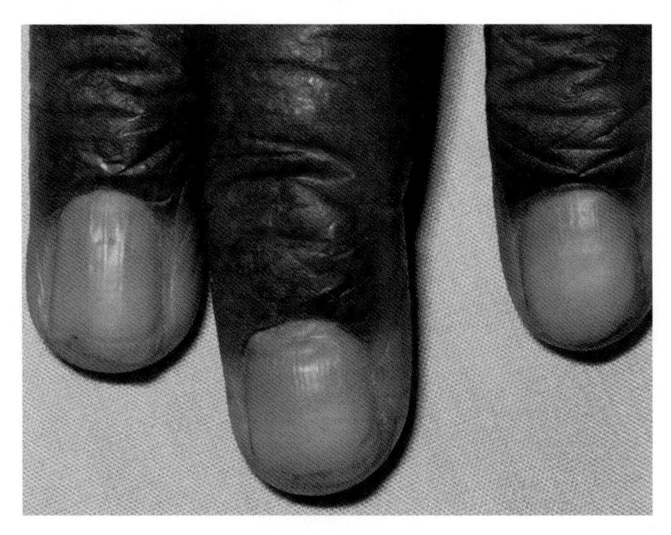

**Figure 446** Beau's lines. These are transverse lines in the same place in all the nails due to cessation of growth in the nail matrix at the time of a severe illness (especially one associated with a high fever). On recovery, the matrix will begin to function normally again and the nail will grow out with a line in it. Finger nails grow at a rate of approximately 1mm/week (toenails at about half that speed), so you can tell how long ago the illness was.

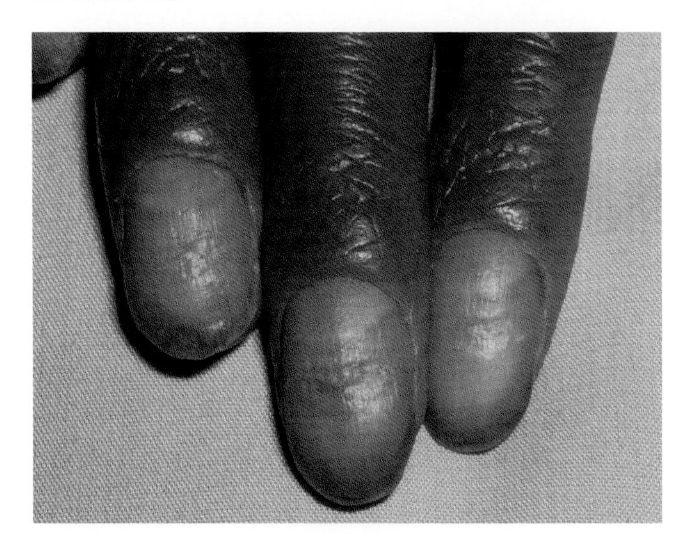

## Abnormalities of the nail bed and hyponychium

The nail bed is the epidermis underneath the nail. In normal circumstances the nail is firmly stuck onto it so it is unable to produce keratin. The hyponychium is the nail bed under the free edge of the nail. The nail is less firmly attached to the nail bed here than to the rest of the nail bed.

**Figure 447** Onycholysis and salmon patches. Onycholysis is the lifting up of the nail from the nail bed due to a problem at the hyponychium. It can occur in psoriasis as here, and after vigorous work with a nail file under the nail. Salmon patches are orange coloured macules under the nail due to psoriasis of the nail bed.

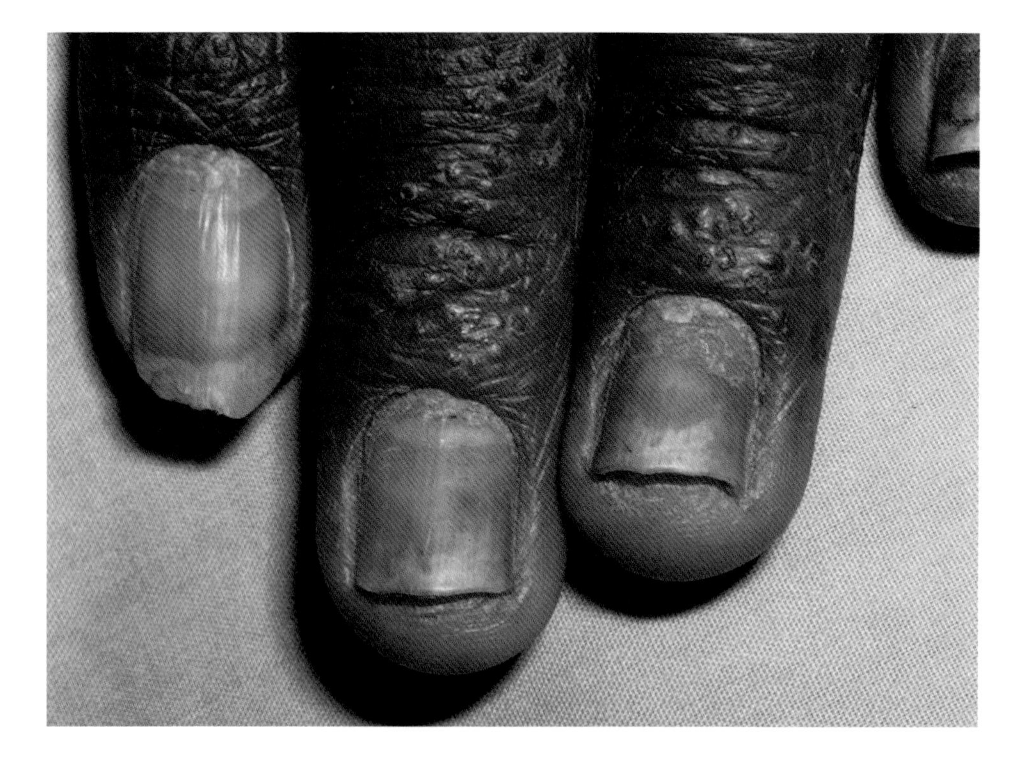

**Figures 448, 449** Subungual hyperkeratosis. Once the nail has lifted off the nail bed in psoriasis, an accumulation of keratin underneath is possible.

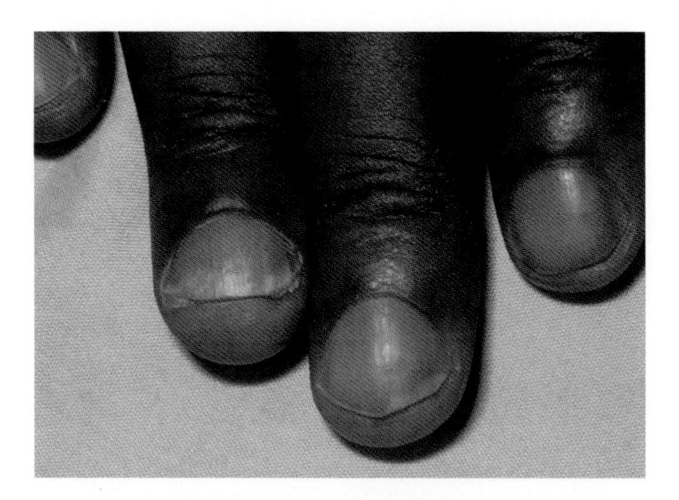

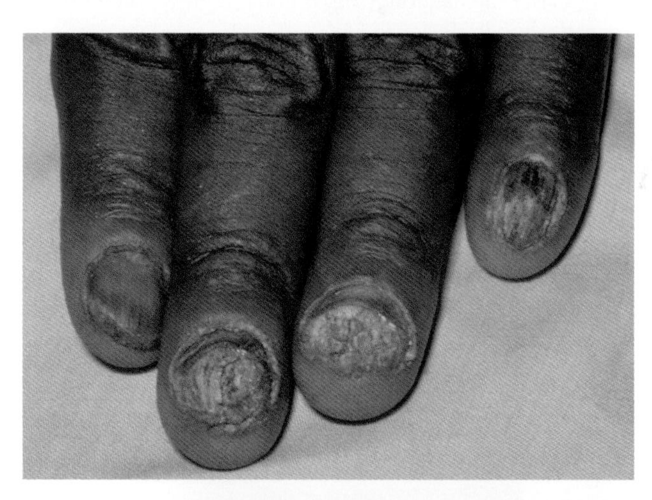

**Figure 450** Most abnormalities of the nail bed cause discolouration under the nail. White discolouration under the nail is due to hypoproteinaemia or chronic renal failure.

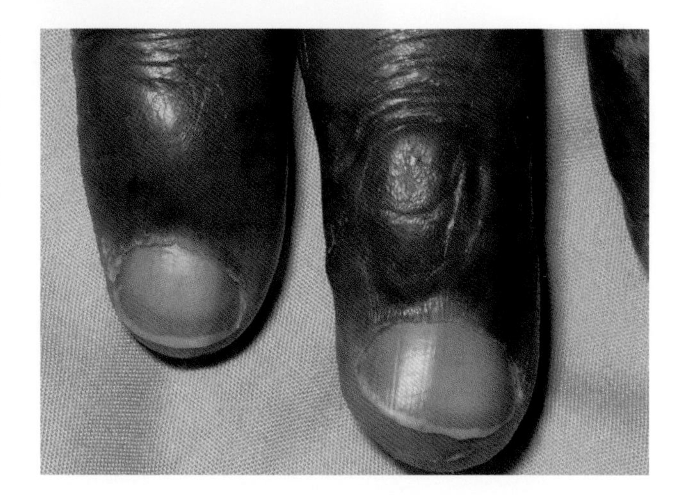

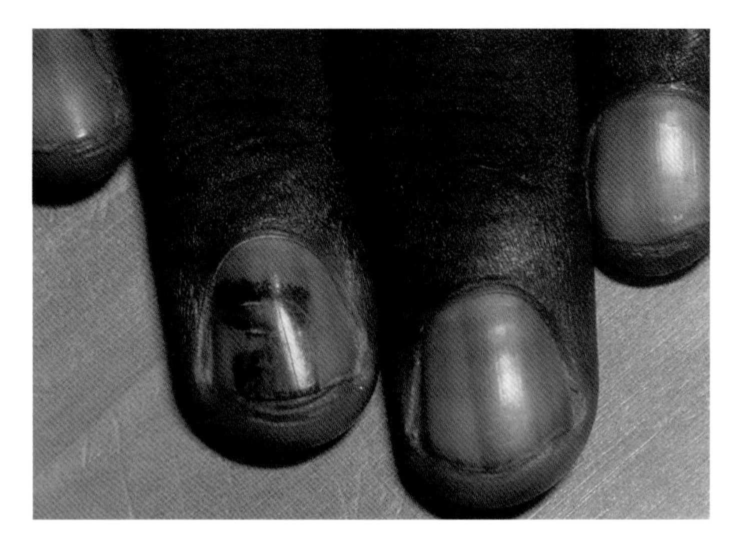

**Figure 451** Subungual haematoma. A red or black mark due to bleeding under the nail following trauma. It grows out at the same speed as the nail itself.

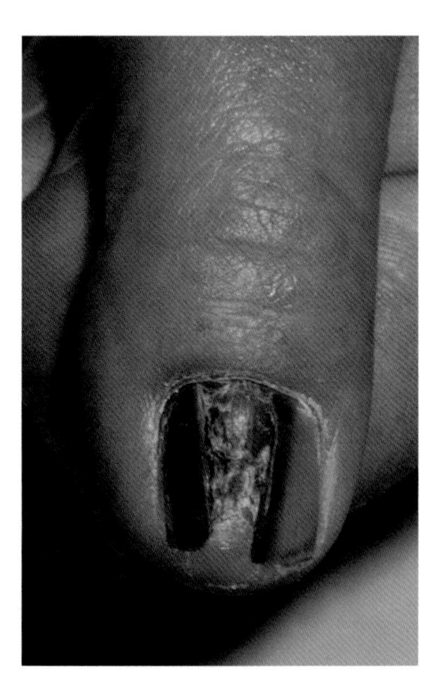

**Figure 452** Subungual malignant melanoma. A round or oval brown macule under the nail is a junctional naevus of the nail bed. If it is growing, or made up of different colours, or growing through the nail think of a malignant melanoma.

# Abnormalities of the nail plate

## Discolouration of the nail plate

**Figures 453, 454** Blue nails. This is a sign of HIV infection. The blue discolouration begins proximally and then becomes diffuse.

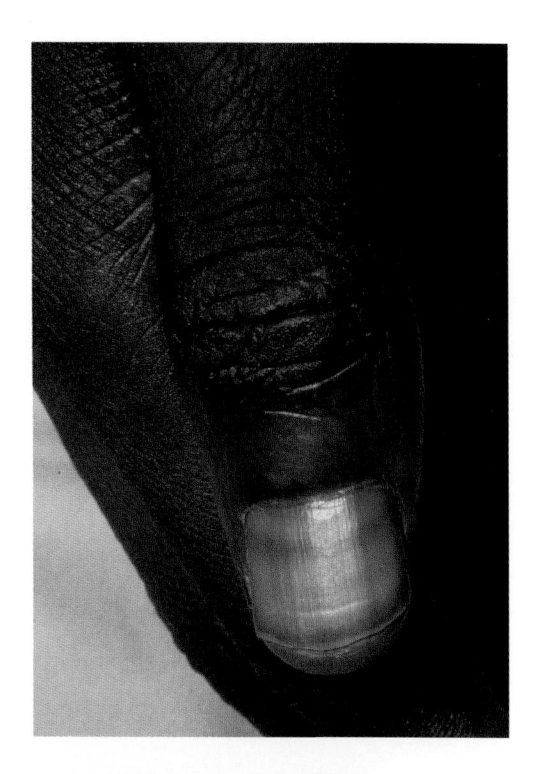

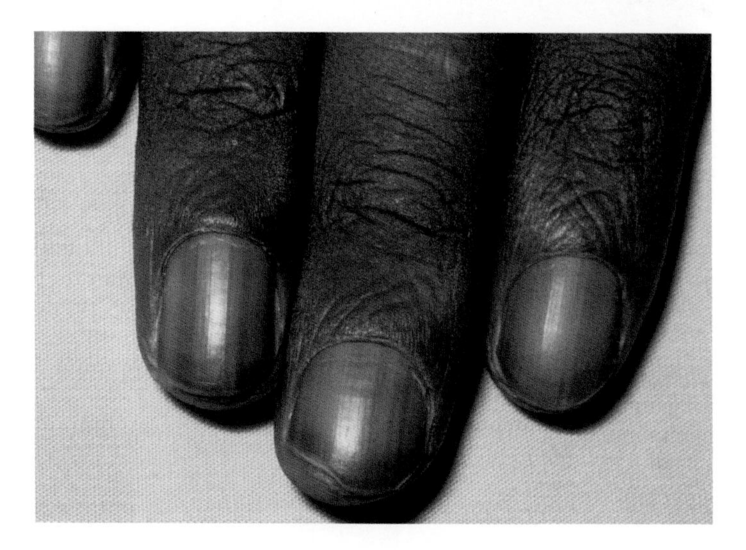

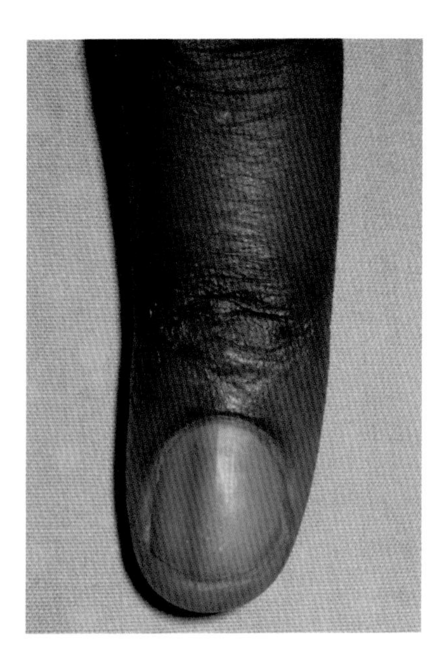

**Figure 455** Brown lines in the nails. Longitudinal brown lines in the nails are due to junctional naevi in the nail matrix.

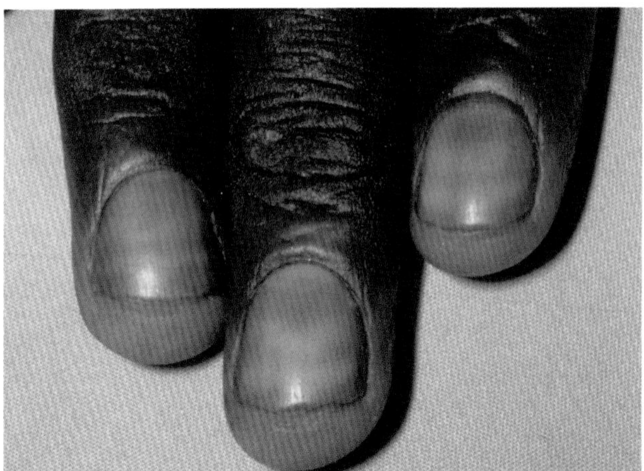

**Figure 456** Red and white stripes across the nails. This is a sign of HIV infection. Its cause is unknown.

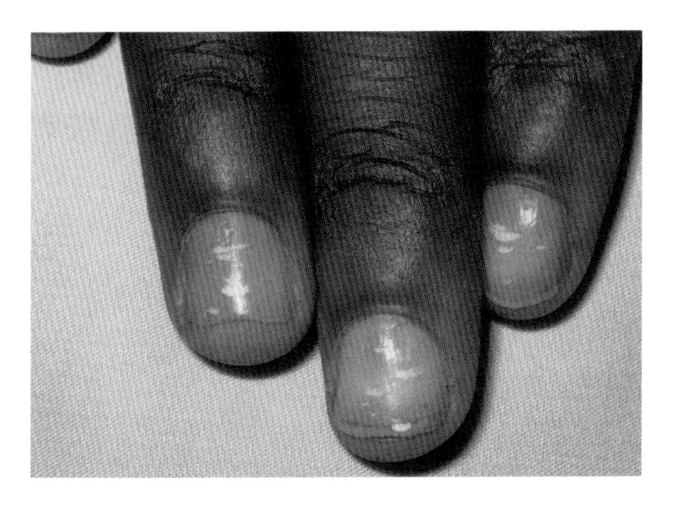

**Figure 457** White nails. Small white patches in the nails are a normal finding after minor trauma.

## Thickening of the nail plate

**Figures 458, 459** Tinea unguium. The nail is discoloured (white or yellow), thickened and slow growing. The toenails are mainly involved because fingernails generally grow too fast for the fungus to become established in them. It may be difficult to distinguish from subungual hyperkeratosis in psoriasis (*see* Figure 449).

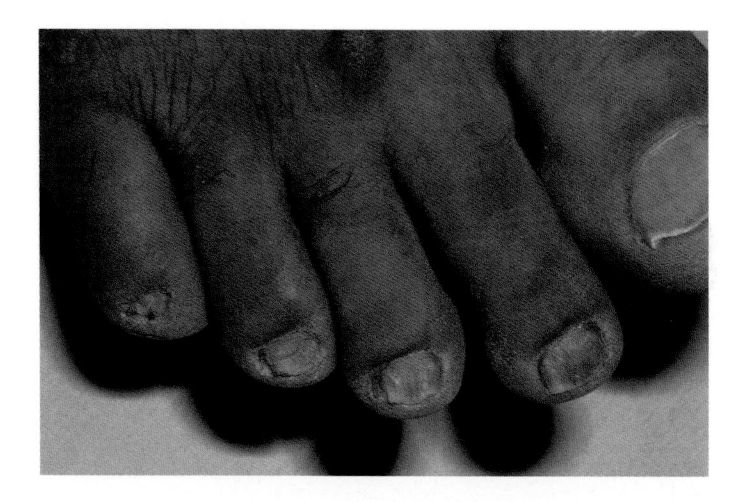

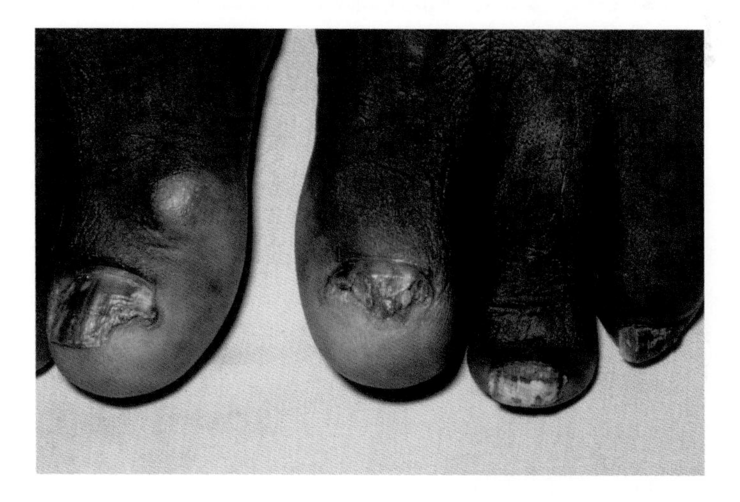

*Treatment:* Most infections are asymptomatic and not noticed by the patient. Do not attempt to treat these patients. If the patient is complaining, use oral terbinafine 250mg/day after food for 3 months. This works well but is very expensive.

## Abnormalities of the cuticle

The cuticle is a specialised form of keratin joining the skin of the posterior nail fold to the nail plate (*see* Figure 441) to prevent bacteria and yeasts from getting into the soft tissues around the nail. If the cuticle is lost (usually in people whose hands are in water all day), infection can enter through the gap which is left. This is called paronychia. There are two types.

**Figure 460** Acute paronychia. This is due to infection with *Staphylococcus aureus* or *Streptococcus pyogenes*. There is a very painful red swelling around the nail and formation of pus.

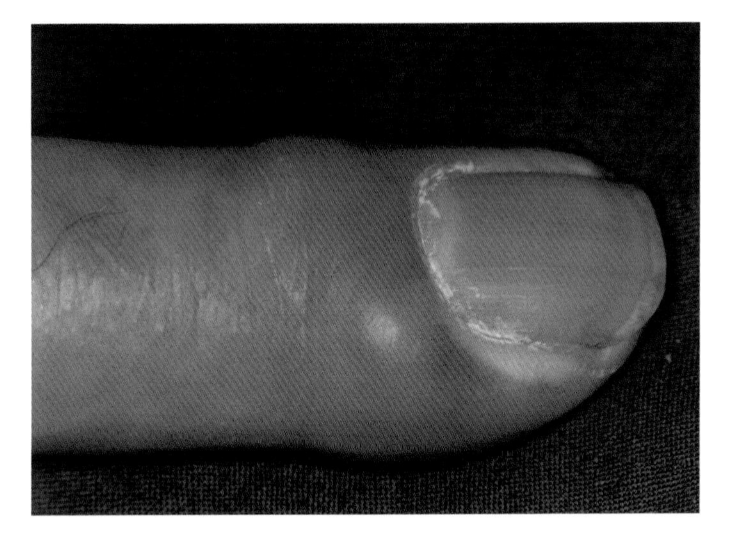

*Treatment:* Incise to release the pus. If pus has not yet formed, antibiotics to cover both staphylococci and streptococci are needed (e.g. erythromycin 500mg qds for 7 days).

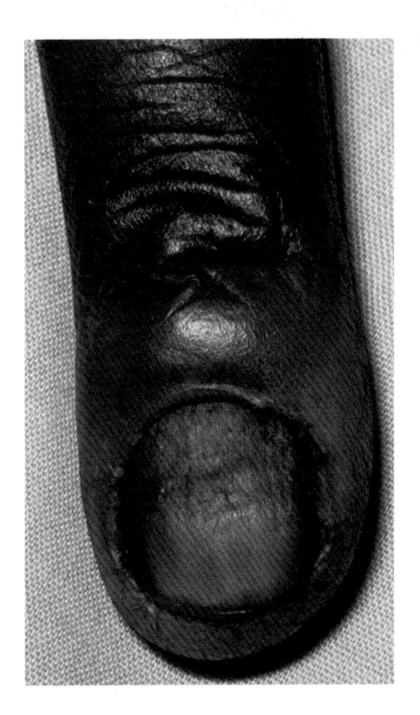

**Figure 461** Chronic paronychia. This is due to *Candida albicans*. It causes a chronic swelling around the nail with transverse ridges and pits in the nail.

*Treatment:* Keep the hands dry until a new cuticle grows. Specific treatment for the candida is not necessary.

## NECROTISING FASCIITIS

**Figure 462** This is an infection of the subcutaneous fat and fascia due to *Streptococcus pyogenes* (*see* Figure 124). The organism produces a toxin which causes thrombosis of dermal blood vessels and necrosis of the skin. Initially, it looks like cellulitis or erysipelas but within 2–3 days necrosis occurs.

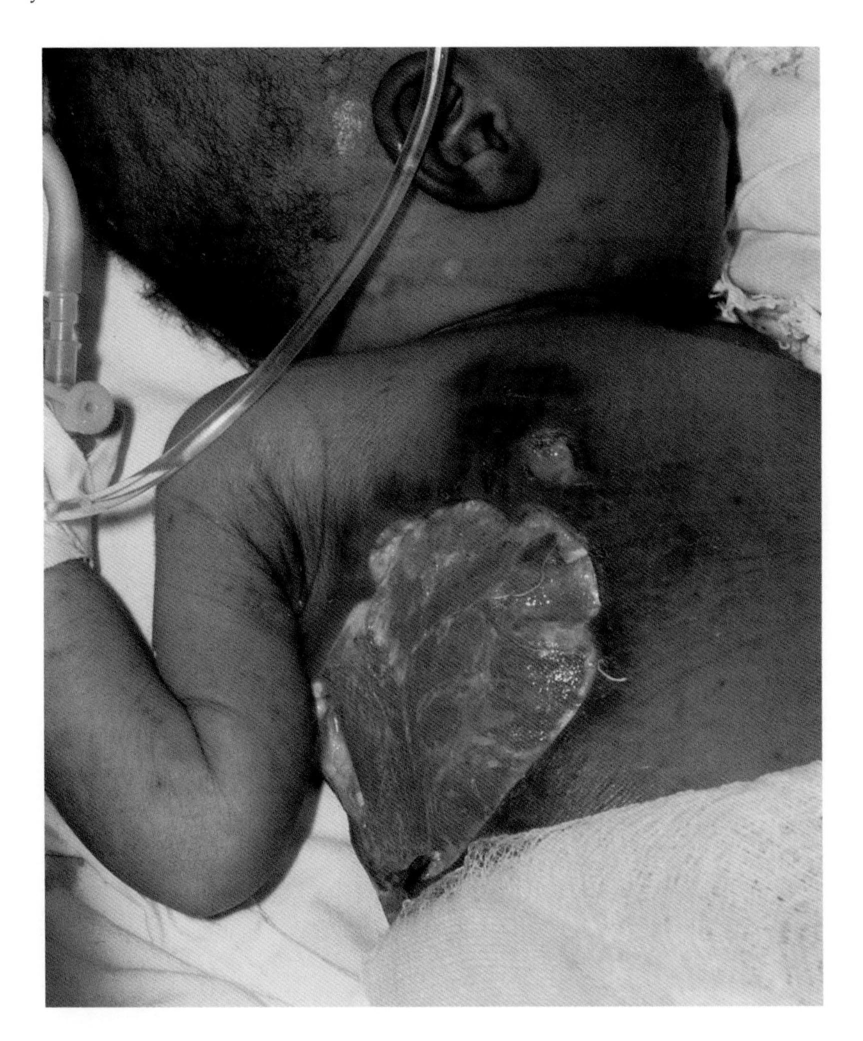

*Treatment:* Surgical excision of all necrotic tissue together with benzyl penicillin intravenously every 6 hours.

## NEUROFIBROMATOSIS (von Recklinghausen's disease)

There are three cardinal signs of this autosomal dominant condition:

- Café-au-lait patches.
- Axillary freckling.
- Multiple neurofibromas.

**Figure 463** Multiple café-au-lait patches. Round or oval hyperpigmented patches which begin in early childhood. More than six of these indicate neurofibromatosis. Less than six may be a normal finding.

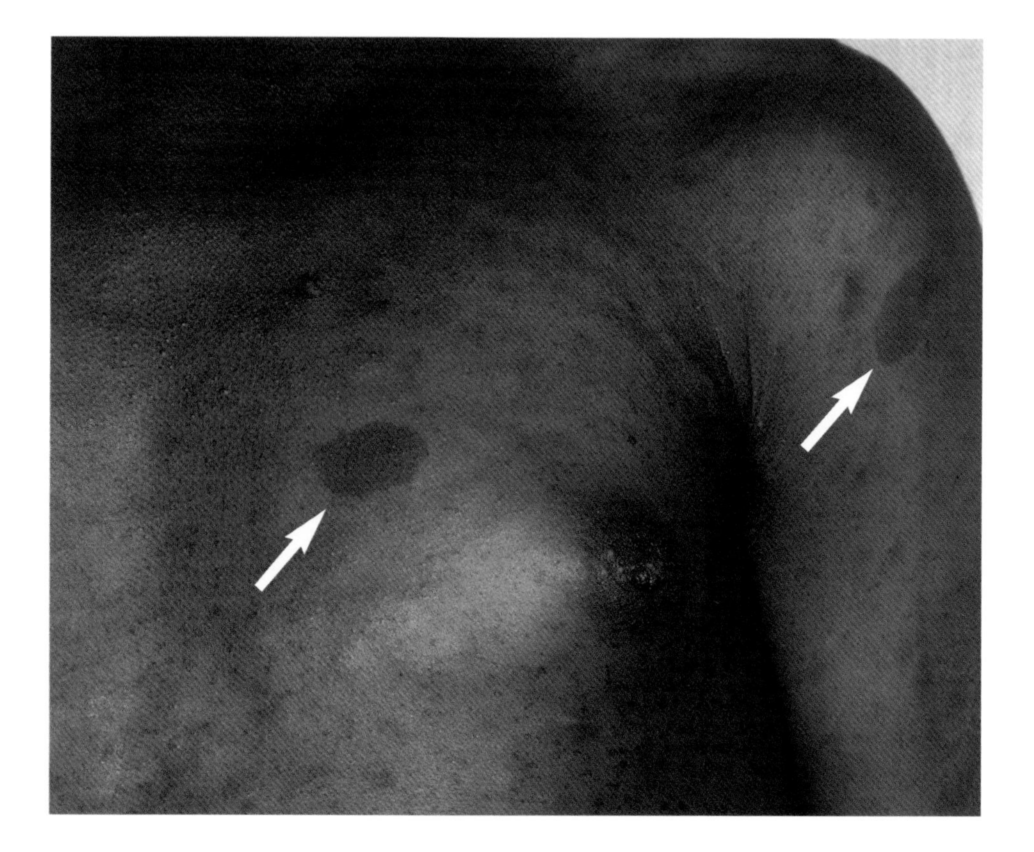

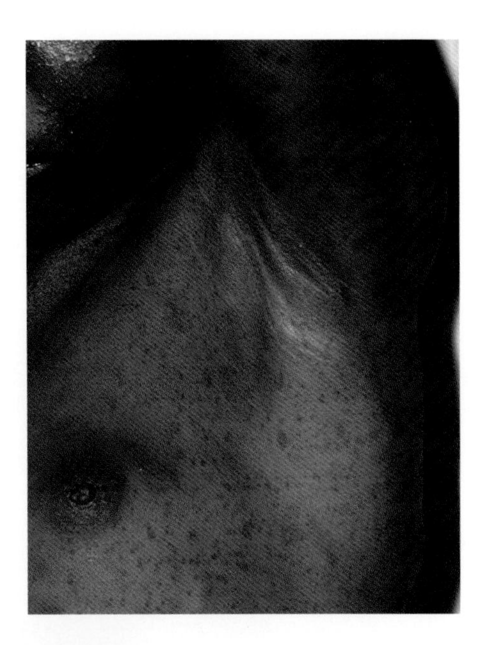

**Figure 464** Axillary freckling.

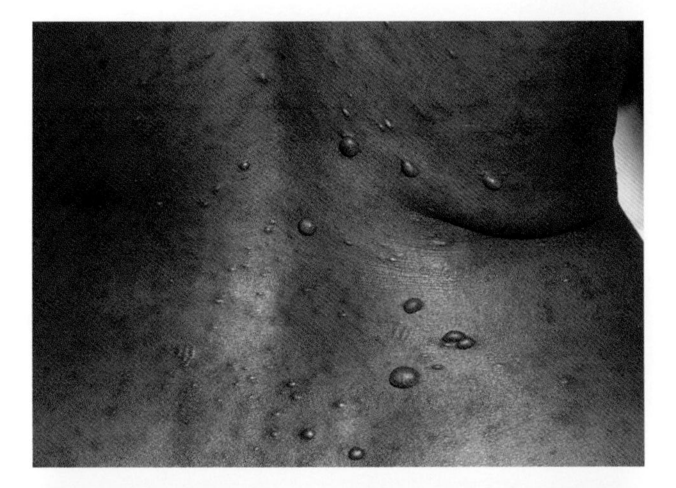

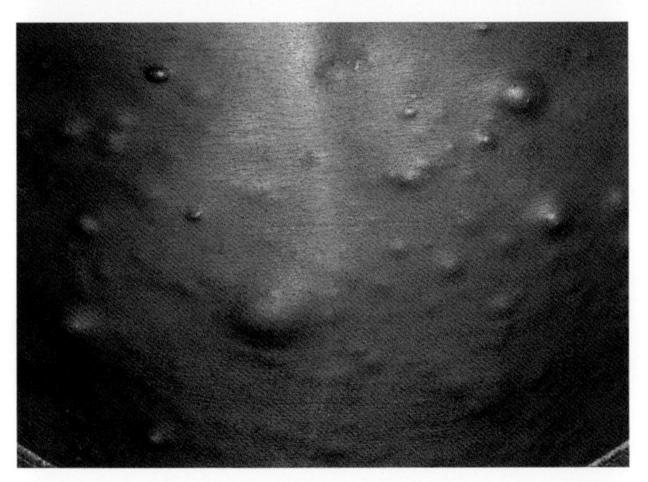

**Figures 465, 466** Multiple neurofibromas. These are soft sessile or pedunculated papules or nodules found anywhere on the body surface. They can be few or very numerous and vary in size from a few millimetres to several centimetres in diameter.

*Treatment:* Excision of unsightly neurofibromas. Otherwise explain the disease and the genetic implications (*see* Figure 295).

**Figure 467** Plexiform neuromas are diffuse linear neuromas along the course of a nerve.

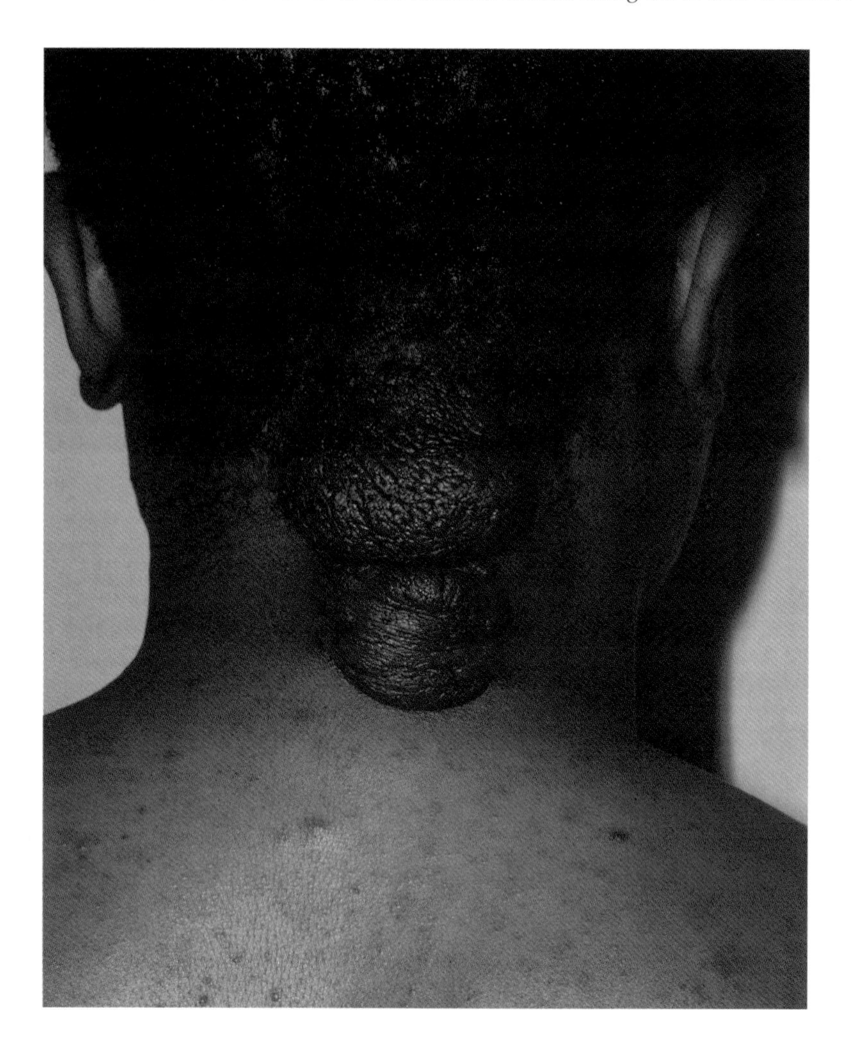

## NIPPLE ECZEMA

**Figure 468** This is eczema confined to the nipple and areola of one or both breasts in young women. It can occur any time after the mid-teens. Do not confuse it with Paget's disease of the nipple which is much more serious (*see* Figure 483).

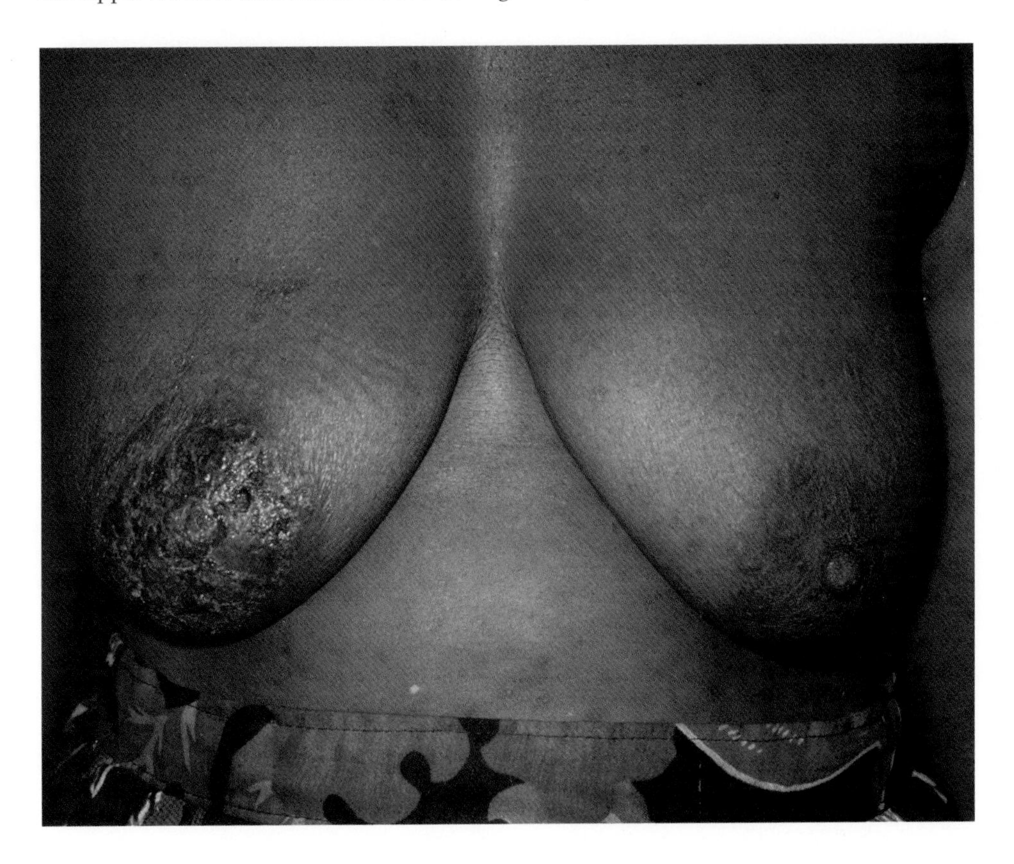

*Treatment:* Reassurance that it is harmless and will get better spontaneously after a time. Meanwhile, 1% hydrocortisone ointment can be applied bd.

## NODULAR PRURIGO

**Figure 469** Discrete, intensely itchy papules and nodules due to scratching and picking. May be found in association with atopic eczema and in patients with HIV infection.

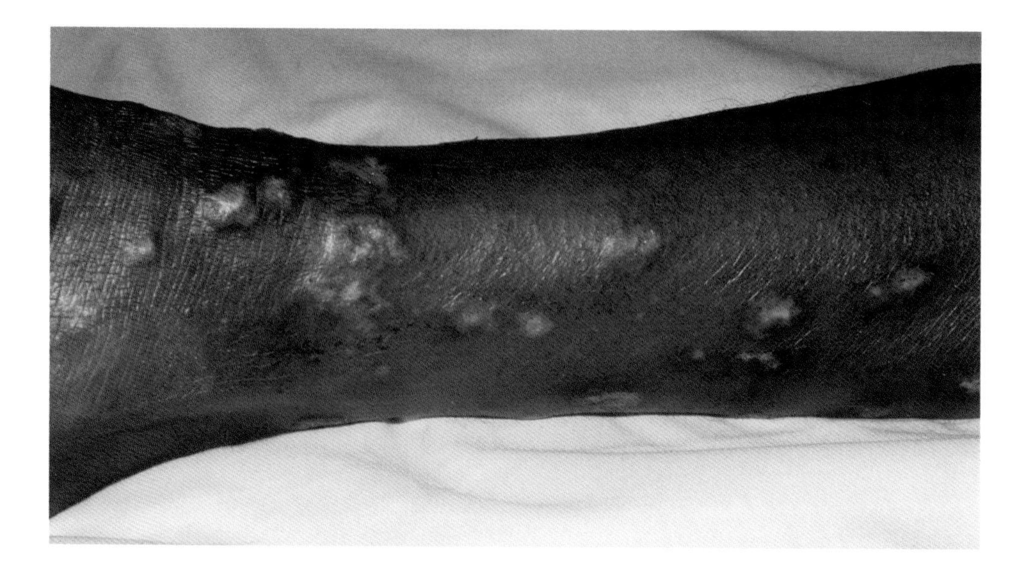

*Treatment:* Potent topical steroid ointments (e.g. 0.1% betamethasone 17-valerate ointment) applied bd.

## NOMA (Cancrum oris)

**Figure 470** This is an acute necrotising gingivitis which progresses to a mutilating ulceration of the mouth and face due to fusiform bacteria and *Treponema vincenti.* It is a disease of poverty and is found in malnourished young children (under 6 years), often after measles, malaria or some other infectious disease. Without treatment, 70–90% of these children will die.

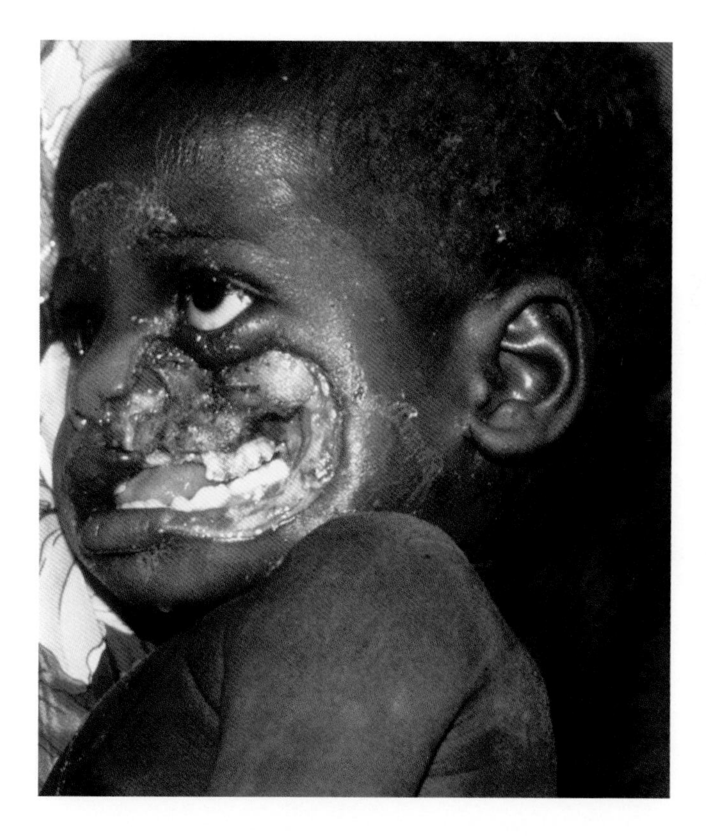

*Treatment:* If it is recognised and treated at the necrotising gingivitis stage it can be treated with antibiotics (ampicillin or a cephalosporin) and a high protein diet. Once ulceration has occurred plastic reconstructive surgery will be needed.

## ONCHOCERCIASIS

Onchocerciasis is due to the filarial worm, *Onchocerca volvulus*. It is transmitted by the bite of black flies, *Simulium damnosum* in West Africa and *Simulium neavei* in East Africa. The flies suck human blood containing microfilaria and then inject the larvae into the next victim. Numerous bites over many years are needed for infestation to occur. The flies breed near fast flowing rivers, so humans who live, work or play near these rivers are most at risk. The injected larvae mature to adult worms in about 3 months and these live in nodules in the dermis, mainly around the pelvic girdle. The female may be 50–60cm long and can produce more than 1000 microfilaria/day which go to the skin and eyes.

**Figure 471** In the skin the microfilaria produce a very itchy rash. In endemic areas everyone scatches themselves or each other with a stick. In time the skin becomes lichenified and so thick that it is likened to elephant skin.

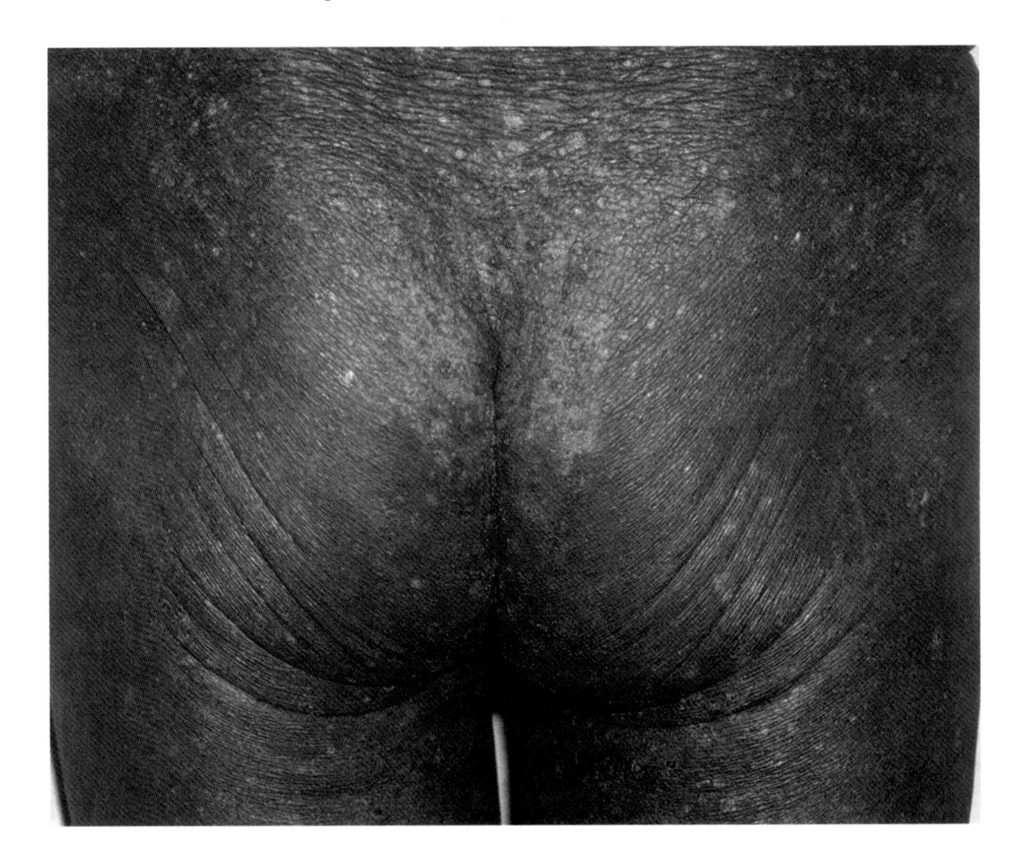

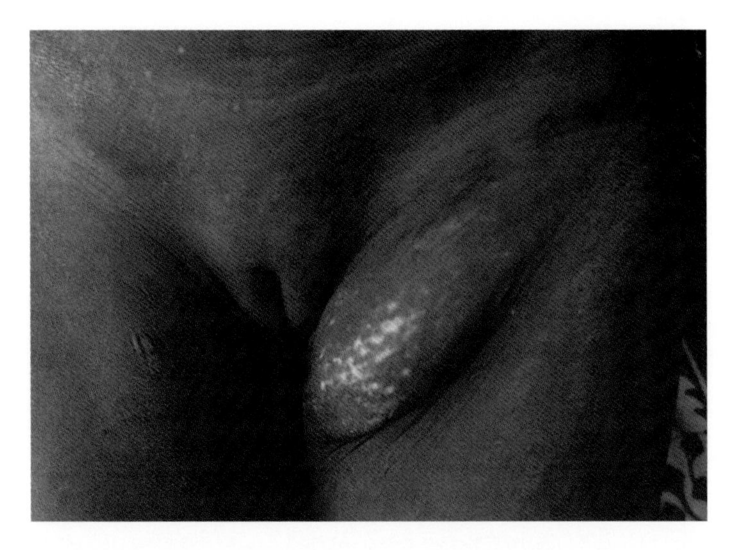

**Figure 472** After some years the loss of elastic fibres in the dermis leaves the skin wrinkled like tissue paper. This, together with inguinal lymphadenopathy, gives rise to the typical 'hanging groin'.

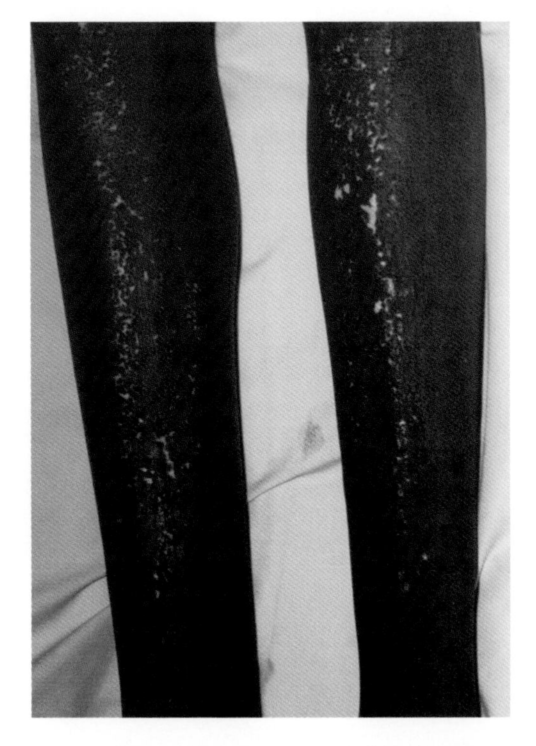

**Figure 473** On the shins there is spotty depigmentation known as 'leopard shins'. This is not pathognomonic for onchocerciasis as it is a fairly common finding on the shins of elderly men.

**Figures 474, 475** The diagnosis of onchocerciasis can be confirmed by doing an oncho snip. Remove a small snip of skin with a scalpel blade and place it on a glass slide with a drop of normal saline. Cover the slide and leave it for half an hour.

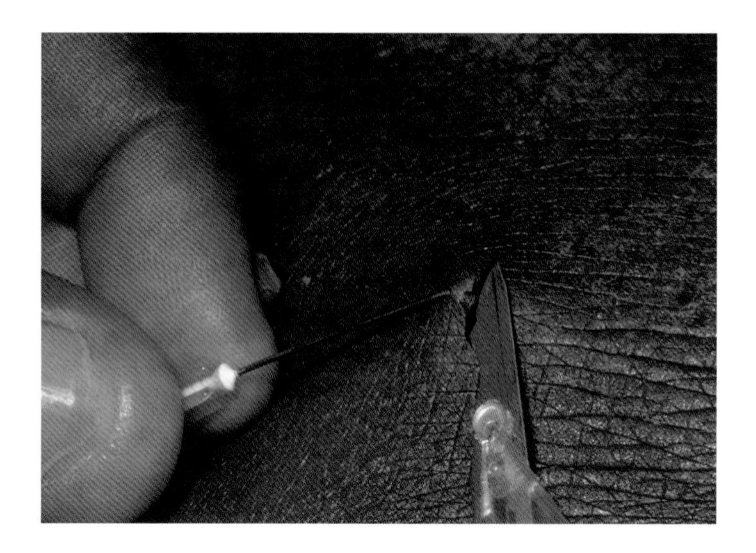

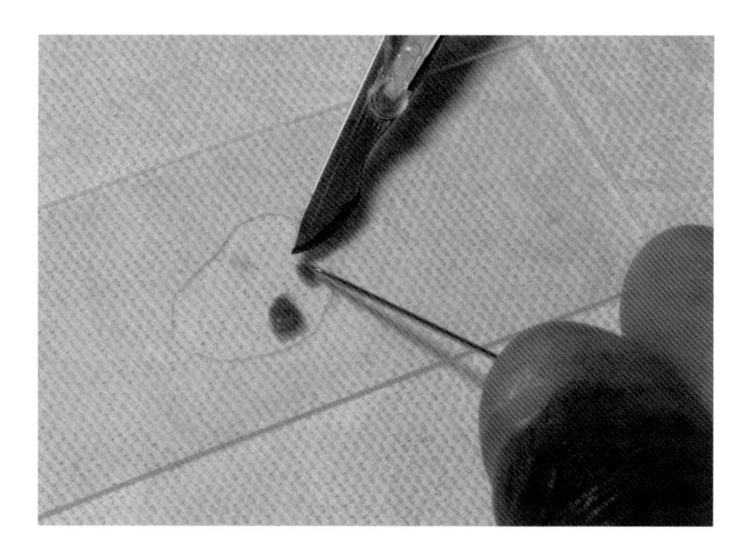

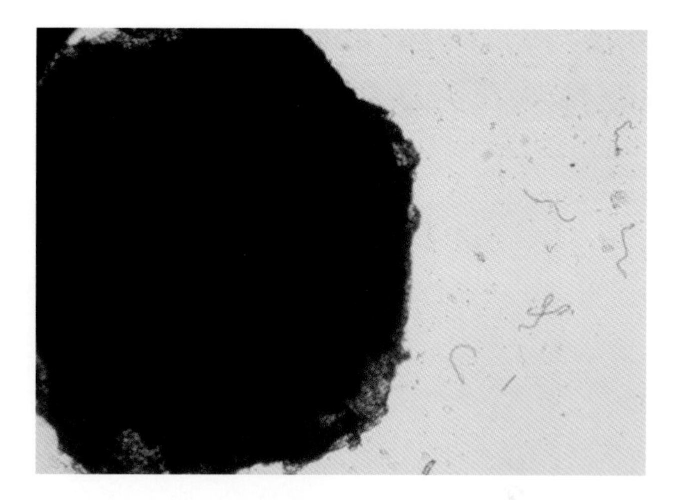

**Figure 476** Positive oncho snip. You can see the microfilaria in the normal saline.

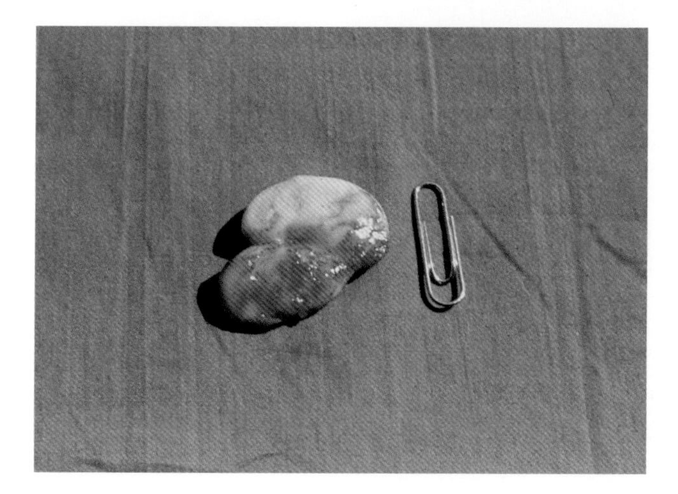

**Figure 477** The diagnosis can also be confirmed by removing one of the onchocercal nodules from around the hips, cutting it across and seeing the adult worms.

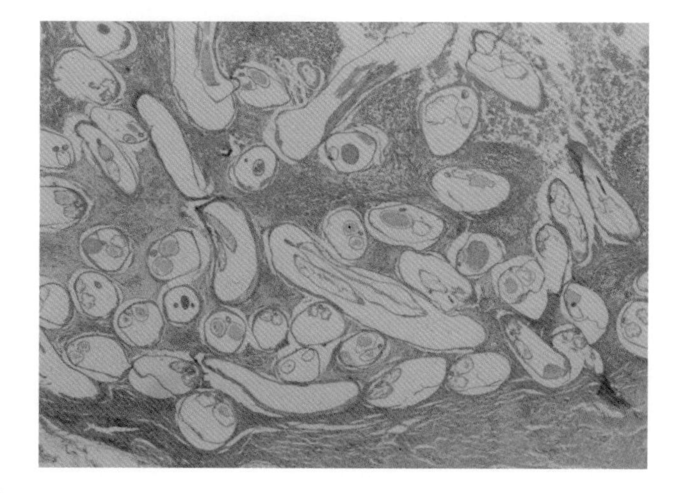

**Figure 478** Alternatively, an onchocercal nodule can be sent for histological examination. The adult worms can be seen on cross section as shown here.

*Treatment:* A single dose of ivermectin, 200$\mu$g/kg body weight, once a year. This makes the microfilaria leave the skin and go to the lymph nodes where they die. The adult worms are not affected so the drug needs to be given once a year until the adult worms die (10–15 years).

## ORAL HAIRY LEUKOPLAKIA

**Figure 479** Viral infection due to the *Epstein–Barr* virus. It causes white linear papules (which look like hairs) along the side of the tongue in patients with HIV infection.

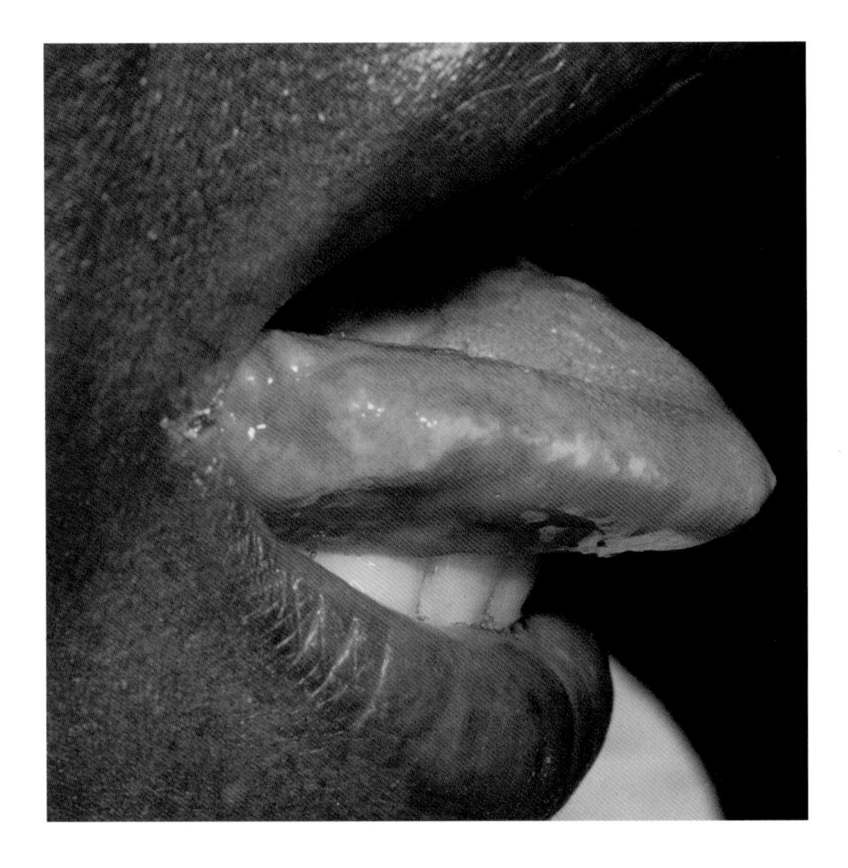

*Treatment:* It is usually asymptomatic so no treatment is needed. Check for HIV infection.

## ORF

**Figure 480** Pox virus infection of young sheep and goats. Sores around the mouth lead to difficulty in suckling so that the young animals have to be fed by humans.

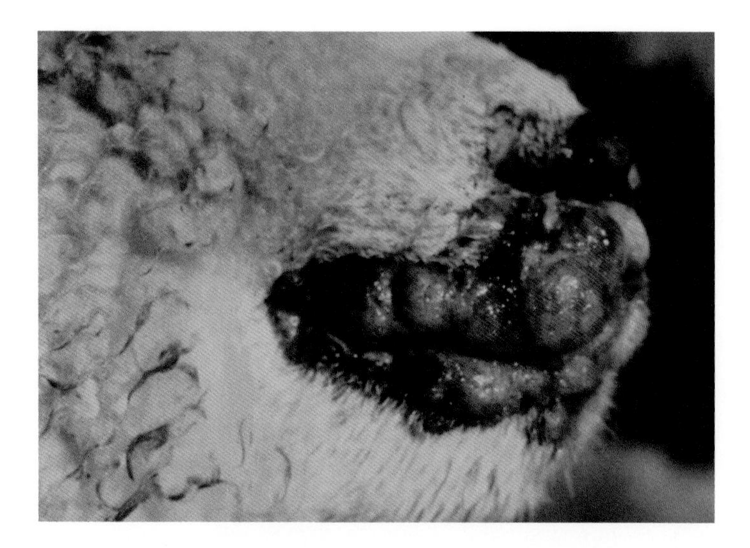

**Figure 481** Reddish papule on a finger with what looks like a blister in the centre in someone who has been hand feeding a young sheep or goat.

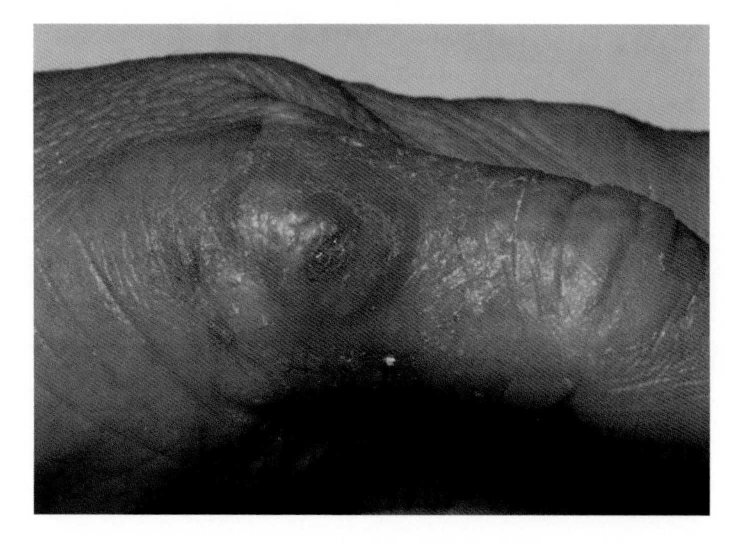

*Treatment:* None is needed because it heals spontaneously after 3–4 weeks.

## OSTEOMYELITIS

**Figure 482** This is a bacterial infection of bone. It may present with a swelling of the skin or multiple discharging sinuses. Confirm the diagnosis by X-raying the underlying bone.

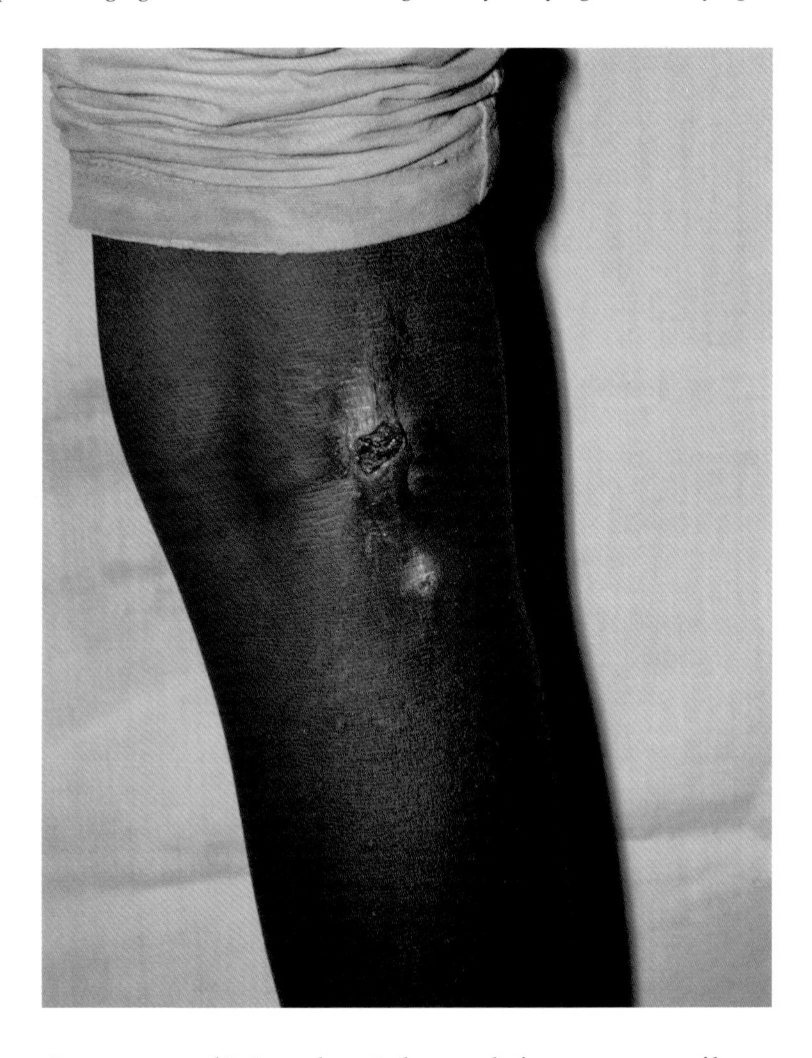

*Treatment:* Intravenous antibiotics and surgical removal of any sequestrae of bone.

## PAGET'S DISEASE OF THE NIPPLE

**Figure 483** An itchy eczematous looking plaque involving the nipple and areola of the breast. It is due to an intraduct carcinoma and should not be confused with the harmless, and much more common, nipple eczema of young women (*see* Figure 468).

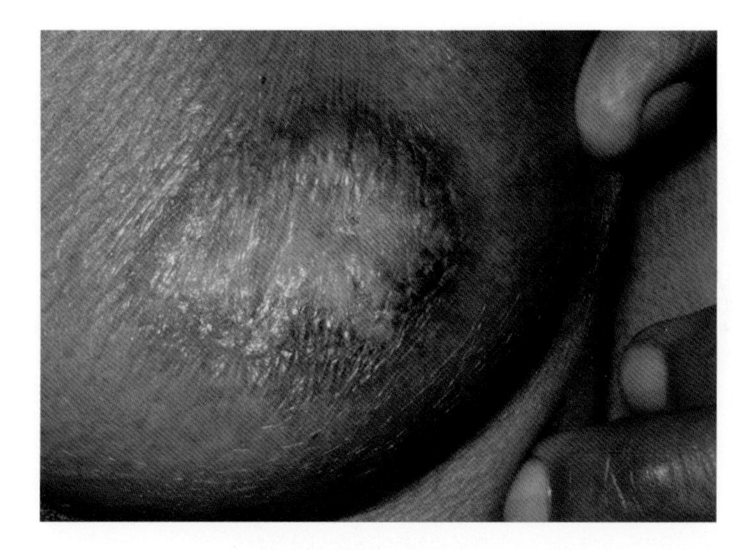

*Treatment:* Mastectomy.

**Figure 484** A biopsy will confirm the diagnosis. Malignant cells can be seen invading the epidermis.

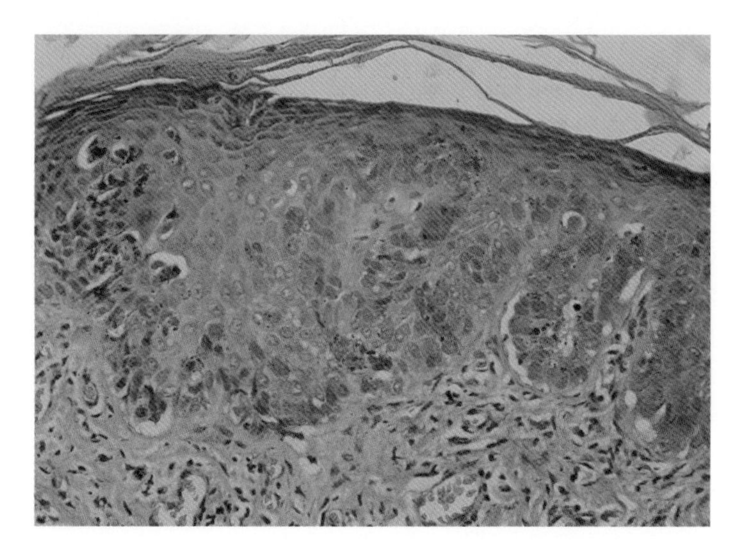

## PALISADING ENCAPSULATED NEUROMA (PEN)

**Figure 485** Small skin-coloured papules which are usually solitary. They may be confused with intradermal naevi clinically (*see* Figure 67) and neurofibromatosis histologically, but they are a distinct entity.

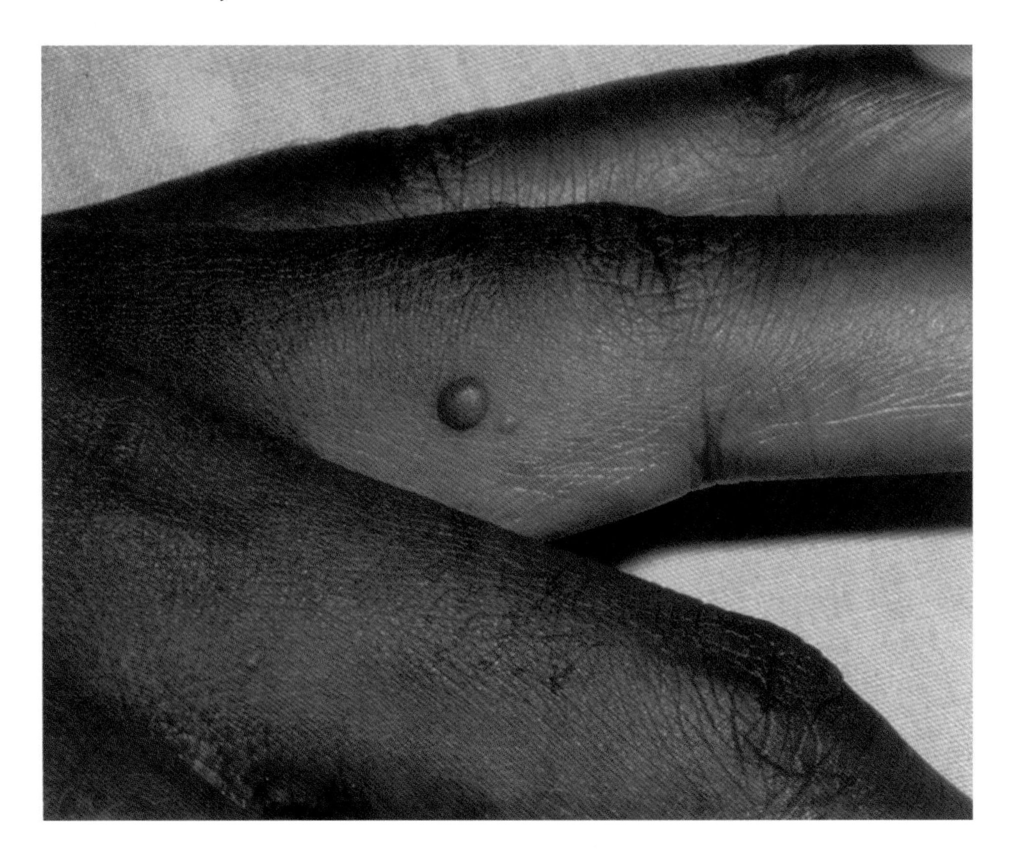

*Treatment:* Reassurance that they are harmless.

## PAPULAR PRURITIC ERUPTION ASSOCIATED WITH HIV INFECTION

**Figure 486** Very itchy symmetrical rash made up of papules and excoriations. Histology shows an eosinophilic folliculitis. Associated with HIV infection.

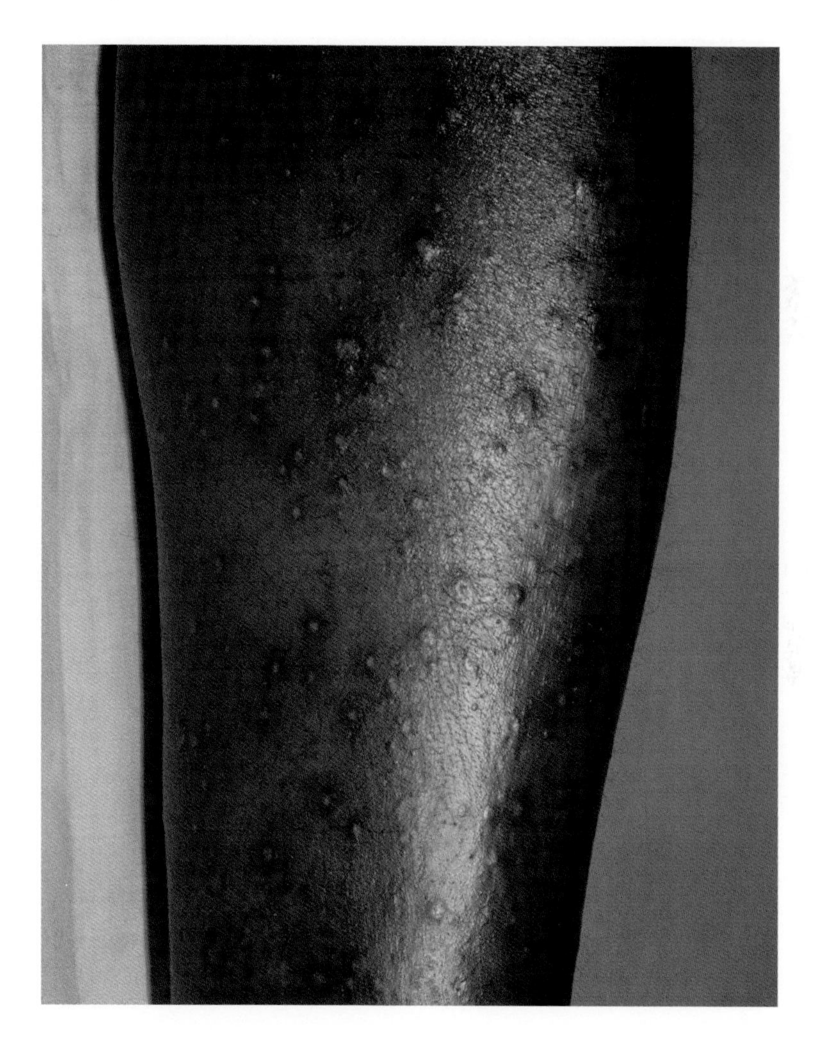

*Treatment:* Exposing the skin to sunlight may help. Otherwise use a moderately potent topical steroid ointment such as 0.1% betamethasone 17-valerate bd to help the itching.

## PAPULAR URTICARIA

**Figure 487** Discrete itchy papular rash which looks like the rash of scabies but without any burrows. It can be a generalised reaction to insect bites in children or a manifestation of internal parasites such as intestinal worms.

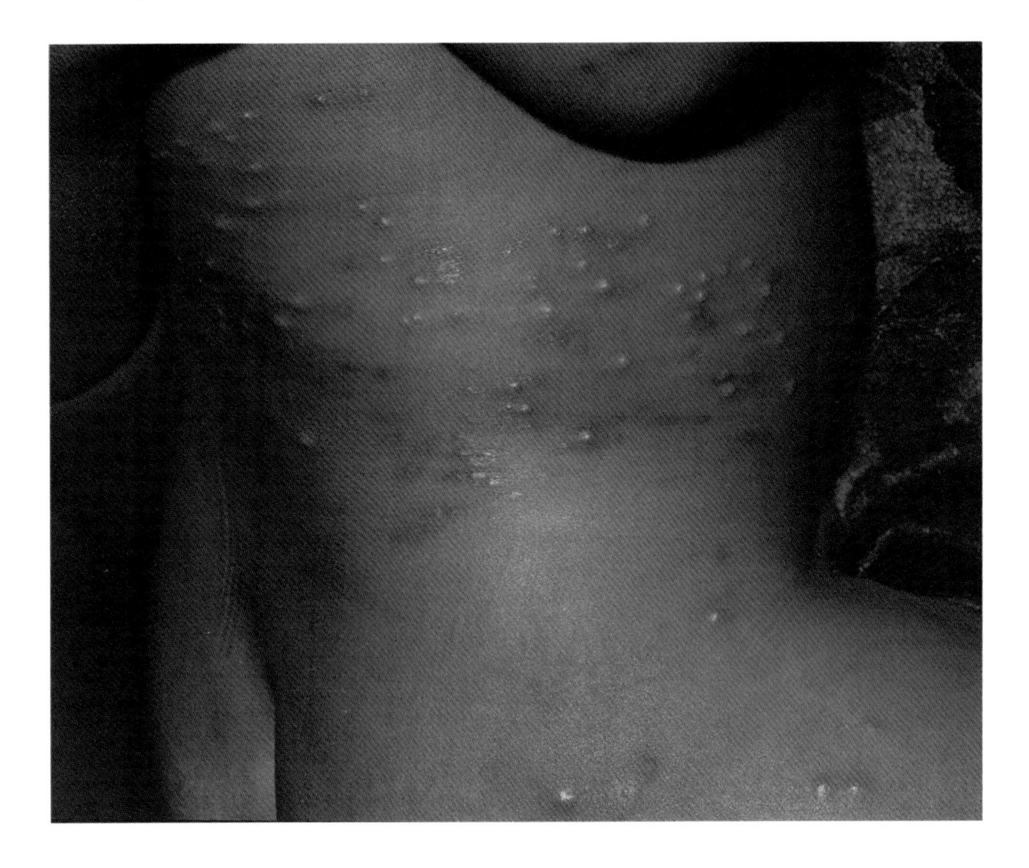

*Treatment:* Check the stool for parasites and ova, and treat the underlying worm infestation.

## PAROTID SWELLING IN HIV INFECTION

**Figure 488** Bilateral parotid swelling in a child is mumps until proved otherwise. In an adult it is usually due to HIV infection but it can also be due to lymphoma as in this patient.

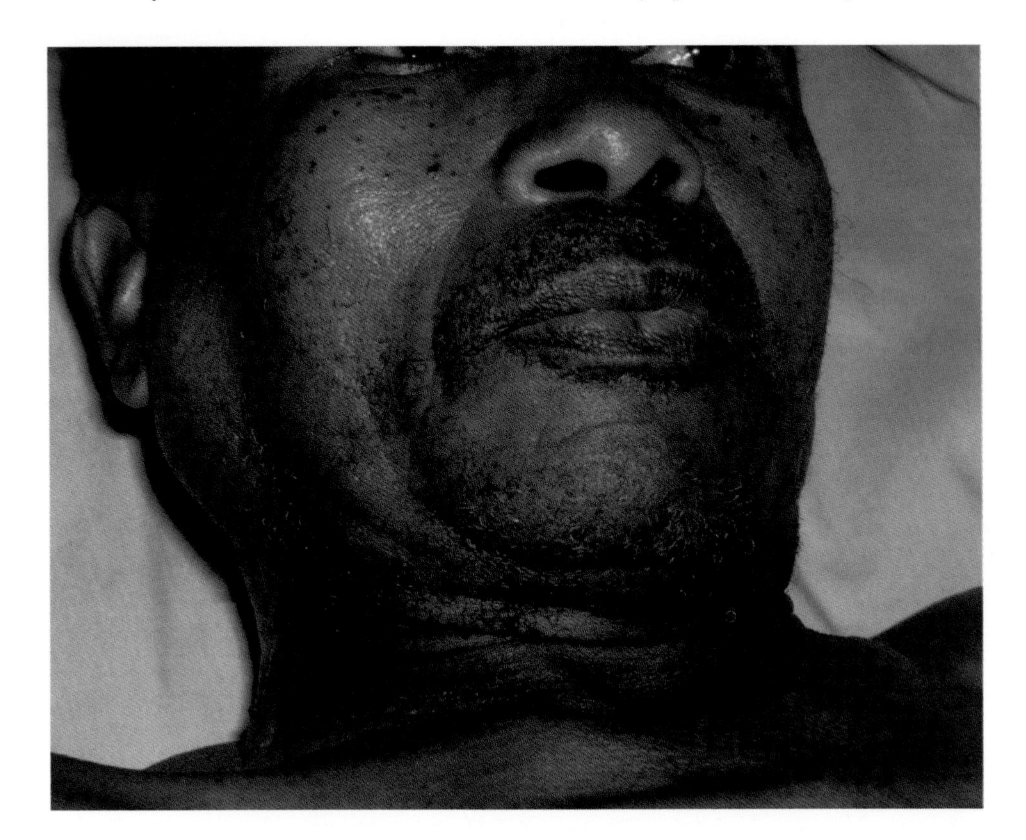

## PELLAGRA

**Figures 489, 490, 491, 492** Disease of the three Ds – dermatitis, diarrhoea and dementia – due to a dietary deficiency in niacin. It occurs mainly in communities where maize is the staple diet and there is no other source of protein, or in alcoholics who spend all their money on alcohol and do not eat properly.

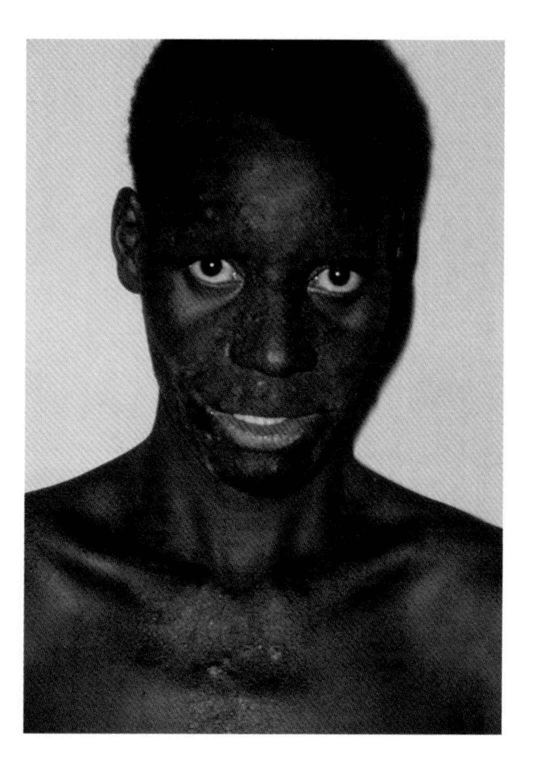

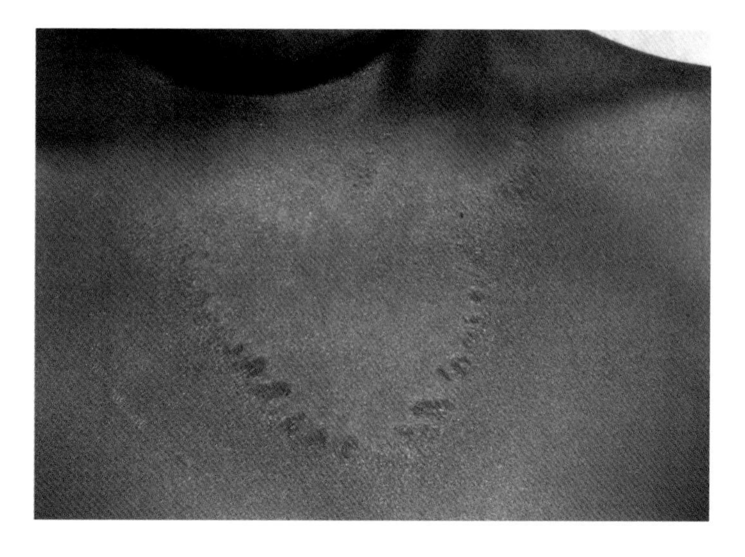

Maize contains little tryptophan, an essential amino acid which is needed as a substrate for niacin production.

The rash characteristically occurs on sun-exposed sites – the face, the 'V' of the neck (it is called Casal's necklace here – Figure 490), the dorsum of the hands and forearms, and the dorsum of the feet. It can also be induced by taking isoniazid and/or pyridoxine.

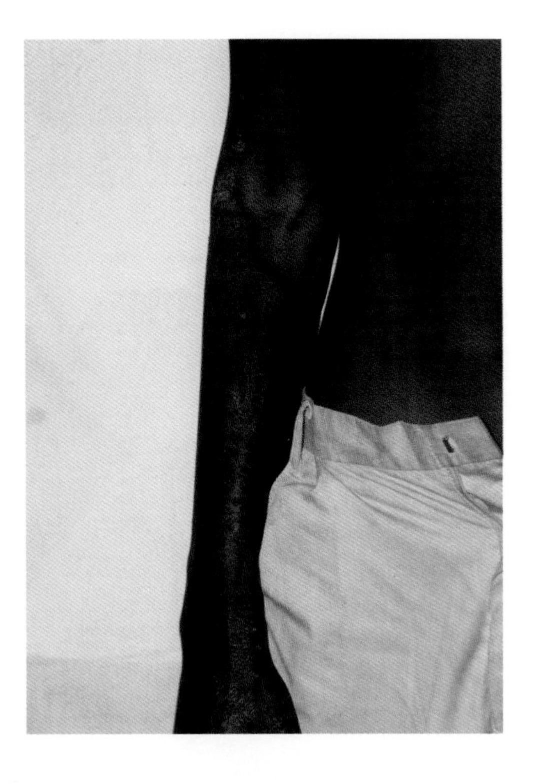

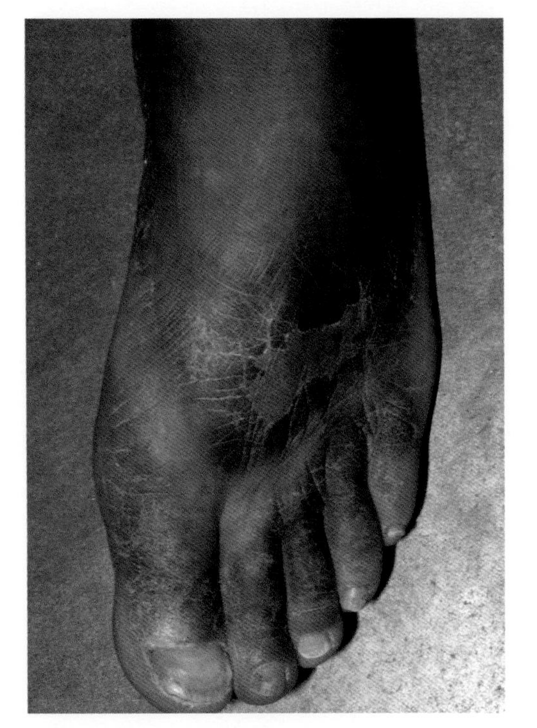

*Treatment:* Niacin 500mg/day orally together with a high protein diet.

## PEMPHIGOID

**Figure 493** A group of autoimmune blistering conditions characterised histologically by blisters at the dermo–epidermal junction.

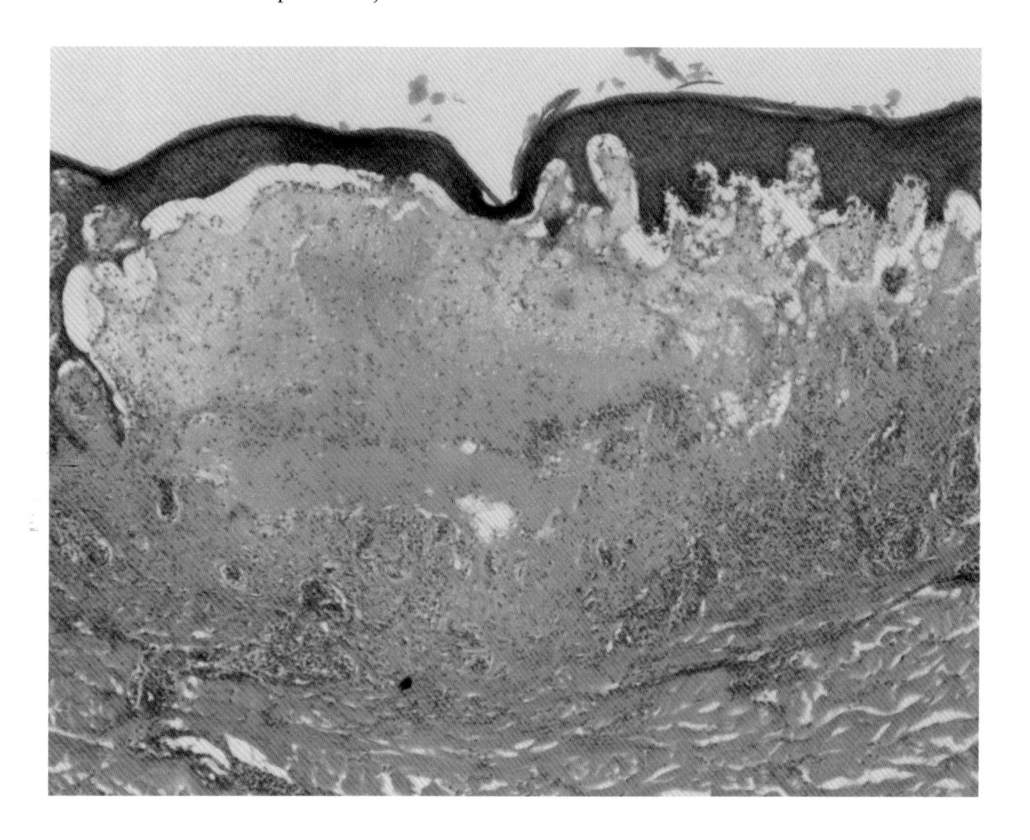

## Bullous pemphigoid

**Figure 494** A very itchy disease of the elderly (mostly age >70 years) in which there are large intact blisters, some of which may be haemorrhagic.

*Treatment:* Prednisolone 30–40mg/day until new blisters stop appearing, then gradually decrease to a maintenance dose of 7.5–10mg/day.

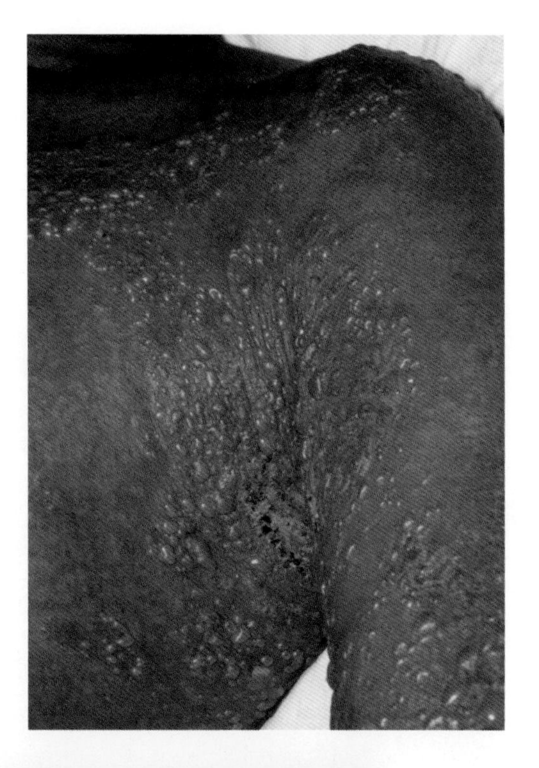

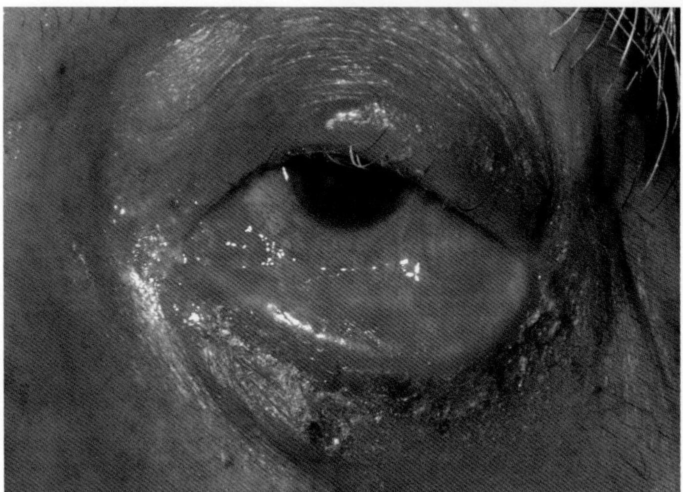

## Cicatricial pemphigoid

**Figure 495** Blisters of mucous membranes – mouth, conjunctiva, urethra and perianal area. The main problems are to do with difficulties in swallowing and scarring of the conjunctivae, which can lead to blindness.

*Treatment:* It does not respond well to oral steroids. Use cyclophosphamide 50–100mg/day.

## PEMPHIGUS

A group of autoimmune blistering eruptions where the blister is intraepidermal.

### Pemphigus foliaceus

**Figure 496** This is the most common type of pemphigus in Africa. The blistering is very superficial, just below the granular layer.

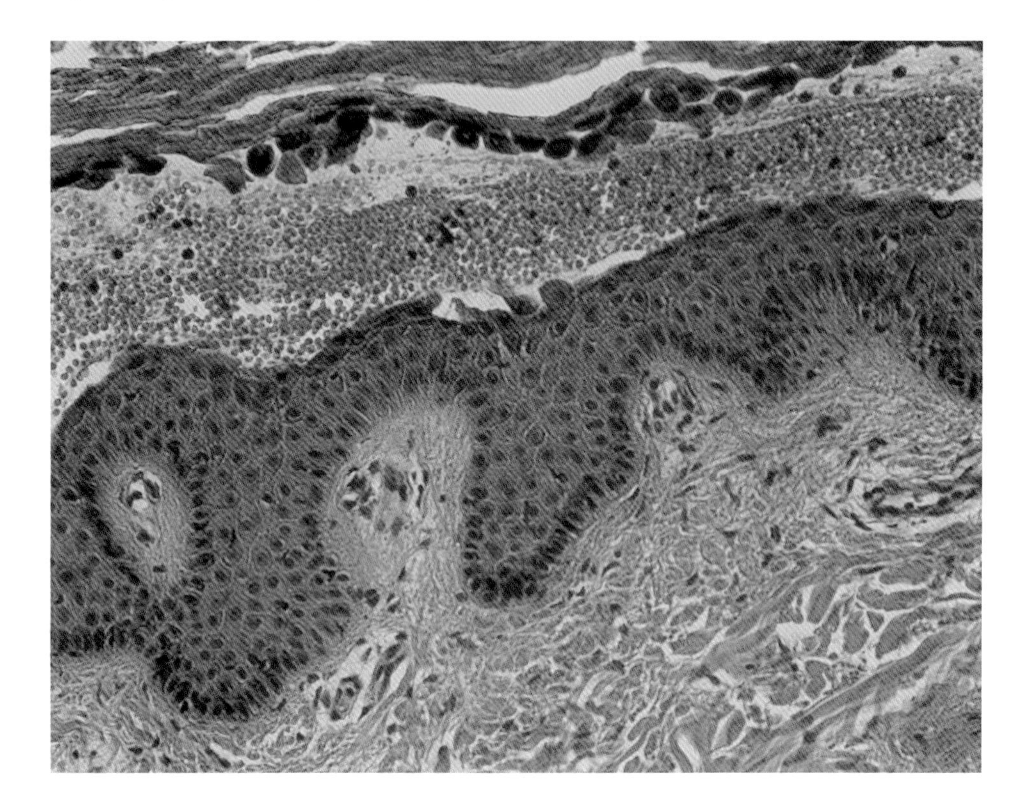

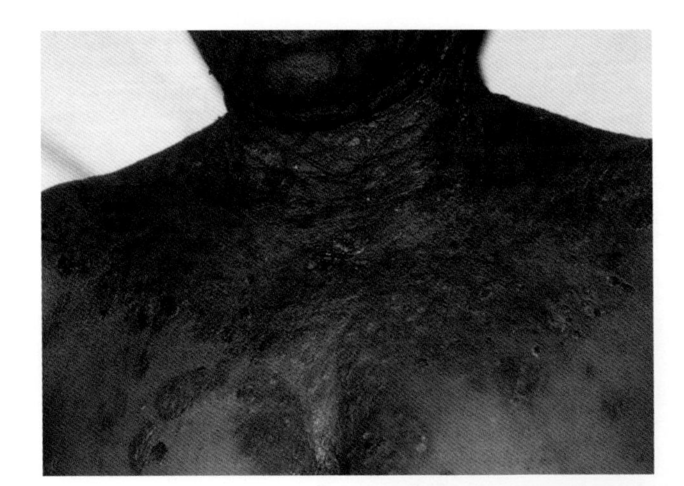

**Figures 497, 498, 499** The rash is mainly on the face, scalp and upper trunk. It often looks scaly although it is actually a blistering disorder.

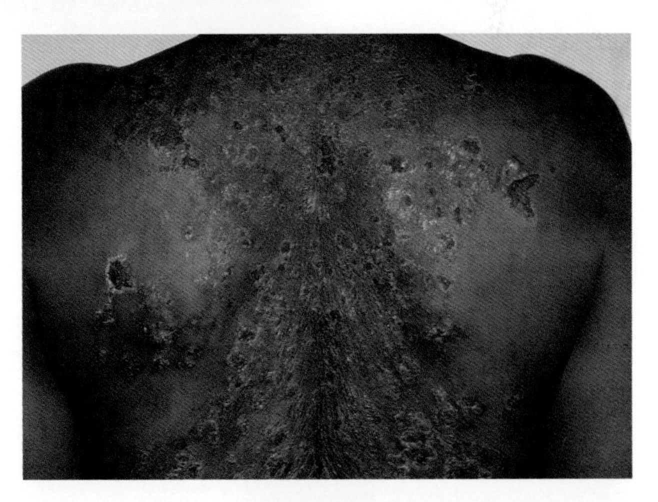

*Treatment:* Prednisolone 60mg/day until the blistering stops and then gradually reduce to a maintenance dose of 7.5–10mg/day.

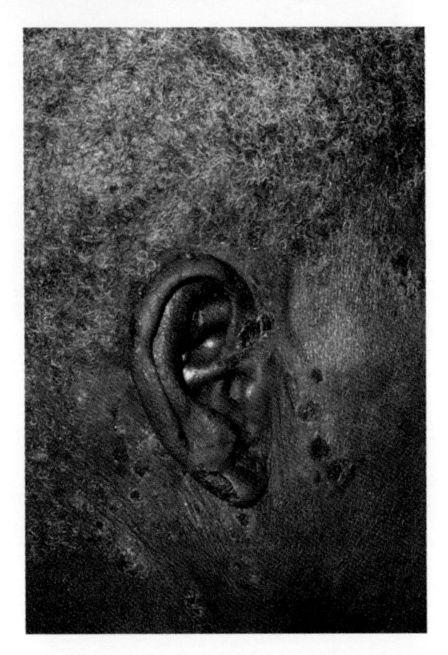

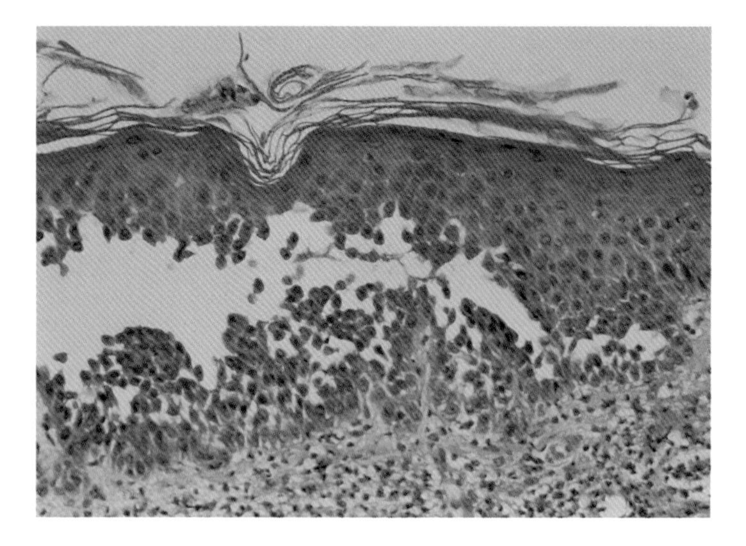

## Pemphigus vulgaris

**Figure 500** This is the most common type of pemphigus in Europe but is rare in Africa. The blister is just above the basal cells in the epidermis.

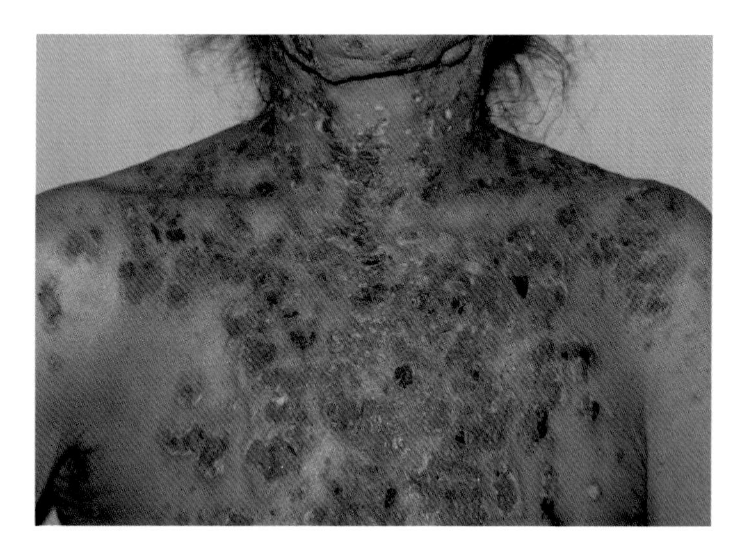

**Figure 501** It often starts with blisters in the mouth for weeks or months before numerous flaccid blisters appear on the skin, which break very quickly leaving erosions.

*Treatment:* Prednisolone 60mg/day. Reduce the dose when the blistering stops and gradually reduce to a maintenance dose of 7.5–10mg/day for the rest of the patient's life.

## Pemphigus vegetans

**Figures 502, 503** This is probably a variant of pemphigus vulgaris in which the flexural lesions become very thick and almost warty.

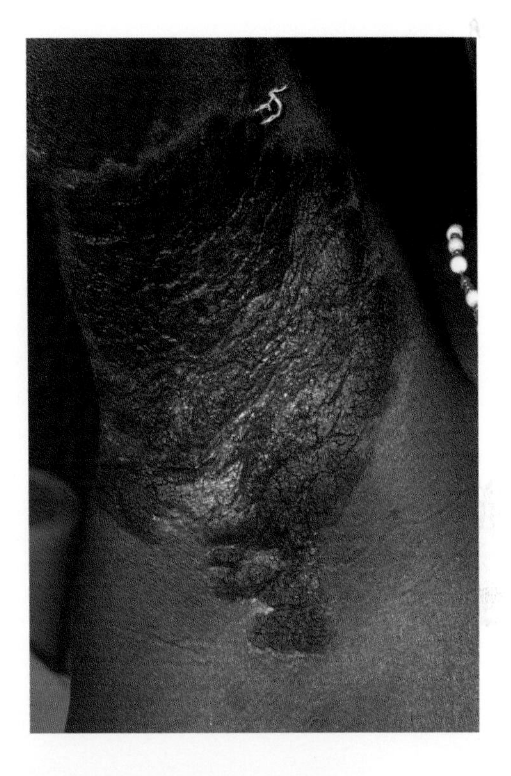

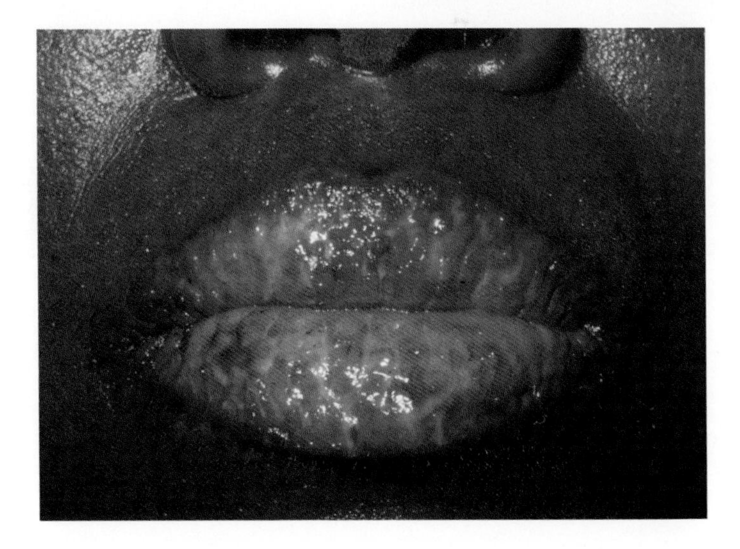

*Treatment:* Prednisolone 60mg / day. Reduce the dose when the blistering stops and gradually reduce to a maintenance dose of 7.5–10mg / day for the rest of the patient's life.

## PEUTZ-JEGHER SYNDROME

**Figure 504** A rare genetic disorder inherited as an autosomal dominant trait (*see* Figure 295). Small hyperpigmented macules are present on the lips, the skin around the mouth and on the fingers and toes from birth or early childhood. They are associated with hamartomatous polyps of the small bowel which can cause intususseption in children.

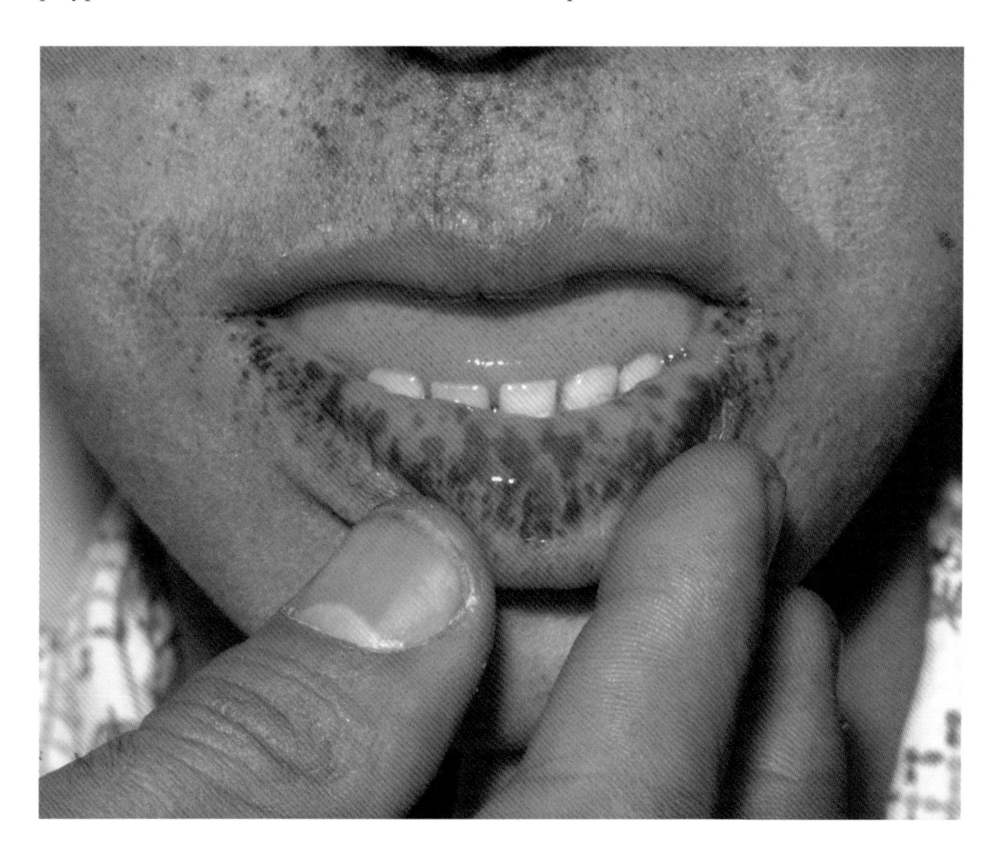

## PHOTOSENSITIVE ECZEMA

**Figures 505, 506** Eczematous rash on sun-exposed sites, i.e. the face, 'V' of neck, back of neck and the dorsum of the hands and forearms. It can be caused by drugs such as dimethylchlortetracycline or chlorpromazine, but is more commonly a manifestation of HIV infection.

*Treatment:* Apply 1% hydrocortisone ointment bd and keep out of the sun. Check for HIV infection.

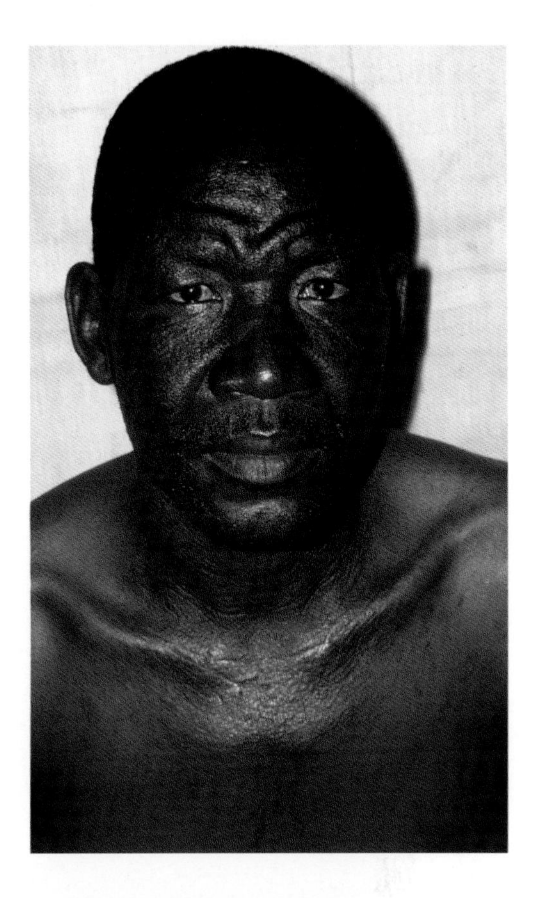

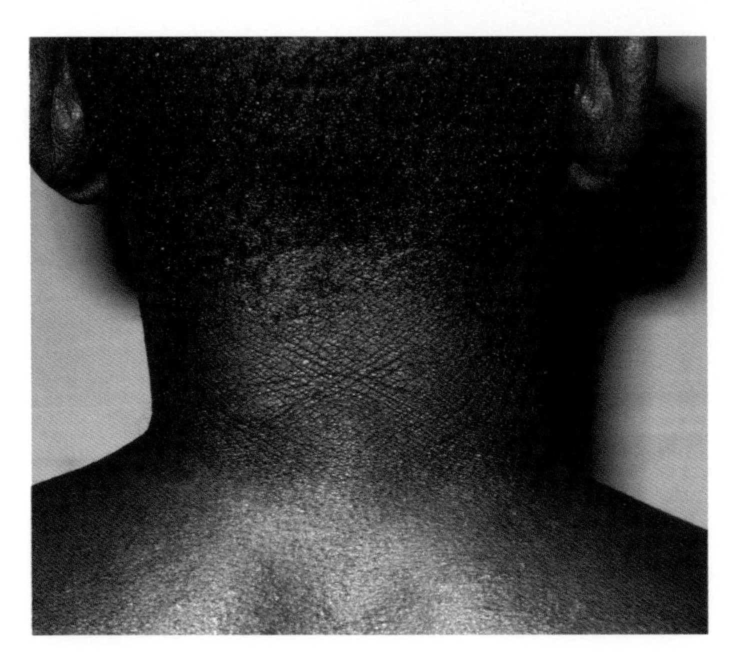

## PHRYNODERMA

**Figure 507** Follicular hyperkeratosis on the elbows, knees and buttocks in children with vitamin A deficiency.

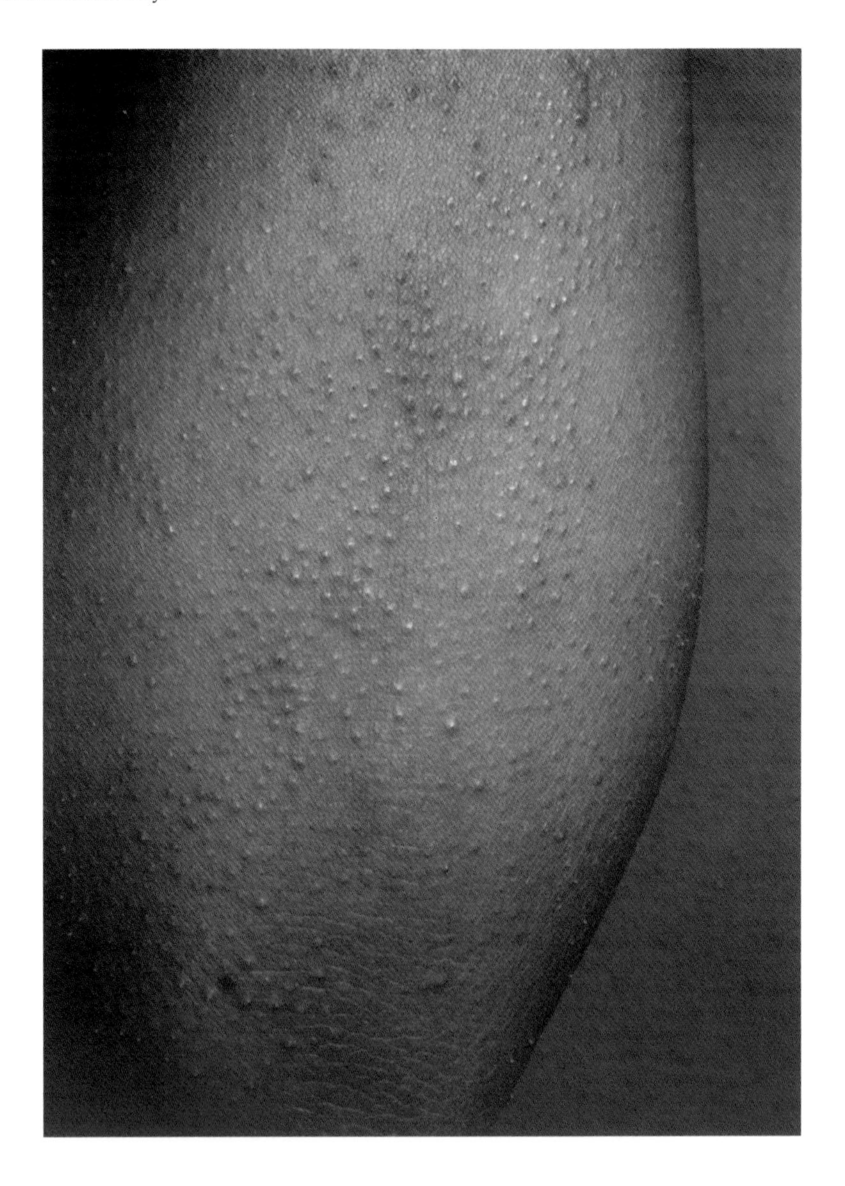

*Treatment:* Improve the diet generally and add multivitamins.

## PHYTOPHOTODERMATITIS

**Figure 508** This is a phototoxic reaction following contact with a variety of photosensitising compounds in plants, plus long-wave ultraviolet light. It presents typically as a linear rash on sun-exposed skin. The most common phototoxic compounds are the furocoumarins (psoralens) contained in a wide variety of plants, especially the *Umbelliferae*, *Rutaceae* and *Moracea* families. These include citrus fruits such as limes and oranges and many vegetables and herbs such as celery, carrots, parsnips, parsley and dill.

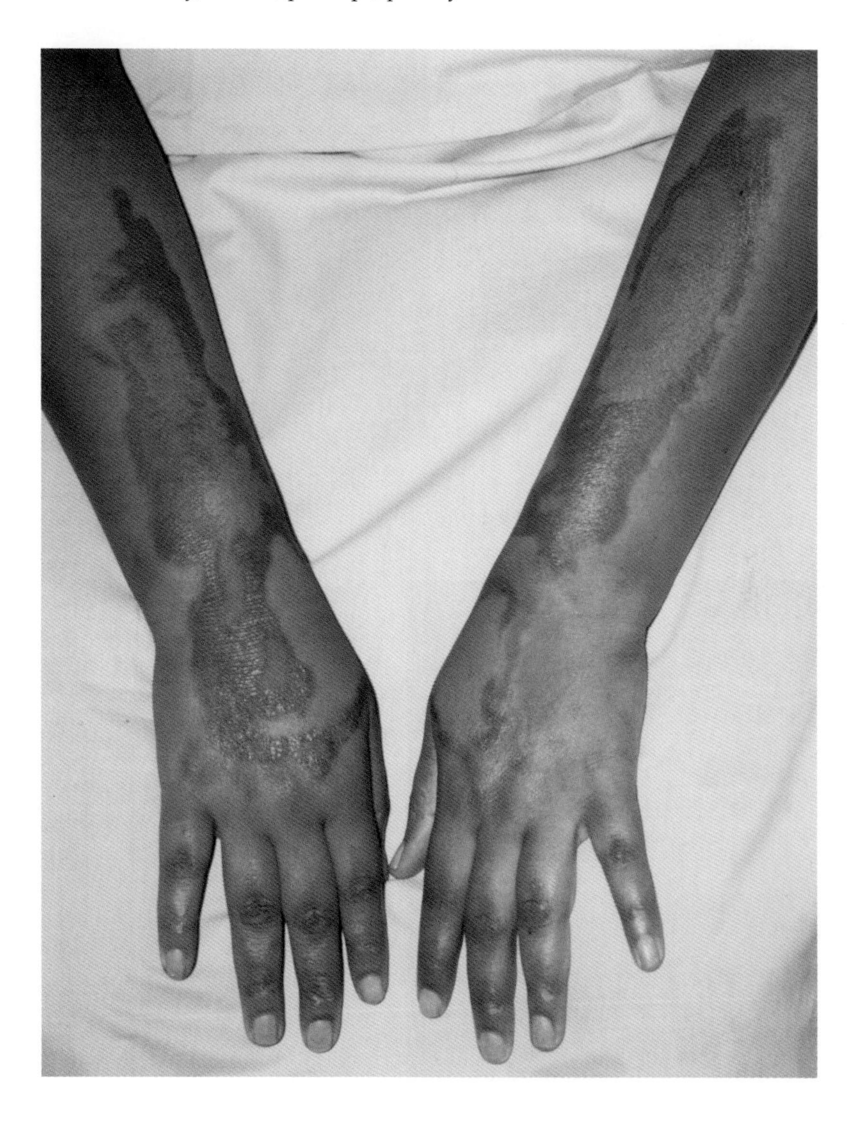

*Treatment:* Avoid future contact with the offending plant.

## PITYRIASIS ALBA

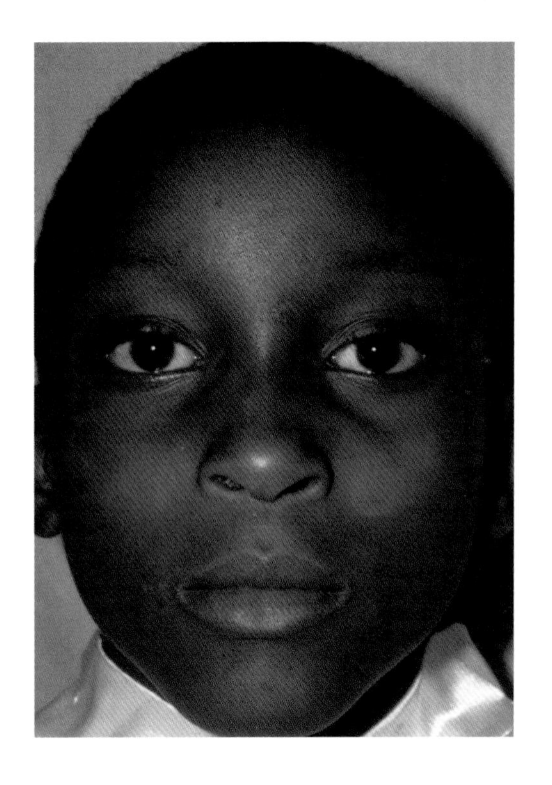

**Figure 509** White, slightly scaly patches on the face of a young child. It can sometimes also be seen on the upper arms. It is very common and can be considered a normal finding.

*Treatment:* Reassurance that it is harmless and that it will get better on its own.

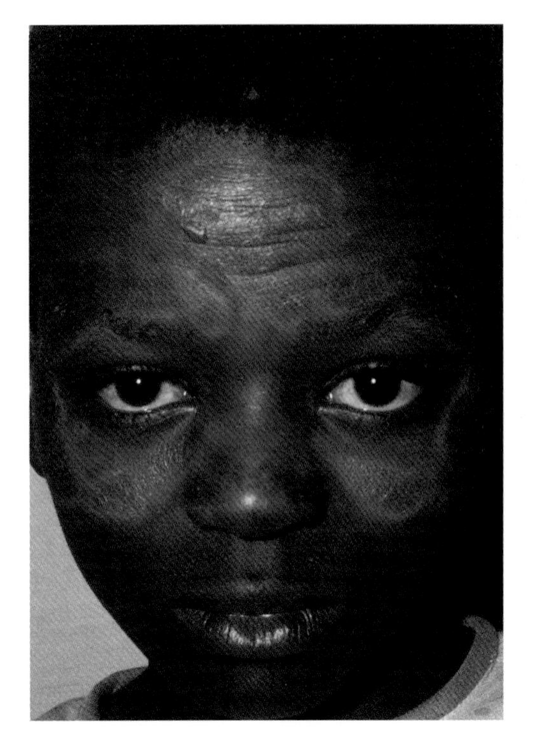

### Melanoderma lichenoides

**Figure 510** This is a variant of pityriasis alba in which there is hyperpigmentation surrounded by hypopigmentation. It is more unsightly than the common pattern of pityriasis alba (*see* Figure 509), but it is also common in children and gets better spontaneously.

*Treatment:* Reassurance only.

## PITYRIASIS ROSEA

**Figure 511** Common viral infection of children and young adults due to human herpes virus-7 (HHV-7). It begins with a herald patch, an oval scaly plaque 2–3cm in diameter, usually on the trunk, although it can be anywhere. Within a few days the rest of the rash appears on the vest and pants area (trunk and proximal limbs), following Langer's lines. There are two types of lesions in the rash:

- Small follicular papules.
- Petaloid lesions. These look like the herald patch but are smaller. They are oval in shape and have a scalloped scale just inside the border of the plaque.

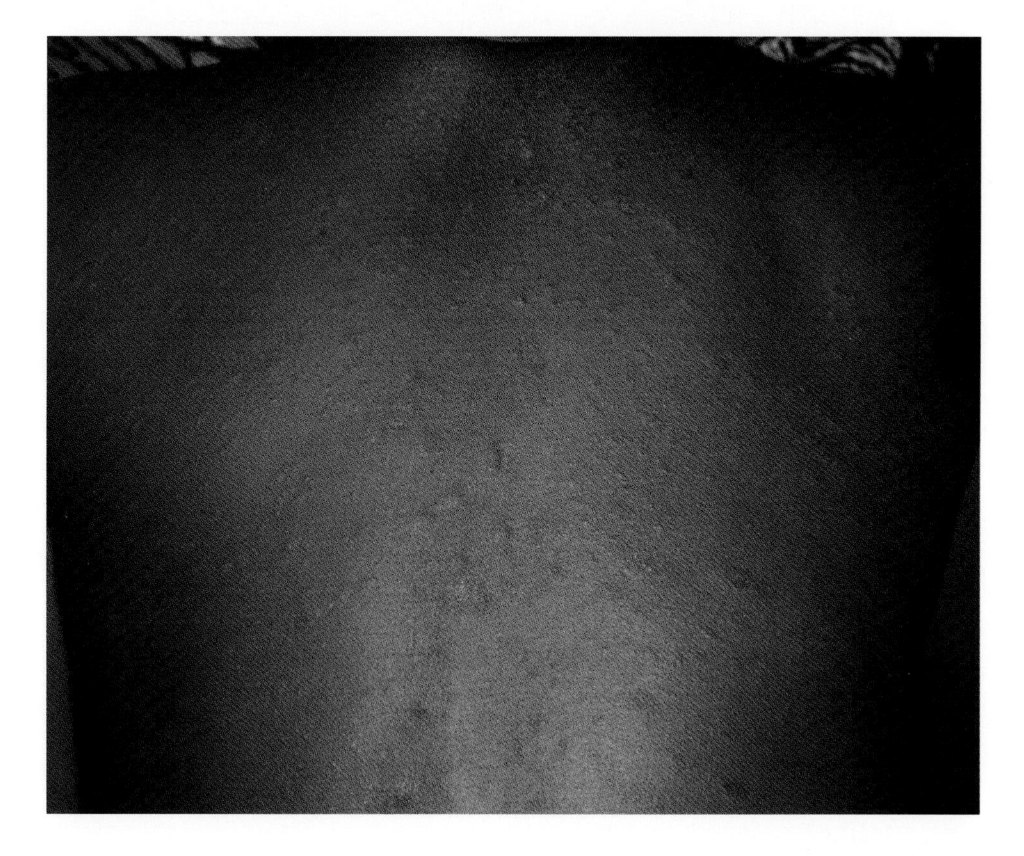

*Treatment:* It is not itchy and therefore needs no treatment. It gets better spontaneously after 6 weeks.

## PITYRIASIS ROTUNDA

**Figure 512** Uncommon non-itchy rash which looks like large plaques of pityriasis versicolor in a funny distribution. Usually found on the lower trunk or limbs. Occasionally associated with malignant disease or HIV infection, but most patients are otherwise fit and well.

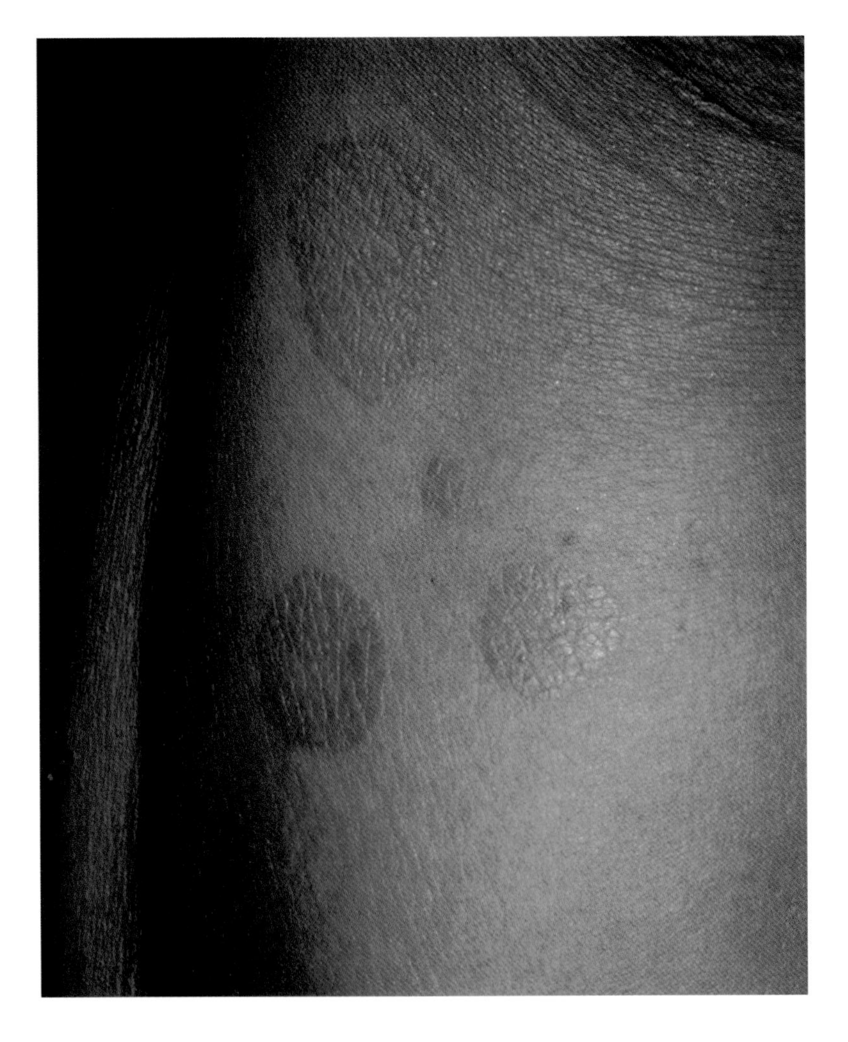

*Treatment:* Nothing is known to make the rash go away. Look for underlying malignancy or HIV infection.

## PITYRIASIS RUBRA PILARIS

**Figure 513** A group of diseases characterised by erythroderma, follicular hyperkeratosis and palmoplantar keratoderma. The rash is red and can be confused with psoriasis (*see* Figure 544), but when it becomes erythrodermic, it characteristically leaves a few well defined islands of normal skin.

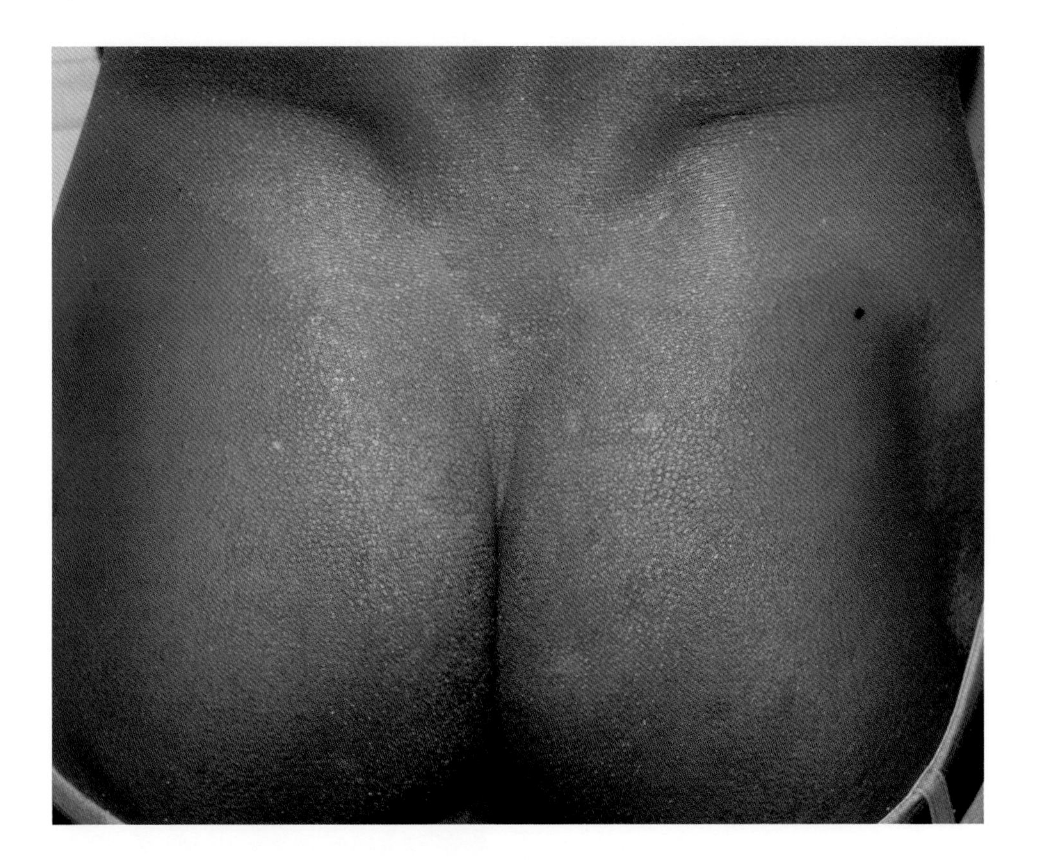

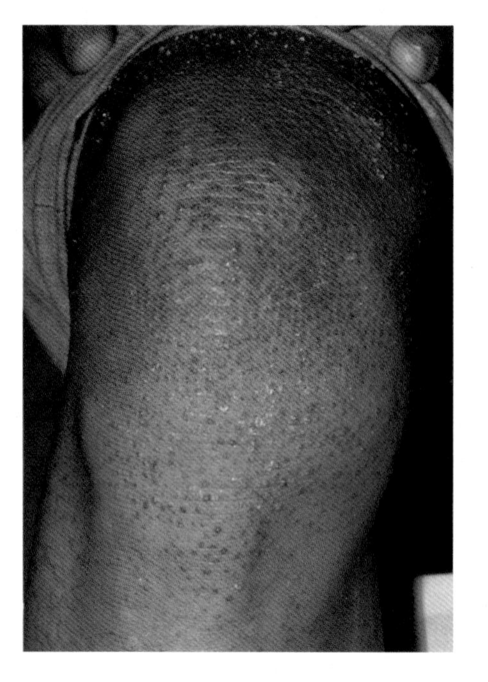

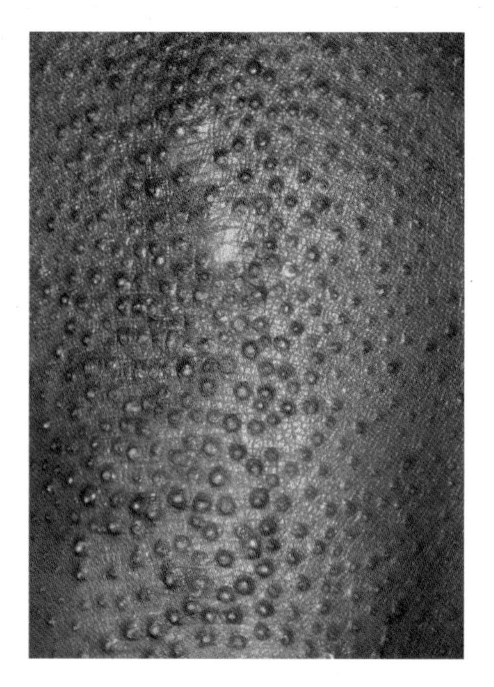

**Figures 514, 515** In pityriasis rubra pilaris the follicular hyperkeratosis is best seen on the backs of the fingers and on the elbows and knees.

**Figure 516** The palmoplantar keratoderma is bright orange in colour. The nails are usually involved and show onycholysis and subungual hyperkeratosis very similar to the changes seen in psoriasis (*see* Figures 447–9).

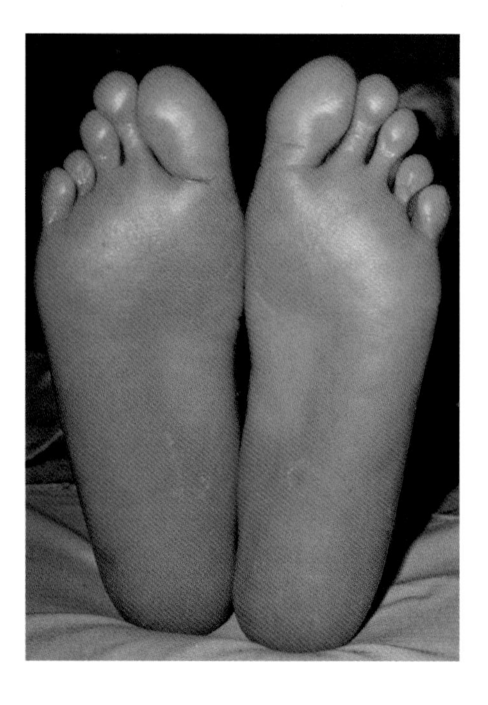

*Treatment:* Oral retinoids if they are available, e.g. acetretin 0.5mg/kg/day. Most varieties get better spontaneously in 1–3 years; some are permanent.

## PITYRIASIS VERSICOLOR

**Figure 517** Very common yeast infection due to *Malassezia furfur*. The word pityriasis means 'bran-like', and versicolor means 'different colours'. Pityriasis versicolor is therefore a scaly rash of different colours. The lesions are small (less than 1cm), usually round and always scaly when scratched. Some may join together to form larger confluent plaques. It is a disease mainly of teenagers and young adults, and the rash occurs predominantly on the upper trunk. This is the white variety.

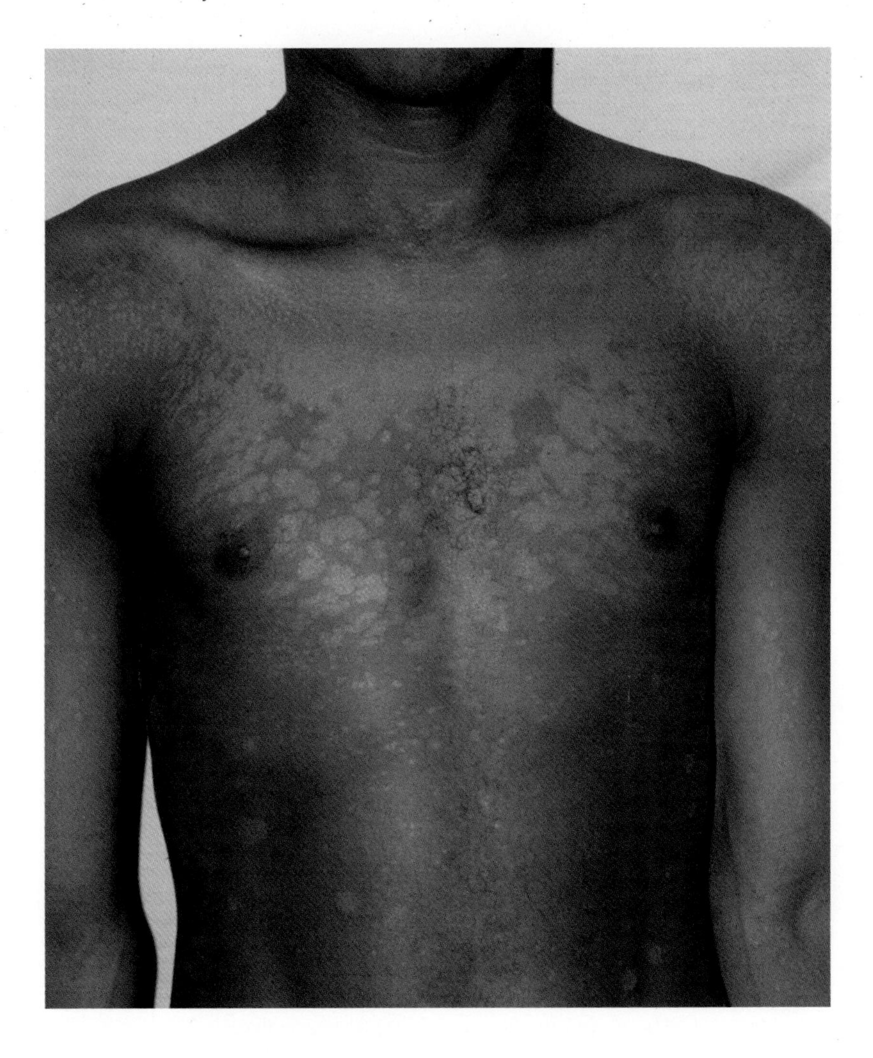

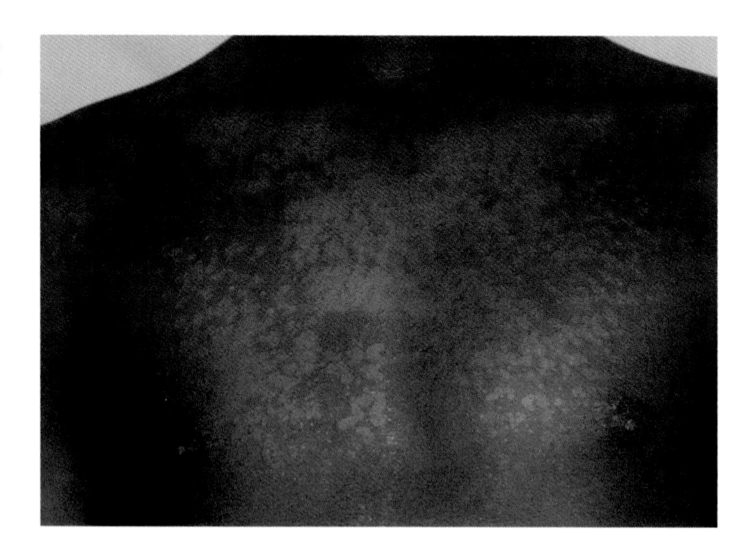

**Figure 518** Pityriasis versicolor on upper chest.

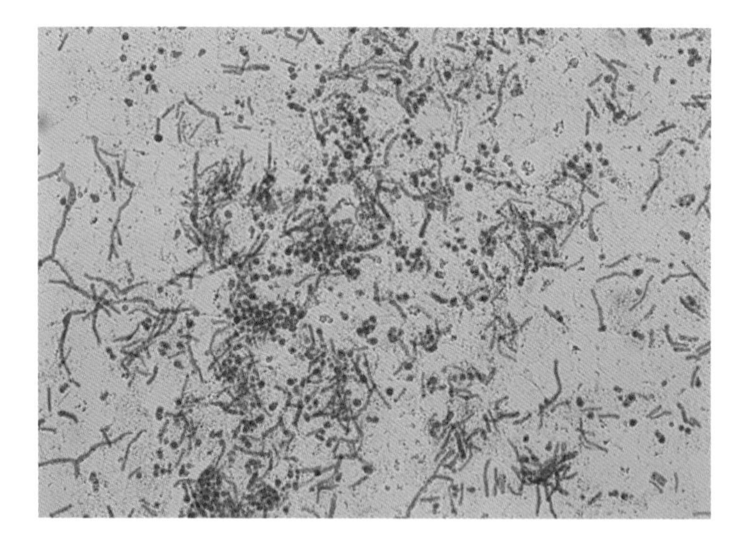

**Figure 519** The diagnosis can be confirmed by scraping off the scales and mixing them on a slide with equal parts of 20% KOH and Parker blue black ink. The organism takes up the blue colour from the ink and both spores and hyphae can be seen.

*Treatment:* Ketaconazole orally 400mg as a stat dose, or 200mg/day for 7 days. Topical alternatives are 20% sodium thiosulphate solution applied nightly for 6 weeks, 2.5% selenium sulphide shampoo (Selsun shampoo) applied bd for 2 weeks, or a topical imidazole cream (clotrimazole, econazole, ketaconazole or miconazole) applied bd for 2 weeks.

## POLYARTERITIS NODOSA

**Figure 520** The cutaneous variety of polyarteritis nodosa is a benign vasculitis of small and medium-sized arteries. It presents with painful subcutaneous nodules on the lower legs and feet, which may ulcerate. There is no systemic involvement. The diagnosis can be confirmed by biopsy.

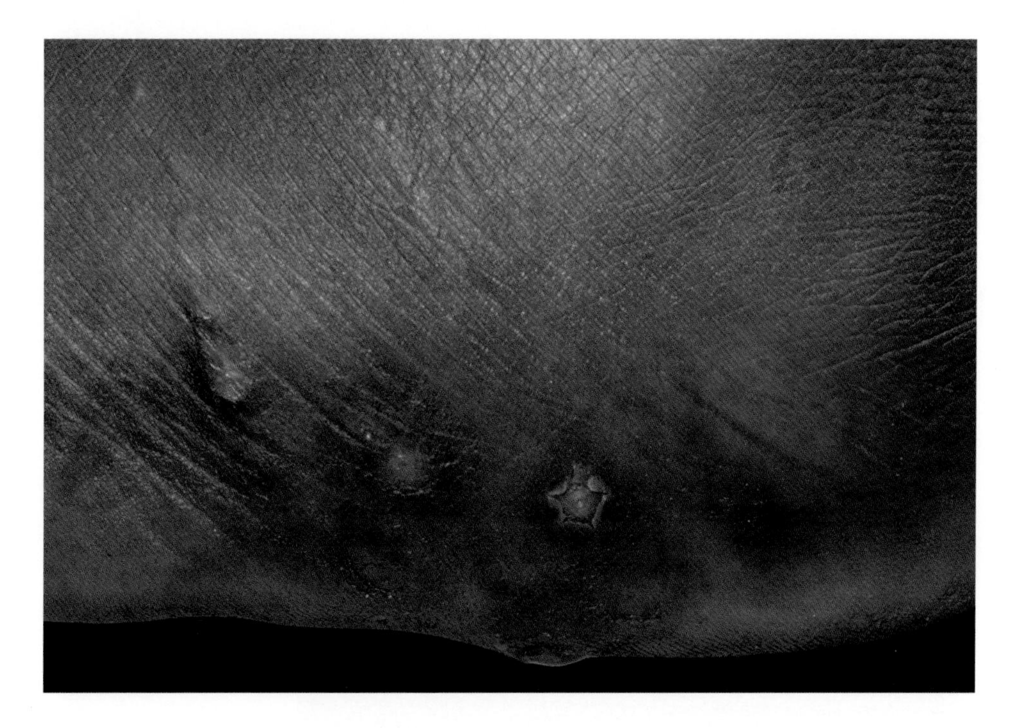

*Treatment:* Prednisolone 10mg/day orally.

## POROKERATOSIS OF MIBELLI

**Figures 521, 522** Rare disease inherited as an autosomal dominant trait (*see* Figure 295). Linear, annular or serpiginous plaques with central atrophy and a peripheral keratotic ridge. Usually present from early childhood although it can occur in adult life in association with HIV infection. A biopsy from the edge shows what is called a 'cornoid lamella', a column of parakeratosis in the middle of hyperkeratosis.

*Treatment:* Surgical excision if possible as they sometimes develop squamous cell carcinomas in later life.

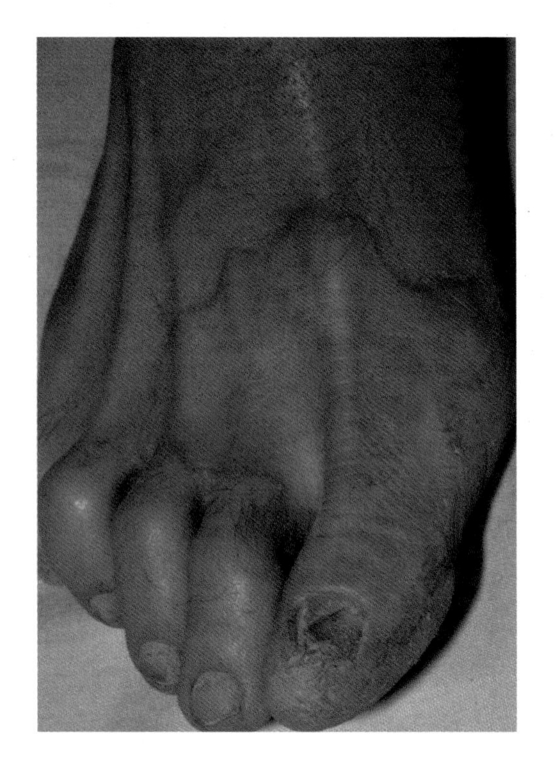

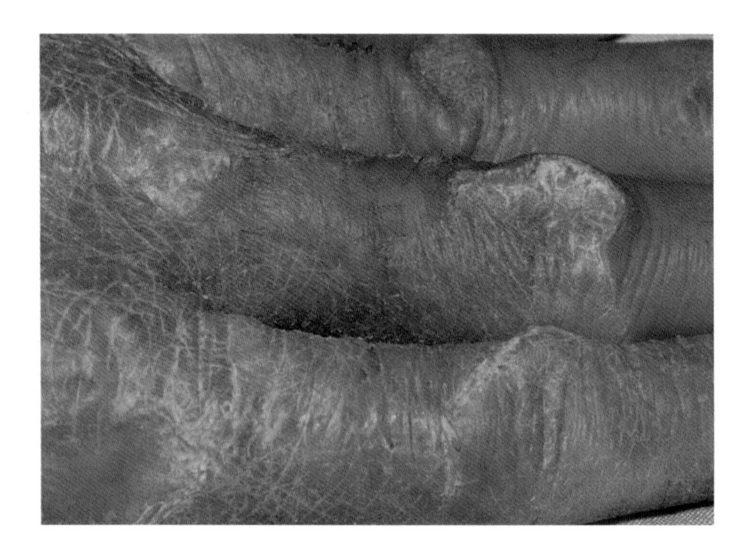

## POST-INFLAMMATORY PIGMENT CHANGE

**Figure 523** Post-inflammatory hypopigmentation. Any inflammatory condition in the epidermis can result in a change in pigment as the condition improves. This is a 2-year-old boy who has had nappy rash. There is hypopigmentation where the rash was.

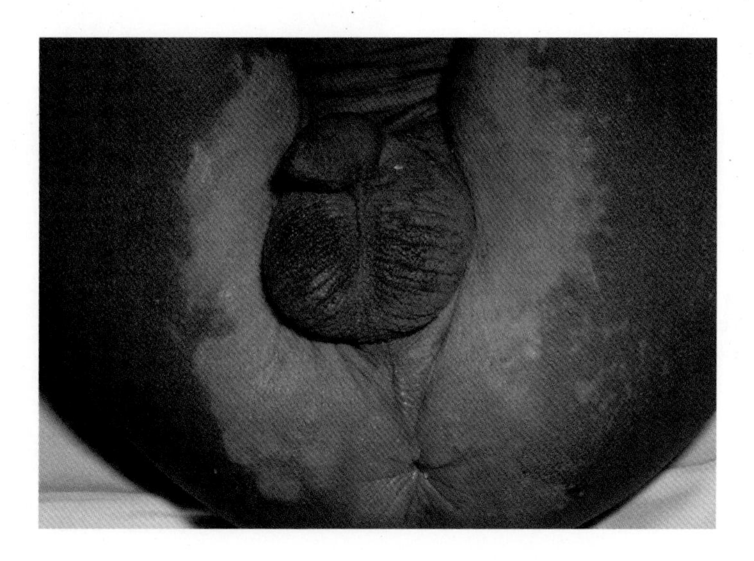

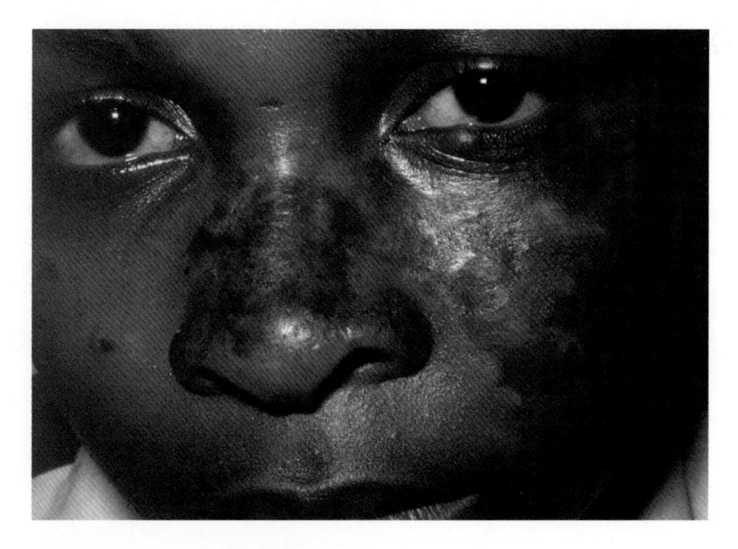

**Figure 524** Post-inflammatory hyperpigmentation. Discoid lupus erythematosus on the face has healed leaving hyperpigmentation.

**Figures 525, 526** Hyperpigmentation after taking minocycline. Blue-black pigmentation due to the deposition of iron in the skin in individuals taking long-term minocycline. The pigmentation may be on sun-exposed areas (Figure 525) or elsewhere. May resolve when the drug is stopped, but may not.

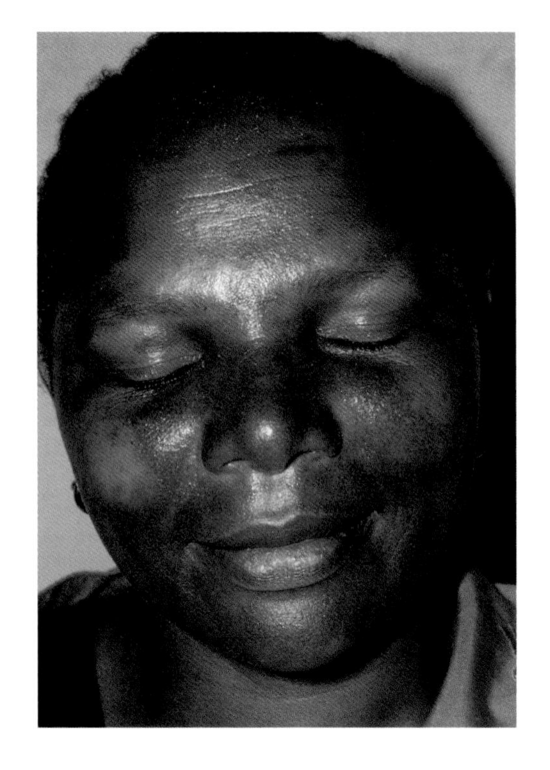

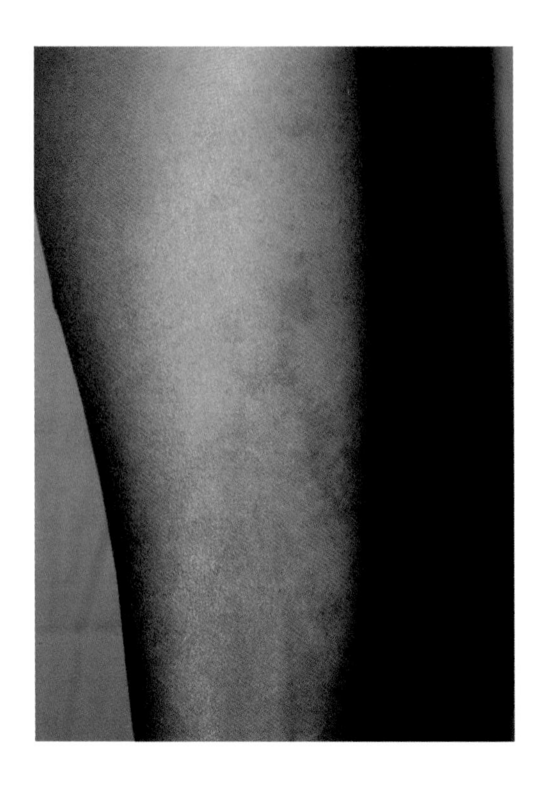

**Figure 527** Post-inflammatory hypo- and hyperpigmentation in the same patient. In this case the pigment change has followed eczema.

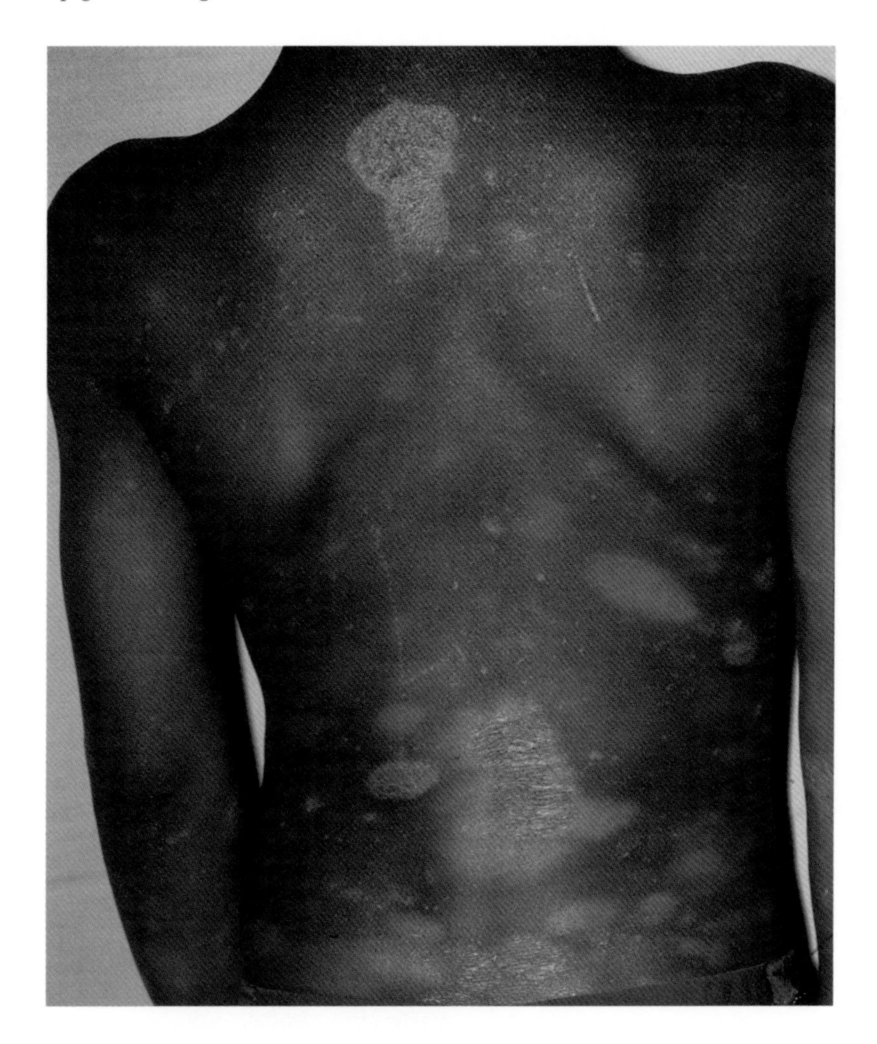

## PRAYER NODULES

**Figure 528** Hyperkeratotic plaques from repeatedly touching forehead on prayer stone.

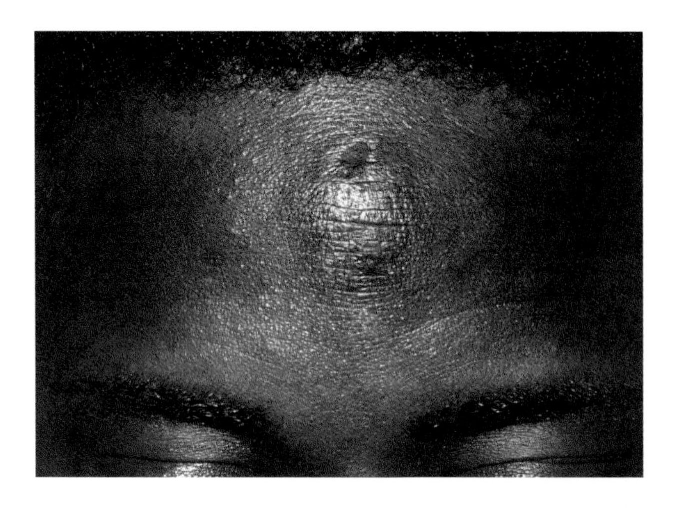

**Figures 529, 530** Hyperkeratotic plaque on dorsum of foot in Moslem man from squatting to pray.

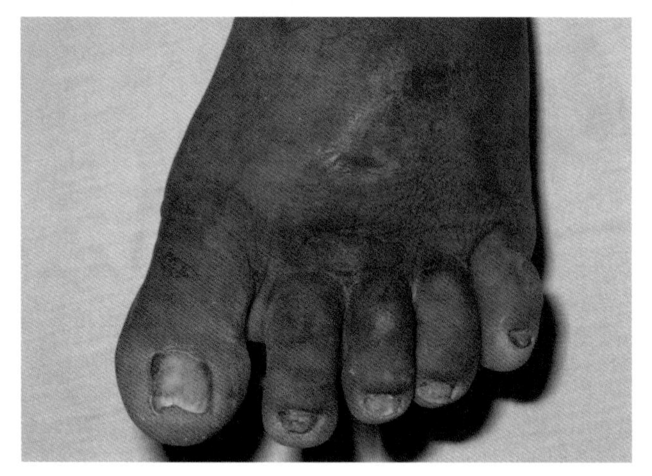

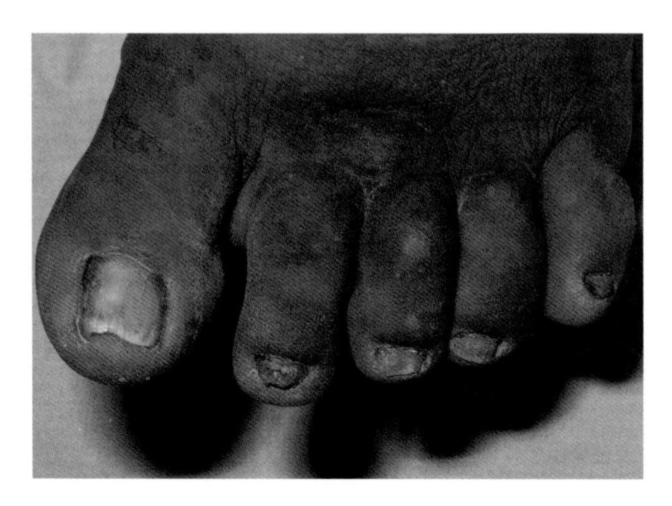

## PRETIBIAL MYXOEDEMA

**Figure 531** Diffuse oedematous plaques on the front of the shins, with prominent hair follicles giving a *peau d'orange* effect. Occurs in patients with hyperthyroidism.

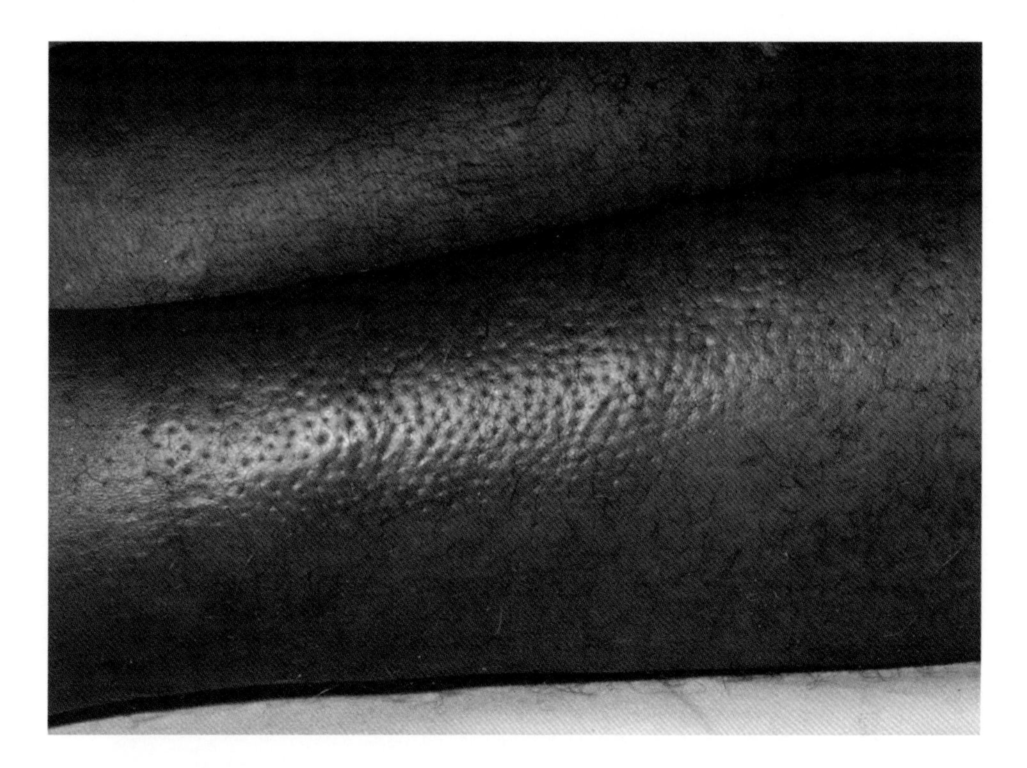

*Treatment:* Treat the hyperthyroidism. For the skin apply a very potent topical steroid (0.05% clobetasol propionate) under polythene occlusion once a week.

## PROGERIA

**Figure 532** Rare premature aging syndrome, inherited as an autosomal recessive trait (*see* Figure 18). Affected children look normal at birth, but by the second year of life show the characteristic features of a large bald head with a bird-like face, loss of subcutaneous fat, dry, thin, transparent and wrinkled skin, especially on the hands and feet, prominent veins, telangiectasia and mottled hyperpigmentation. Extensive atheroma causes early death from myocardial infarction.

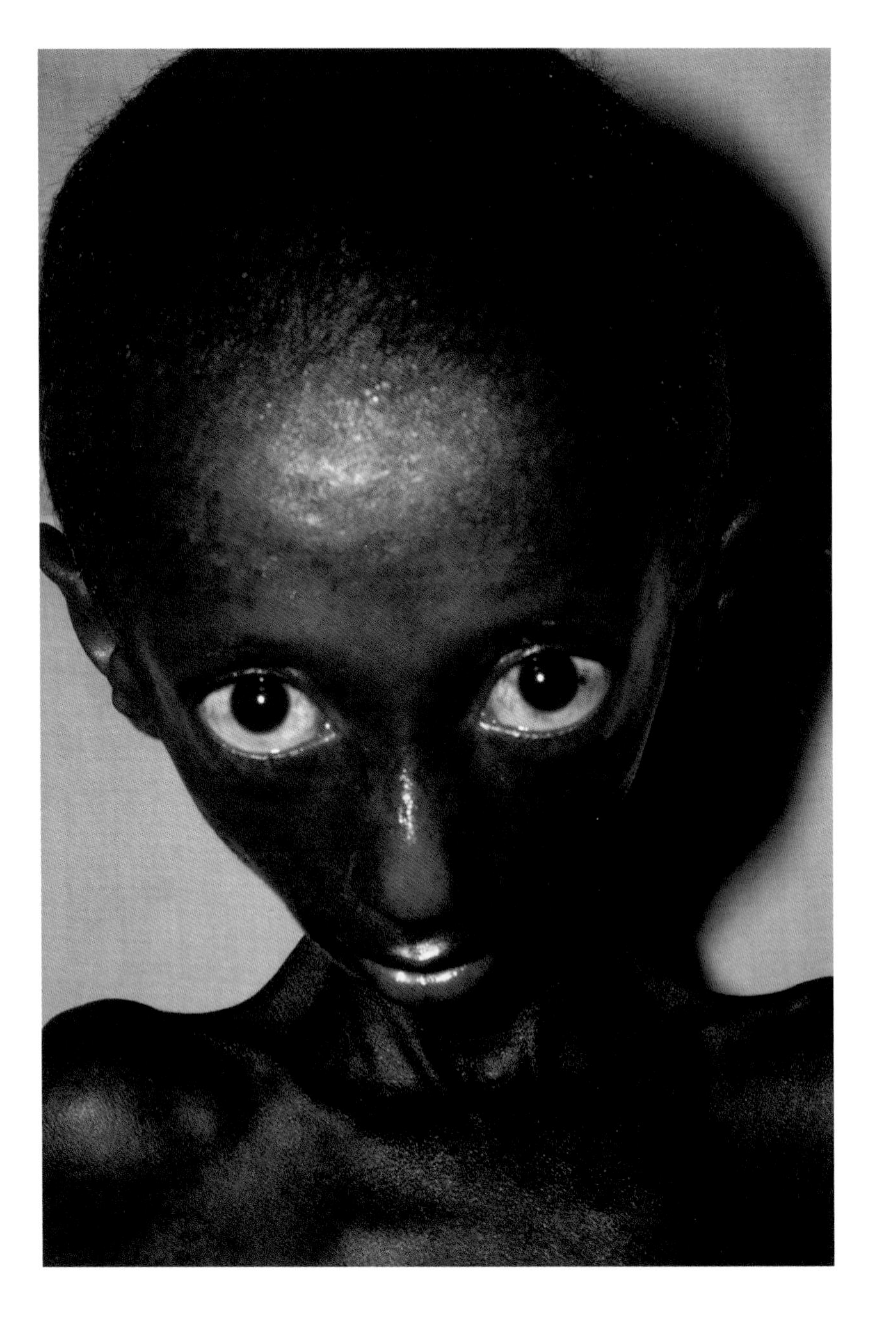

## PSEUDOXANTHOMA ELASTICUM

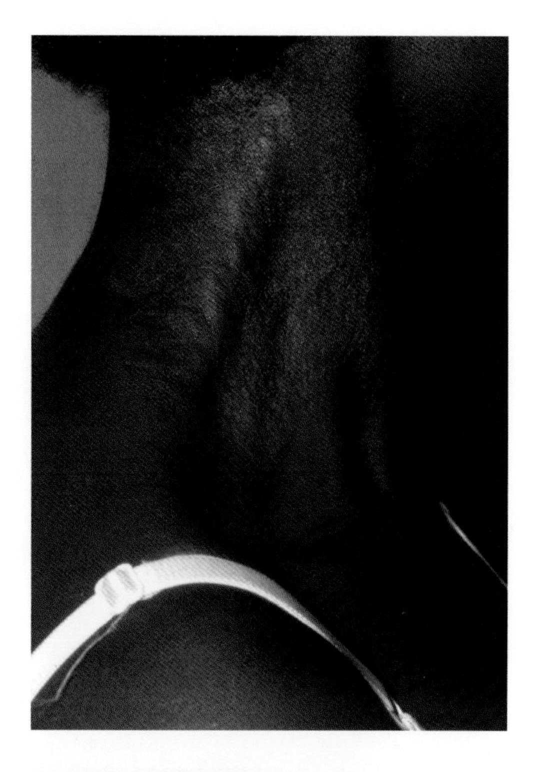

**Figure 533** A rare group of connective tissue disorders involving the skin, eyes and blood vessels. There are both autosomal dominant and recessive forms. The skin lesions are quite distinctive and appear in childhood or early adult life. Plaques of lax, wrinkled skin looking like a brown crêpe bandage are seen on the neck, axillae and groins.

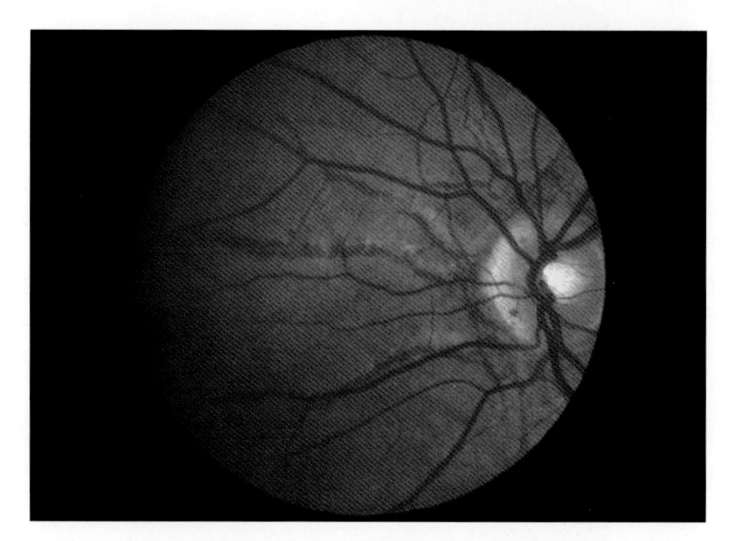

**Figure 534** The retina shows angioid streaks – greyish and yellowish streaks radiating out from a grey ring around the optic nerve. The vascular abnormalities cause hypertension, intermittent claudication, coronary thrombosis, cerebrovascular accidents and gastrointestinal bleeding.

## PSORIASIS

**Figure 535** Red, well defined, scaly plaques occur anywhere on the body surface.

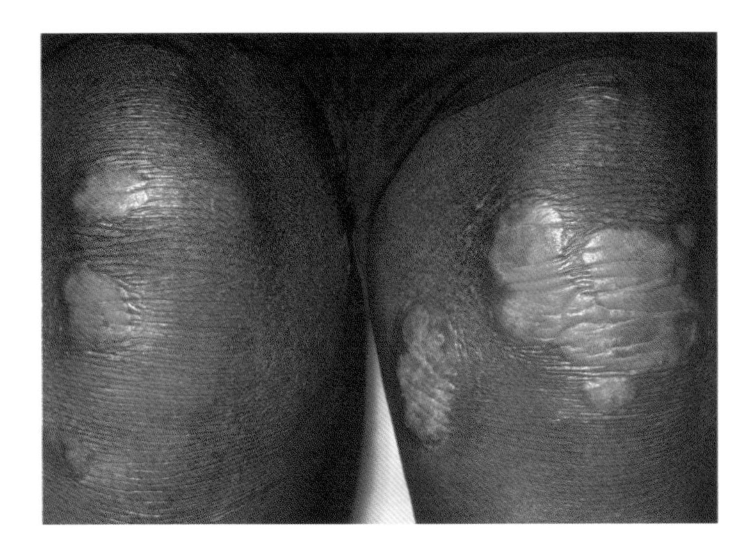

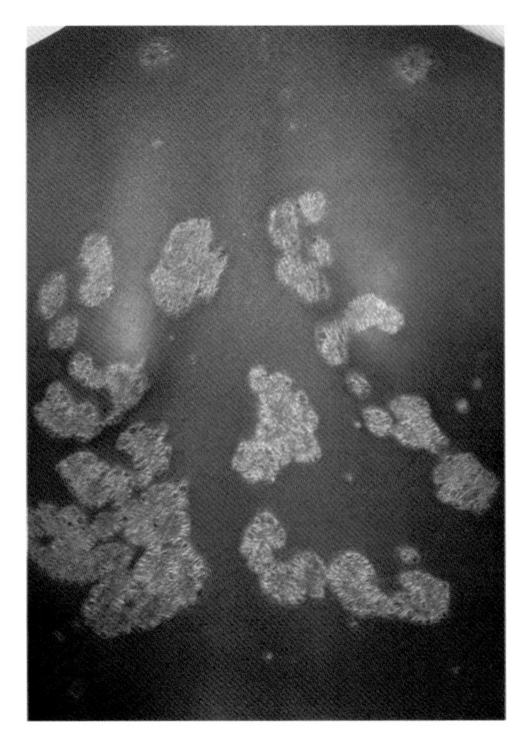

**Figure 536** The plaques characteristically have white or silvery scales which come off easily on scratching.

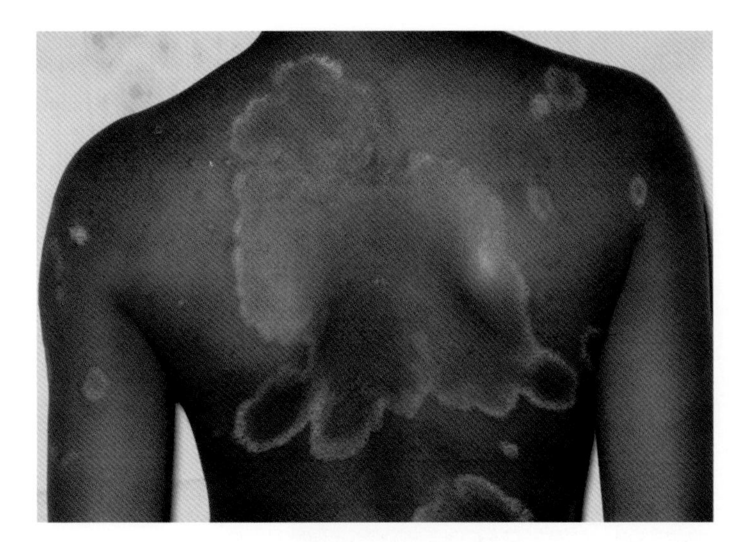

**Figure 537** Sometimes the plaques are annular.

*Treatment:* Ultraviolet light often improves psoriasis, so exposing the affected skin to the sun for half an hour a day may be all that is needed. Otherwise, apply 3% crude coal tar ointment in the morning and then expose the skin to sunlight for half an hour.

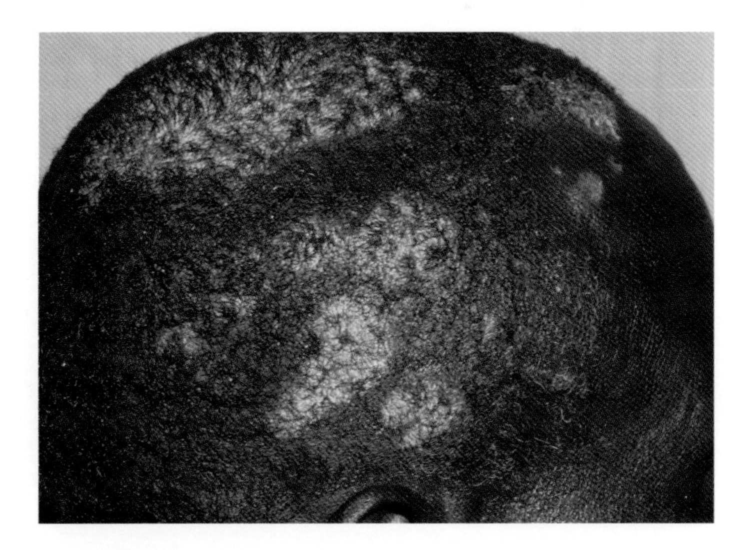

**Figure 538** The scalp is often involved with well defined, red, scaly plaques. The hair usually hides them, but at the same time stops the scales from falling off. This results in thick, heaped up plaques which can be better felt than seen.

*Treatment:* Apply 3% crude coal tar in Vaseline at night and wash it off in the morning.

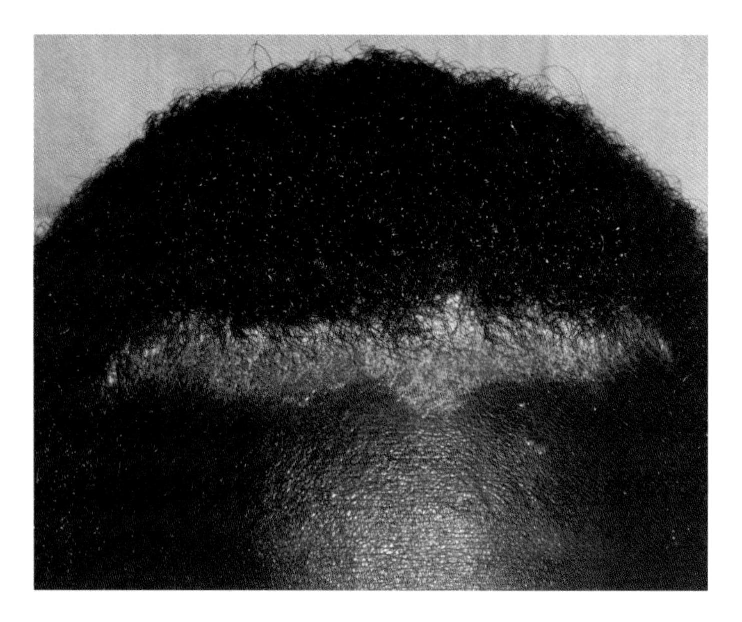

**Figure 539** Corona psoriatica. Psoriasis of the scalp often extends out of the hair margin onto the forehead.

*Treatment:* Apply 3% crude coal tar in Lassar's paste to the forehead at night.

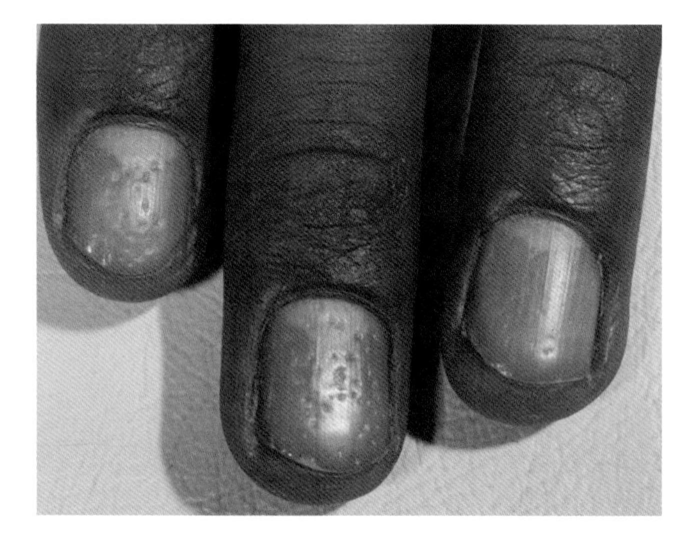

**Figure 540** The nails show pitting (shown here), salmon patches, onycholysis and subungual hyperkeratosis (*see also* Figures 447–9).

*Treatment:* None available for nails.

**Figures 541, 542** In the flexures the characteristic white scale is not seen, but the plaques remain red and well defined.

*Treatment:* Apply a moderately potent topical steroid (e.g. 0.05% clobetasone butyrate) ointment or cream bd. Tar will make the skin of the flexures sore, so do not use it.

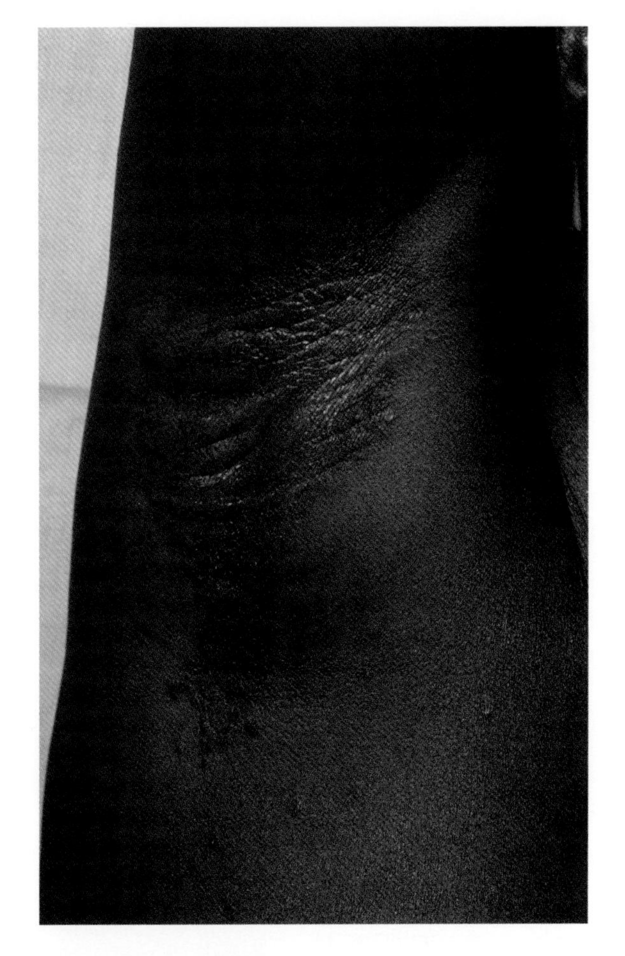

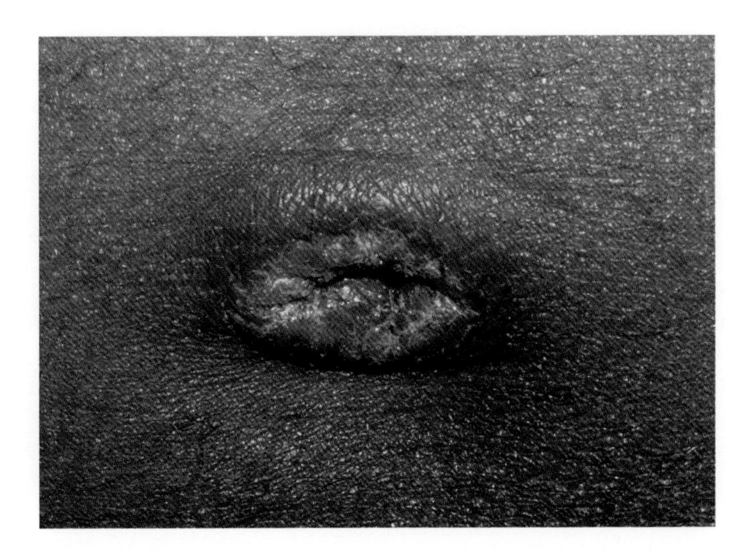

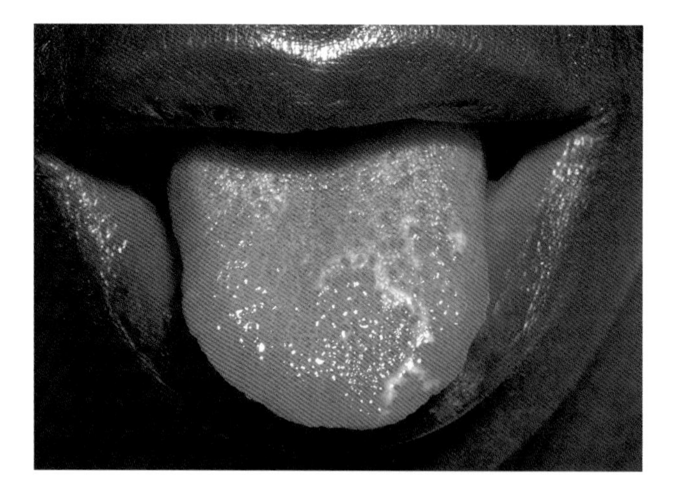

**Figure 543** On the tongue, psoriasis looks similar to geographic tongue (*see* Figure 631).

*Treatment:* It is asymptomatic and needs no treatment.

## Erythrodermic psoriasis

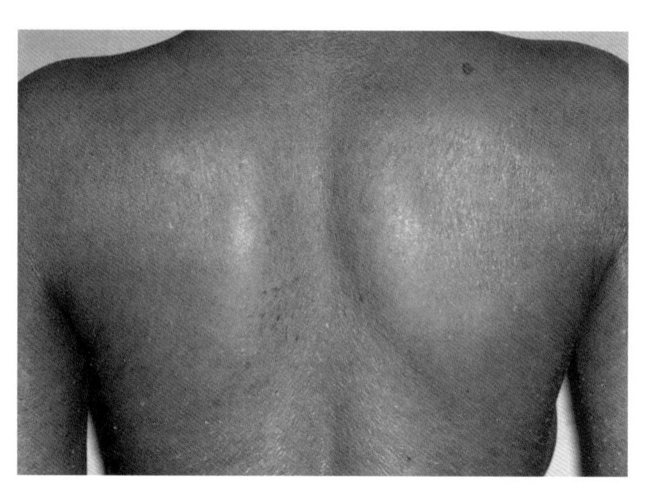

**Figure 544** Psoriasis can be universal. The whole body is red and scaly, or hyperpigmented and scaly (*see also* Figure 238). The scales make a mess in the bed or on the floor (*see* Figure 239).

*Treatment:* Use only bland ointments as tar or dithranol will make it worse. If it does not settle, consider weekly methotrexate orally or by intramuscular injection. Check for HIV infection.

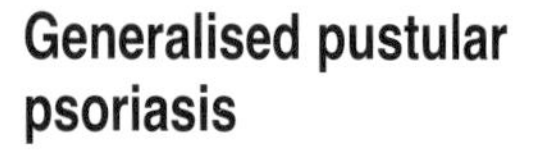

## Generalised pustular psoriasis

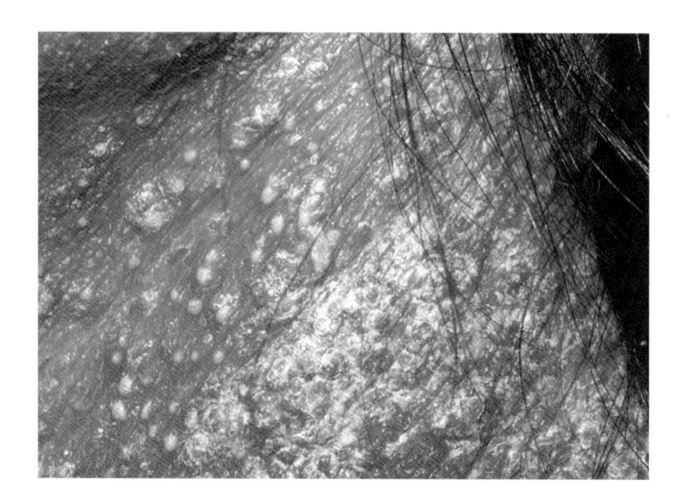

**Figure 545** This usually occurs in patients with psoriasis who have been treated with potent topical steroids or systemic steroids. The patient develops crops of tiny pustules all over the body together with a swinging fever.

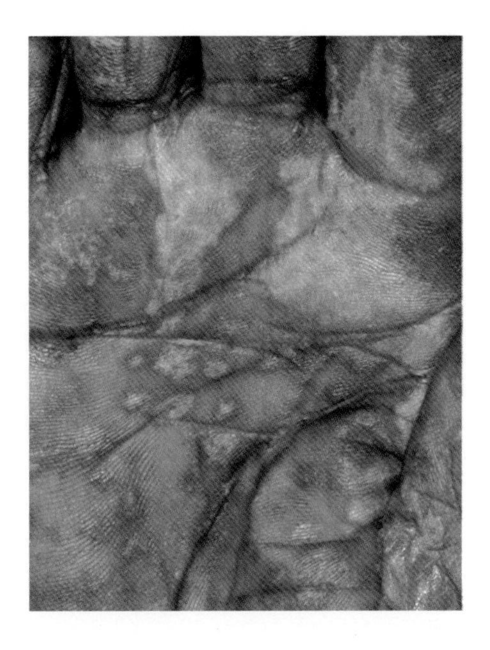

**Figure 546** Sometimes the pustules become confluent to give 'lakes' of pus.

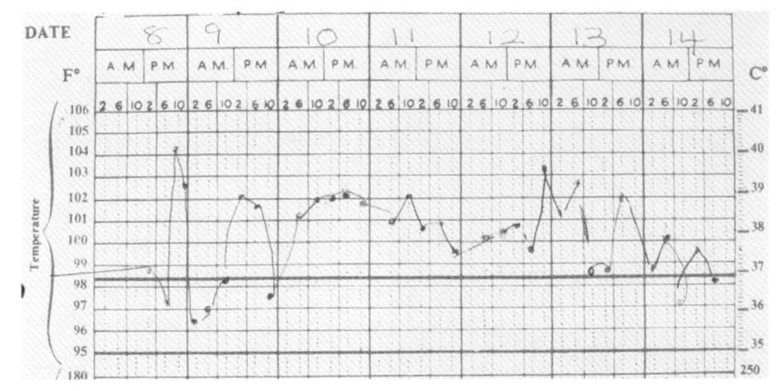


**Figure 547** Each time the temperature rises, new pustules appear. This is a serious illness which may cause the patient's death.

*Treatment:* Stop the steroids. Bed rest and bland ointments (e.g. Vaseline or Vaseline mixed in equal parts with liquid paraffin). If it does not settle consider oral or intramuscular methotrexate once a week.

## Psoriatic arthritis

**Figure 548** This is an erosive arthritis similar to rheumatoid arthritis occurring in patients with psoriasis. It is very uncommon in Africa. Check for HIV infection if you see it.

*Treatment:* Non-steroidal anti-inflammatory drugs as for rheumatoid arthritis.

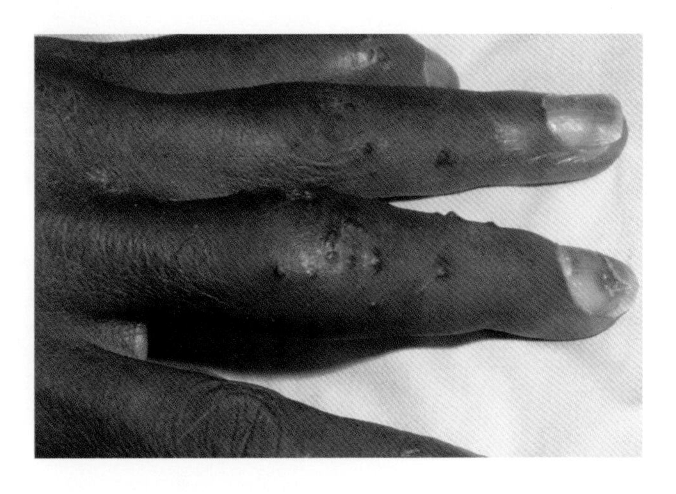

## Psoriasis and HIV infection

**Figures 549, 550, 551** Patients with HIV infection often have unusual patterns of psoriasis, particularly thick hyperkeratotic plaques. They may have ordinary psoriasis (*see* Figures 535–43), or erythrodermic or generalised pustular psoriasis (*see* Figures 544–6).

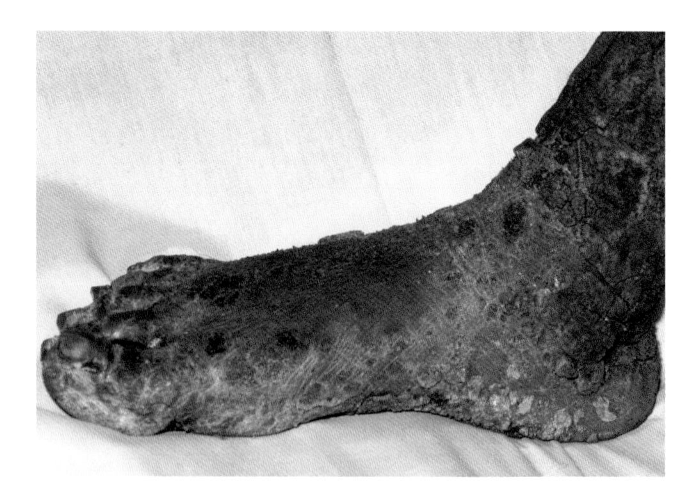

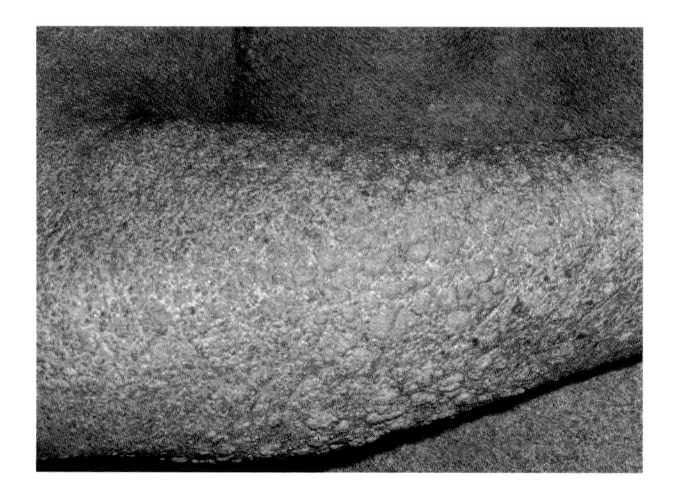

*Treatment:* This is the same whether the patient is HIV positive or not (*see* Figures 537–48).

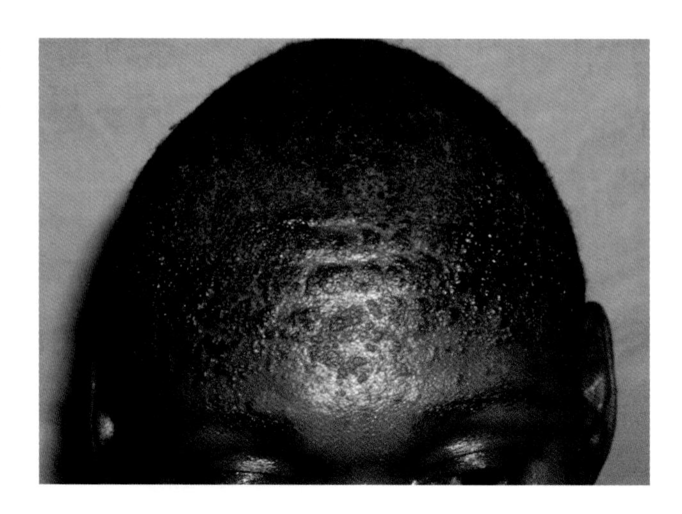

## PURPURA

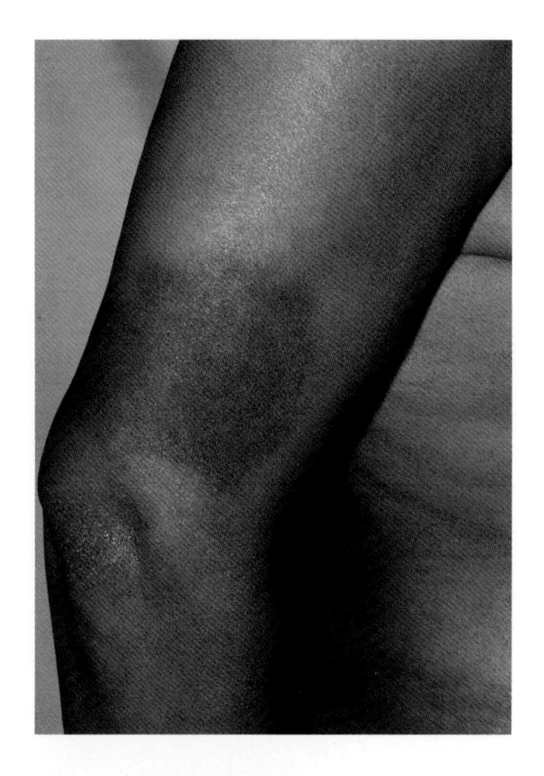

**Figures 552, 553** Purpura is discolouration of the skin due to extravasation of RBCs (*see also* Figure 660). Small (<2mm) lesions are called petechiae, larger lesions (as shown here), ecchymoses or bruises. Large ecchymoses like this can be due to thrombocytopaenia or coagulation defects.

*Treatment:* Look for the underlying cause (check platelet count and clotting screen) and treat that.

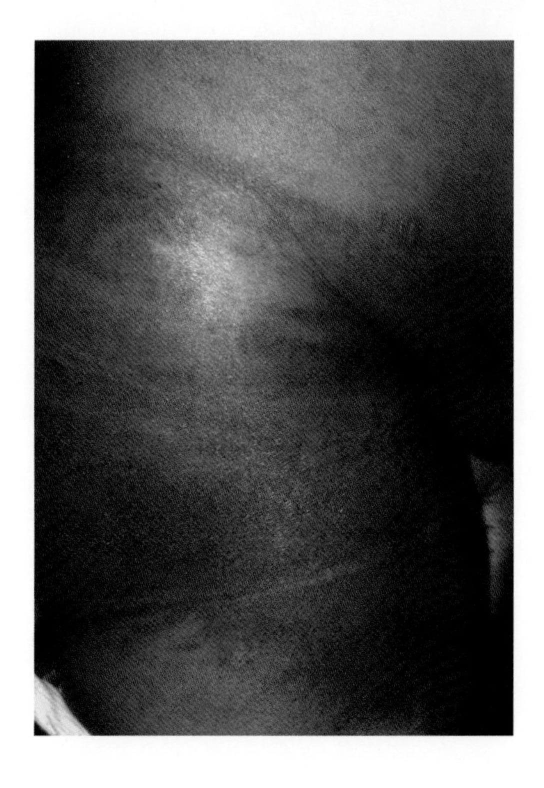

## PYODERMA

**Figure 554** This is the term for a superficial bacterial infection of the skin which does not fit into the usual classification of staphylococcal and streptococcal infections (*see* Figures 124 and 309). It is usually a secondary bacterial infection on top of atopic eczema or scabies.

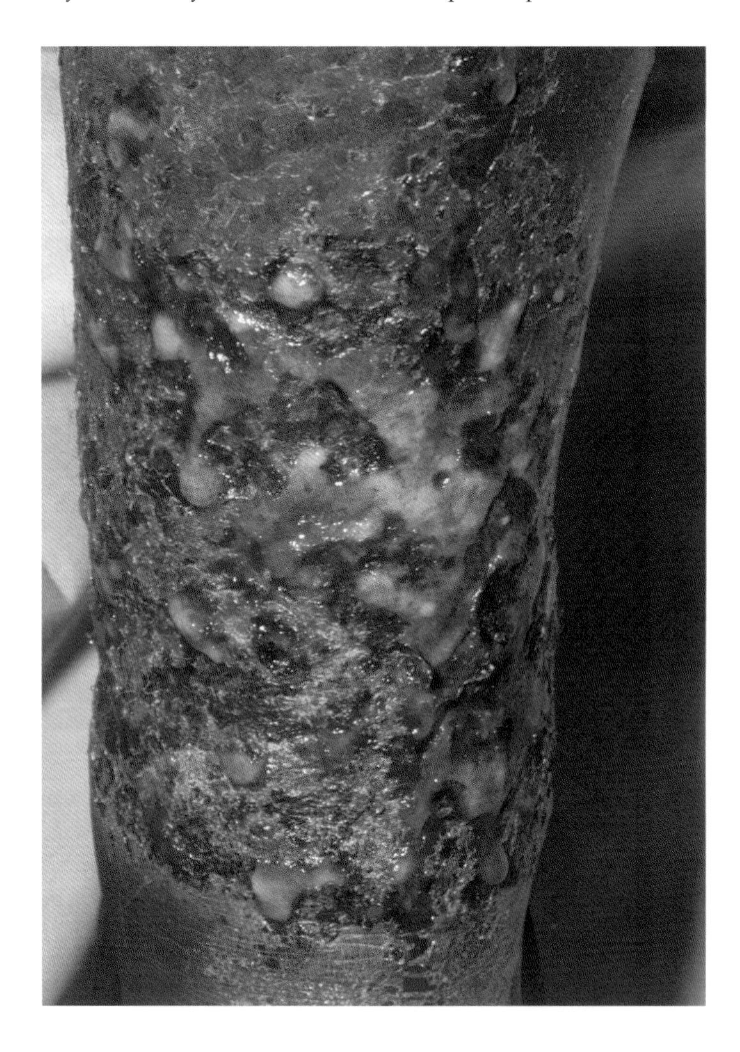

*Treatment:* Treat the underlying disease and at the same time give an oral antibiotic, cloxacillin if it is due to *Staphylococcus aureus*, or phenoxymethylpenicillin (Penicillin V) if it is due to *Streptococcus pyogenes*.

## PYODERMA GANGRENOSUM

**Figure 555** Begins with a pustule which rapidly enlarges and breaks down to form an ulcer. The ulcer has a raised, hyperpigmented, overhanging edge and a necrotic base. It can grow to 10cm in diameter or more in a few days. In the West it is often associated with ulcerative colitis, Crohn's disease, rheumatoid arthritis or multiple myeloma, but in Africa it usually occurs in a patient who is otherwise well.

*Treatment:* High doses of systemic steroids; 60mg prednisolone/day for an adult. Reduce the dose once the ulcer shows signs of healing. Alternatives are clofazamine or minocycline.

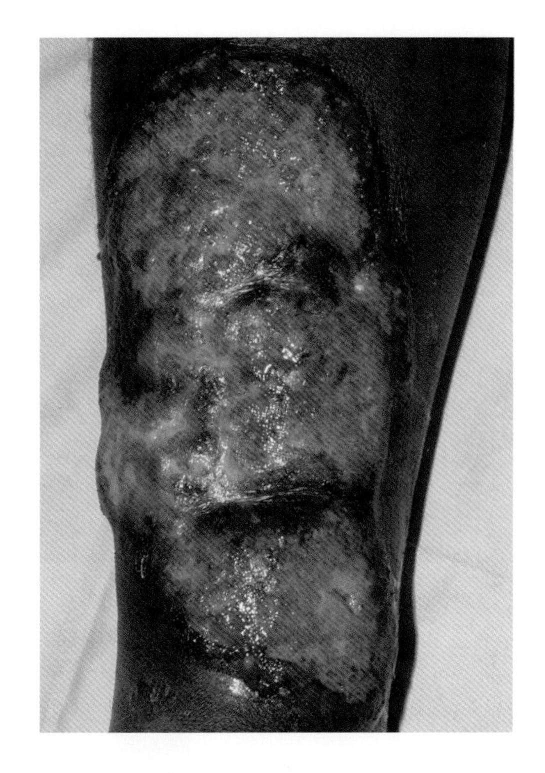

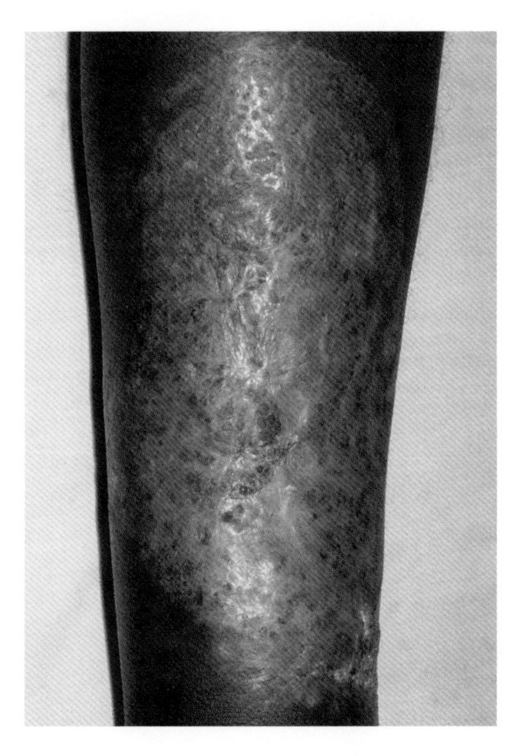

**Figure 556** The ulcer heals leaving a cribriform scar (same patient as in Figure 555).

## PYOGENIC GRANULOMA

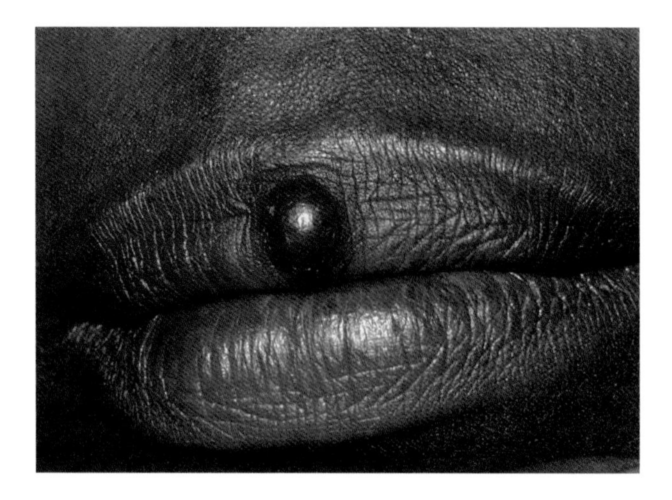

**Figure 557** A rapidly growing vascular nodule which appears after trauma (usually a prick with a thorn). It occurs most commonly in children on the fingers, toes or face, but it can occur at any age and at any site. It is bright red in colour, surrounded by a hyperkeratotic collar and it can bleed. Left to its own devices it will heal after 9–12 months.

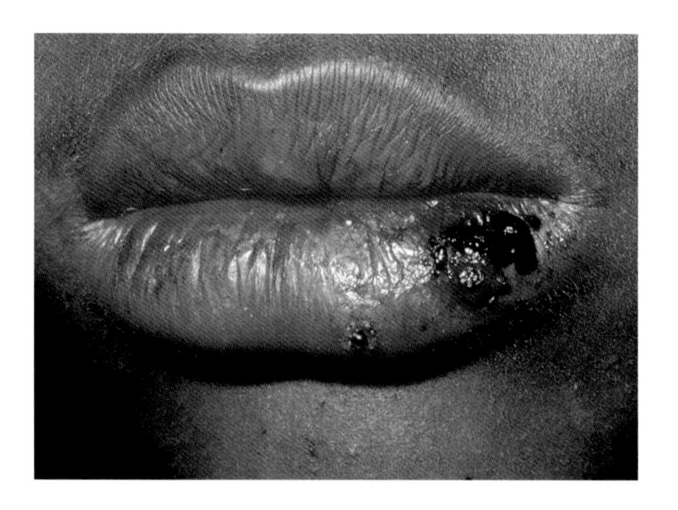

**Figure 558** Bleeding and crusting may mask the diagnosis. Do not confuse it with Kaposi's sarcoma (*see* Figure 321) or an amelanotic melanoma (*see* Figure 121).

*Treatment:* It can be removed by curettage and cautery under local anaesthesia if it is causing a nuisance by bleeding. Otherwise leave it alone until it resolves spontaneously.

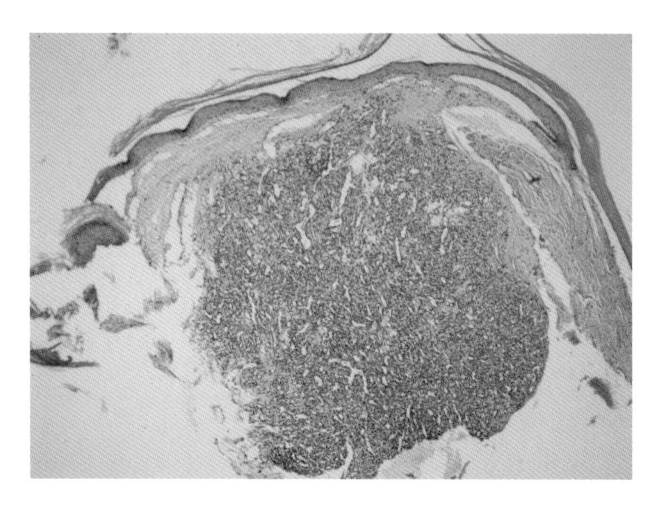

**Figure 559** The histology shows a lobulated dermal mass made up of innumerable small capillaries in a loose oedematous matrix.

## RACIAL HYPERPIGMENTATION OF THE SOLES

**Figure 560** Hyperpigmented macules on the soles is a normal finding in Africans. They should not be confused with the macules of secondary syphilis which occur on both palms and soles (*see* Figure 601).

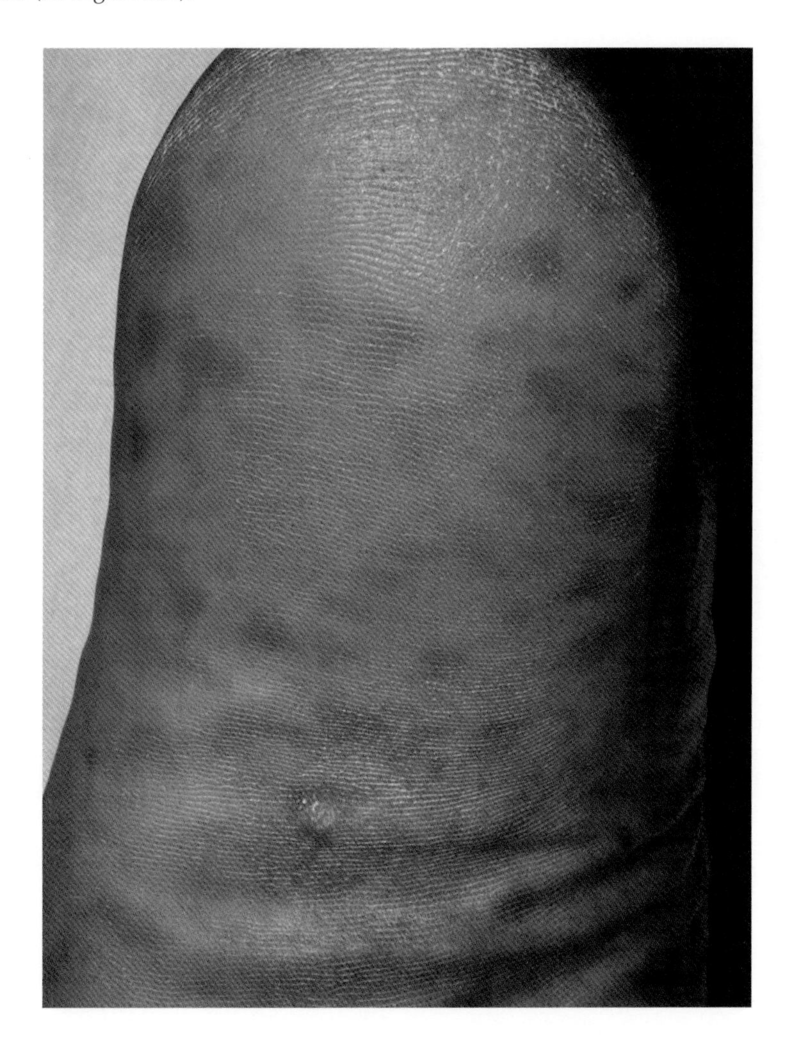

## RHINOPHYMA

**Figure 561** Massive sebaceous gland hyperplasia on the nose. In the West it is seen in association with rosacea, but rosacea is very rare in Africans.

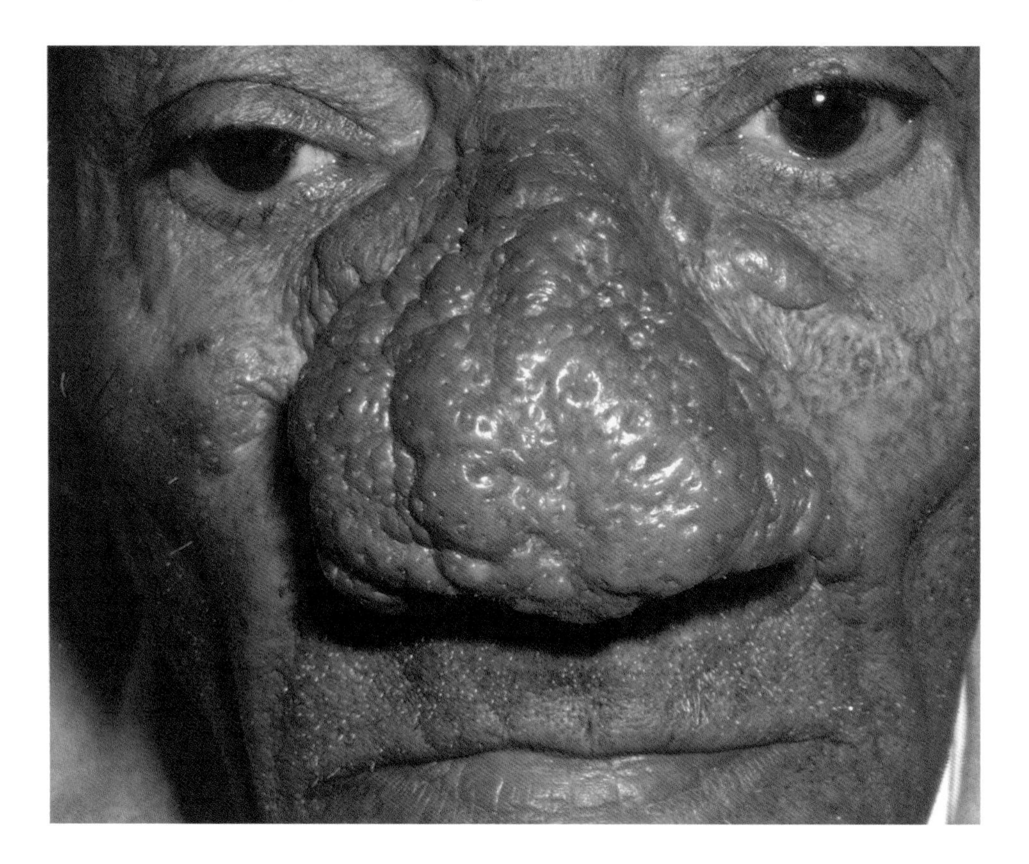

*Treatment:* The excessive bulk can be shaved off the nose under a nerve block if it is very unsightly.

## RUBELLA

**Figure 562** Common viral infection of children due to a rubivirus. After an incubation period of 14–21 days, a macular rash begins on the face and neck. It spreads down the body over 24–48 hours and then clears from the face downwards over 2–3 days without any scaling. The child is infectious from 5 days before to 3 days after the rash appears. The major problem with rubella is the risk to the foetus if the mother is infected in the first trimester of pregnancy. It causes multiple congenital abnormalities in the foetus, of the eyes (cataract, glaucoma, microphthalmia), ears (deafness) and heart (patent ductus arteriosus, atrial septal defect, ventricular septal defect, pulmonary stenosis).

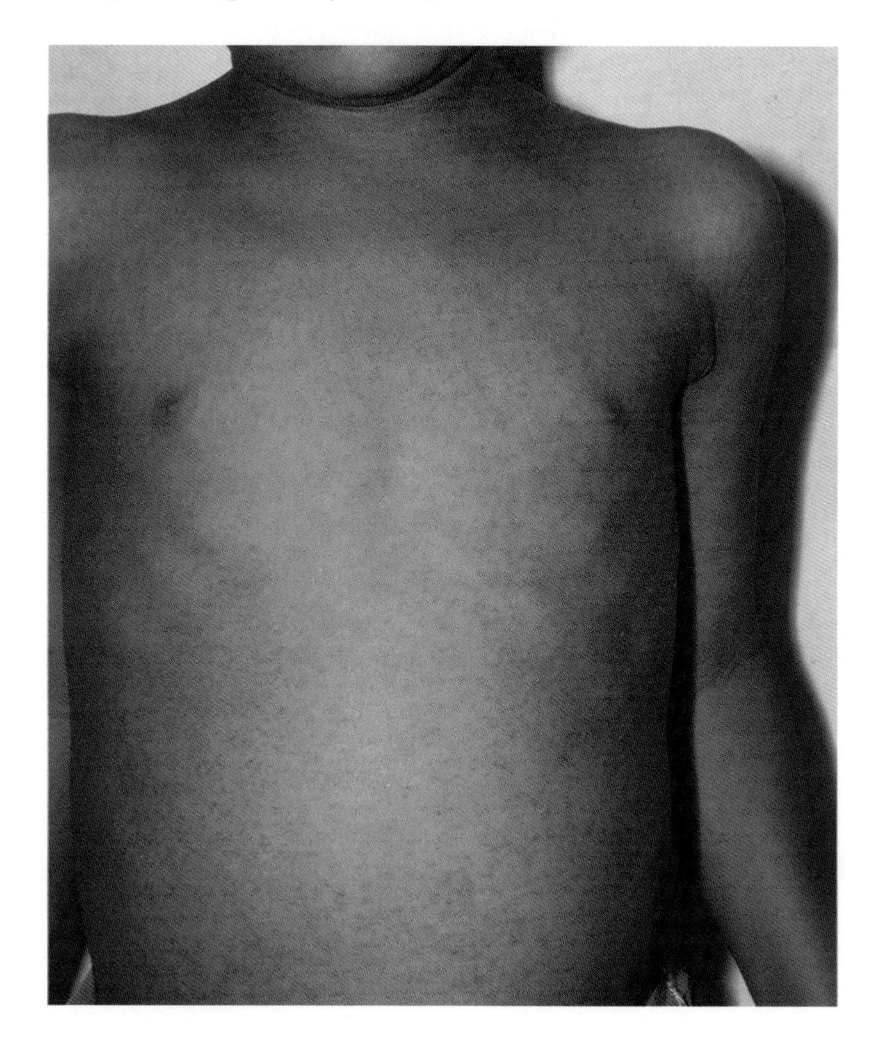

## SCABIES

**Figure 563** Scabies is an infestation with the human scabies mite, *Sarcoptes scabei*.

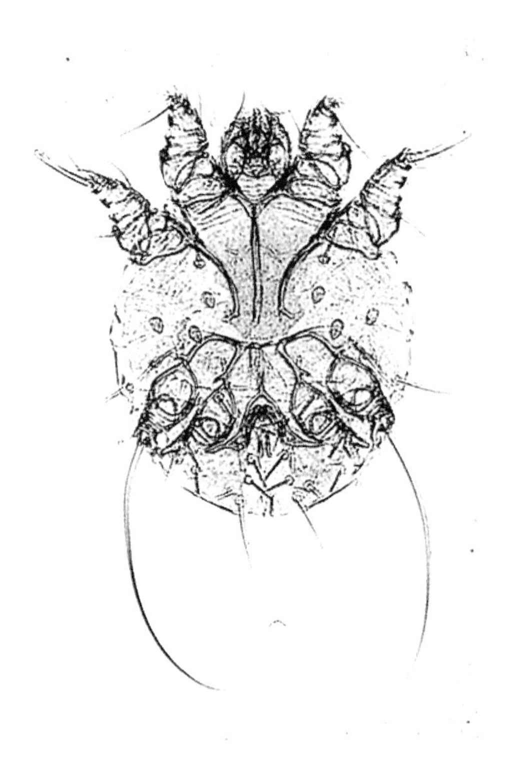

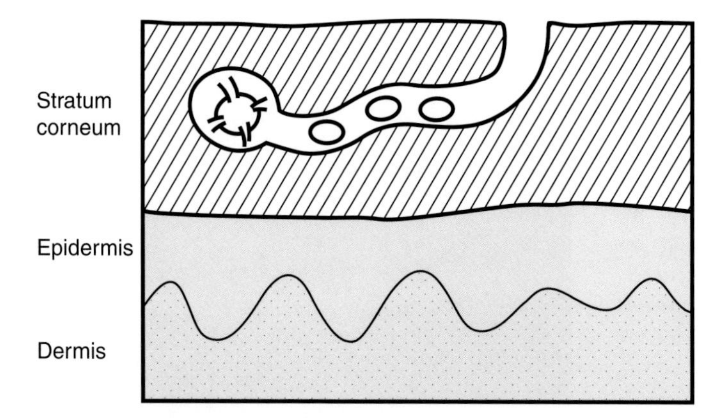


**Figure 564** A newly fertilised female mite walks from one person to another at a time of prolonged physical contact (e.g. sleeping in the same bed). The mite will then look for a place to burrow and lay its eggs. The burrow is within the stratum corneum, usually in the finger webs, along the sides of the fingers, or on the front of the wrists.

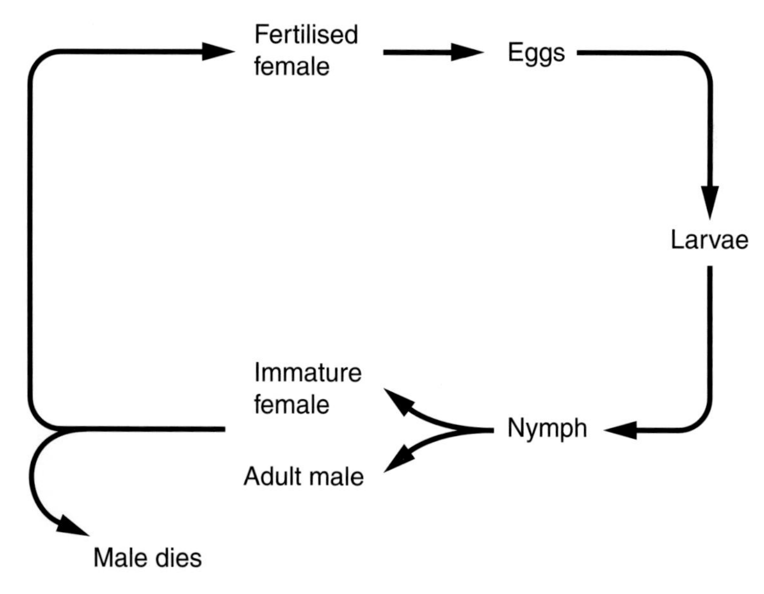


**Figure 565** Life cycle of the scabies mite. The fertilised female lays 2–3 eggs/day for about 2 months. The whole cycle from egg to adult mite takes 10–14 days. The male and female adult mites have to find each other on the skin surface in order to mate. As they are only pinhead size, most (>90%) do not find a partner and die.

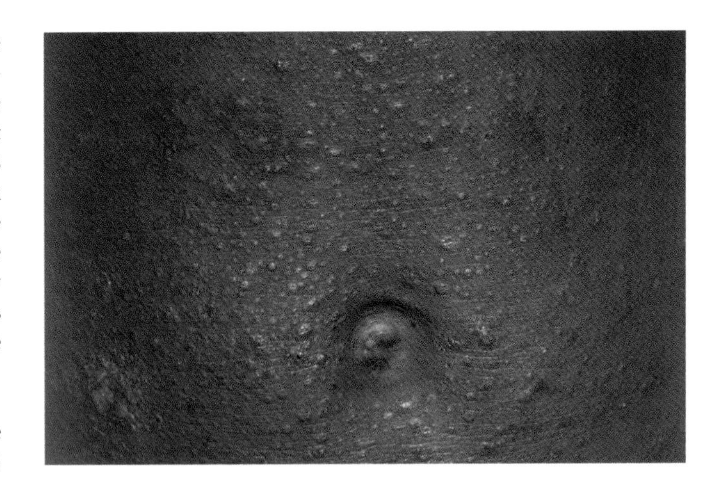

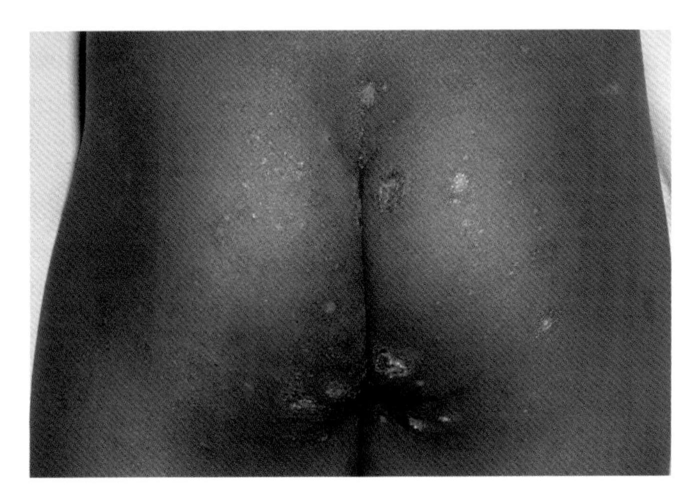

**Figures 566, 567** The rash is an allergic reaction to having the mites in the skin. It develops 4–6 weeks after infestation. It is an itchy rash all over the body, but sparing the face. There are nearly always other members of the family who are also itching.

*Treatment:* 1% Lindane cream or lotion, 25% benzyl benzoate emulsion, 5% permethrin cream or 10% sulphur ointment are the topical options. They should be applied to the whole body except the face and scalp, and left on the skin for 24 hours. All close contacts, particularly all those sharing a bed, must be treated at the same time.

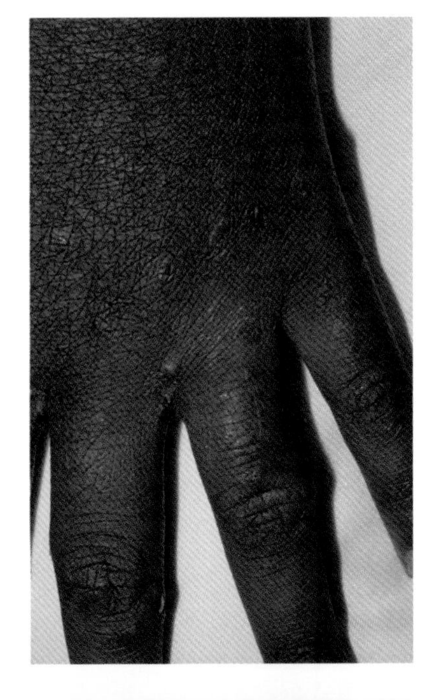

**Figure 568** There is always a rash on the hands, especially in the finger webs. Here also the burrows can be found – linear 'S'-shaped papules, 3–5mm in length, along the sides of the fingers or on the front of the wrists. Small vesicles may be more easily seen than the burrows.

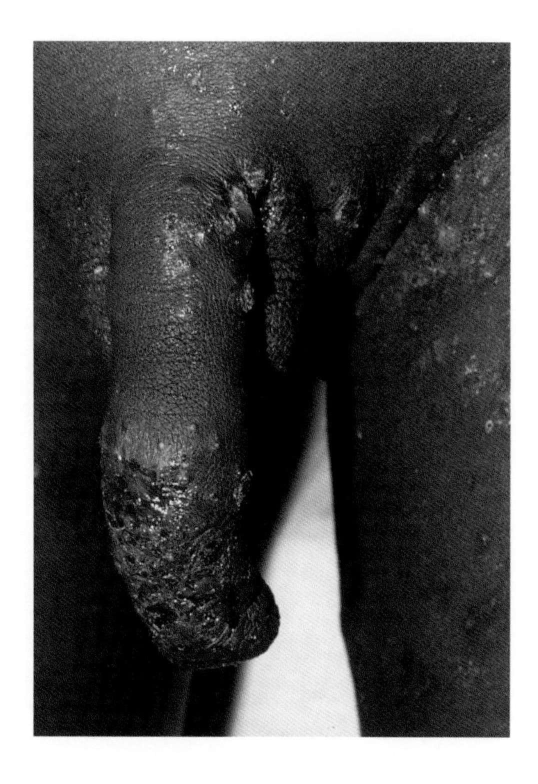

**Figure 569** In males there is always a rash on the genitalia, itchy papules, burrows or secondary infection.

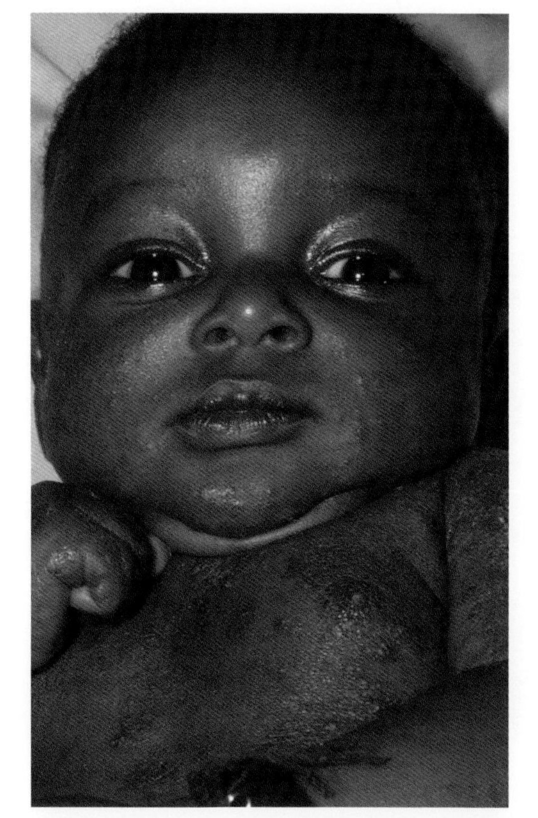

**Figure 570** In infants the rash may be present on the face as well as the rest of the body.

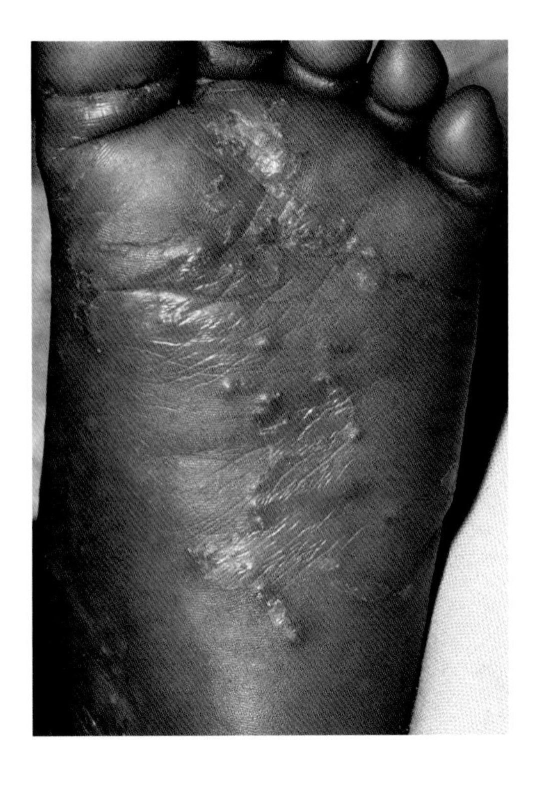

**Figure 571** In infants the burrows are on the palms and soles, instead of the finger webs. They are easily seen.

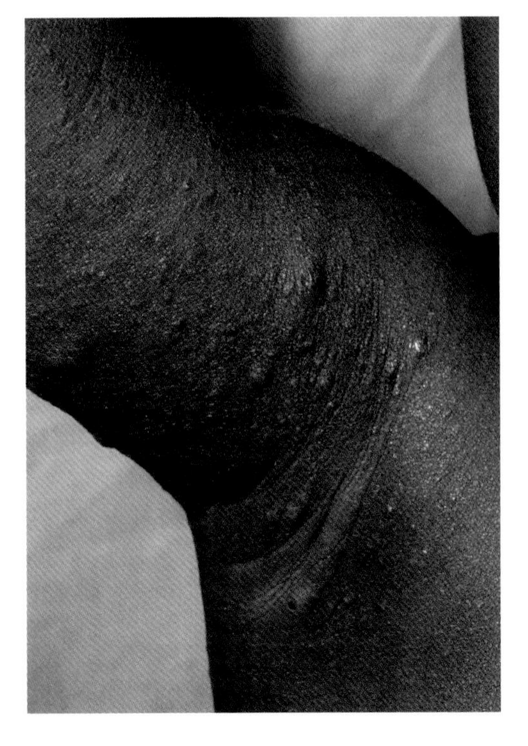

**Figure 572** Scabetic nodules. In some people itchy papules remain after scabies has been treated, especially around the axillae.

*Treatment of scabetic nodules:* Apply a topical steroid, such as 0.025% betamethasone 17-valerate bd, until the itching stops. Retreatment of the scabies is not necessary.

## Crusted scabies

**Figures 573, 574** Crusted scabies (also called Norwegian scabies) is scabies in an immunocompromised host or in someone with mental retardation or sensory loss. It is most commonly found in individuals who are HIV positive. It is an infestation with the scabies mite, *Sarcoptes scabei,* but with a different host response. Instead of only having a few mites in the skin there may be thousands or even millions. The rash often looks like eczema (Figure 573), but there may be thick hyperkeratotic scale (Figure 574). This type of scabies is very infectious to other people around the patient.

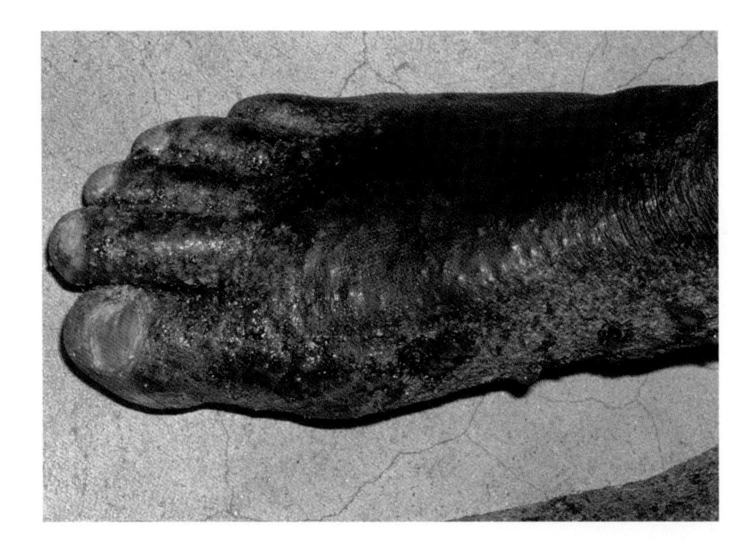

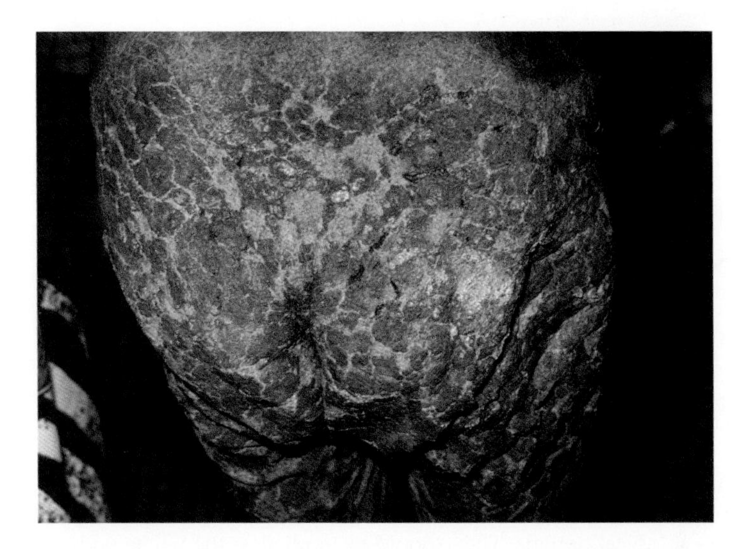

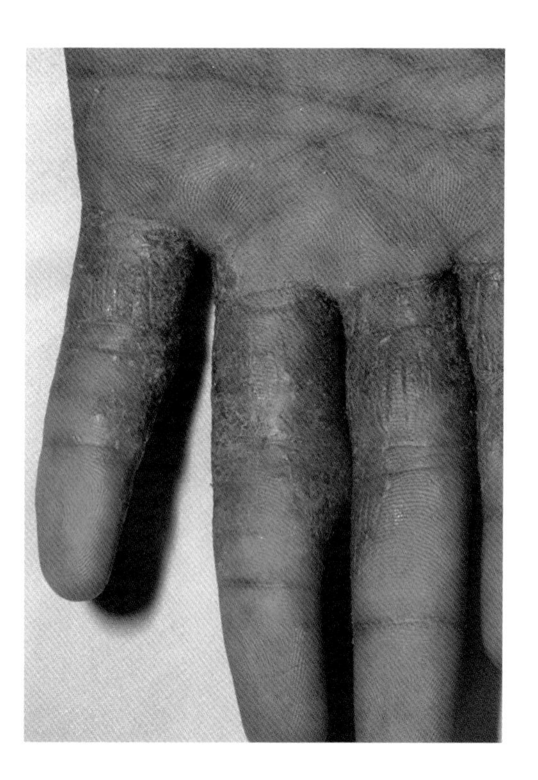

**Figure 575** Numerous burrows may be seen on the palms and soles in crusted scabies, even in adults.

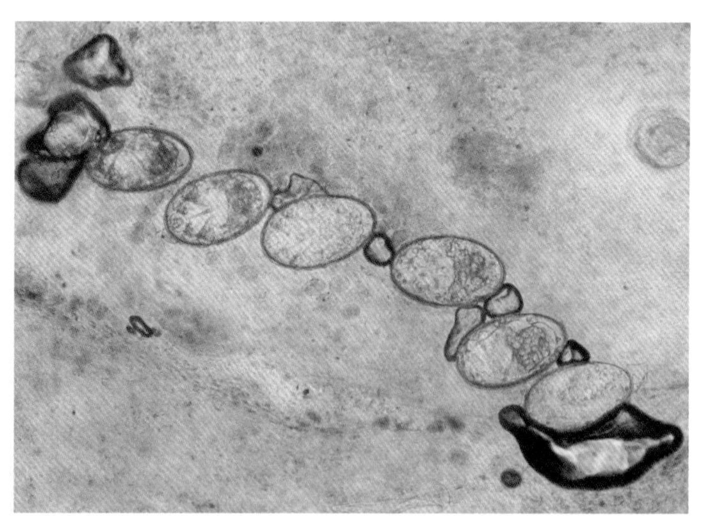

**Figure 576** Scabies eggs in skin scales. Scraping the scaly rash and mixing the scales on a slide with KOH will reveal multiple eggs, larvae, nymphs and adult mites.

*Treatment:* As for ordinary scabies but repeated a second time after 24 hours. 1% Lindane cream or lotion, 25% benzyl benzoate emulsion, 5% permethrin cream or 10% sulphur ointment are the topical options. They should be applied to the whole body except the face and scalp, and left on the skin for 24 hours. All members of the family and other close contacts must be treated at the same time. In addition, the floor and walls of the house should be treated with an emulsifiable concentrate of Actellic 50 EC (pirimiphos methyl) 80mg diluted in 20 litres of water. The bedding should be taken outside and left in the hot sun for 1 hour.

## SCHISTOSOMIASIS (Bilharzia)

**Figure 577** Schistosomiasis of the labia minora. Small granulomas, erosions, ulcers, warty papules or nodules can occur on the skin or genitalia from schistosomiasis which are due to the blood flukes *Schistosoma haematobium* or *S. mansoni*. The skin lesions arise from a granulomatous reaction to eggs in the dermis, which have found their way there from the pelvic veins. Infestation occurs from contact with fresh water snails, which are the intermediate hosts. Free swimming cercariae are released from the snails and penetrate human skin. These pass through the skin into the veins, mature to flukes in the intrahepatic portal veins and then pass to the pelvic veins where they lay their eggs.

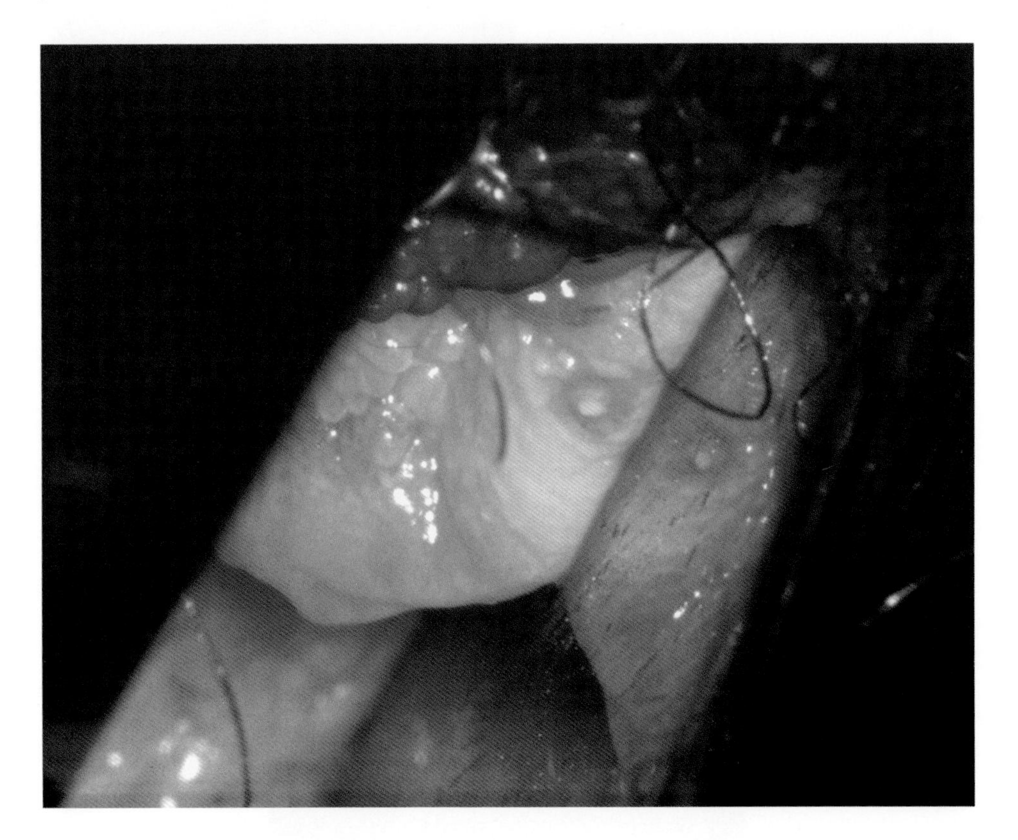

*Diagnosis:* Find eggs in the urine (*S. haematobium*), or stool (*S. mansoni),* or in a skin biopsy.

*Treatment:* Prazaquantil 40mg/kg body weight as a single dose. Advise the patient not to bathe or swim in fresh water rivers or lakes.

## SCLERODERMA (Systemic sclerosis)

**Figures 578, 579** Multisystem disorder in which the skin of the face becomes tight. It is difficult for the patient to open the mouth wide.

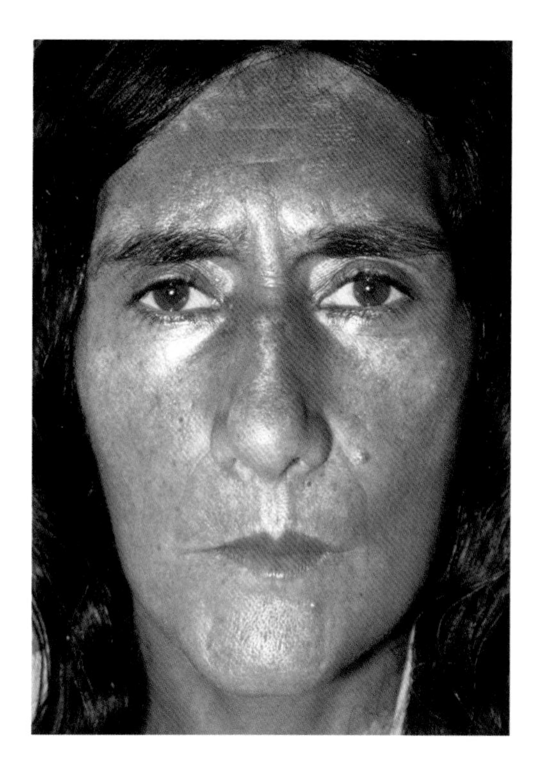

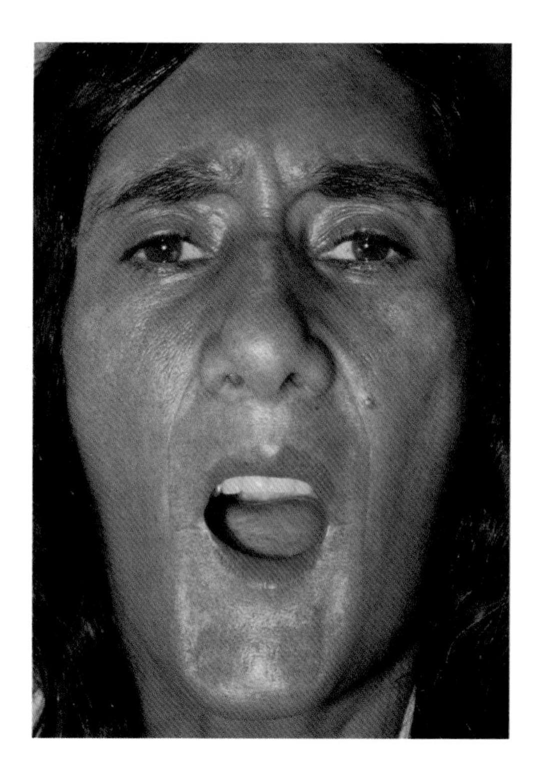

**Figure 580** The skin of the fingers is also tight and there may be calcification in the dermis and subcutaneous fat which can ulcerate through the skin.

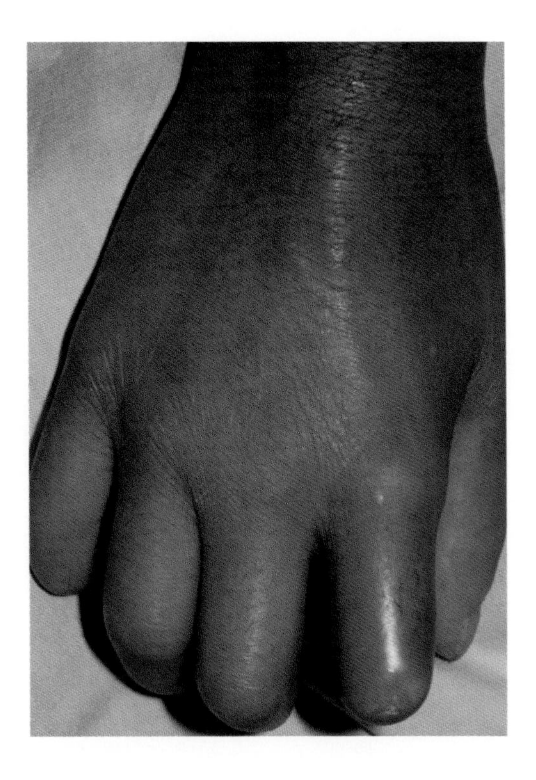

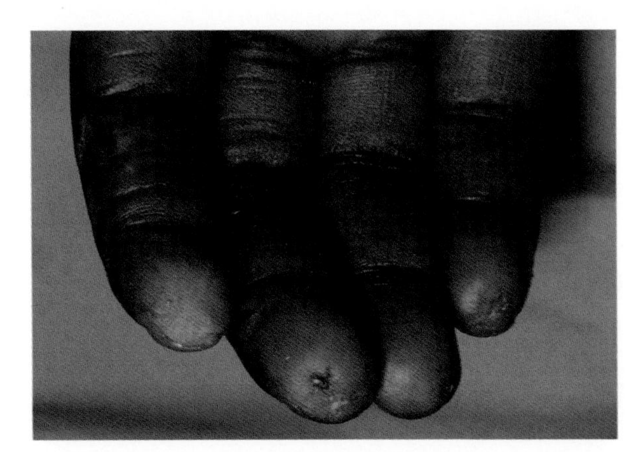

**Figure 581** There may be loss of the tips of the fingers due to vasculitis. There is also nail fold telangiectasia as in dermatomyositis (*see* Figure 178) and systemic lupus erythematosus. There may also be problems in swallowing from involvement of the oesophagus; steatorrhoea from involvement of the small bowel; constipation or diarrhoea from involvement of the colon; dyspnoea from fibrosis of the lungs; cardiac arrhythmias from involvement of the myocardium; and proteinuria and renal failure from involvement of the kidneys.

*Treatment:* Unsatisfactory. Nothing works well.

## SEBACEOUS GLAND HYPERPLASIA

**Figure 582** Yellowish papule with a central punctum. Due to enlargement of the sebaceous glands attached to a single hair follicle. These are much more common in Europeans than in Africans and are quite harmless.

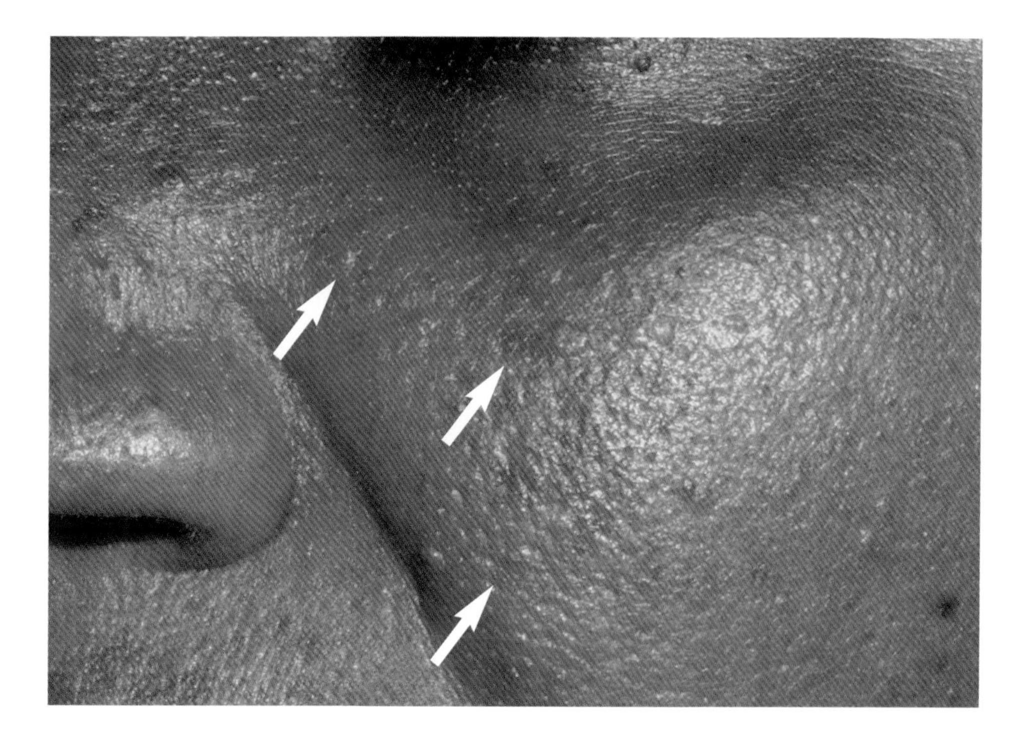

## SEBORRHOEIC WART

**Figure 583** Common hyperpigmented papules on the face and trunk in the elderly. They have a warty appearance and look as if they are 'stuck on' the skin.

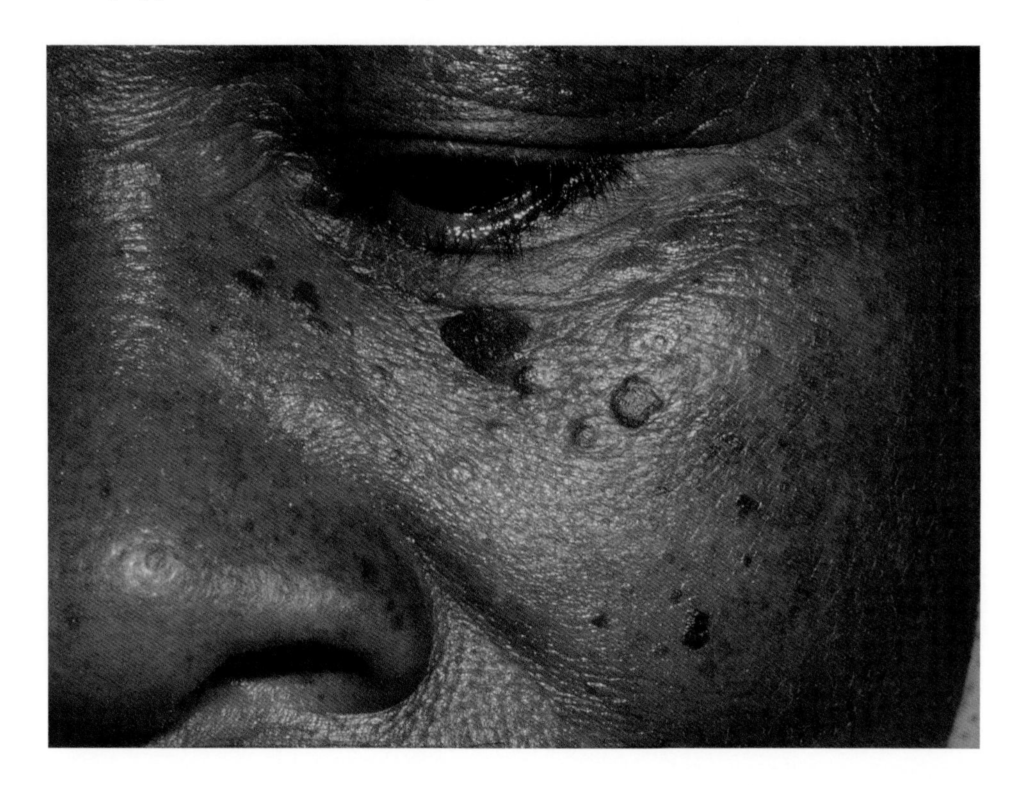

*Treatment:* None is needed since they are a normal finding in older people.

## SIDE EFFECTS OF TOPICAL STEROIDS

**Figure 584** Perioral dermatitis. The application of topical steroids (stronger than 1% hydrocortisone) to the face of young adults results in perioral dermatitis. This is a rash around the mouth, made up of small papules and vesicles, which spares the area immediately around the lips.

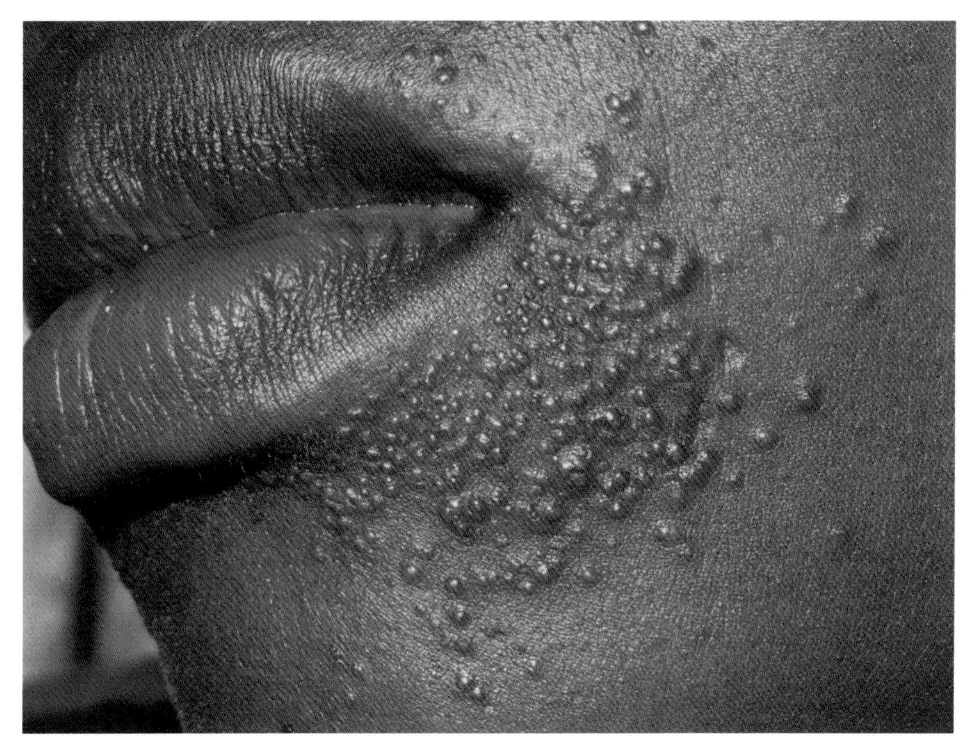

*Treatment:* The topical steroids must be stopped. The rash will then resolve but it may take several months. Oral tetracycline 250mg bd (on an empty stomach) for 6 weeks may speed up its resolution.

**Figures 585, 586** Steroid facies. The application of topical steroids (stronger than 1% hydrocortisone) to the face of adults over the age of 30 years will result in telangiectasia, and later tearing of the skin and scarring.

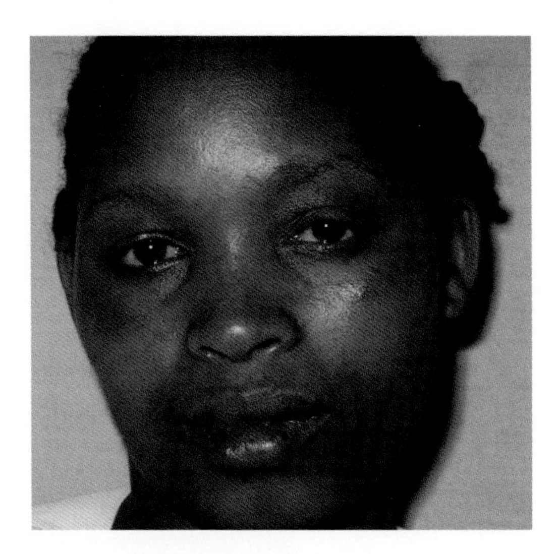

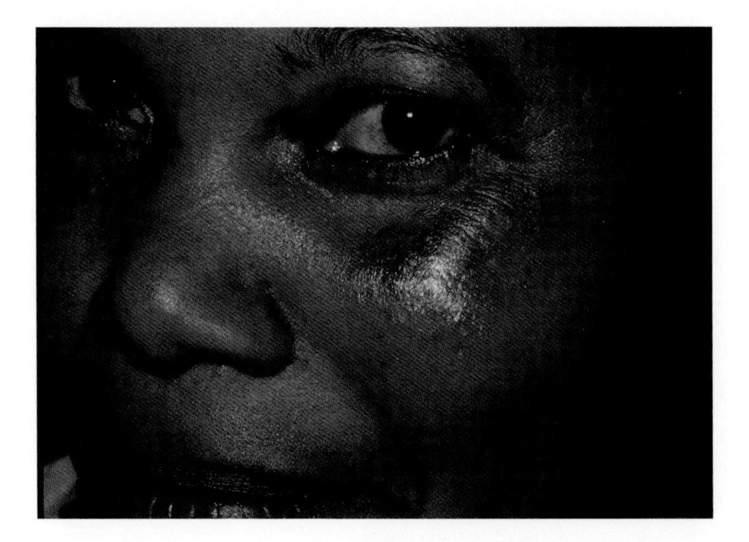

*Treatment:* Stop the topical steroids. Topical steroids stronger than 1% hydrocortisone should not be used on the face. The only exception to this rule is for the treatment of discoid lupus erythematosus (*see* Figure 402).

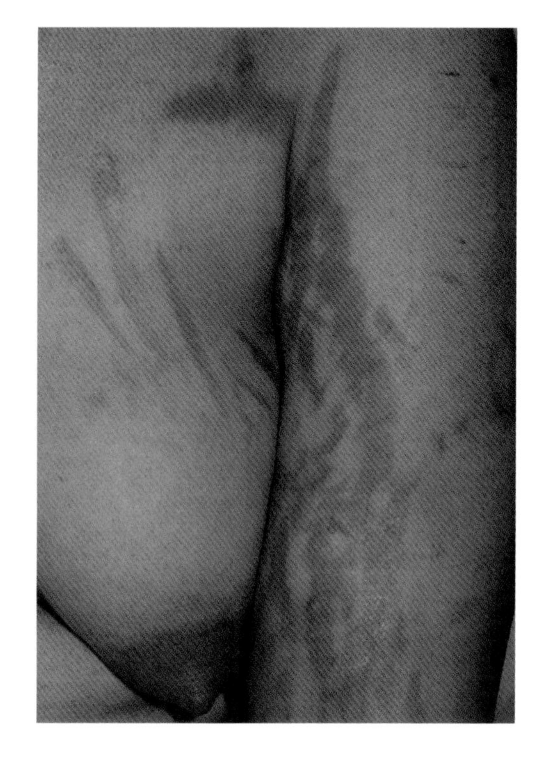

**Figure 587** Striae are due to loss of dermal collagen. This lady had been applying potent topical steroids in an attempt to lighten her skin colour.

*Treatment:* Stop topical steroids to prevent even more skin damage. The striae are likely to be permanent.

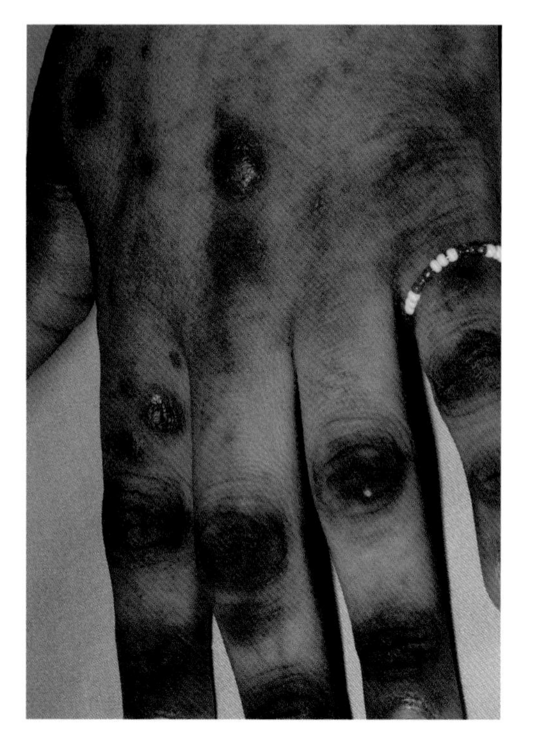

**Figure 588** Loss of pigment due to inhibition of melanocyte activity. Although this was what the patient wanted, the uneven pigmentation that resulted was unsightly.

*Treatment:* Stop the topical steroids.

## SKIN TAGS

**Figure 589** Small hyperpigmented, pedunculated papules on the neck and other flexures.

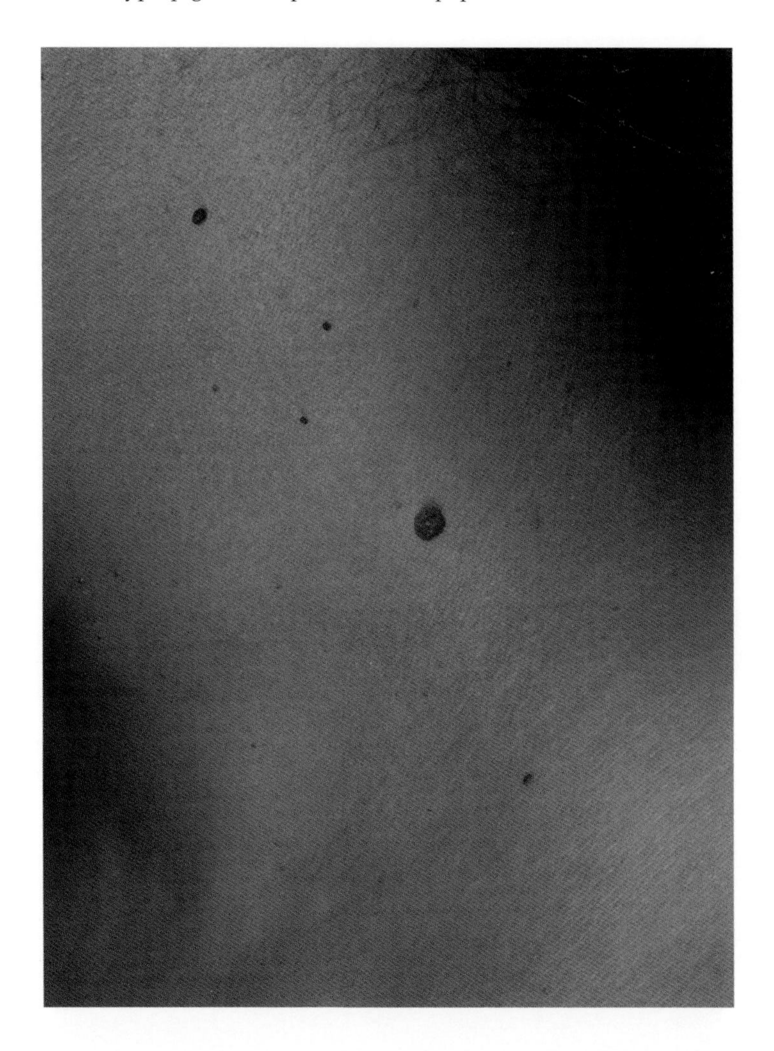

*Treatment:* They are a normal finding and quite harmless. If they are unsightly they can be snipped off with a pair of sharp scissors and the bleeding stopped with a silver nitrate stick or a cautery.

## STAPHYLOCOCCAL SCALDED SKIN SYNDROME

**Figure 590** A disease caused by *Staphylococcus aureus*, mainly in infants. Older children in the same family may have impetigo from infection with the same organism. An exotoxin produced by the staphylococcus causes necrosis of the upper epidermis, which shears off through the granular layer. If you remove the blister roof you will find that it is made up only of keratin (compare this with the blister roof in TEN, *see* Figure 194).

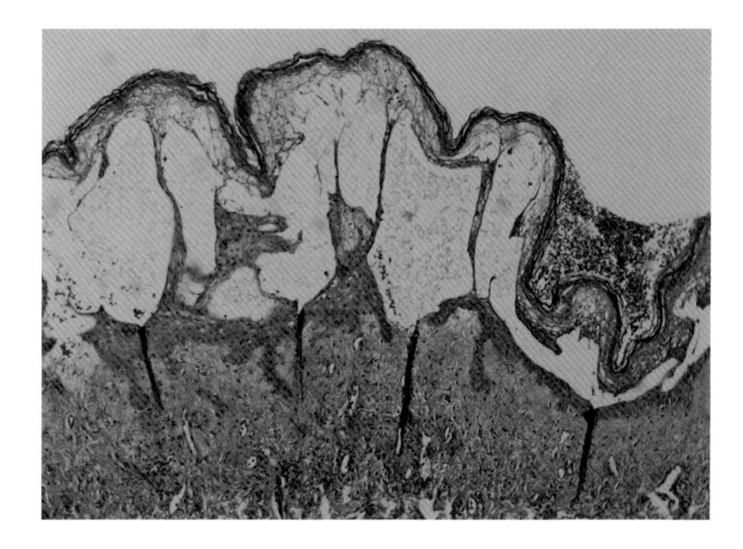

**Figure 591** The skin changes are like those of a scald. The skin becomes red and very painful, so the child may cry before there is anything to see. The skin then slides off leaving superficial erosions like those in toxic epidermal necrolysis (*see* Figure 193).

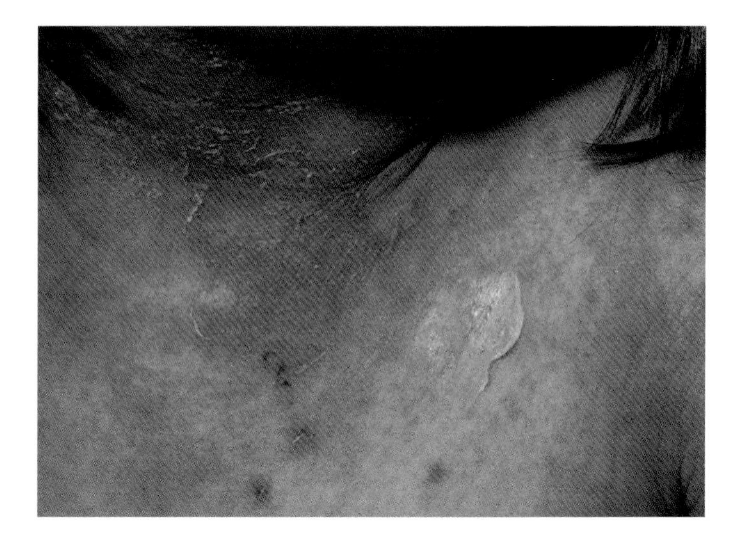

*Treatment:* Oral cloxacillin elixir 62.5mg orally qds for 7 days.

## SUBCORNEAL PUSTULAR DERMATOSIS

**Figures 592, 593** Disease of middle-aged and elderly patients (mainly women) in which crops of small pustules occur, mainly in the flexures. The histology shows a subcorneal pustule but no bacteria. The cause is unknown.

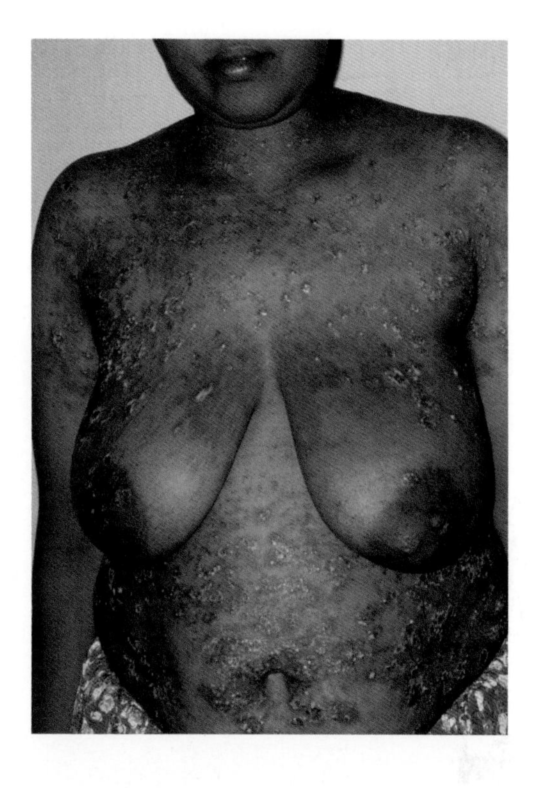

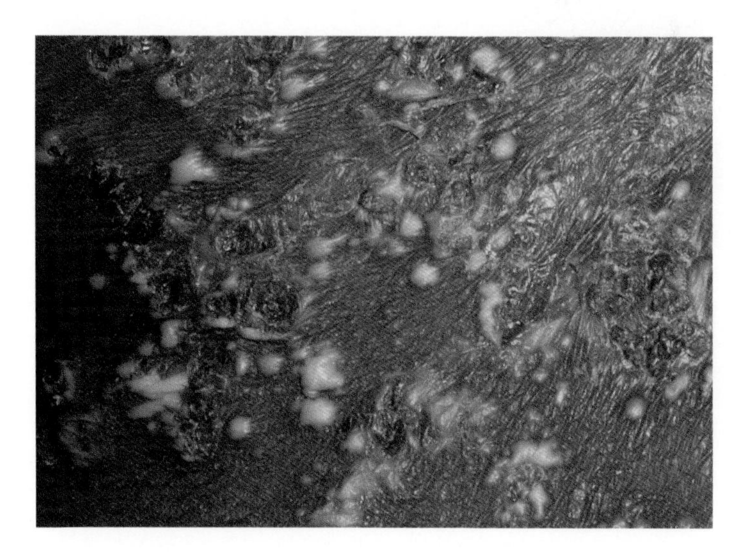

*Treatment:* Dapsone (diaminodiphenylsulphone) 50–150mg/day orally usually works well.

## SWEET'S DISEASE (Acute febrile neutrophilic dermatosis)

**Figure 594** An acute illness in which the patient develops a fever together with painful, red, oedematous plaques on the skin. A blood count shows a leukocytosis with a high neutrophil count and a high ESR. Most patients are middle-aged females. The diagnosis can be confirmed by doing a skin biopsy. There is a neutrophilic infiltrate in the reticular dermis together with marked oedema but no vasculitis. Some patients with Sweet's disease have acute myeloid leukaemia or some other form of myelodysplasia.

*Treatment:* Prednisolone 30mg/day until all signs and symptoms disappear. Then gradually taper it off. If it recurs, repeat the treatment.

# SYPHILIS

Syphilis is a sexually transmitted disease due to *Treponema pallidum*.

## Primary syphilis

**Figure 595** The primary chancre appears 14–21 days after infection. It begins as a painless papule at the site of inoculation, which then ulcerates. The ulcer is clean, round in shape and has an indurated margin. There is usually bilateral inguinal lymphadenopathy. Without treatment the ulcer heals in 3–6 weeks.

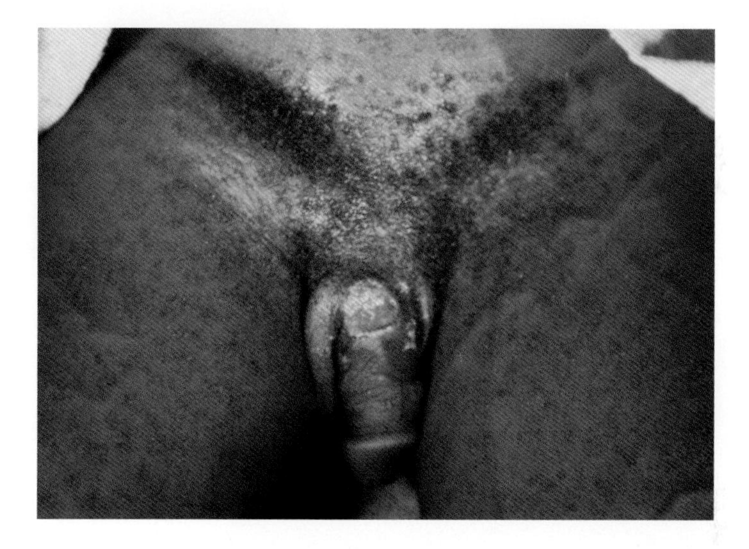

*Treatment:* Benzathine penicillin 2.4 megaunits im as a single dose. Always check for HIV infection too.

**Figure 596** The diagnosis is made by dark field examination of fluid obtained from the surface of the ulcer. Magnify x100 and use a dark field condenser to see the spirochaetes.

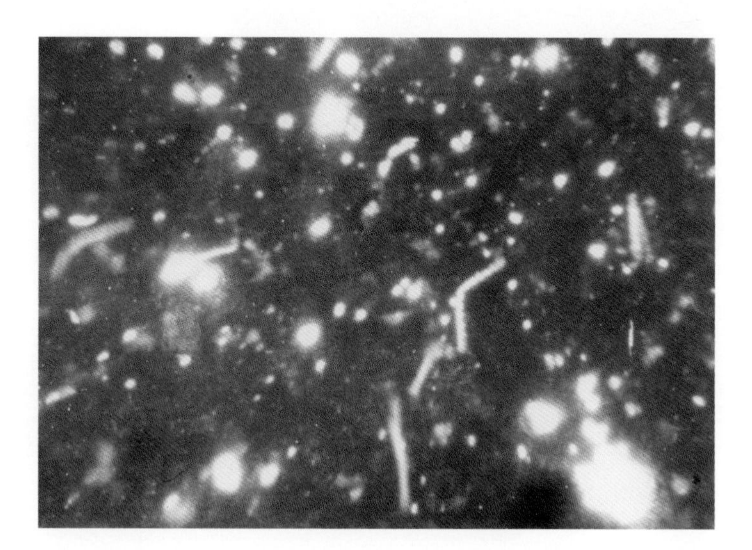

## Secondary syphilis

**Figures 597, 598** 4–10 weeks after infection with *Treponema pallidum* the signs of secondary syphilis appear. General malaise (fever, headache, sore throat and non-specific aches and pains), widespread lymphadenopathy and a rash occur. The rash is usually made up of widespread macules or scaly papules which are not itchy. This kind of rash can be confused with pityriasis rosea (*see* Figure 511).

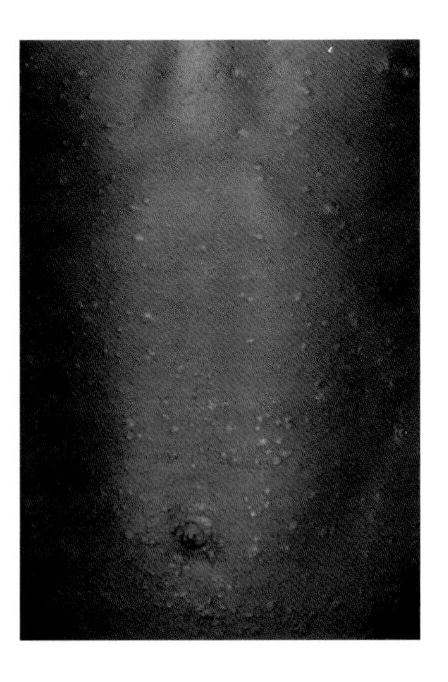

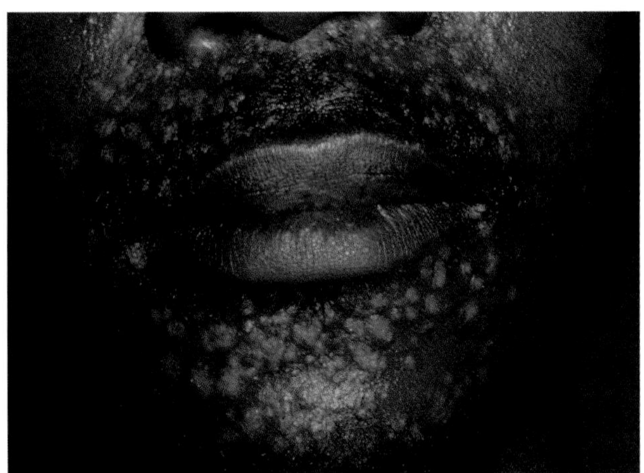

**Figure 599** The rash is very variable and it can mimic almost any skin disease. Annular plaques like this are a common pattern.

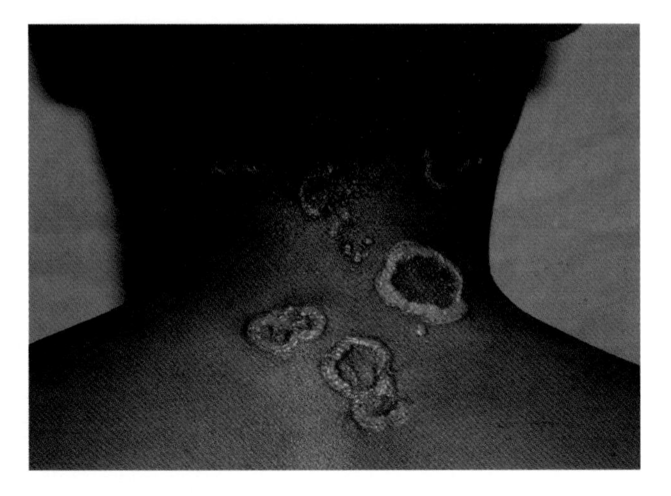

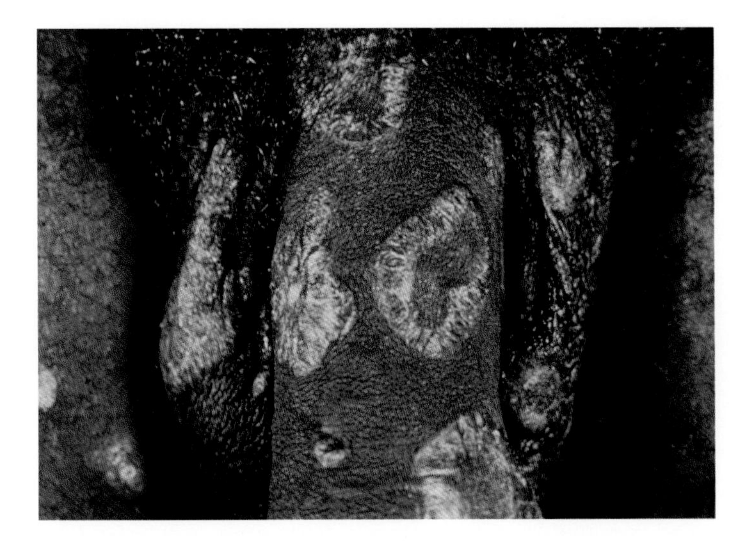

**Figure 600** Scaly plaques mimicking psoriasis (*see* Figures 535–6).

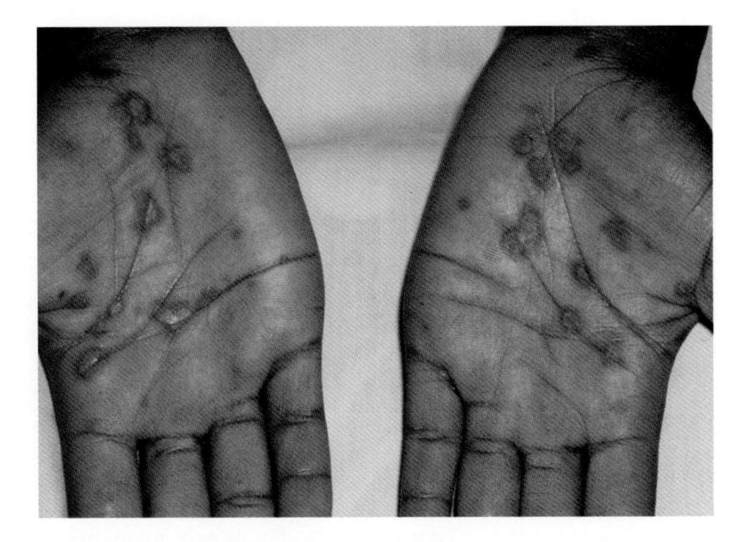

**Figure 601** Macules or papules on the palms and soles are typical but are not always present. They should not be confused with the normal racial hyperpigmentation that occurs on the soles (*see* Figure 560).

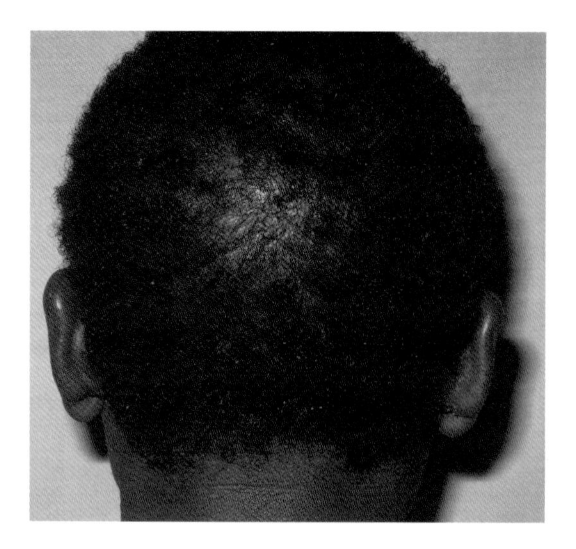

**Figure 602** Patchy alopecia is a common finding.

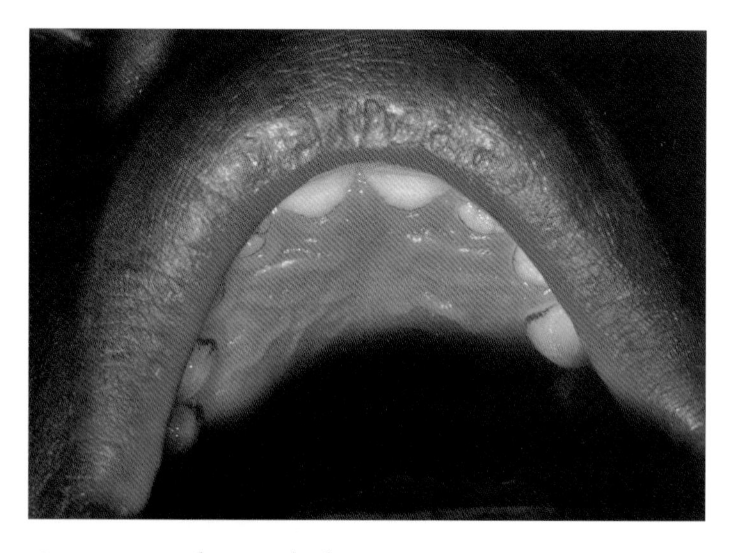

**Figure 603** In the mouth there may be 'snail track' ulcers – superficial erosions with a slimy surface.

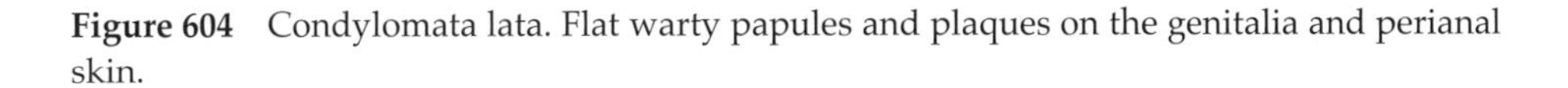

**Figure 604** Condylomata lata. Flat warty papules and plaques on the genitalia and perianal skin.

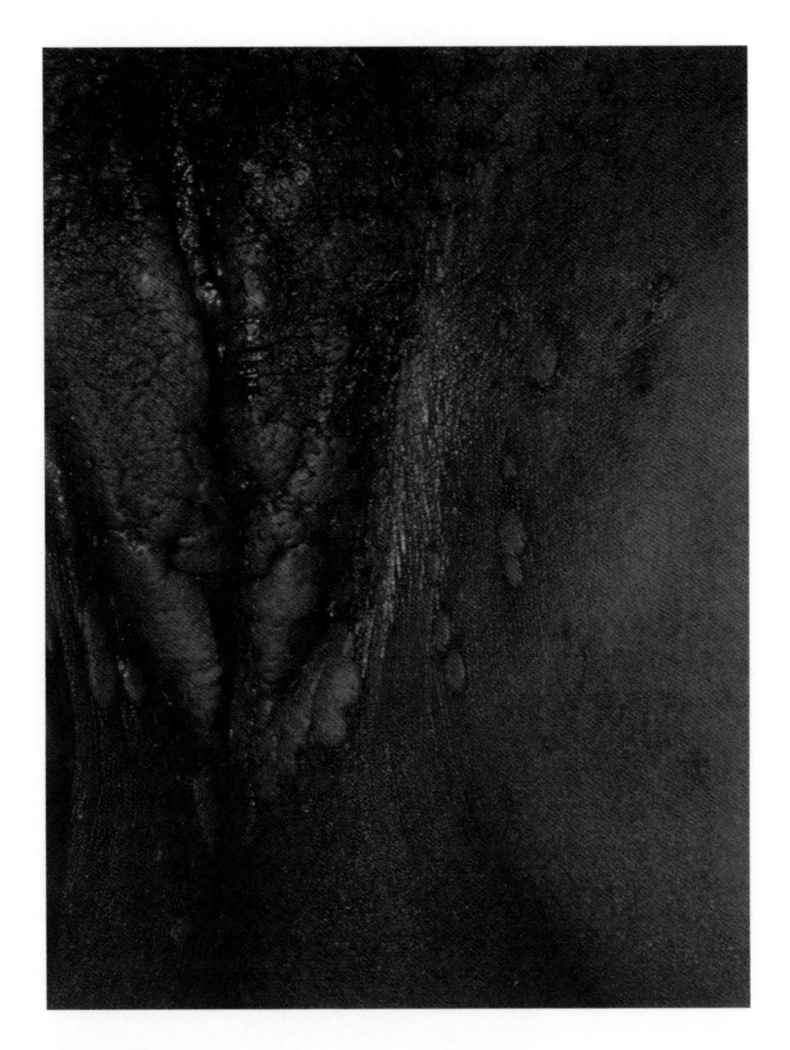

*Diagnosis:* The diagnosis of secondary syphilis can be confirmed by finding spirochaetes on dark field examination of the skin lesions. Remove the surface scale and scrape the exudate from underneath onto a glass slide and examine with a dark field condenser (*see* Figure 596). Serological tests for syphilis are always positive at this stage. Check the RPR or VDRL.

*Treatment:* Benzathine penicillin 2.4 megaunits im as a single dose. Always check for HIV infection too. If the patient is HIV positive give three doses of benzathine penicillin at weekly intervals.

## SYRINGOMA

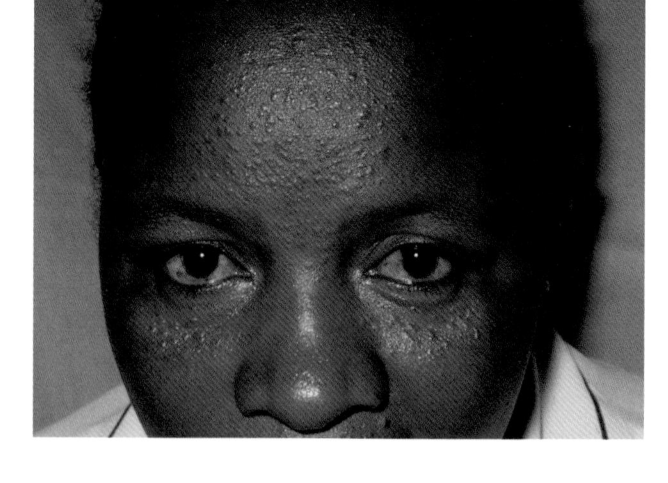

**Figure 605** Benign tumour of eccrine sweat ducts, inherited as an autosomal dominant trait (*see* Figure 295). Symmetrical small, skin-coloured papules appear on the lower eyelids and upper cheeks after puberty. Occasionally more extensive on the forehead too, as here.

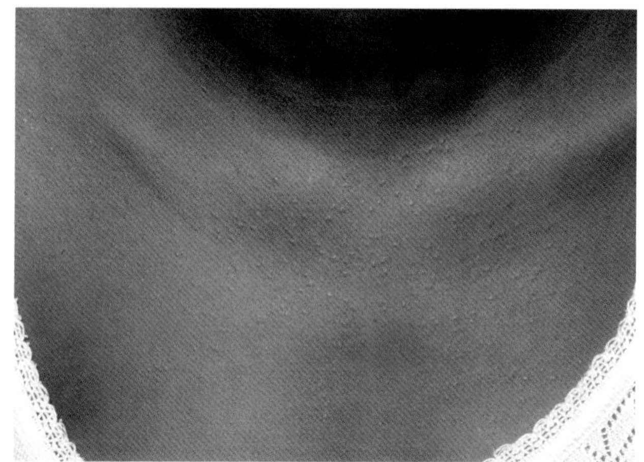

**Figures 606, 607** Syringomas are occasionally widely disseminated on the trunk as well as being present on the lower eyelids.

*Treatment:* They are quite harmless and can be left alone.

## TANAPOX

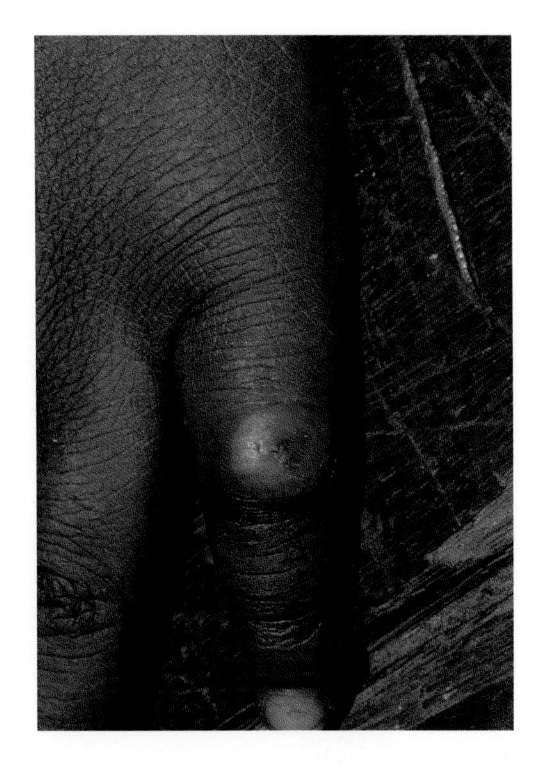

**Figure 608** This is a pox virus infection of monkeys which is transmitted to humans through mosquito bites. There is usually clustering of cases geographically but no human-to-human transmission. The skin lesions are usually single and often found on the lower legs (although they can be found anywhere). They begin as a non-itchy papule which becomes vesicular, then necroses and heals spontaneously after 3–4 weeks. If the lesion is on the face there may be marked oedema around it. This is an early lesion – 3 days old – in a 4-year-old child.

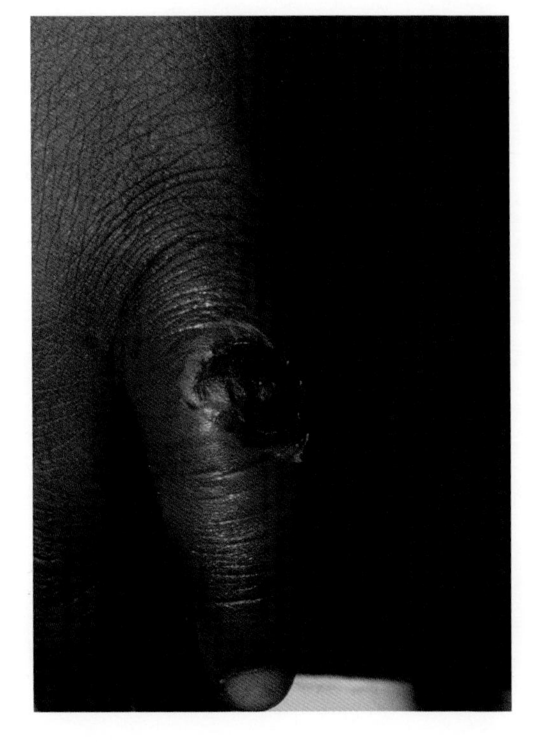

**Figure 609** Late lesion – 3 weeks old (same patient as in Figure 608).

*Treatment:* Reassurance that it is not serious. The lesions heal after 4 weeks.

## THREAD VEINS

**Figure 610** Symmetrical dilatation of venules on the lower legs and thighs, looking like branches of a tree.

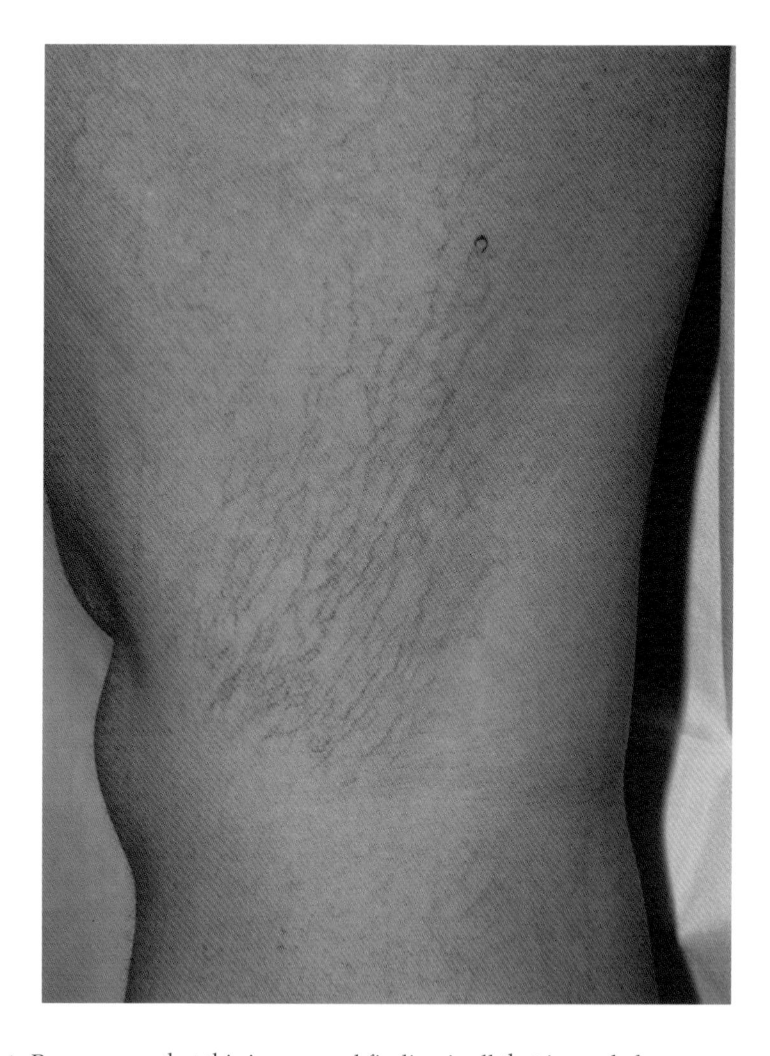

*Treatment:* Reassurance that this is a normal finding is all that is needed.

## TINEA

**Figure 611** Tinea or ringworm is the name given to superficial fungal infections of the skin. These fungi live in the stratum corneum and feed on keratin. They are called dermatophytes and belong to three genera of fungi:

- Microsporum.
- Trichophyton.
- Epidermophyton.

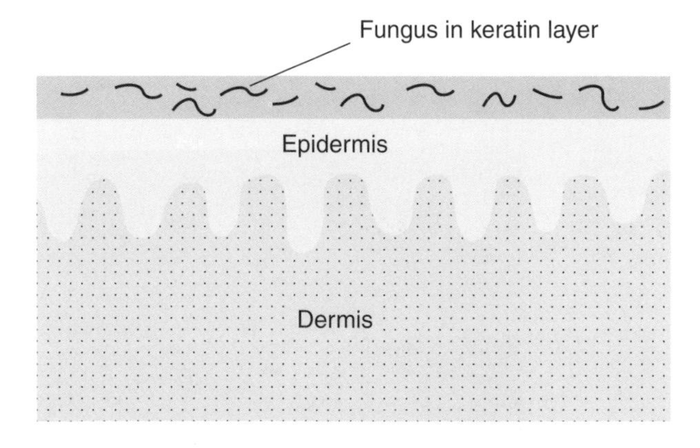


### Tinea corporis (ringworm on the face, trunk or limbs)

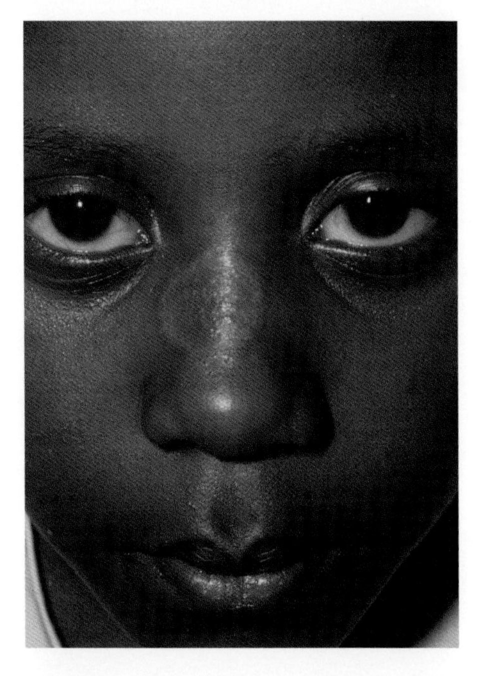

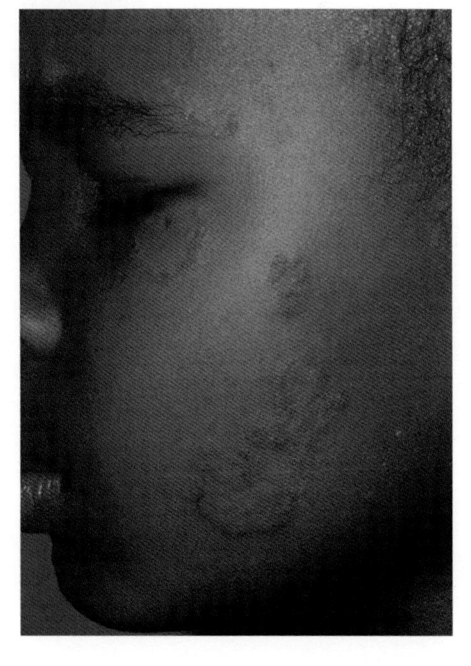

**Figures 612, 613** Single or multiple plaque(s) with a raised scaly border. Very common in children, but can occur at any age.

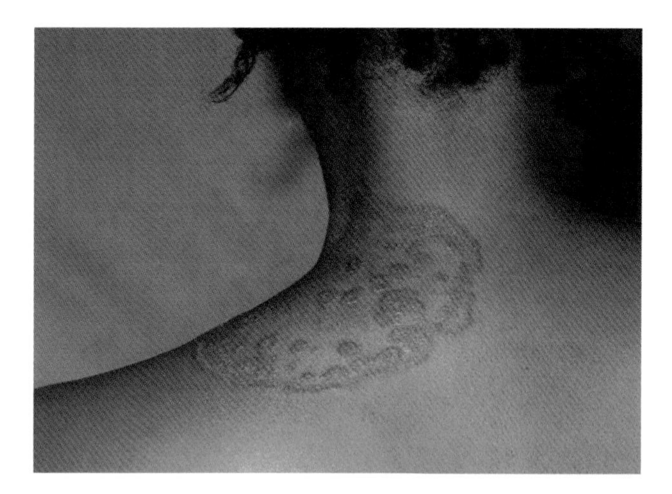

**Figure 614** Usually unilateral or asymmetrical. Always think of tinea if there is a unilateral scaly rash.

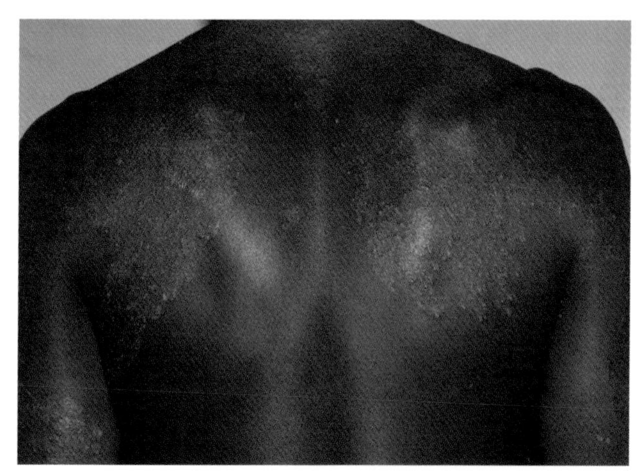

**Figure 615** May be extensive and symmetrical in hot and humid areas, or in patients with HIV infection.

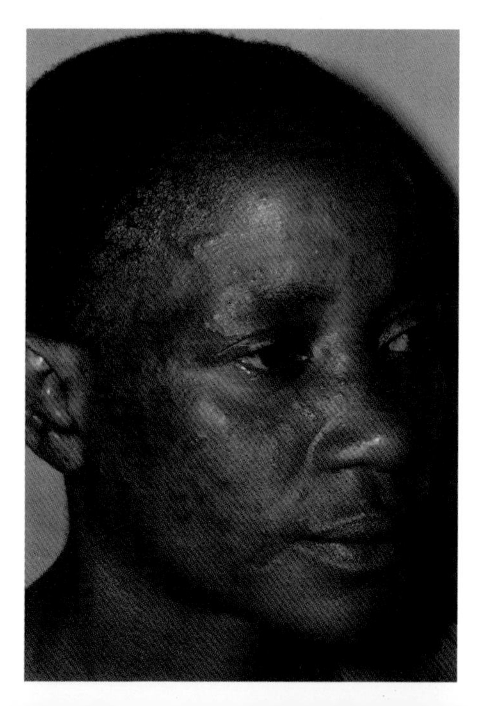

**Figure 616** Applying topical steroids by mistake to tinea can make it look very different (red in colour and more extensive). This pattern is called 'tinea incognito'.

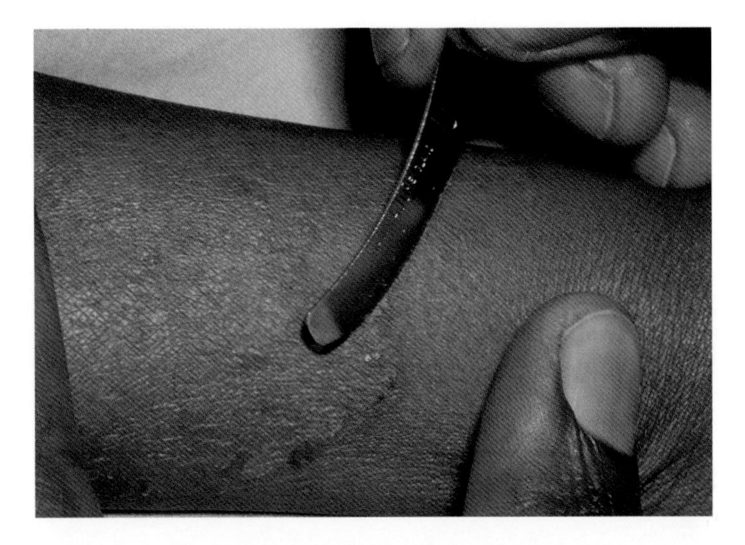

**Figure 617** The diagnosis of tinea can be confirmed by scraping the scales from the edge of the plaque with a blunt scalpel and putting them on a glass slide with a drop of 20% KOH.

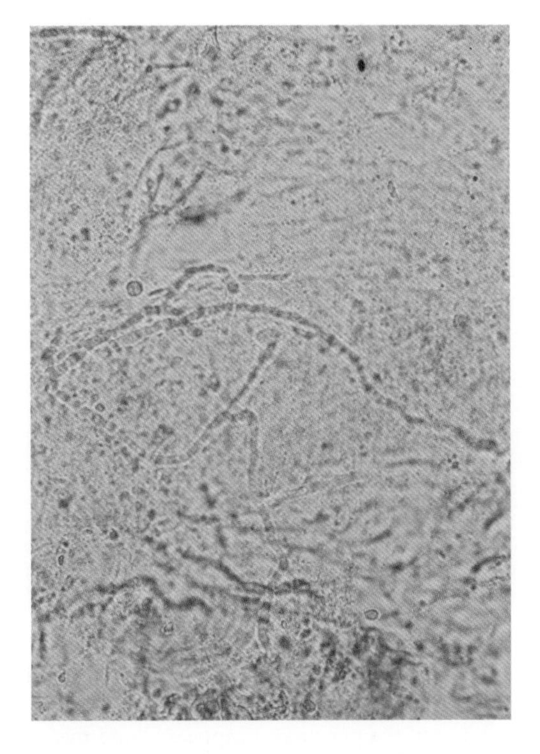

**Figure 618** KOH preparation. Branching fungal hyphae can be seen all over the slide.

**Figure 619** The scales can also be cultured on Sabouraud's dextrose agar containing chloramphenicol and cyclohexamide. *Trichophyton rubrum* (top surface) after 14 days.

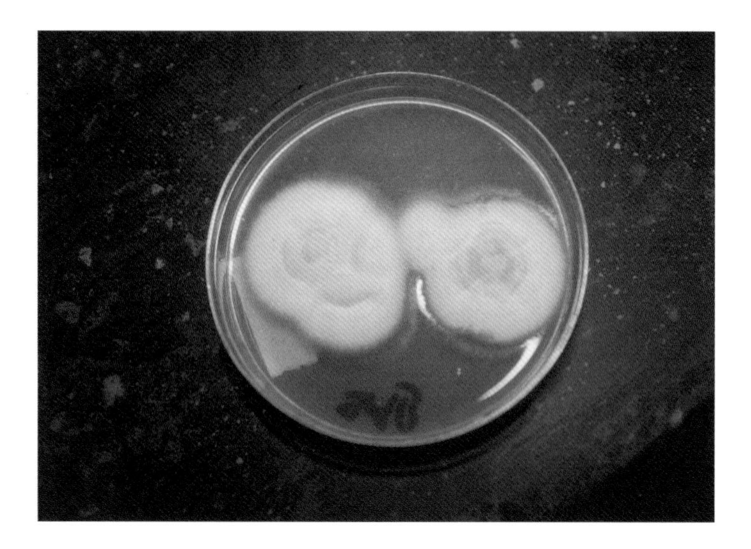

**Figure 620** *Trichophyton rubrum* (under surface) after 14 days.

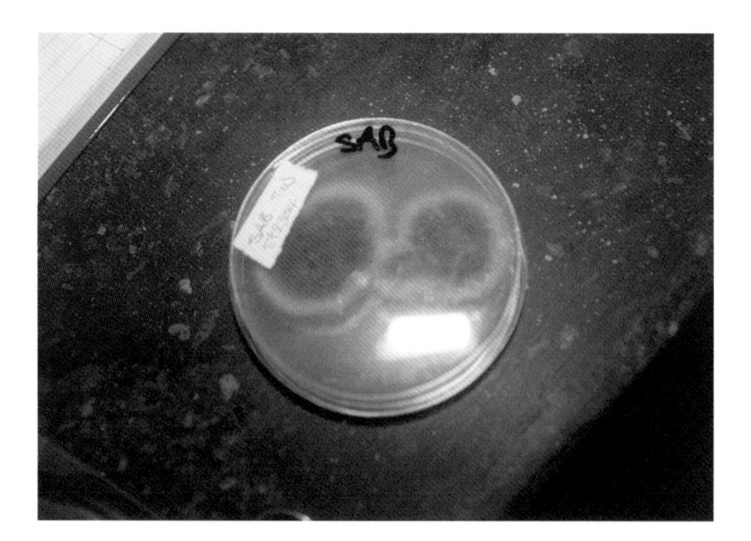


*Treatment of tinea corporis:* Compound benzoic acid ointment (Whitfield's ointment) is a mixture of 6% benzoic acid with 3% salicylic acid in emulsifying ointment. It is cheap and widely available. Apply bd until the tinea has disappeared and then for a further 2 weeks. It is a keratolytic agent, which means that it removes the keratin on which the fungus feeds rather than killing the actual fungus. More expensive topical anti-fungal agents like the imidazole creams can also be used. They are applied bd for 2–3 weeks.

## Tinea capitis (scalp ringworm)

**Figure 621** This is the most common cause of hair loss in children. There are discrete bald patches and the underlying scalp is scaly. However, if you look carefully the hairs are there, but broken off very short. Without treatment it gets better spontaneously at puberty. It only occurs after puberty in patients with HIV infection. In adults with tinea capitis always check for HIV.

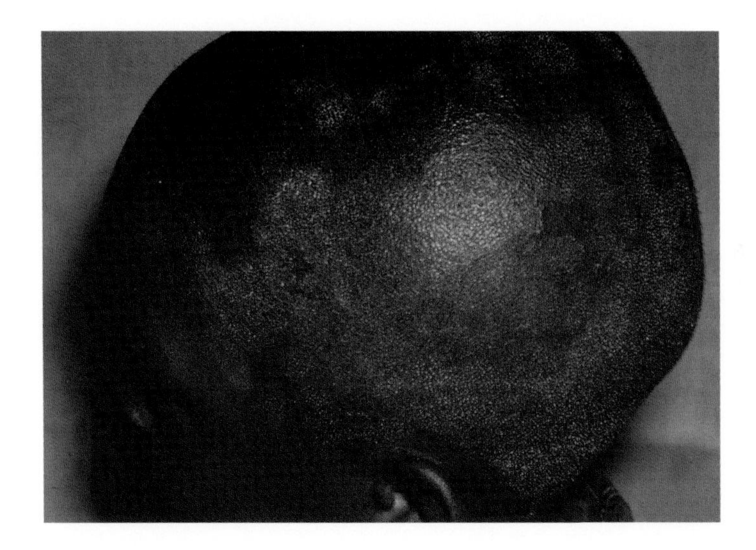

**Figure 622** Animal ringworm can cause an inflammatory reaction so that the scalp is red and scaly, and not just scaly. Marked inflammation with boggy swelling and multiple pustules is called a kerion.

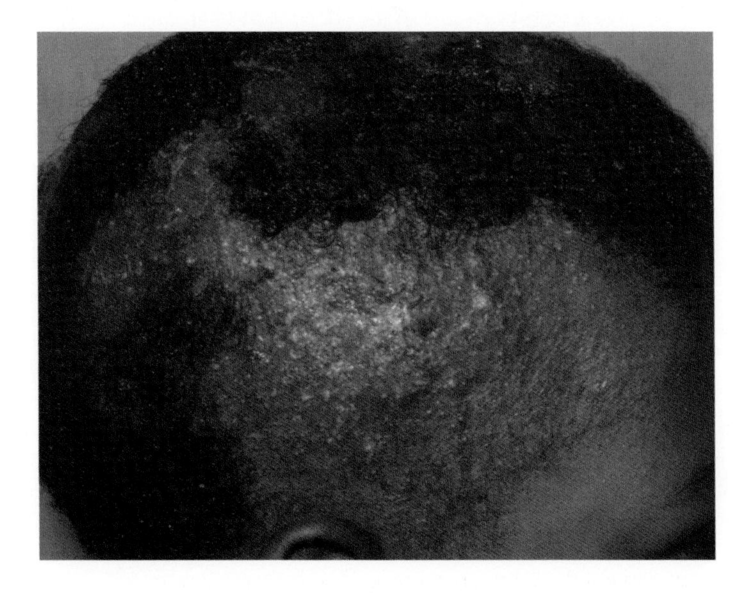

**Figure 623** The diagnosis of tinea capitis can be confirmed by removing one of the short broken hairs and putting it on a slide with 20% KOH. The hair shaft is full of fungal spores.

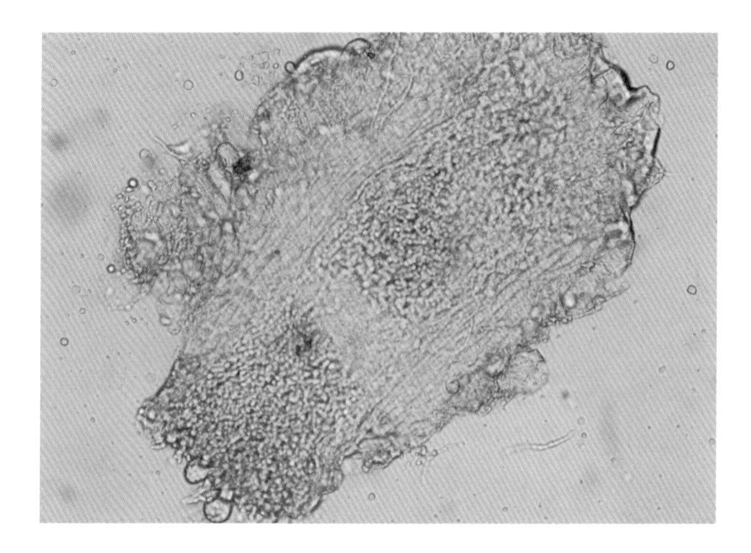

**Figure 624** *Treatment:* Oral griseofulvin, 10mg/kg body weight/day, as a single dose with food for 6 weeks. Treat all affected children in the house, school or village. Do not treat with topical anti-fungal agents as they cannot get to the site of the infection.

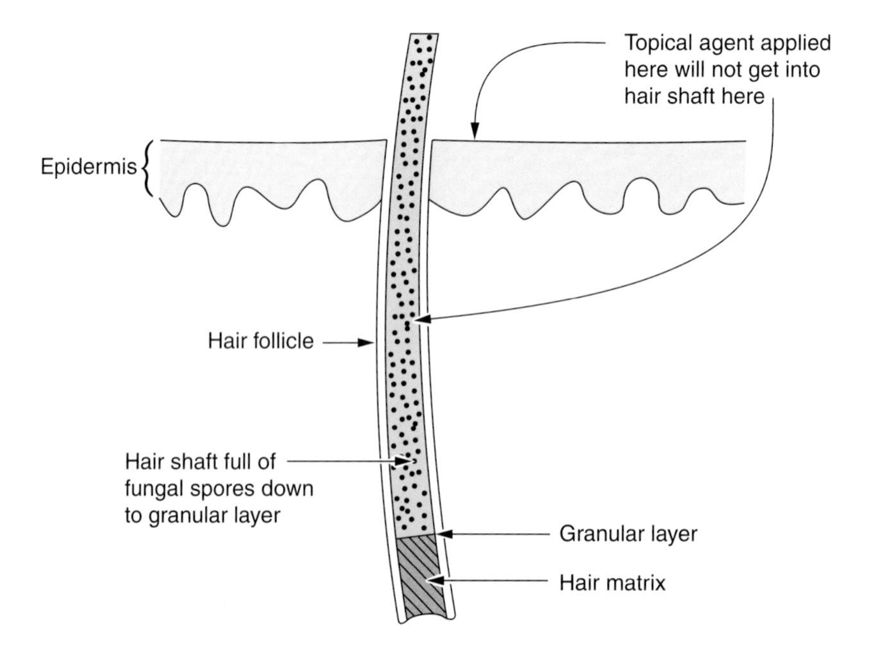

## Tinea pedis

**Figure 625** Common fungal infection in adults, not children. White scaling between the 4th and 5th toes, or between the 3rd and 4th toes on one foot only. The other diseases which look similar – candida, erythrasma, eczema, psoriasis and lichen planus – are all bilateral and symmetrical from the beginning.

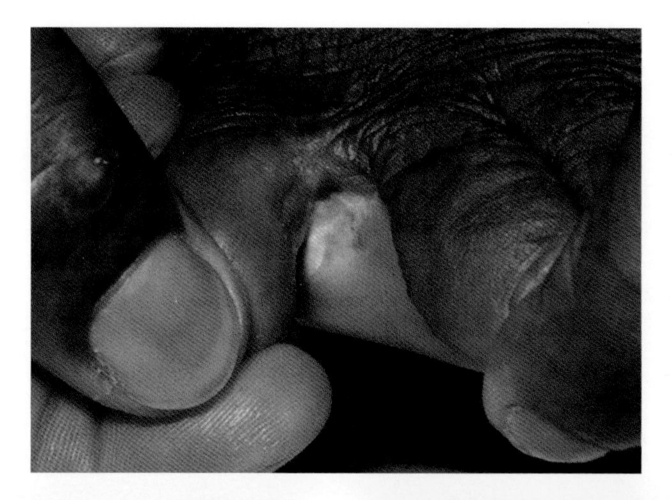

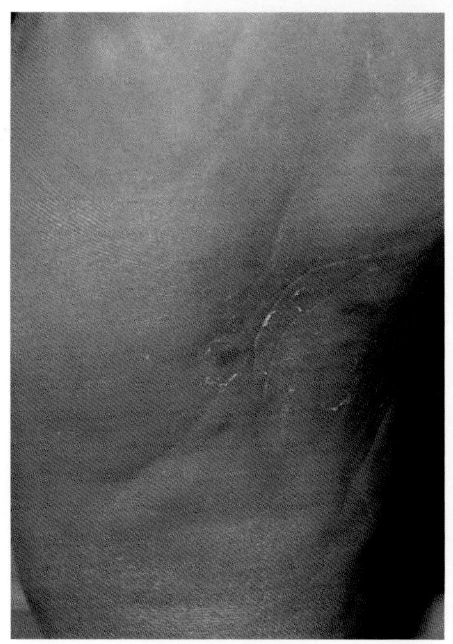

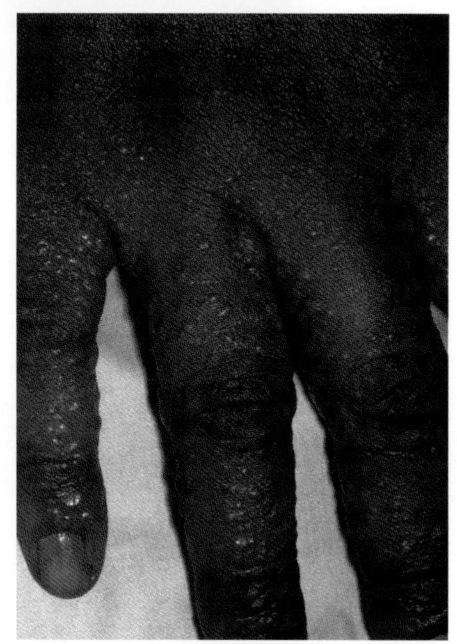

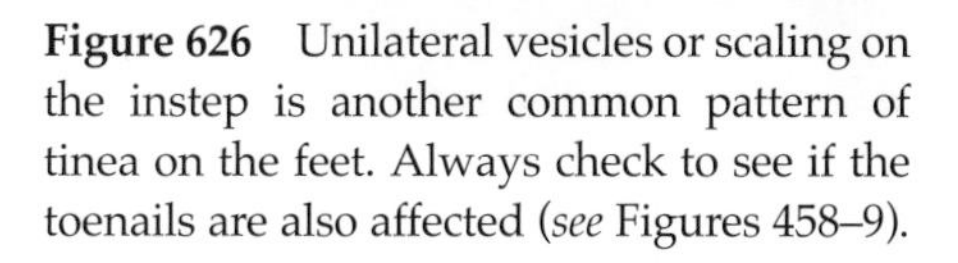

**Figure 626** Unilateral vesicles or scaling on the instep is another common pattern of tinea on the feet. Always check to see if the toenails are also affected (*see* Figures 458–9).

*Treatment:* Whitfield's ointment applied bd until it is clear.

**Figure 627** Some patients with tinea pedis develop vesicles on the palms and the sides of the fingers and soles. This is called an 'id' reaction (there is no fungus in the vesicles). It gets better when the tinea is treated.

## Tinea cruris

**Figures 628, 629** A fungal infection of the groin, buttocks and upper thighs, usually acquired from the patient's own feet (i.e. he also has tinea pedis). A scaly plaque grows out from the groin crease which, like tinea corporis, has a raised scaly edge. It is usually asymmetrical, but can be bilateral and symmetrical in patients who live in a hot, humid environment or those with HIV infection.

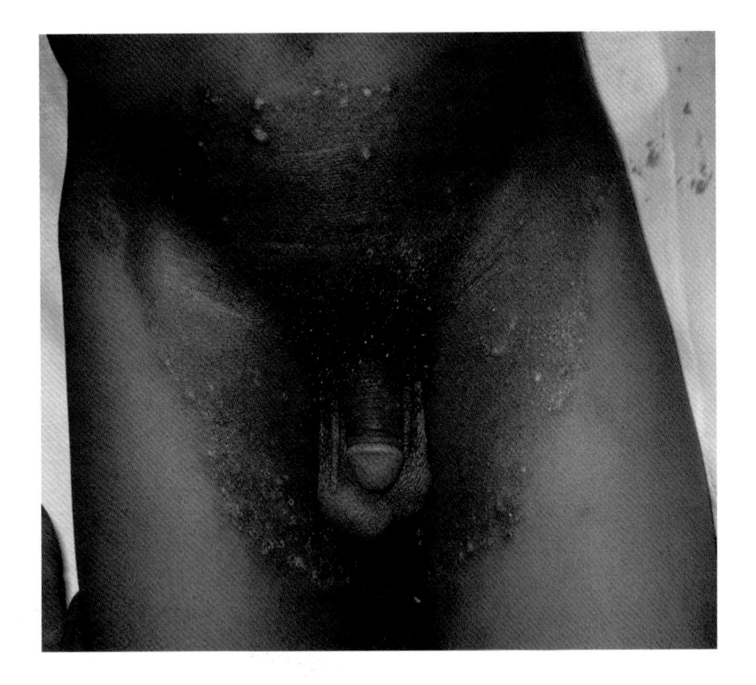

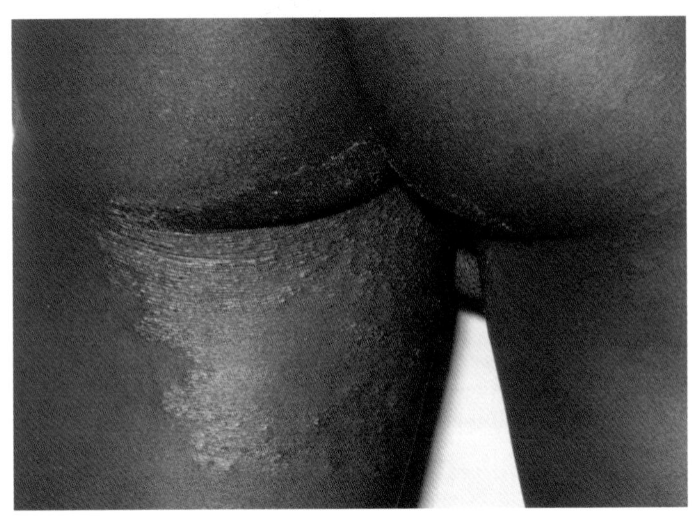

*Treatment:* Whitfield's ointment applied bd to the groin and toewebs until they are clear. Whitfield's ointment may make the patient sore in the groin. Alternative treatments are Castellani's paint applied bd, or an imidazole cream applied bd for 2 weeks.

## TONGUE ABNORMALITIES

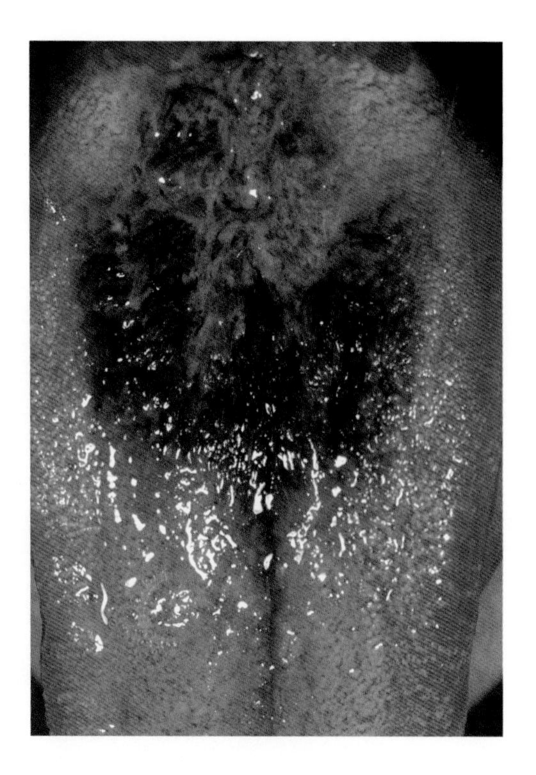

**Figure 630** Black hairy tongue. This is due to overgrowth of the filiform papillae of the tongue. It is not of any significance and needs no treatment.

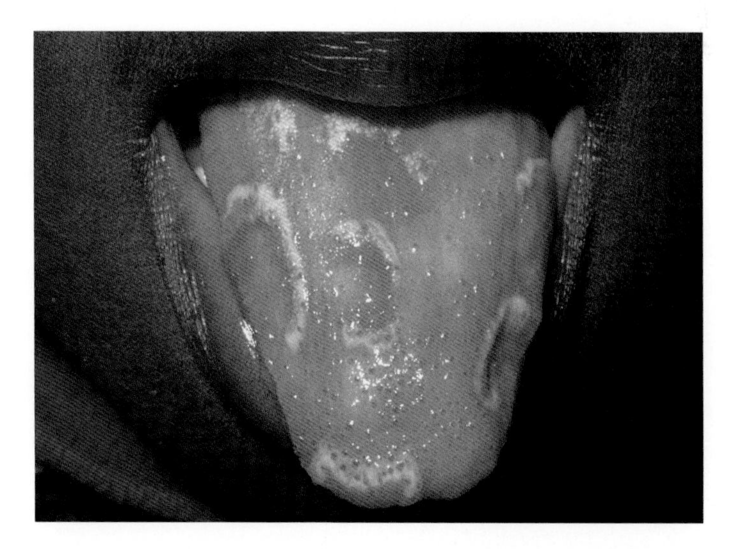

**Figure 631** Geographical tongue. Very common normal finding which is usually asymptomatic. There are smooth red patches with raised white edges, which are constantly changing size and shape.

*Treatment:* Reassurance that it is harmless is all that is required.

**Figures 632, 633** Hyperpigmentation of the tongue, buccal mucosa and palate is a normal finding in black Africans. It should not be confused with Kaposi's sarcoma in the mouth, which is red or purple coloured not brown (*see* Figure 324). Similar hyperpigmentation can occur on the soles of the feet (*see* Figure 560).

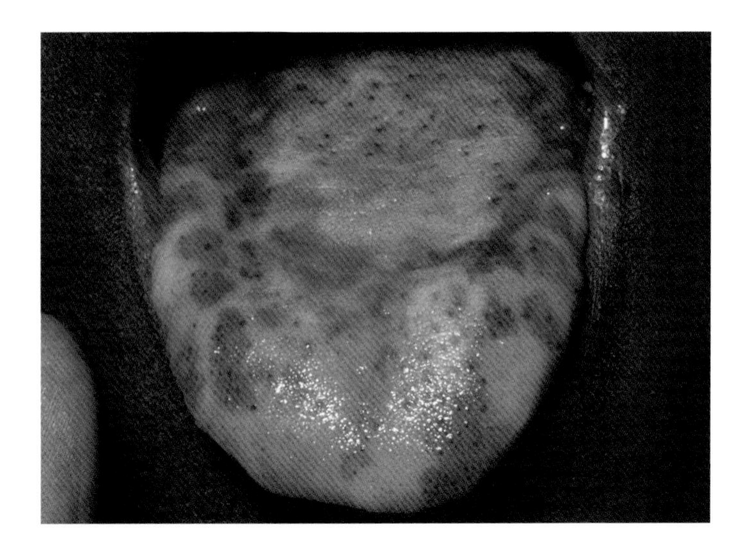

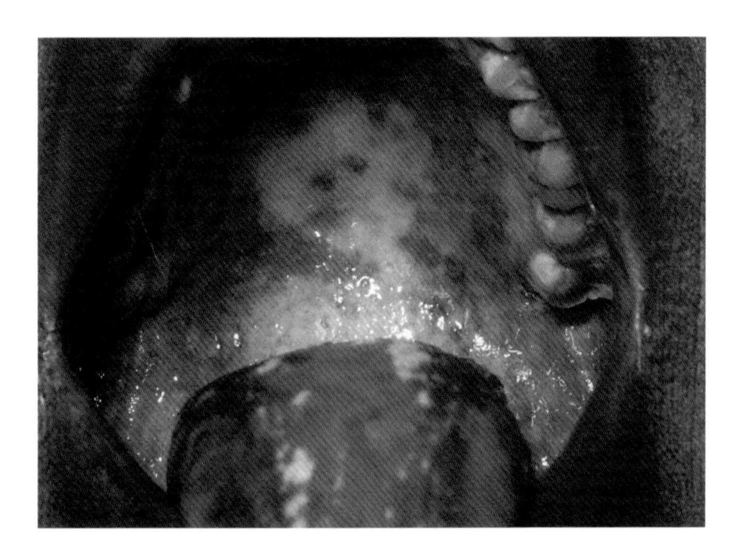

*Treatment:* Reassurance that it is a normal finding.

## TRICHOEPITHELIOMA (Epithelioma adenoides cysticum)

**Figures 634, 635** Rare genetic disorder inherited as an autosomal dominant trait (*see* Figure 295). Multiple small, round, translucent papules occur around the nose and eyes after puberty.

*Treatment:* Normally leave them alone. If they are very unsightly they can be curetted off under a general anaesthetic.

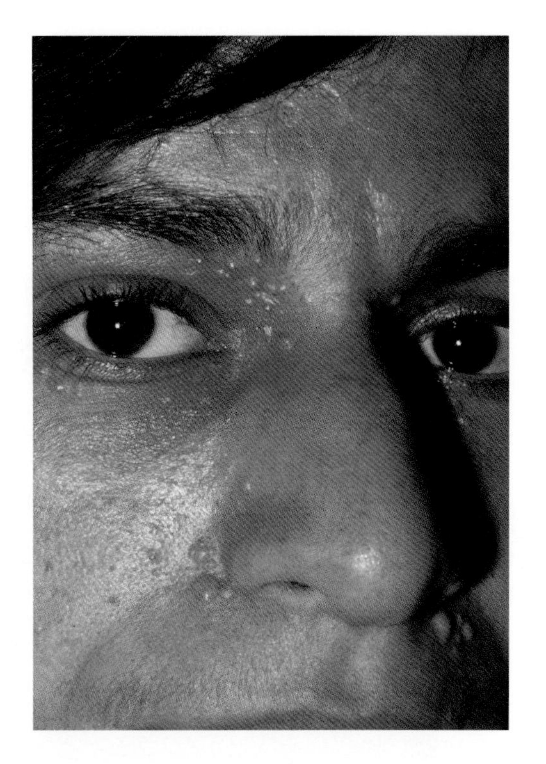

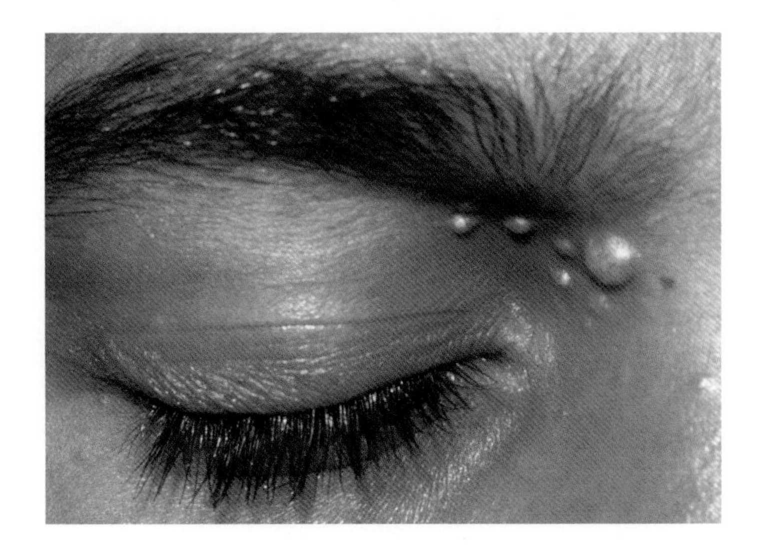

## TRICHOMYCOSIS AXILLARIS

**Figure 636** Pale concretions stuck to axillary hairs. These are made up of colonies of corynebacteria. They are usually asymptomatic.

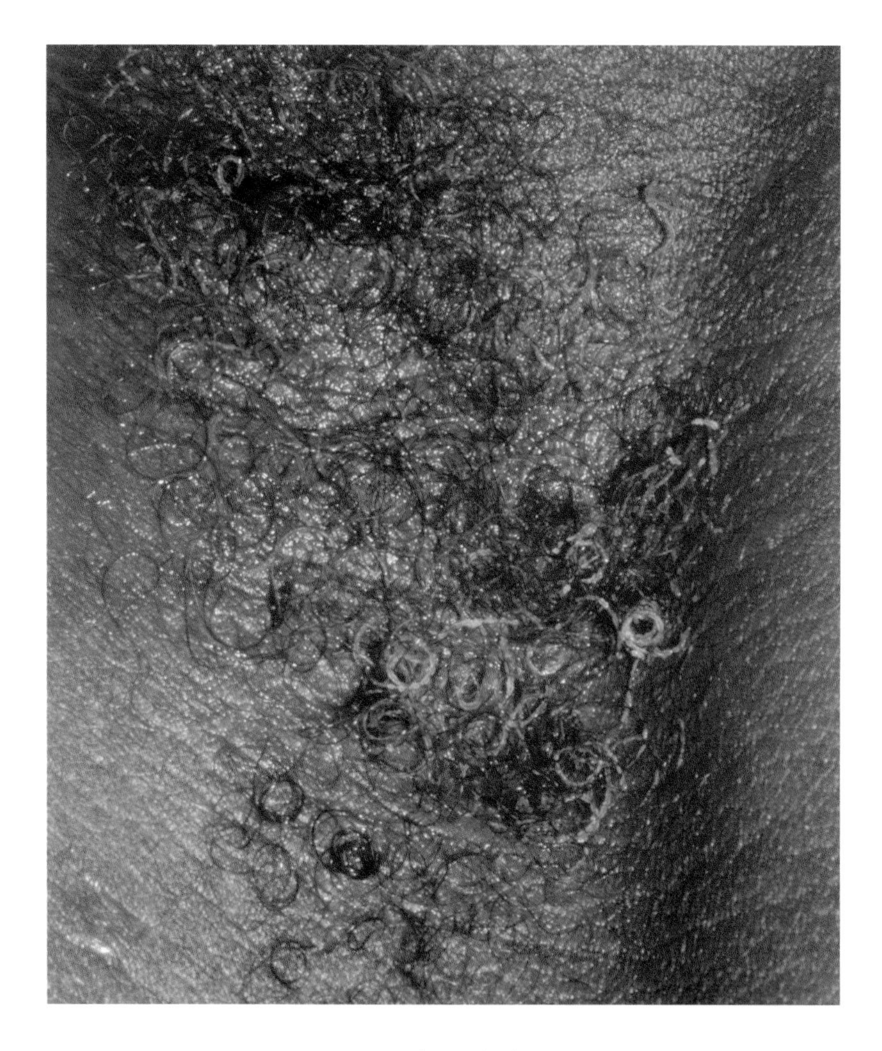

*Treatment:* None needed; if it is a problem, shave the hairs off.

## TRIPE PALMS

**Figure 637** Thickening of the palms and soles but with a curious rugose surface like the lining of the small bowel. It can be associated with acanthosis nigricans (*see* Figures 2–3) and internal malignancy, as in this man, or it can occur alone.

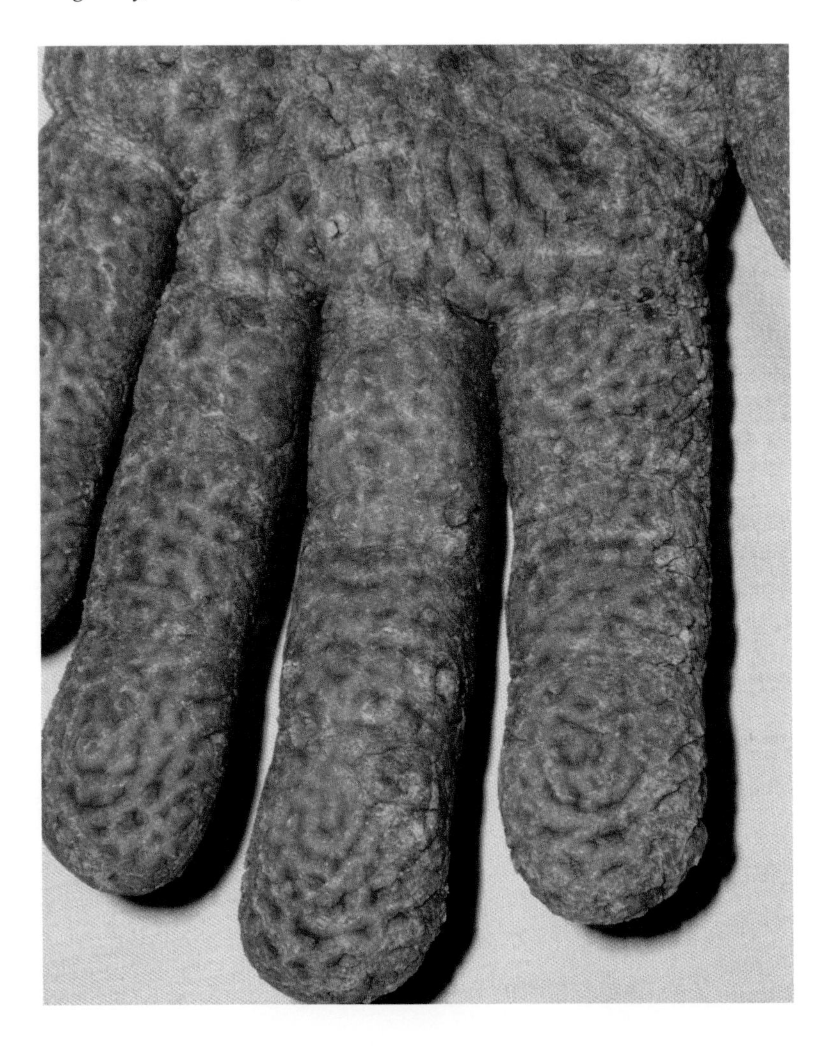

# TUBERCULOSIS

Tuberculosis is a chronic infection with *Mycobacterium tuberculosis*. Skin tuberculosis is not common despite the rise in HIV infection and the increase in pulmonary and glandular TB. There are several different patterns.

## Lupus vulgaris

**Figure 638** This is tuberculosis in the skin of a patient with good cell-mediated immunity to the organism. It starts as small translucent or skin-coloured papules, which join together to form plaques. These extend very slowly over many years.

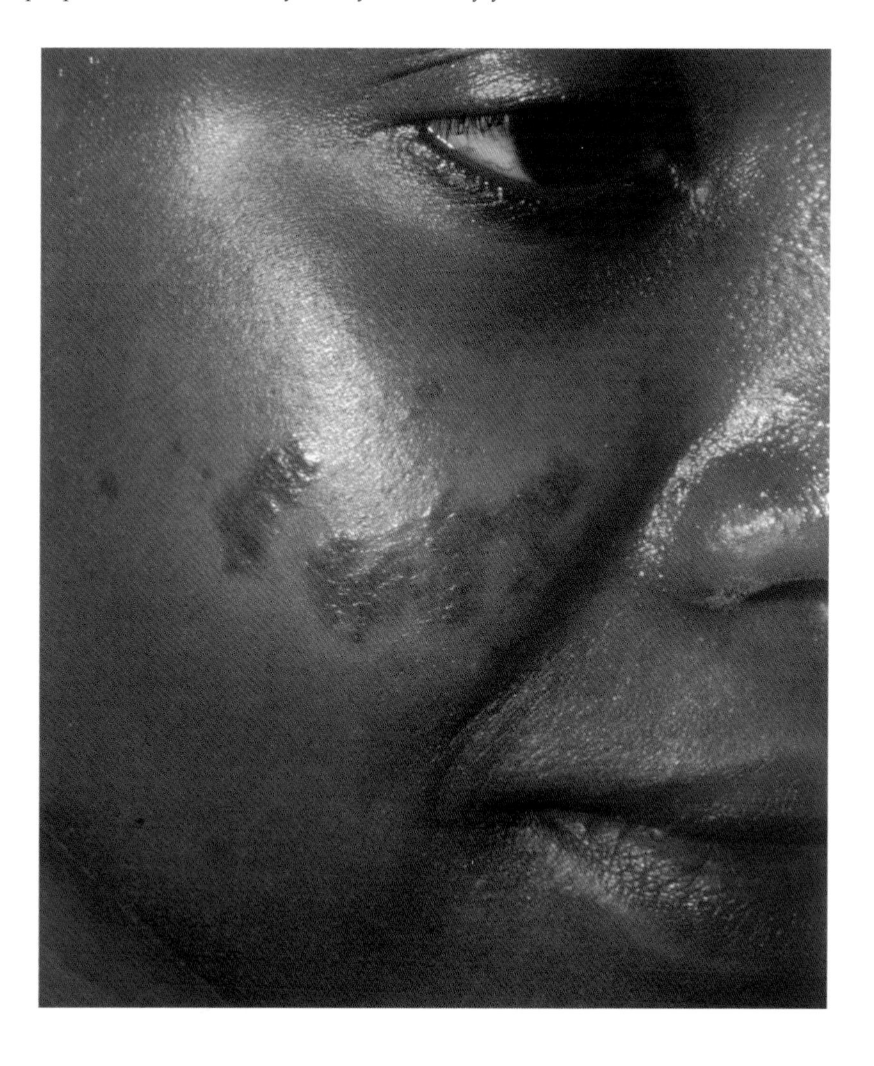

## Orificial tuberculosis

**Figure 639** This is tuberculosis of the skin around the mouth, nose or anus in a patient with tuberculosis elsewhere (in this case of the spine). Small papules or nodules break down to form ulcers. Normally, there is a bluish edge to the ulcers.

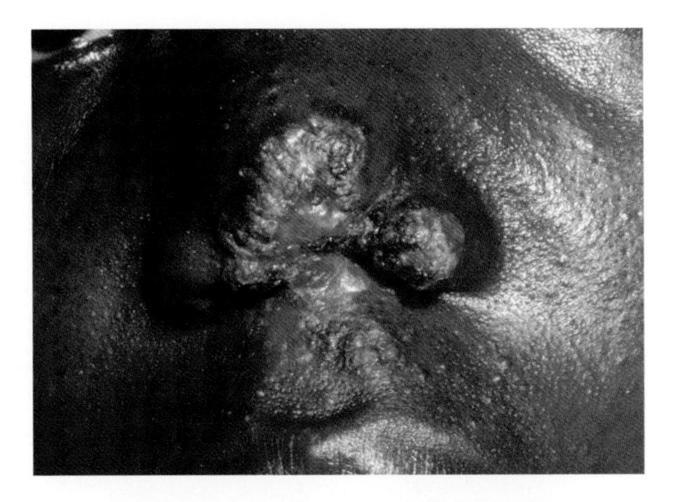

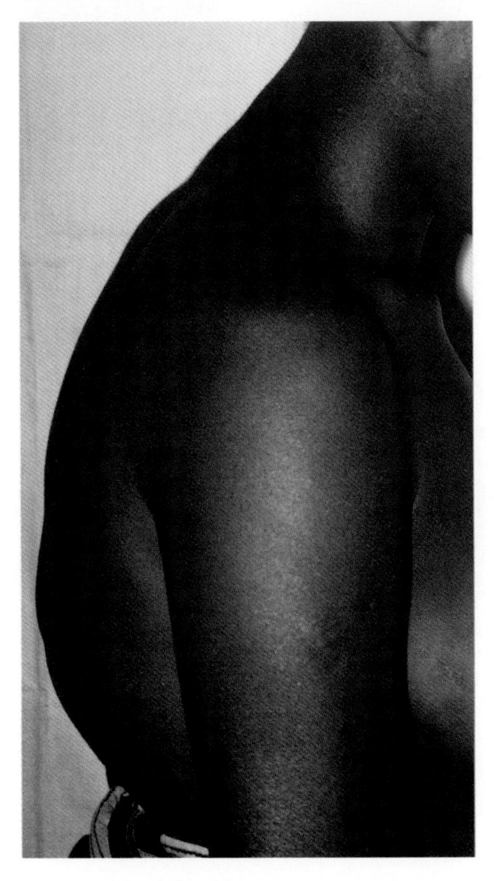

**Figure 640** Tuberculosis of the spine (same patient as in Figure 639).

## Papulonecrotic tuberculide

**Figures 641, 642** Necrotising papules on the extremities in a patient with a tuberculous focus elsewhere. Due to haematogenous spread of tubercle bacilli in a patient with good cell-mediated immunity.

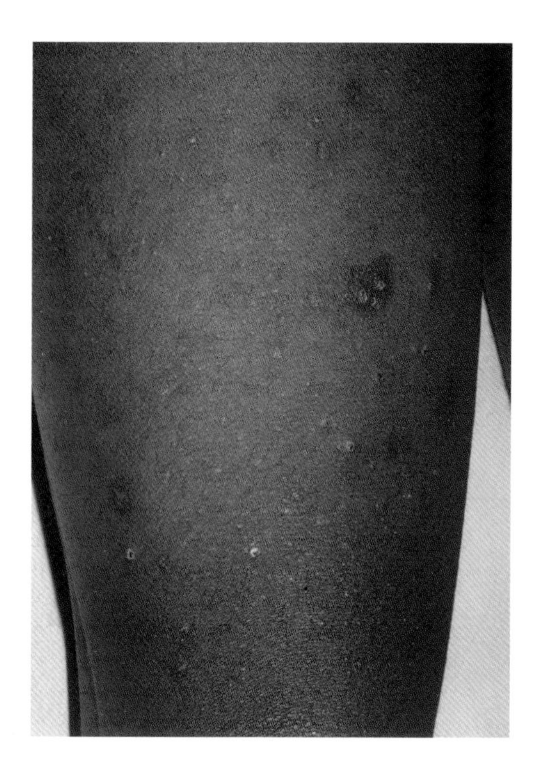

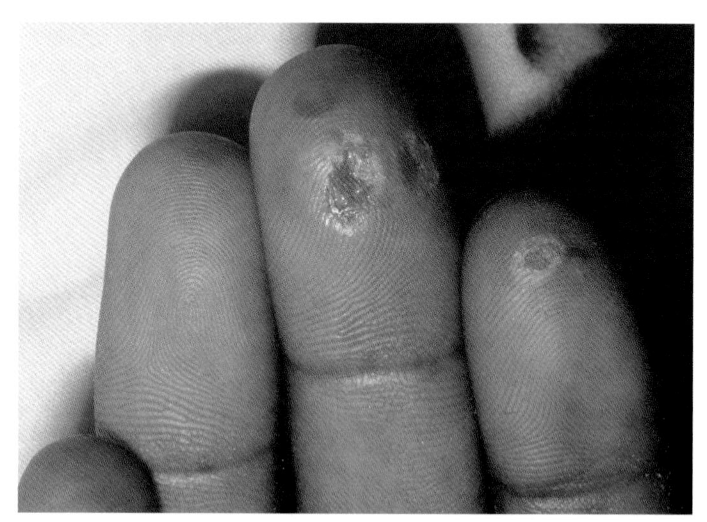

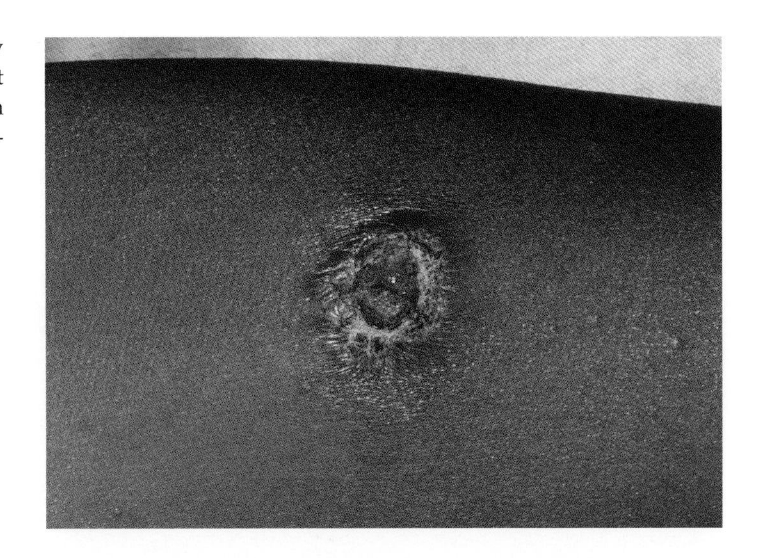

**Figure 643** Strongly positive Mantoux test in a patient with papulonecrotic tuberculide.

## Scrofuloderma

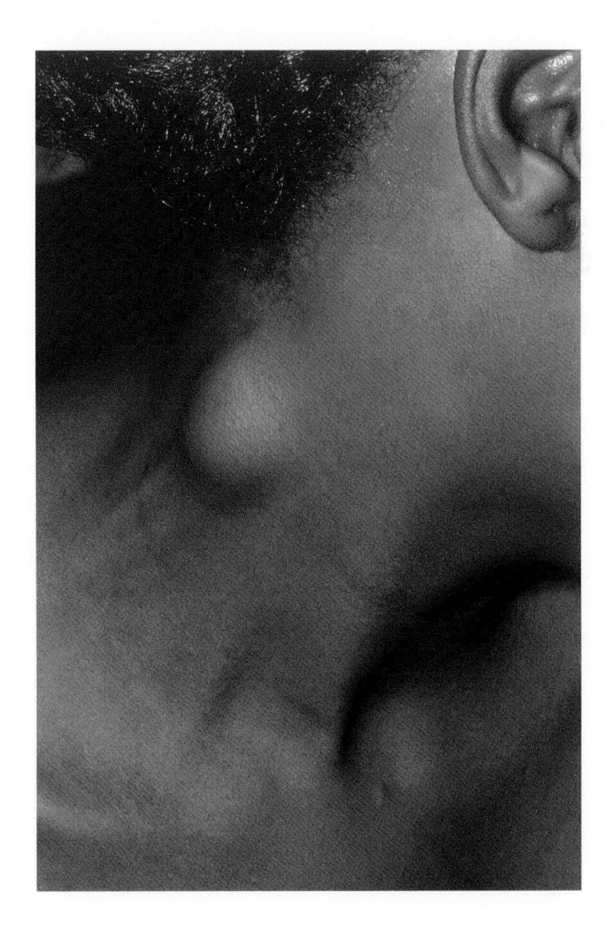

**Figure 644** Tuberculous glands in the neck are usually unilateral and painless.

**Figure 645** The breakdown of tuberculous glands with multiple skin sinuses is known as scrofuloderma. The diagnosis can be confirmed by seeing caseating granulomas and acid fast bacilli in a biopsy or needle aspiration from the underlying gland.

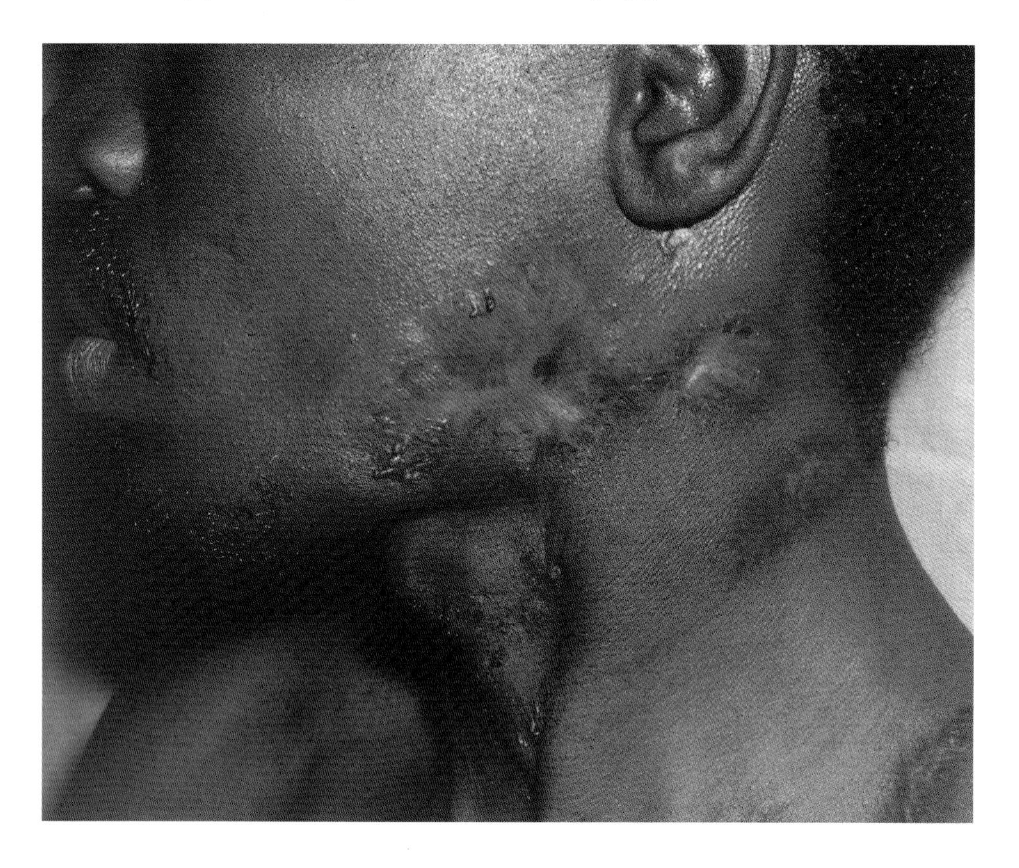

*Treatment of all kinds of cutaneous TB:* Anti-tuberculous chemotherapy for 9 months. Check for HIV infection.

## TUBEROUS SCLEROSIS (Epiloia)

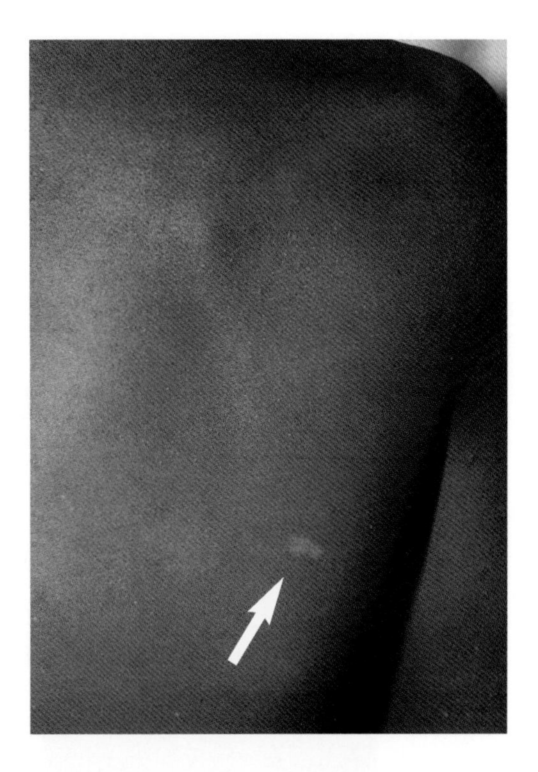

**Figure 646** Rare genetic disorder inherited as an autosomal dominant trait (*see* Figure 295). Hamartomas occur in the skin, brain, eye, kidney and heart. The first skin lesion to appear is the ash leaf macule. This is a white ovoid macule or patch which is present from birth. These can be single or multiple. They are usually found on the trunk or limbs.

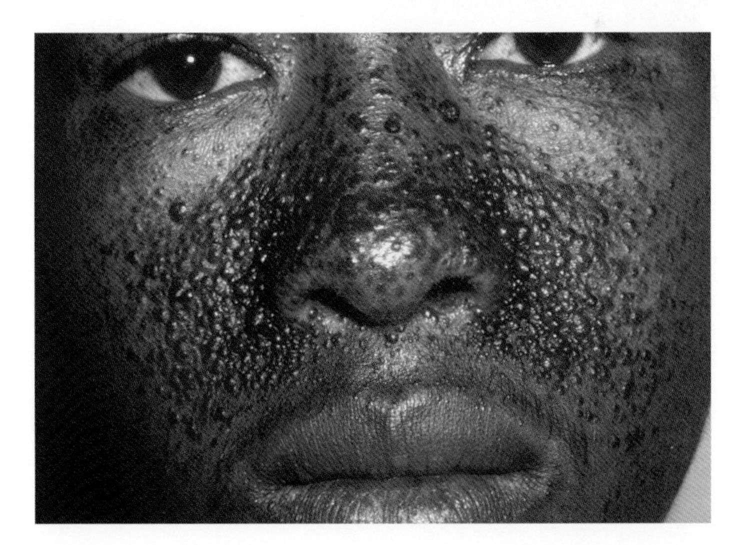

**Figure 647** Angiofibromas begin in the nasolabial folds and then spread out to the cheeks and chin. They appear around the age of 3–4 years. They are also known as adenoma sebaceum. Other skin lesions which occur in this condition are the shagreen patch (an irregularly thickened plaque usually in the lumbosacral area) and periungual and subungual fibromas (skin-coloured papules around and under the nails (fingernails and toenails) which appear at puberty). Patients also have epilepsy and mental retardation due to hamartomas in the brain.

*Treatment:* The disease needs to be explained to the patient and the family. The epilepsy should be controlled with anti-epileptic drugs. Nothing can be done for the skin lesions.

## TUNGIASIS (Jiggers)

**Figures 648, 649** Due to invasion of the skin by a newly fertilised female sand flea, *Tunga penetrans*. It lives in sandy soil in areas where people and animals are living. Once the female has mated it must find a source of food to feed the developing eggs. It burrows into human or animal skin, head first, to feed on blood from the upper dermal capillaries. Its cloaca is left exposed and through this it breaths and lays its eggs. As it feeds it becomes engorged with blood and the developing eggs. It becomes spherical in shape and squirts out the oval white eggs, which you can see on the skin (Figure 649). The papules containing the sand flea are most commonly found on the feet, especially under the toes or toenails, but they can occur elsewhere.

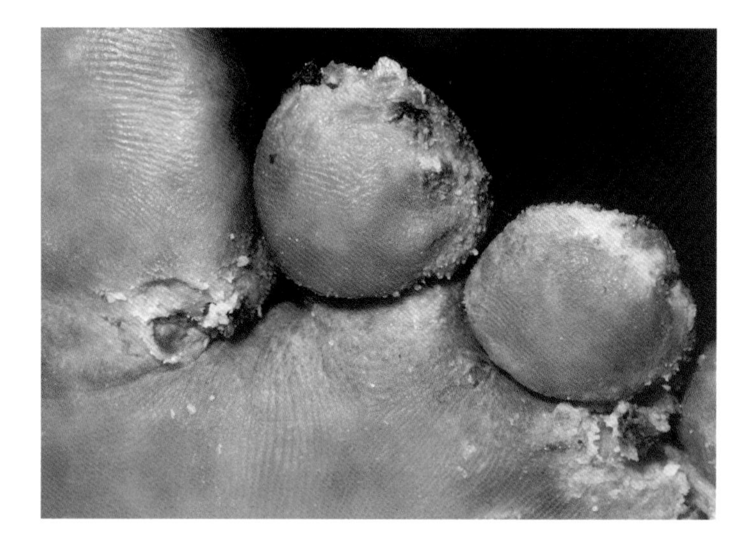

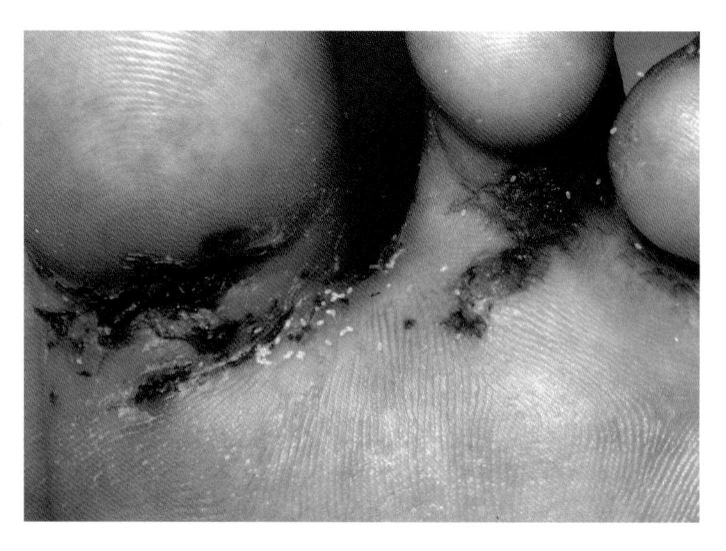

*Prevention:* Since tungiasis occurs in individuals who walk around barefoot or live in houses with dirt floors, it can be prevented by wearing shoes and sweeping the floor regularly.

*Treatment:* Winkle them out carefully with a pin. If they are numerous soak the feet in kerosene or 1% lindane lotion.

# ULCERS ON THE LEGS AND FEET

## Arterial ulcer

**Figure 650** Arterial ulcers are due to poor arterial blood supply to the foot. They occur mainly in elderly patients with arteriosclerosis, or diabetics. Painful ulcers on the tips of the toes, the heel or the front of the shin are typical. They may be deep enough to see the tendons in the base of the ulcer. The patient may give a history of intermittent claudication. Confirm the diagnosis by finding one or more of the arterial pulses in the leg or foot to be missing. Without treatment, many of these patients develop gangrene of the foot or leg (*see* Figure 249).

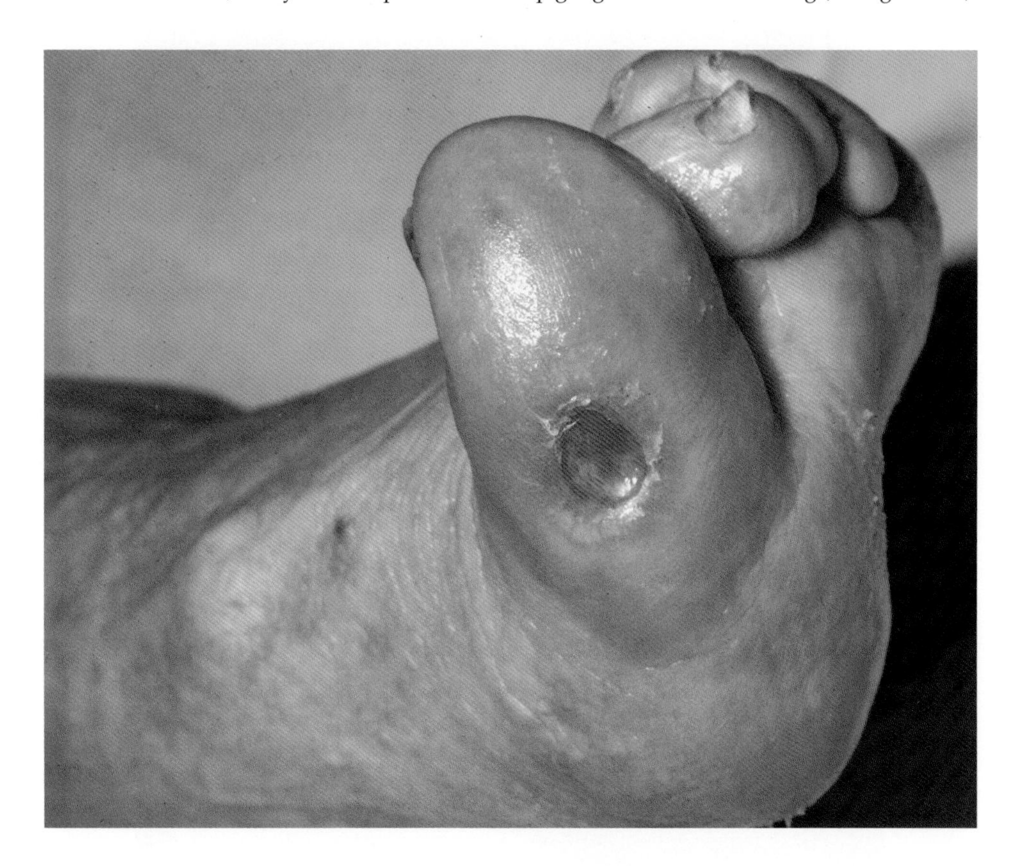

*Treatment:* Improve the blood supply by stopping smoking +/– sympathectomy.

## Buruli ulcer

**Figure 651** Single firm, painless subcutaneous nodule on a limb, which either heals spontaneously or ulcerates. Ulcers can remain small and heal without treatment, or spread rapidly undermining the skin over large areas, even an entire limb. It is due to *Mycobacterium ulcerans* which is found in water bugs deep in the mud of permanent wetlands (swamps). Most patients are children who play in and around swamps. The organism enters the skin through a cut or abrasion. The diagnosis can be confirmed by taking a smear from the necrotic base of an ulcer and finding clumps of acid fast bacilli with a Ziehl-Neelson stain.

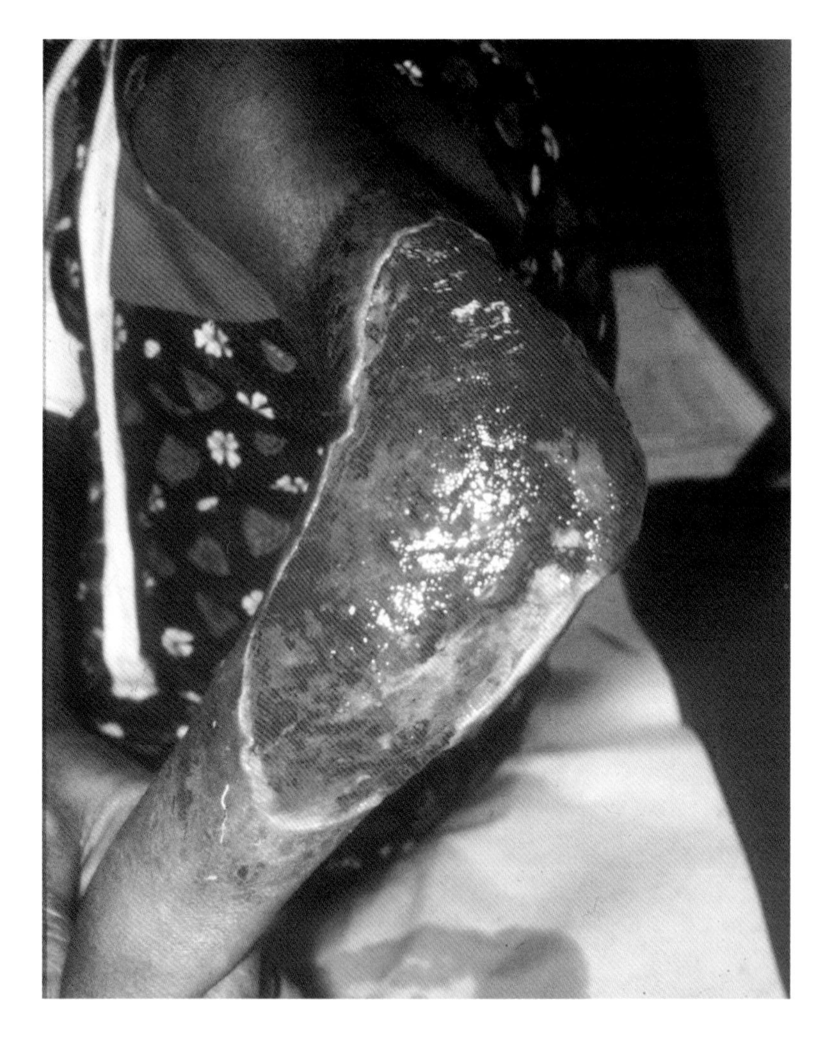

*Treatment:* Early lesions (non-ulcerative) can be healed with oral rifampicin or by surgical excision. Ulcers require wide excision and grafting.

## Neuropathic ulcer

**Figure 652** These are ulcers, mainly on the soles of the feet, caused by trauma to anaesthetic feet. They occur over bony prominences, particularly the first metatarsophalangeal joint, the metatarsal heads or the heel, or at any site of injury. They are deep, painless, and often covered with thick callous. The sensory loss is usually caused by leprosy (*see* Figure 372), paraplegia or diabetes mellitus.

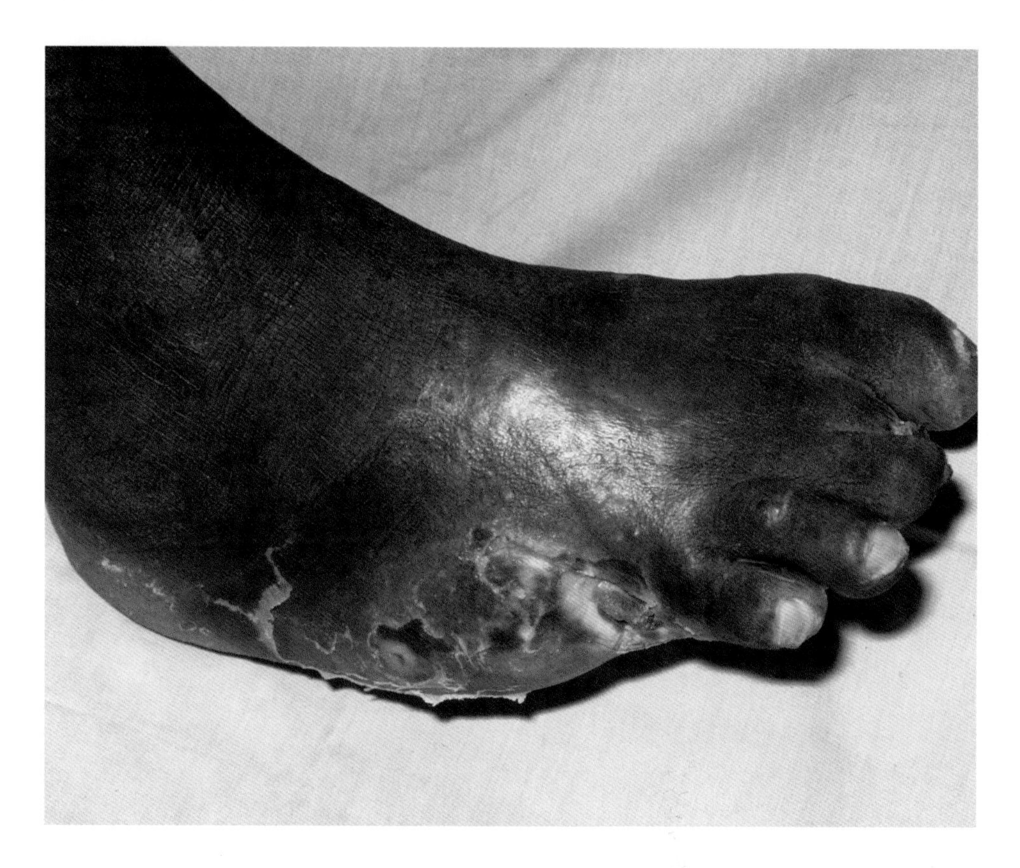

*Treatment:* Keep the skin of the feet soft by soaking in soapy water for half an hour daily, and pare down the hard skin around the ulcer with a sharp scalpel blade. Keep the wound clean and protect from further injury until it has healed. If the ulcer does not heal, consider putting the patient in a walking plaster (Plaster of Paris). Once the ulcer has healed, well fitted shoes with Plastazote insoles should be worn to prevent further injuries.

## Sickle cell ulcer

**Figure 653** Patients with sickle cell anaemia, who are homozygous for the sickle cell gene, develop ischaemic ulcers on the legs and feet in childhood or early adult life. They look like venous ulcers (*see* Figure 655) but are due to the blockage of small arteries in the legs and feet by the sickling red blood cells. The diagnosis should be suspected in any young patient with leg ulcers. A past history of painful swelling of the fingers and toes in infancy, generalised and severe bone pain, episodes of dyspnoea or anaemia may be clues to the diagnosis.

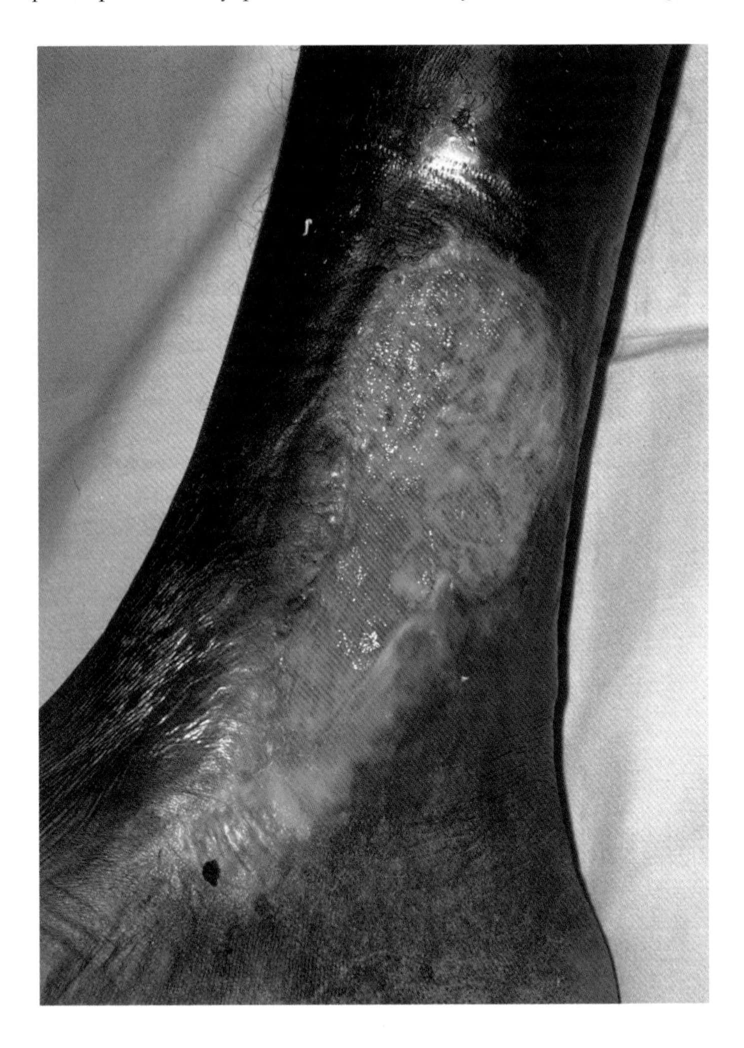

*Diagnosis:* Confirm by haemoglobin electrophoresis.

*Treatment of the leg ulcers:* Keep them clean until they heal.

## Tropical ulcer (tropical phagadenic ulcer)

**Figure 654** Painful, fast growing ulcer with a rolled edge on the lower legs and feet of malnourished children. Due to fusiform bacilli and treponemes. It begins in the rainy season and grows rapidly to 3–7cm over 2–3 weeks. It can last 10–15 years if not treated.

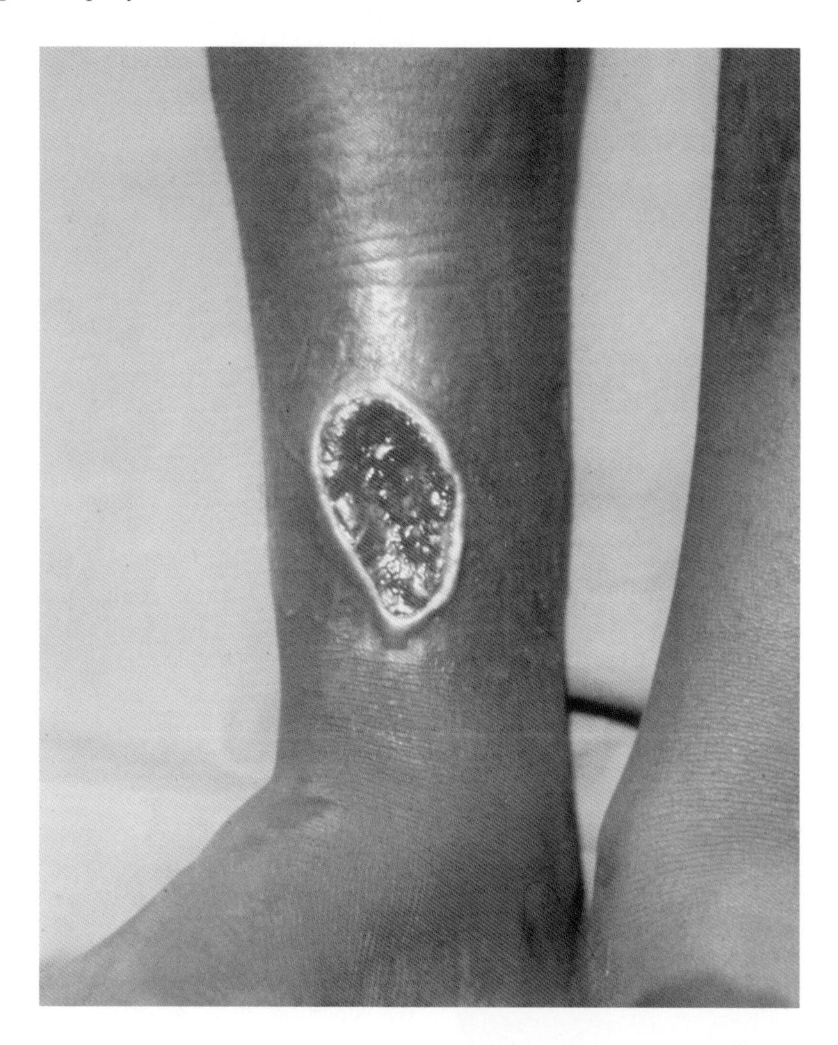

*Treatment:* Clean the ulcer and apply 0.5% Gentian Violet paint bd and improve the patient's diet. Oral antibiotics such as phenoxymethylpenicillin (Penicillin V), erythromycin, tetracycline (not in children <12 years of age) or metronidazole can be given for 1 week.

## Venous ulcer

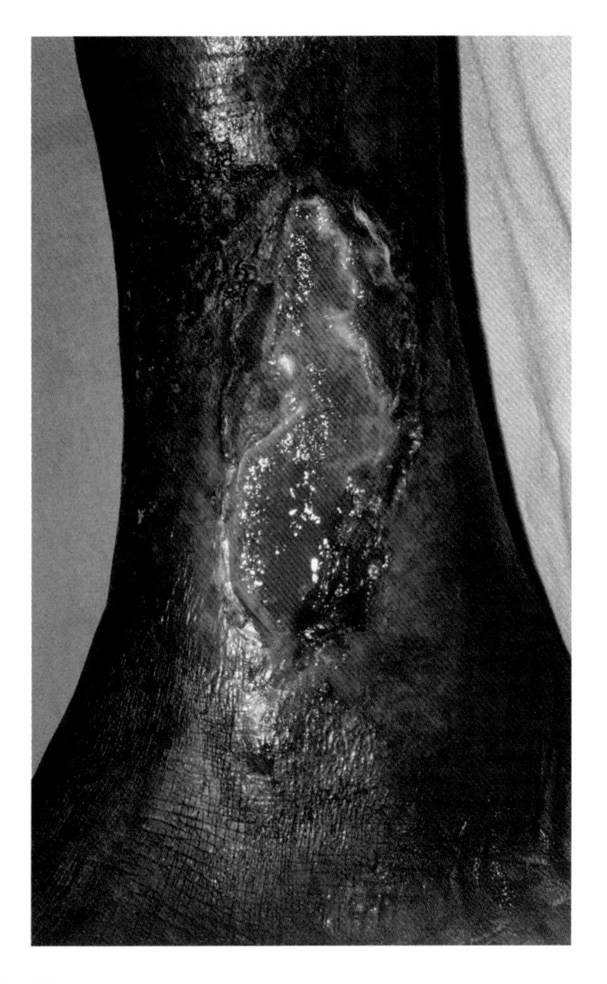

**Figure 655** Large, superficial ulcer over the medial or lateral malleolus. It is due to loss of the valves in the deep veins after a deep vein thrombosis.

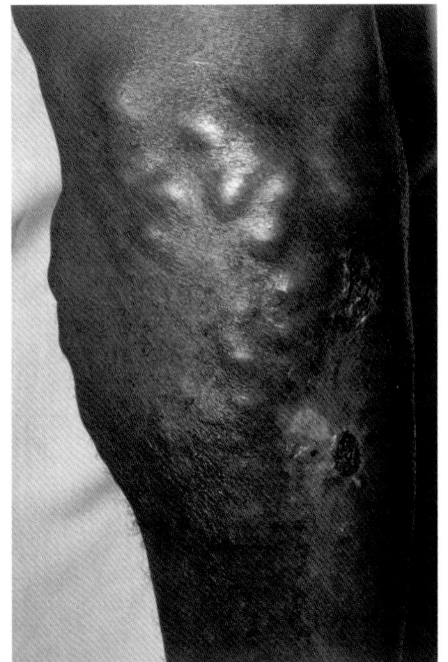

**Figure 656** Varicose veins in a patient with a venous ulcer. Other associated findings are oedema of the leg, hyperpigmentation and eczema.

*Treatment:* Wear elastic bandages to compress the superficial veins to ensure that venous blood is transported back to the heart and lungs for re-oxygenation. Treatment must be life-long. Immobility must be discouraged and, when sitting, the legs should be elevated and the ankles kept moving.

## URTICARIA

**Figure 657** Itchy rash due to the release of histamine in the skin. The features are therefore the same as Lewis's triple response, i.e. erythema, followed by oedema and then an erythematous flare. It can be due to a type I allergic reaction, e.g. after penicillin or certain foods, or, more commonly, it is associated with taking aspirin or having intestinal worms. Sometimes no cause can be found. It is the most common rash where individual lesions come and go within a few hours.

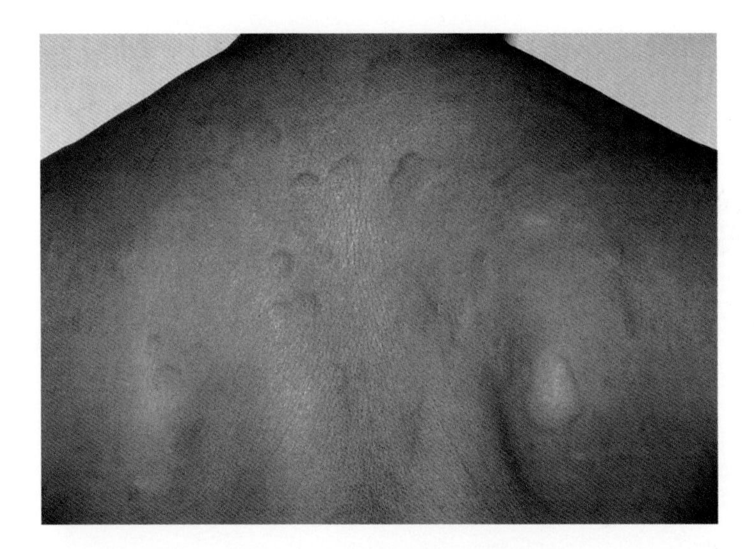

**Figure 658** Angio-oedema is urticaria of the soft tissues of the eyelids, lips or tongue.

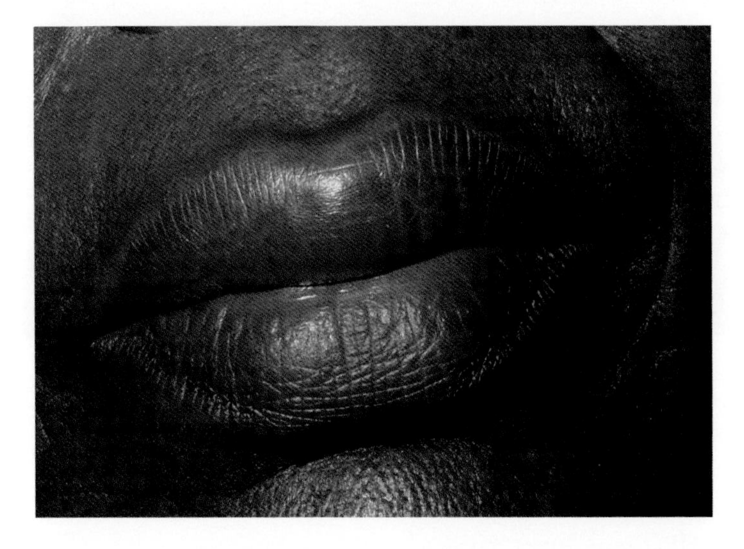

*Treatment:* Treat or remove the underlying cause if possible. If it is due to a drug or food, avoid it in future. If it is due to intestinal worms they can be eradicated with the appropriate treatment. If no cause is found, give a long-acting antihistamine by mouth, e.g. promethazine 25mg nocte, until it gets better spontaneously. Non-sedative long-acting antihistamines, such as cetirazine (10mg nocte) or loratidine (10mg/day), are preferable to promethazine but are much more expensive.

## URTICARIA PIGMENTOSUM

**Figure 659** Disease due to an accumulation of mast cells in the upper dermis. It presents with a widespread hyperpigmented macular rash. If the macules are rubbed or scratched they form wheals as in urticaria. When it begins in childhood it usually gets better spontaneously, but in adults it is usually permanent.

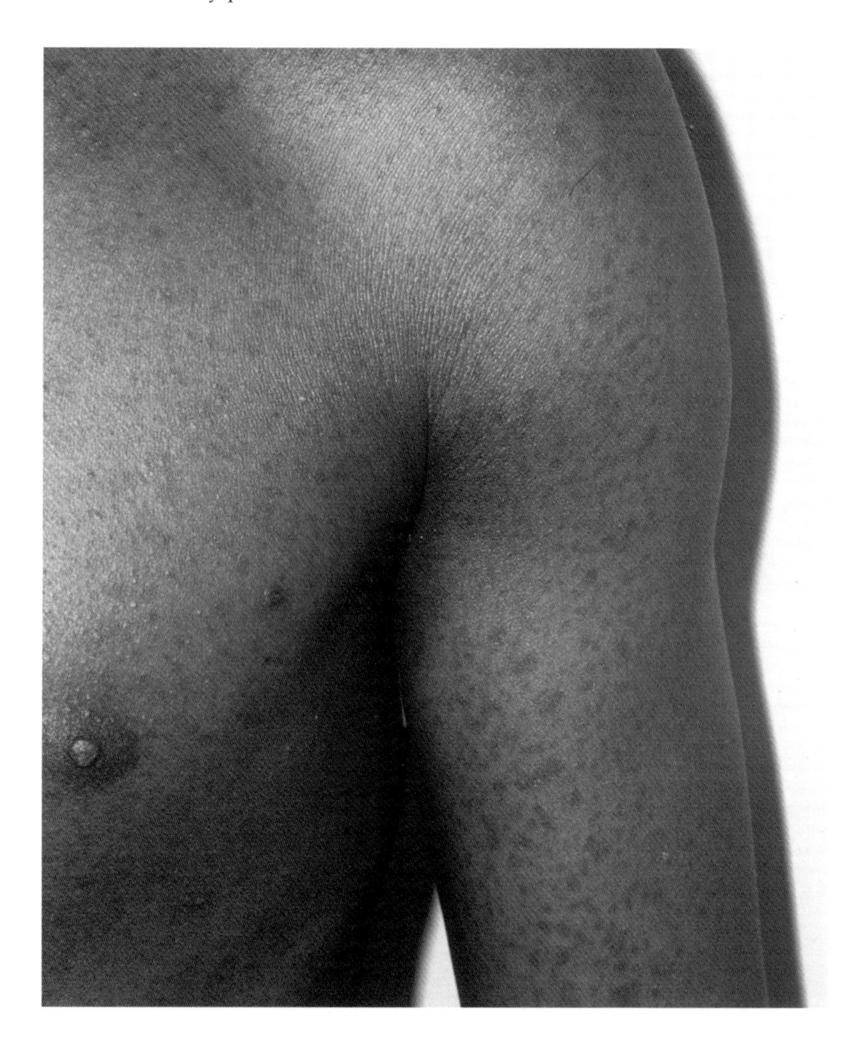

*Treatment:* Usually none is needed as it is just a cosmetic problem. If itching is a problem, a long-acting antihistamine can be given, such as promethazine 25mg nocte or cetirazine 10mg nocte.

## VASCULITIS

**Figure 660** Vasculitis is a group of diseases in which there is deposition of immune complexes in the small blood vessels in the skin. The clinical features include erythema, urticaria, purpura and ischaemic necrosis. The main causes are:

- Infection, e.g. streptococcal sore throat, chronic pyelonephritis, dental abscess, empyema, septicaemia.
- Drugs, e.g. sulphonamides and other antibiotics, thiazide diuretics.

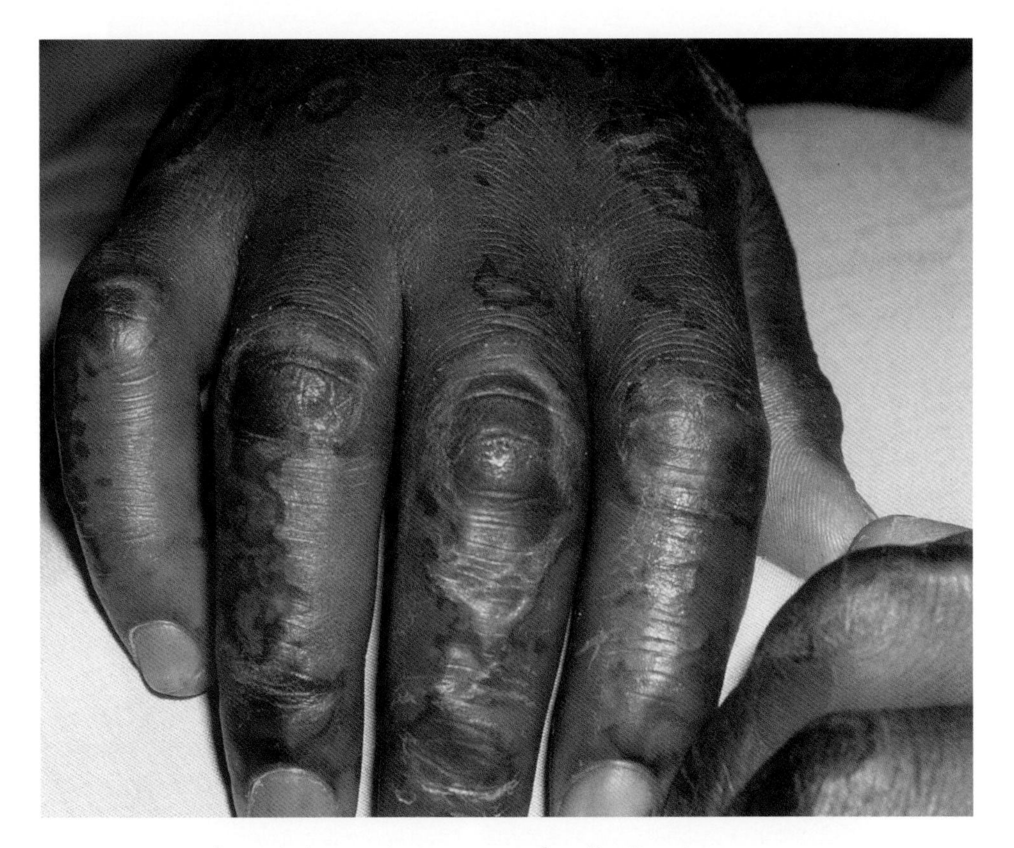

*Treatment:* Treat the underlying infection or stop the offending drug.

## VITILIGO

**Figure 661** Patches of depigmentation of the skin due to loss of melanocytes. Why this happens is unknown. It most commonly begins in childhood with symmetrical patches of white skin on the trunk and limbs.

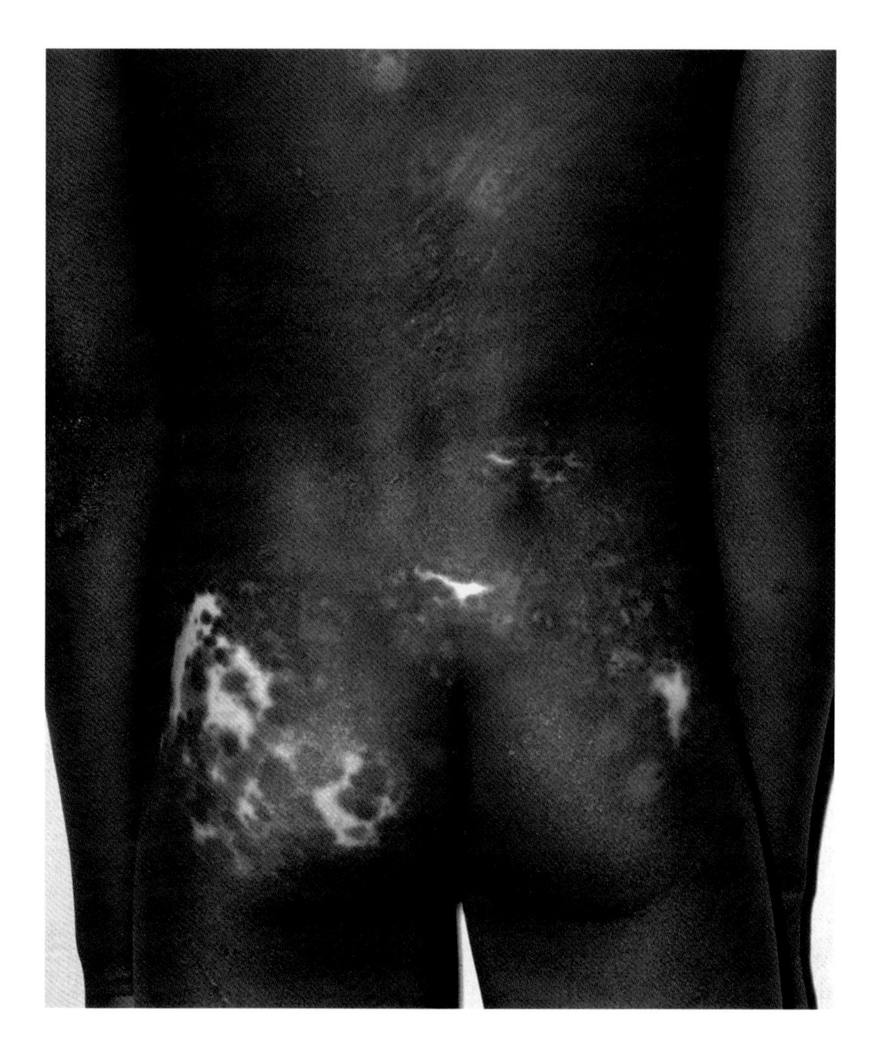

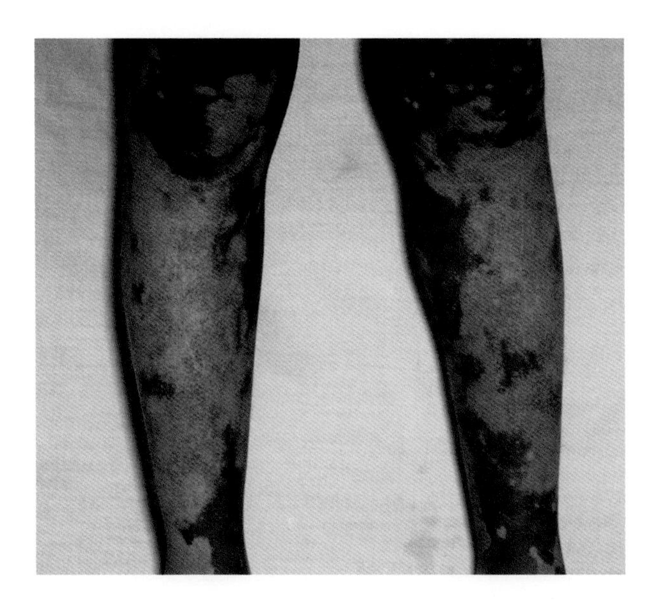

**Figure 662** Vitiligo on the legs of a 7-year-old girl.

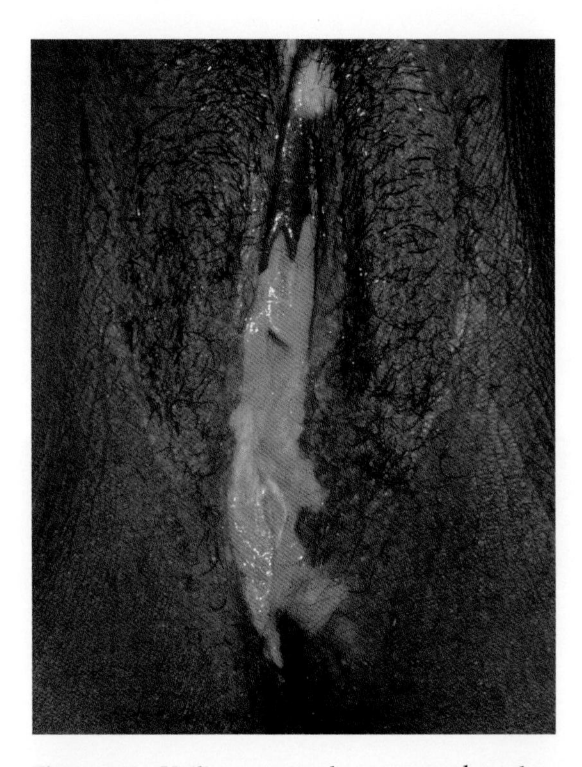

**Figure 663** Vitiligo commonly occurs on the vulva. Do not confuse it with lichen sclerosis et atrophicus (*see* Figure 392) which is itchy and atrophic, whereas vitiligo is simply an area of colour change.

**Figures 664, 665, 666** Other common sites for vitiligo are the ends of the fingers, the lips and the gums.

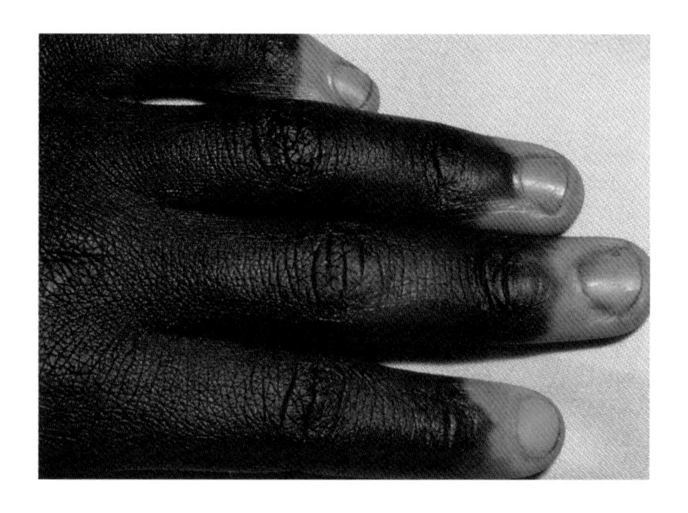

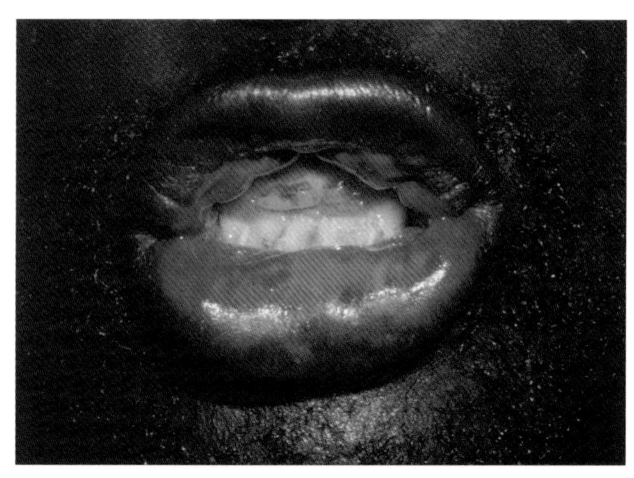

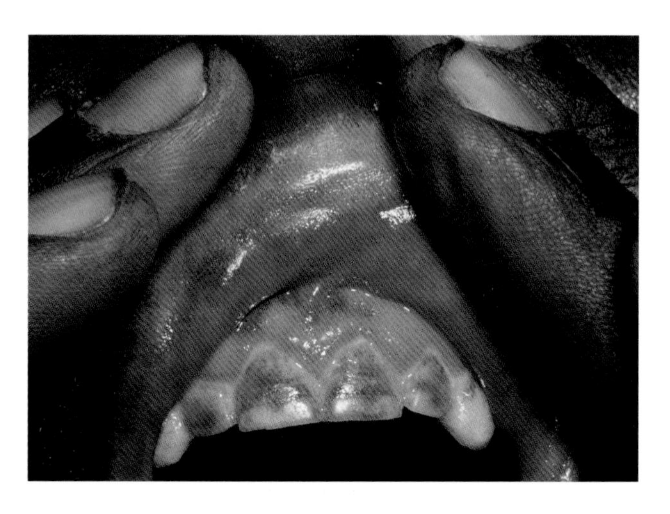

**Figure 667** In hairy areas, the hairs may also be white.

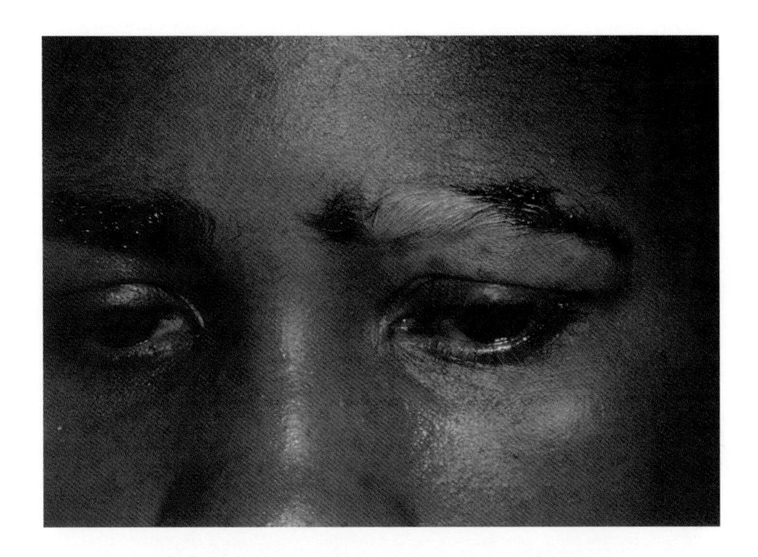

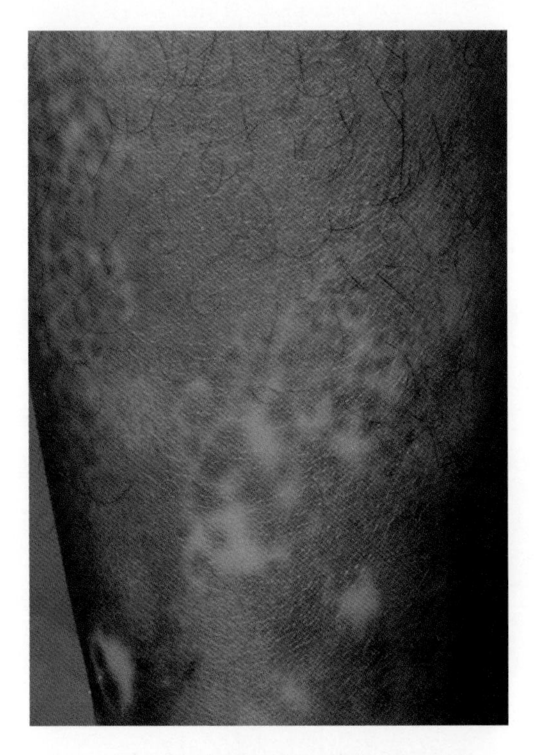

**Figure 668** Repigmentation of the patches can occur from melanocytes in the hair follicles, giving a spotty appearance to begin with.

*Treatment:* Ultraviolet light is helpful, which perhaps explains why vitiligo is not common on the face in Africa. If sunlight alone does not help, apply a moderately potent topical steroid, e.g. 0.05% clobetasone butyrate cream or ointment bd.

## Segmental vitiligo

**Figure 669** This is vitiligo confined to one part of the body only, not usually to a dermatome. It remains segmental and does not progress to the generalised disease. It does not usually repigment spontaneously.

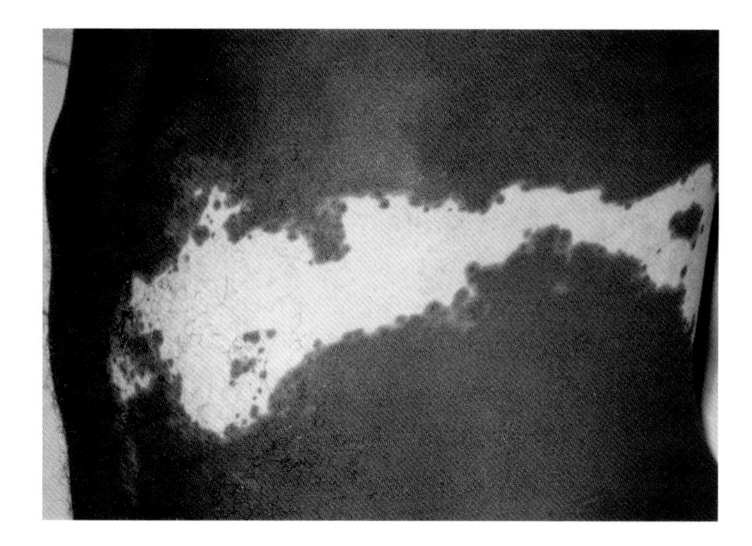

**Figure 670** *Treatment:* Pinch grafts can be applied to the vitiligo to initiate repigmentation.

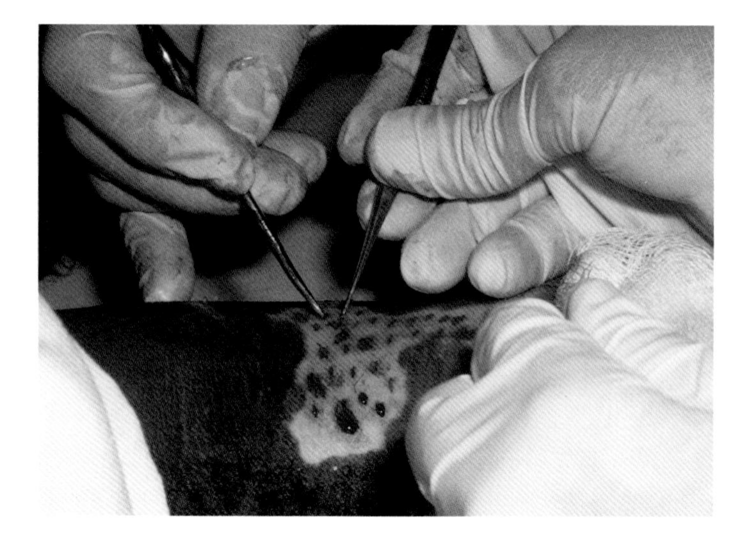

## WARTS (Verrucae)

Warts are an infection of the epidermal cells by one of the numerous human papilloma viruses (HPV). All types of warts are more common in patients with HIV infection.

### Common warts (Verruca vulgaris)

**Figure 671** Small hyperpigmented, rough, warty papules on the hands, mainly of children (although they can be found anywhere). They are transmitted from one child to another through broken skin (cuts, grazes, etc.). Due to HPV 2, 4, 26, 27, 29 or 57.

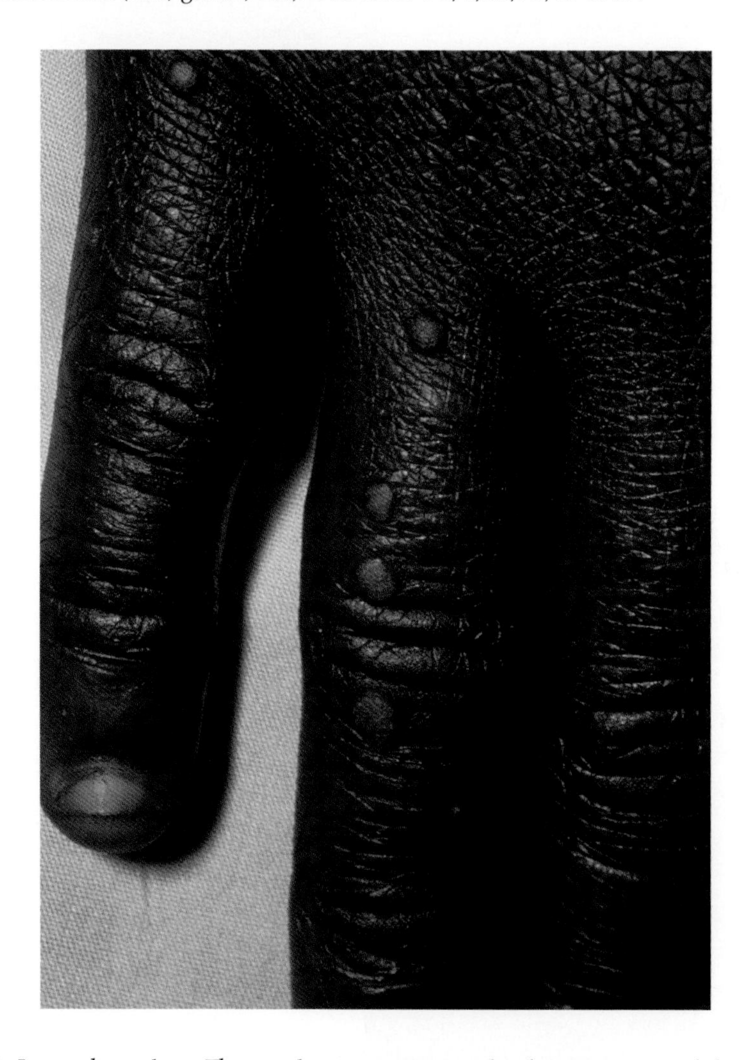

*Treatment:* Leave them alone. They get better spontaneously after an average of about 2 years.

## Plane warts

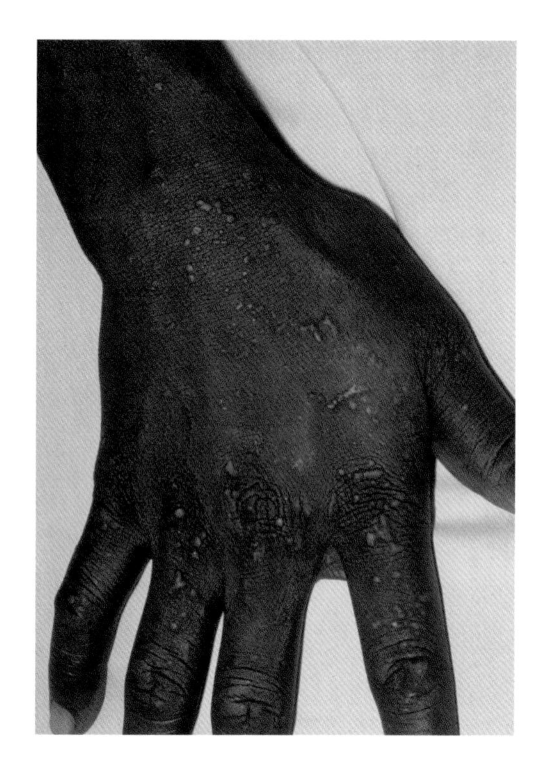

**Figure 672** These are small flat-topped warts which are not rough to the touch. They are most common on the face or backs of hands in children and often show the Koebner phenomenon (*see* Figure 344). In adults think of associated HIV infection. They are due to HPV 3, 10, 26 or 28.

*Treatment:* They are not usually unsightly, so they can be left alone until they resolve spontaneously.

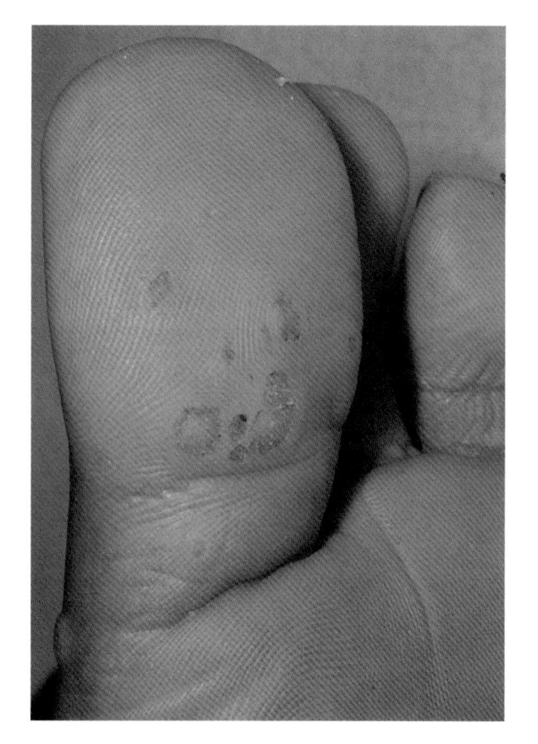

## Plantar warts

**Figure 673** Warts on the soles of the feet due to HPV 1 or 4.

**Figure 674** Plantar warts can be painful due to the hyperkeratosis which occurs around the wart.

*Treatment:* Rub down the hyperkeratosis with a pumice stone so that it is level with the skin to stop the pain. They get better spontaneously.

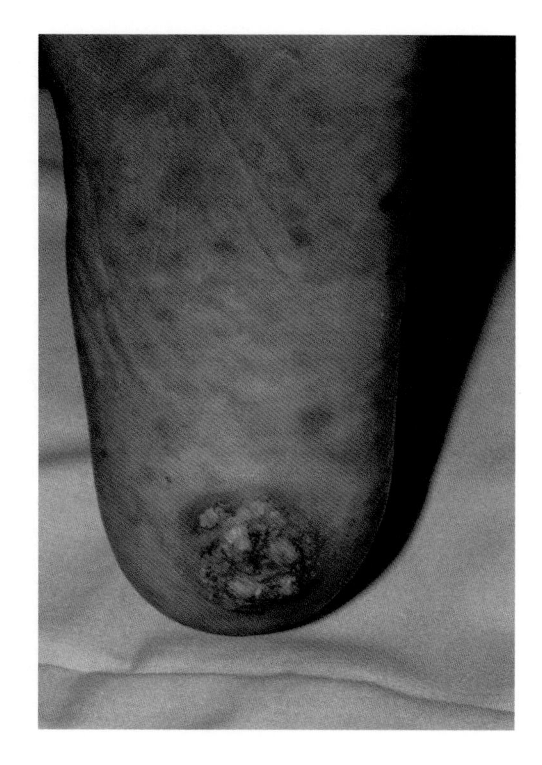

## Genital warts (Condylomata accuminata)

**Figure 675** Warty papules on the genitalia or perianal skin.

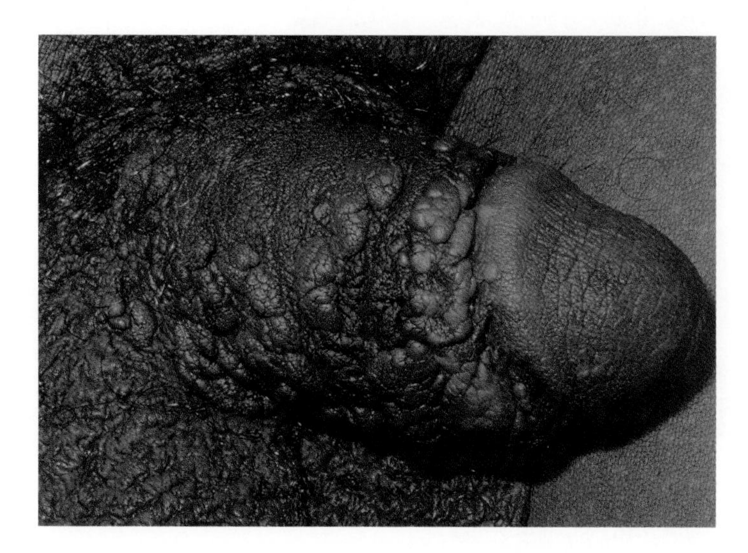

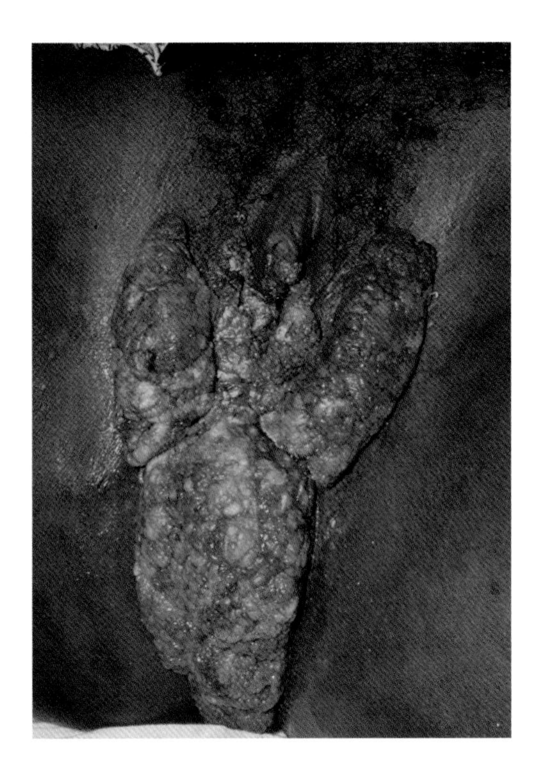

**Figures 676, 677** They may become confluent to form cauliflower-like masses. They are quite different from the flat warts that occur in secondary syphilis – condylomata lata (*see* Figure 604). Genital warts due to HPV 6 and 11 are harmless, but those due to HPV 16 and 18 are associated with malignant and premalignant lesions of the cervix in women.

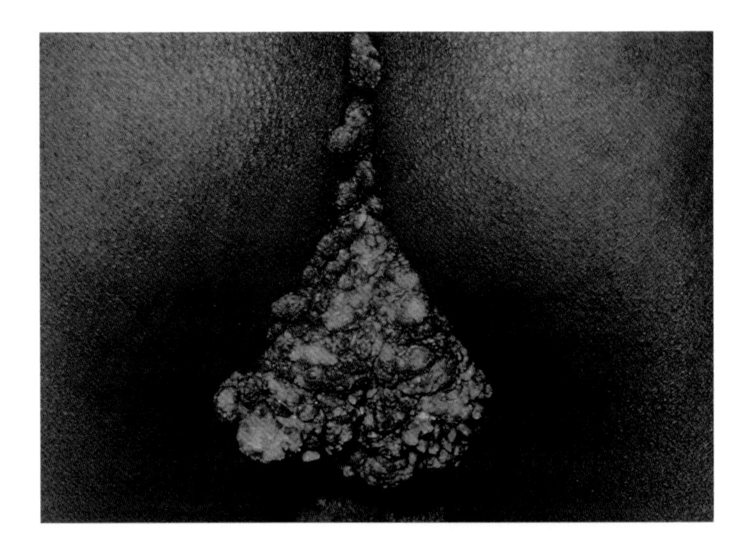

*Treatment of genital warts:* Paint with 20% podophylline once a week; wash it off after 6 hours with soap and water.

## Warts in the mouth

**Figure 678** Warts in the mouth are quite common in children who also have common warts on the fingers. Presumably they are transferred to the mouth by sucking the fingers. In adults think of HIV infection. The common HPV types are 2a and 57.

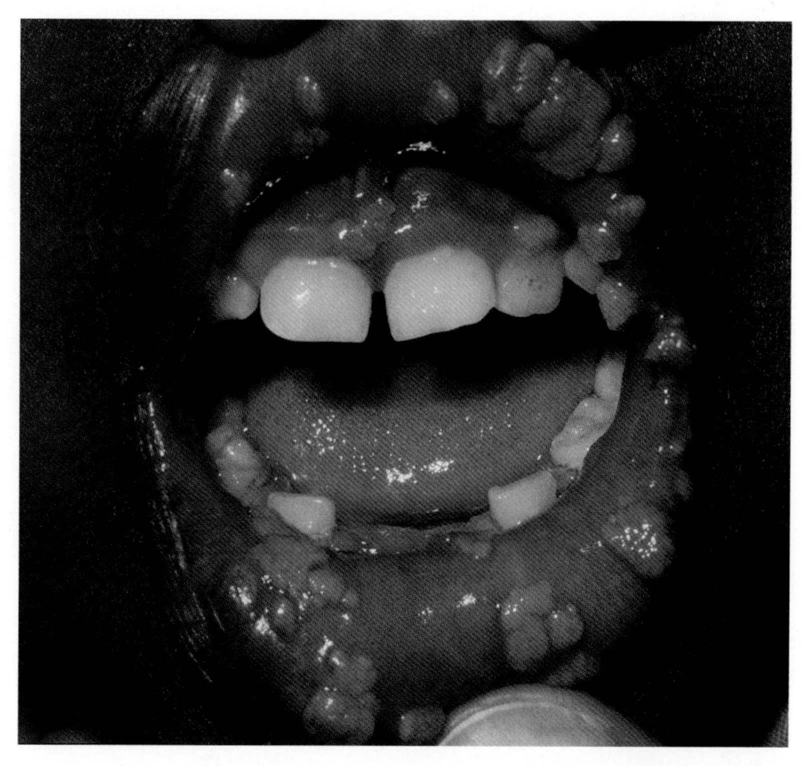

*Treatment:* Leave them alone until they disappear spontaneously. In adults check for HIV.

# XANTHOMAS

## Eruptive xanthomas

**Figure 679** Small hyperpigmented papules on the limbs and buttocks in patients with Fredrickson's Types I, IV and V hyperlipidaemia. Most patients are diabetic.

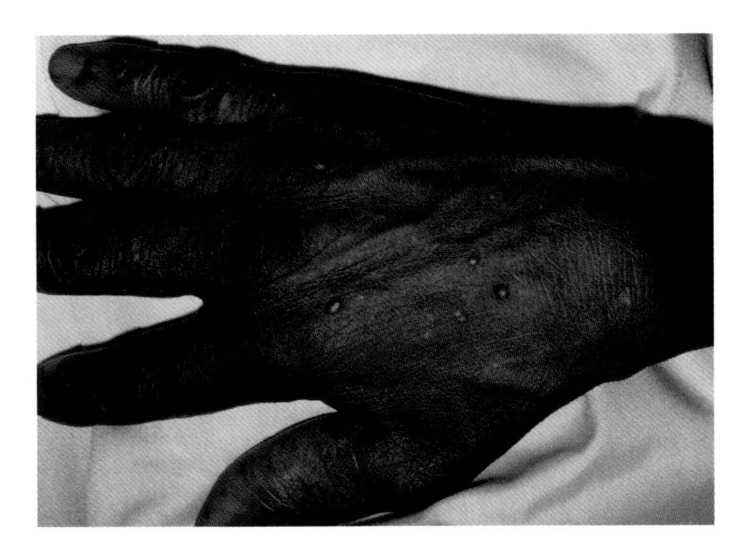

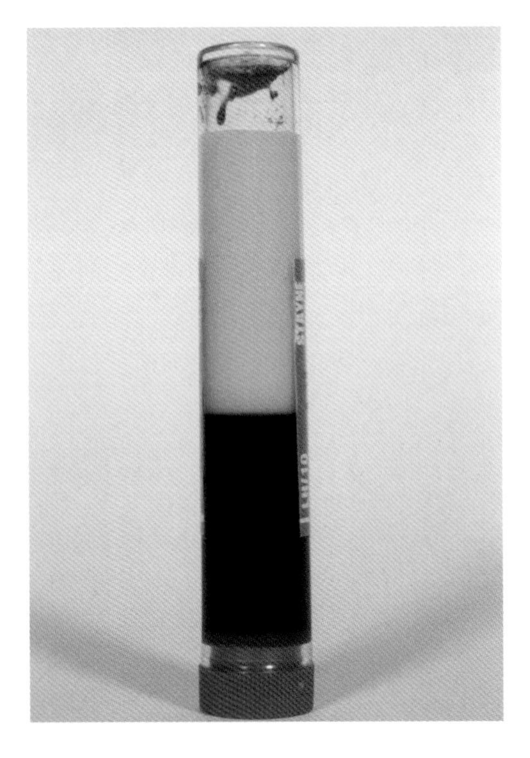

**Figure 680** Blood from these patients will show creamy plasma due to chylomicrons.

*Treatment:* Check for diabetes mellitus and treat that.

## Xanthelasma

**Figure 681** Flat yellowish plaques on the inner aspect of the upper and/or lower eyelids. They are due to the accumulation of lipids in the dermis but are not usually associated with hypercholesterolaemia.

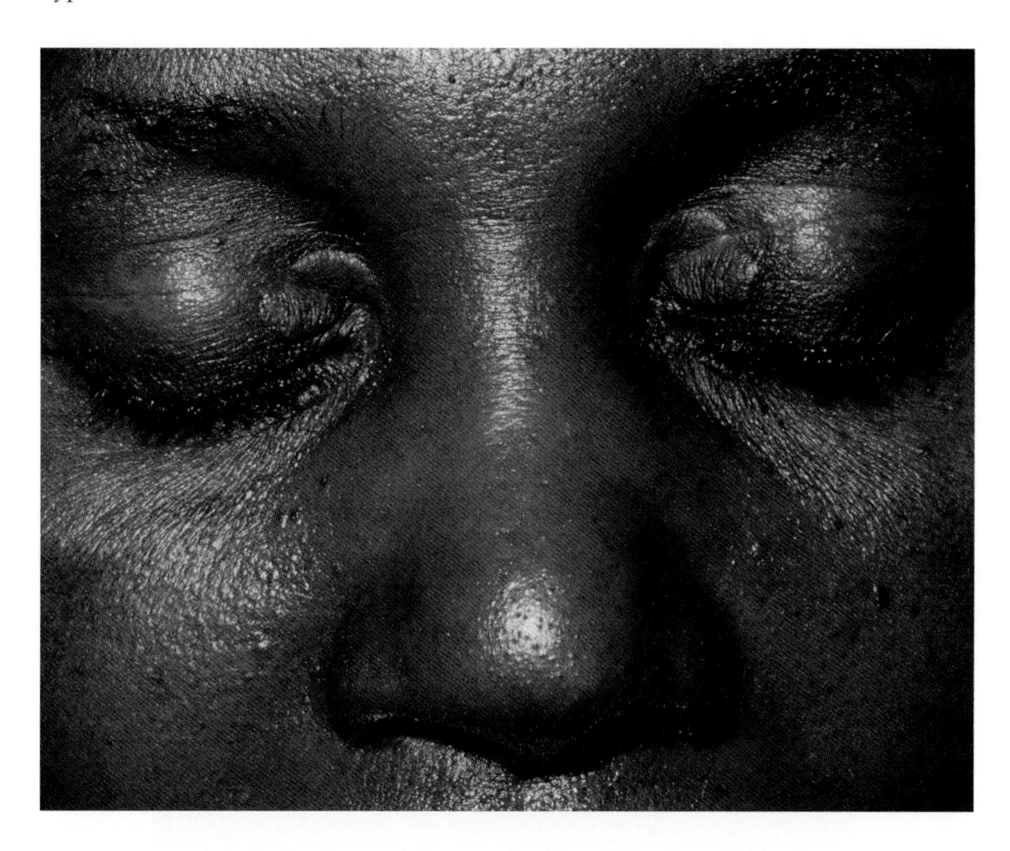

*Treatment:* Reassure the patient that they are harmless. If they are very unsightly they can be excised or painted with a saturated solution of trichloracetic acid (TCA). The TCA should be washed off with surgical spirit as soon as the skin goes white (which will be after a few seconds).

## XERODERMA PIGMENTOSUM

**Figure 682** Rare genetic condition inherited as an autosomal recessive trait (*see* Figure 18). There is a defect in DNA repair resulting in hypersensitivity to ultraviolet light and early, often fatal, skin cancers. The child is normal at birth. By the age of 12–15 months the characteristic hyperpigmented macules appear on sun-exposed sites (the face and backs of hands and forearms), and the child develops photophobia.

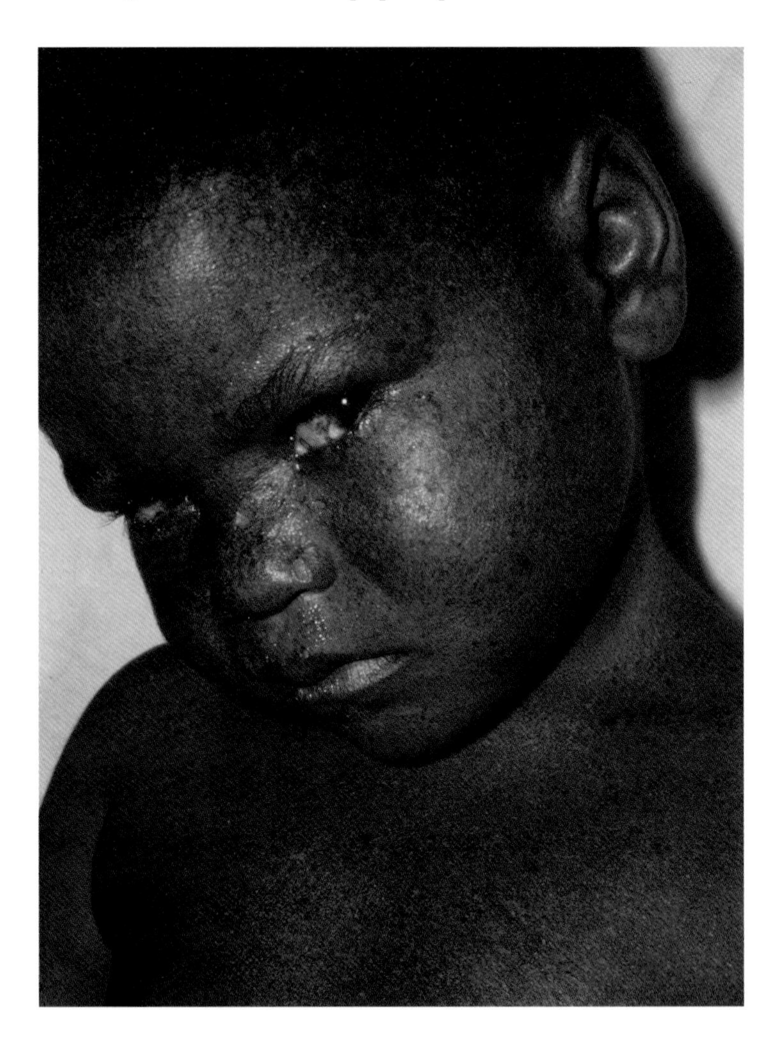

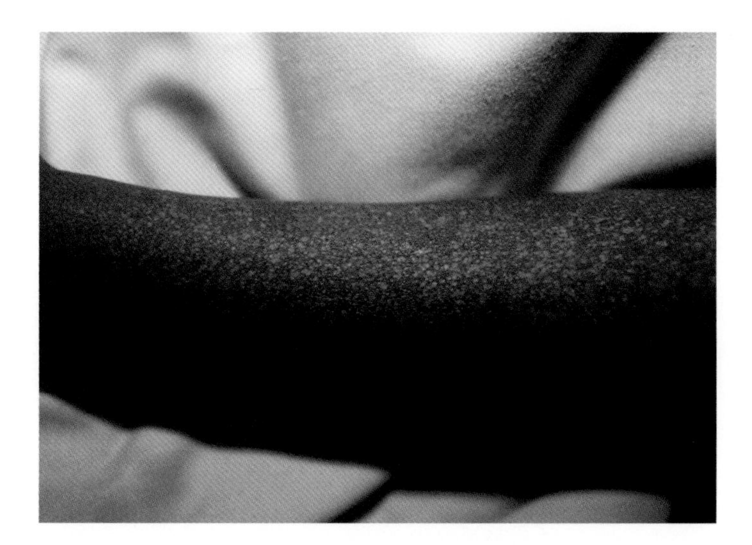

**Figure 683** Later there may be a mixture of hyper- and hypopigmented macules.

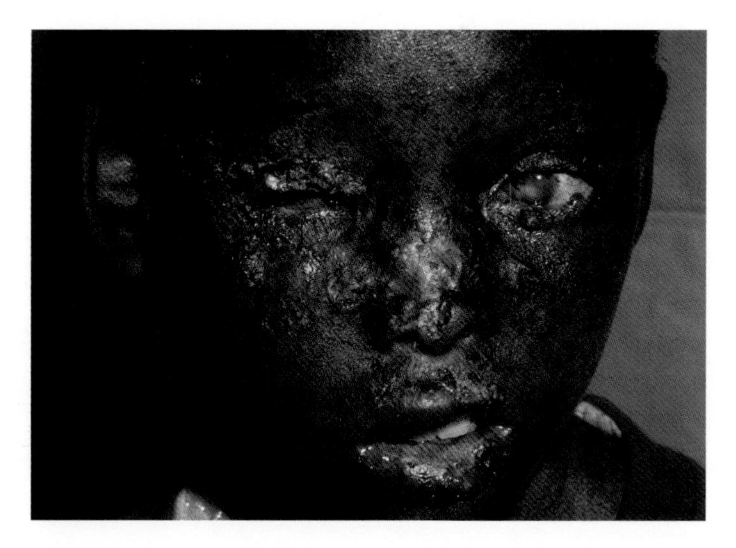

**Figure 684** Multiple skin cancers in a 10-year-old child. Basal cell carcinomas, squamous cell carcinomas and malignant melanomas all occur in this condition.

*Treatment:* Keep the child out of the sun or use protective clothing as soon as the diagnosis is made (as for albinos, *see* Figure 31).

# INDEX